I0832198

Ketsugo Goju-Ryu Karate-Do
Vol. 4: Kumite, Hojo Undo & Stretching

Ketsugo Goju-Ryu Karate-Do
Vol. 4: Kumite, Hojo Undo & Stretching

by Robert Oliver

First Printing
ISBN: 979-8-9896402-8-7

DEDICATION

This book is dedicated to Shodai Jay Trombley, the visionary founder of Ketsugo Goju-Ryu Karate-Do who spent 61 years in the martial arts and will never be forgotten.

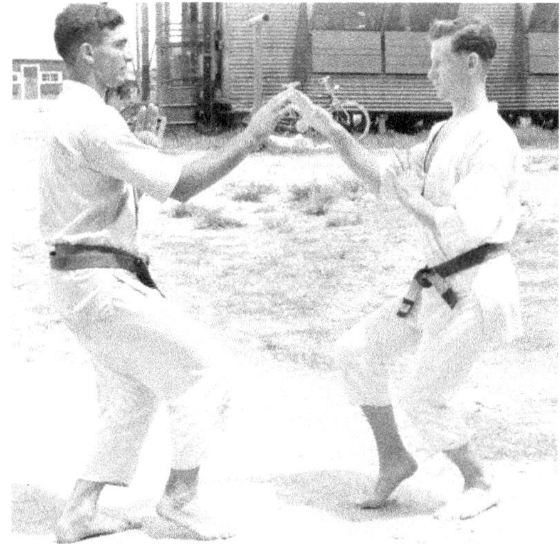

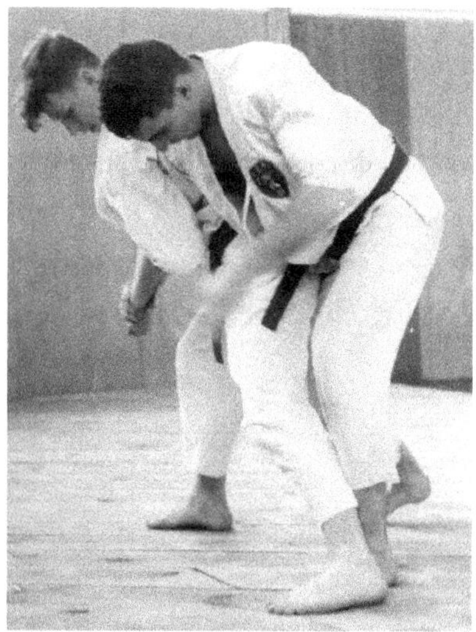

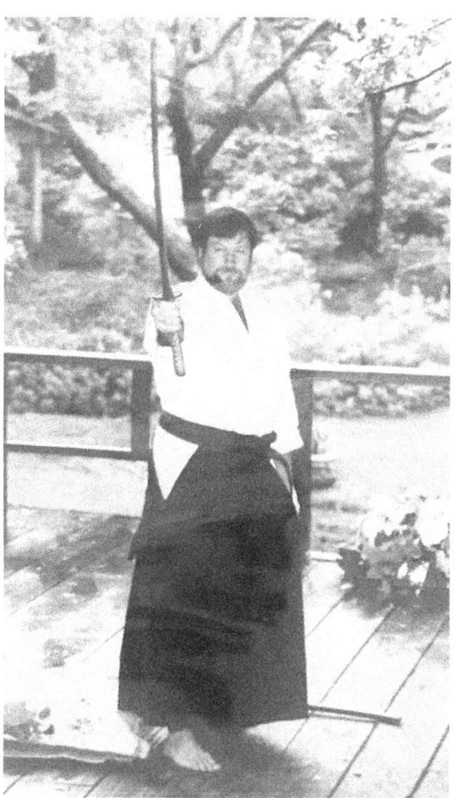

Shodai Jay Trombley (1938 - 2022)

ACKNOWLEDGMENTS

I want to thank my wife, Ashley, for helping me with the demonstrations and modeling for the two-man exercises; my good friend Will for helping me smooth out some of the clunkiness; and, as always, a big thanks to the people who trained before me, who set the path and tradition of Ketsugo Goju-Ryu Karate-Do, which is still around more than 50 years later.

KGJKA Black Belts

Alyce Strickland | Tom Rieber | Rusty Fralia | Todd Kauffman | Lavada White | Shane Facemyer | David Griffin | Ken Johnson | Bob Loewenstein | Mark Ashraf | Sharon Griffin | Marshall Van Norden | Allen Crowley | Christine Landmon | Andrew Smith | Marvin Madison | Kyle Brown | Russell Dare | Chris Collins | Jared Smith | Kenneth Taliaferro | Alan Viengluang | Trent Boe | Mike Perry | Brodie Wolgamott | Ashley Oliver | Robert Oliver | George Eastlick | Cliff Knudson | Tim Bryant | Armando Navarro

FOREWORD

Looking back on the prior books in this series, it is hard to believe I initially wanted the whole system to be one book, including the biography of our founder, Shodai Jay Trombley. That would have meant either tiny pictures or a 2,000-page book. It never fails to amaze me how deep this system really is until I put something like this together. My intention was always to document the system itself for anyone interested, but also to make it somewhat useful for active students. Still, as I have stated in each of these books, it is not intended to replace formal teaching in a dojo, but rather to assist and inform. A student still needs a sensei to demonstrate the flow of these exercises, correct mistakes, and show how certain physical limitations can be adapted.

This book is an important addition to the Ketsugo Goju-Ryu Karate-Do series. Our founder, Shodai Jay Trombley, designed many of the bunkai and kiso kumite exercises contained here, building on what he learned in the 1950s with Seikichi Toguchi as part of the Shoreikan Goju-Ryu system, which was still in its infancy at the time. As for sparring, iri kume was practiced during the last hour of every class in Toguchi's dojo, with no protective gear. Kicks were used, but sparingly, as were punches to the head and face. Leg kicks were allowed, but strikes to the groin were not. The idea was to practice technique, not to seriously injure one another. In the 1960s, while in Florida, Shodai learned boxing techniques, and in the 1970s and 1980s he trained full-contact fighters in Texas, using many of the same training methods found in his karate system.

I have also added a section on stretching, one of the more undervalued aspects of training, but no less important than any of the other material. The stretching section is Shodai's version of Daruma Taiso, an exercise originally created by Chojun Miyagi and further developed by Seikichi Toguchi. In Toguchi's dojo, this exercise took nearly an hour and began every class. I hope the reader will enjoy this catalog of exercises devoted to kumite in the Ketsugo Goju-Ryu Karate-Do system. My wife Ashley, a fellow black belt in KGJKA, worked with me on all of the two-person photographs.

In this fourth volume, we examine all aspects of kumite within the Ketsugo Goju-Ryu Karate-Do system. In this context, kumite is used as an umbrella term for fighting and the training devoted to it outside of kata. The material is divided into two sections: self-defense and sparring. Self-defense drills differ from sparring drills in that they tend to be more directly related to an actual fight. These drills emphasize two or three movements to disable an attacker or escape a hold before creating distance.

They consist of techniques derived from kata, called bunkai kumite, and drills that focus on countering, called kiso kumite. These are prearranged exercises that help students refine technique, but they also provide other benefits.

Bunkai and kiso kumite drills improve body conditioning, particularly of the arms, as well as speed and distance management. One person punches while the partner blocks simultaneously. If one person does not time their block properly, they can be struck. If the defender does not gauge distance properly, the counter will not land, and the student may become accustomed to fully extending punches without contact. However, these drills are only part of training. The student must also spar.

To prepare for sparring, waza exercises were developed to practice offensive combinations more closely related to sparring than self-defense. Freestyle sparring (irikume) involves two people practicing techniques within a set time frame, without stopping after each point of contact, but with rules and protective gear for safety. In sparring, the student must distinguish it from real self-defense. For example, kata may teach a student to break an opponent's arm at the elbow or strike the eyes or throat, but these techniques are not permitted in sparring.

Sparring, for all its benefits, requires a different mindset. Irikume may resemble a fight on the surface, but it is still only a training exercise. The key is to recognize what is gained from sparring: the ability to use offensive and defensive techniques against another person without relying on a choreographed sequence. Most importantly, it helps develop the ability to remain composed amid relative chaos.

- Author

TABLE OF CONTENTS

Self-Defense

Bunkai Kumite

Bunkai Kumite (or Kata Kumite) are two-person exercises in which two people move together, completing both offensive and defensive movements. The participants begin by punching and blocking at the same time, after which the exercise breaks into different sequences, generally derived from a kata. This exercise has many benefits, including timing and speed (punching and blocking at close range simultaneously), distance (gauging the necessary distance to strike and block with the movements), and body conditioning (the offensive person should control punches, while the defensive person must redirect the punch using leverage and strength).

In a standard punching routine, the student practices by punching the air, focusing solely on the punch itself—the technique. In kumite drills, the target is another person and should be adjusted as needed. On defense, the student must adapt to the offensive partner's steps, adjusting as necessary. This helps students work with opponents of any size. Another important benefit is mental. A student must maintain a certain level of calmness to remember each counter, much like remembering each sequence in a kata. However, unlike practicing a kata, Bunkai Kumite drills assist the participant in working with an actual partner, as opposed to imagining a combatant.

Different angles will be referenced in the descriptions, since the drills do not always follow a simple left-and-right, back-and-forth pattern. For illustrative purposes, the angle image used in the kata volumes has been rotated clockwise. When performing kumite exercises, the left side will be considered the shomen side (0°).

Although not shown below, all bunkai and kiso kumite exercises include a bow in and a bow out. Participants begin facing each other in heiko dachi. After the ready command and a bow (rei), each person steps into or sets in a specific kamae. To end each exercise, the participants complete these steps in reverse order, stepping back into heisoku dachi, bowing, and then stepping out into heiko dachi.

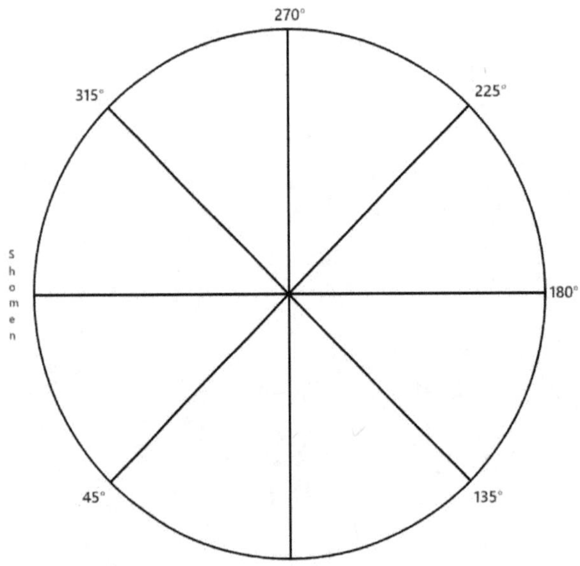

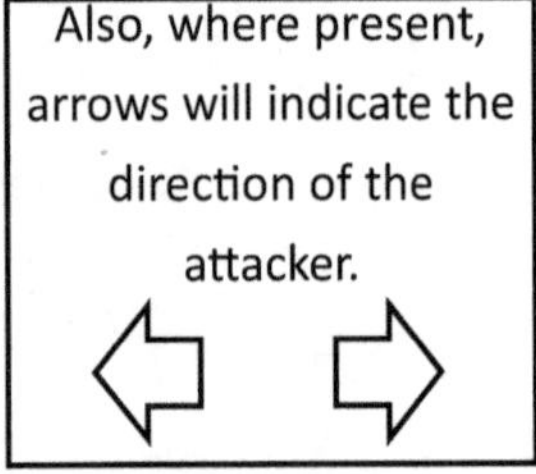

1. Gekisai Kumite Ichi

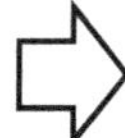

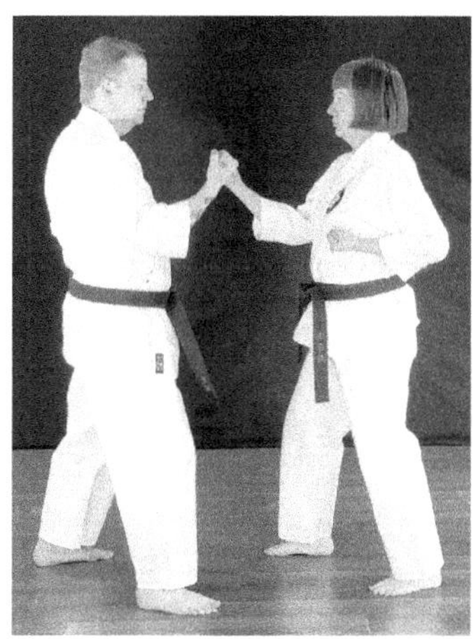

Basic Front Facing Closed Hand Kamae

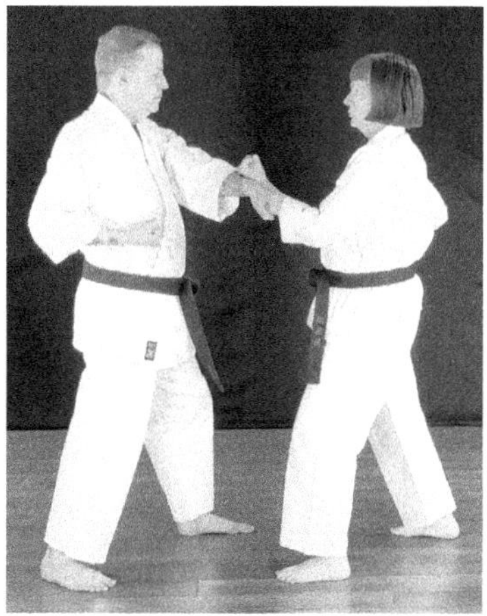

1. Left: Step Forward, Chudan Zuki / Right: Step Back, Chudan Uke

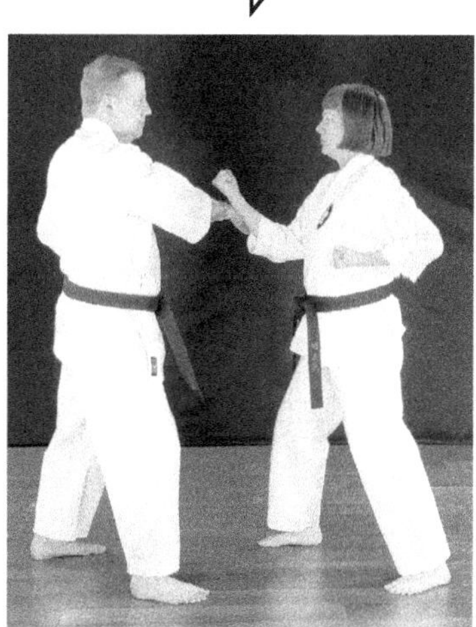

2. Left: Step Forward, Chudan Zuki / Right: Step Back, Chudan Uke

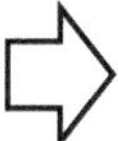

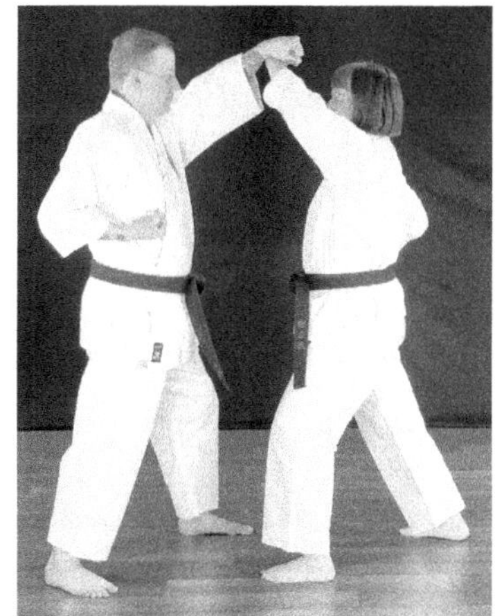

3. Left: Step Forward, Jodan Zuki / Right: Step Back, Jodan Age Uke

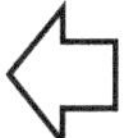

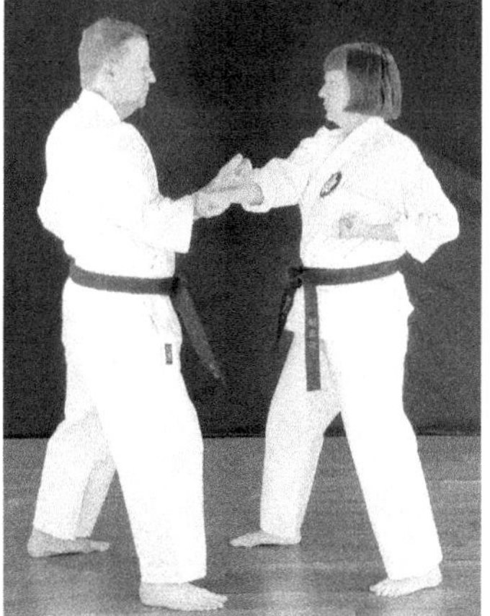

4. Left: Step Back, Chudan Uke / Right: Step Forward, Chudan Zuki

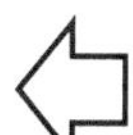

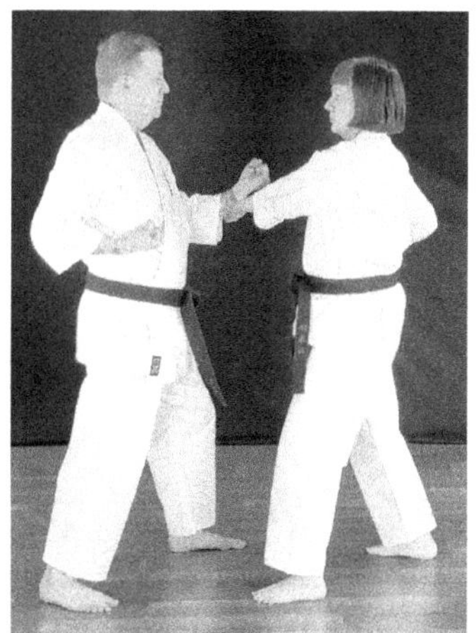

5. Left: Step Back, Chudan Uke / Right: Step Forward, Chudan Zuki

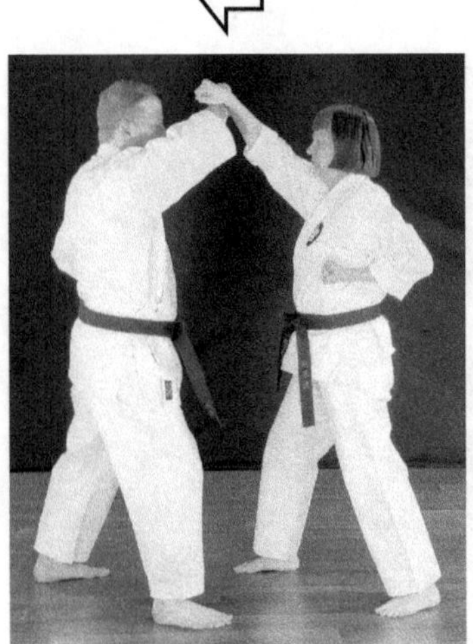

6. Left: Step Back, Jodan Age Uke / Right: Step Forward, Jodan Zuki

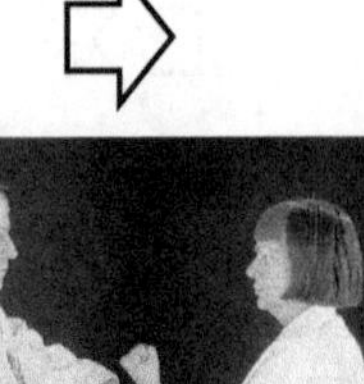

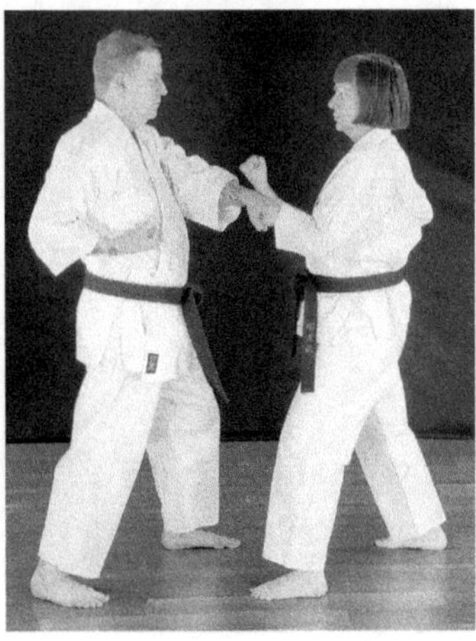

7. Left: Step Forward, Chudan Zuki / Right: Step Back, Chudan Uke

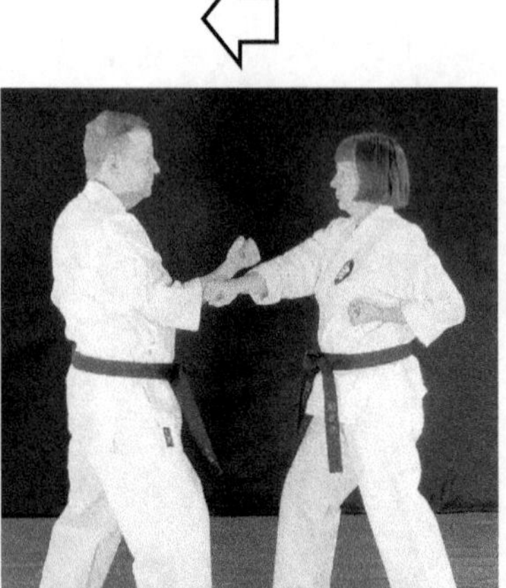

8. Left: Step Back, Chudan Uke / Right: Step Forward, Chudan Zuki

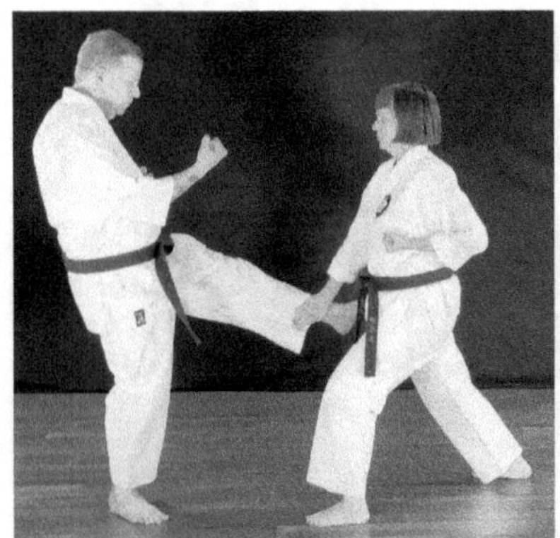

9. Left: Mae Geri Gedan / Right: Step Back into Zenkutsu Dachi, Gedan Shotei Barai

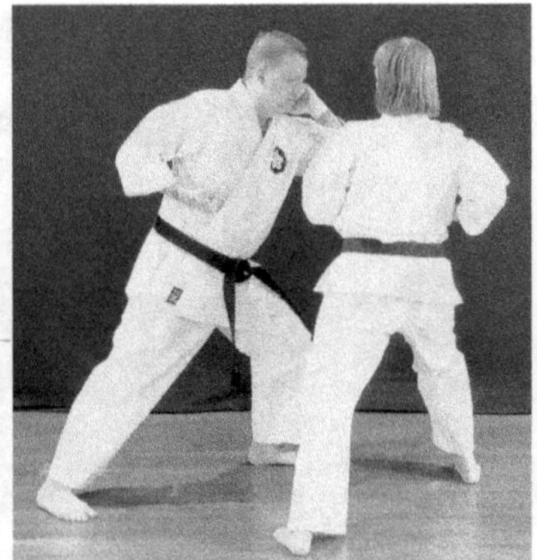

10. Left: Land in Zenkutsu Dachi, Empi Age Uchi / Right: Pivot Right, Shotei Oshi

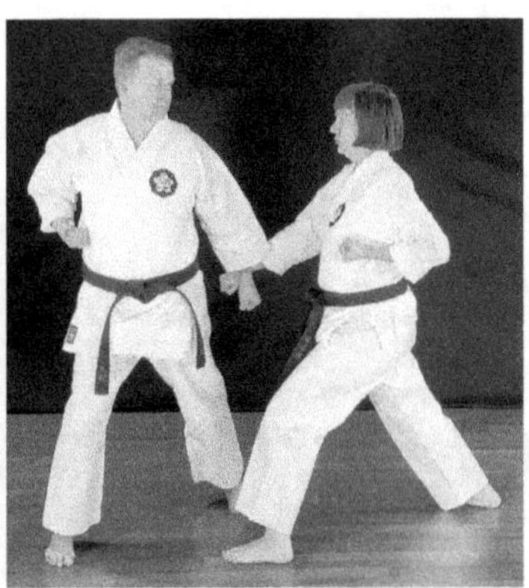

11. Left: Pivot Right, Yoko Gedan Barai / Right: Pivot Left, Gyaku Zuki

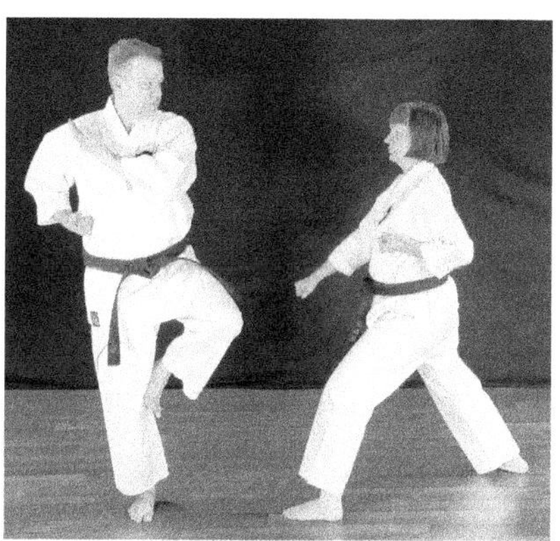

12. Left: Chamber Foot and Hand for Shuto Uchi

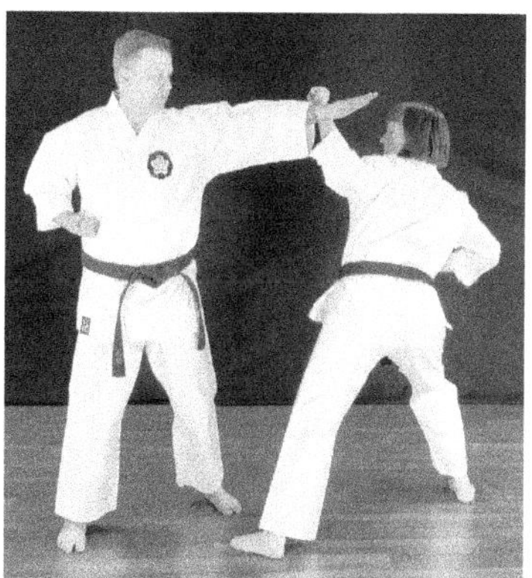

13. Left: Yoko Shuto Uchi and Fumikomi Geri / Right: Pivot Right, Jodan Yoko Age Uke

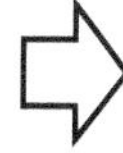

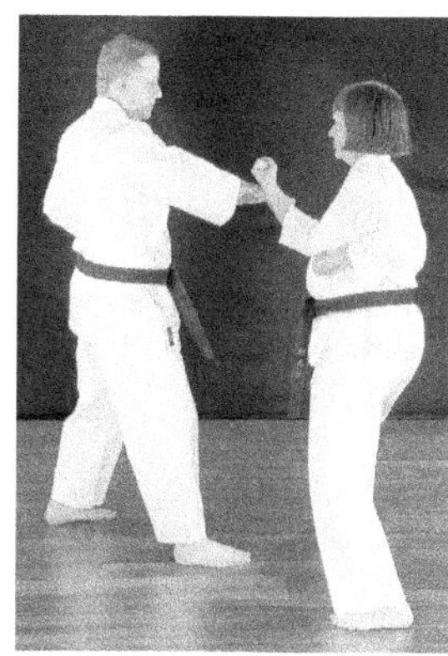

14. Left: Step Forward, Chudan Zuki / Right: Step Back on a 135° Angle into Neko Ashi Dachi with Chudan Uke, Turn Left Fist Over — Palm Down

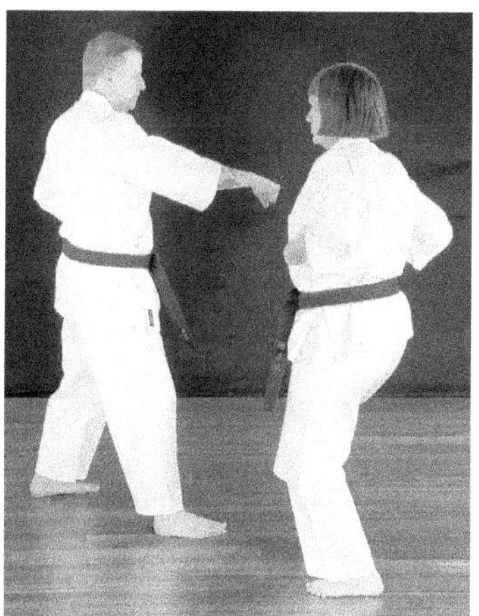

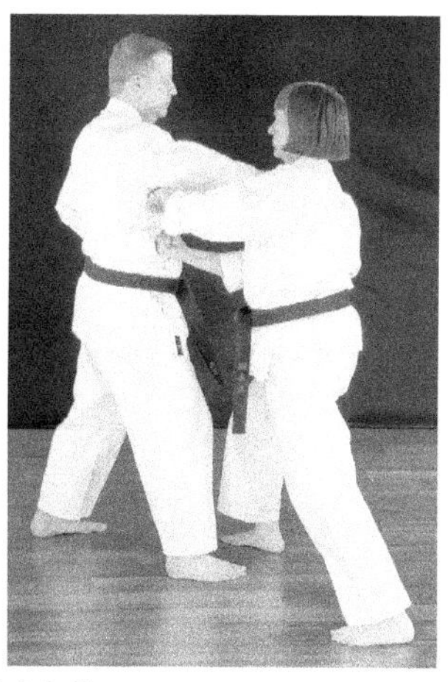

Repeat in Other Direction

15. Right: Awase Zuki (Kiai)

2. Gekisai Kumite Ni

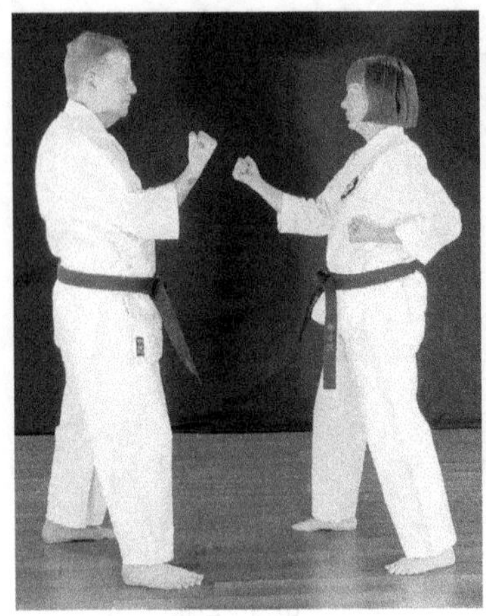

Basic Front Facing Closed Hand Kamae

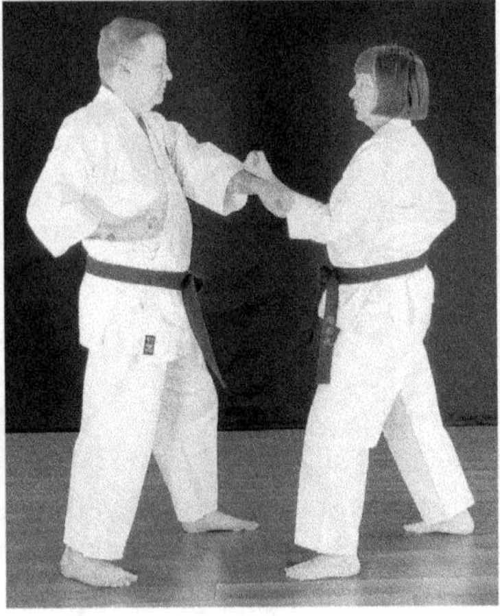

1. Left: Step Forward, Chudan Zuki / Right: Step Back, Chudan Uke

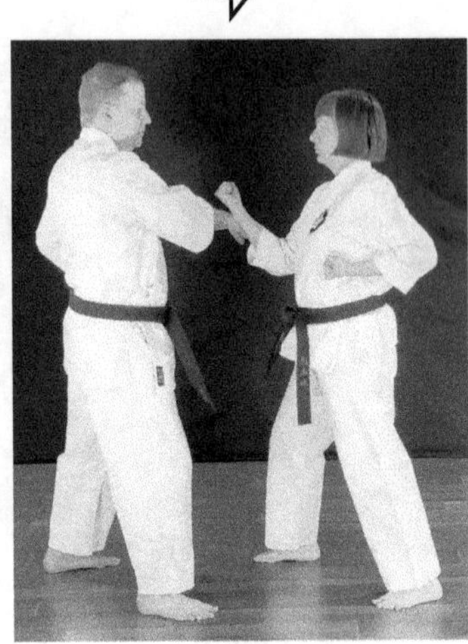

2. Left: Step Forward, Chudan Zuki / Right: Step Back, Chudan Uke

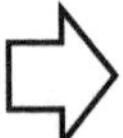

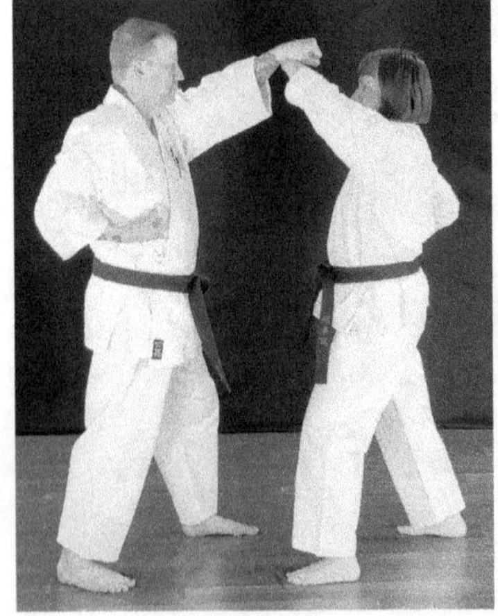

3. Left: Step Forward, Jodan Zuki / Right: Step Back, Jodan Age Uke

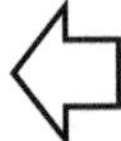

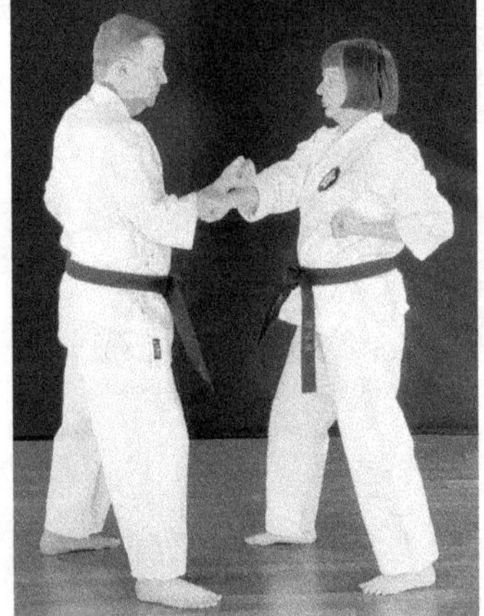

4. Left: Step Back, Chudan Uke / Right: Step Forward, Chudan Zuki

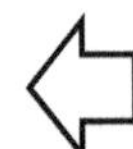

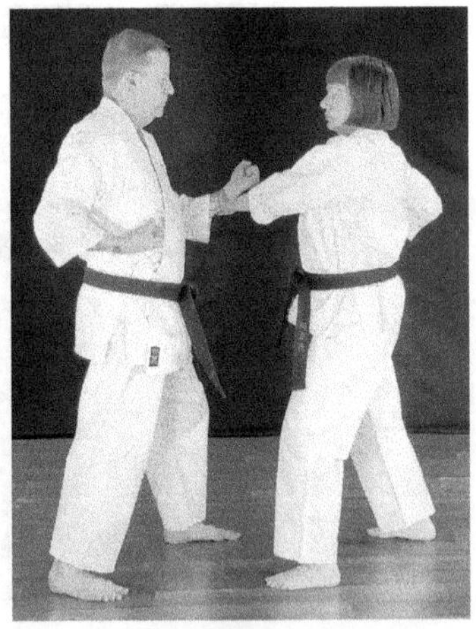

5. Left: Step Back, Chudan Uke / Right: Step Forward, Chudan Zuki

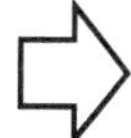

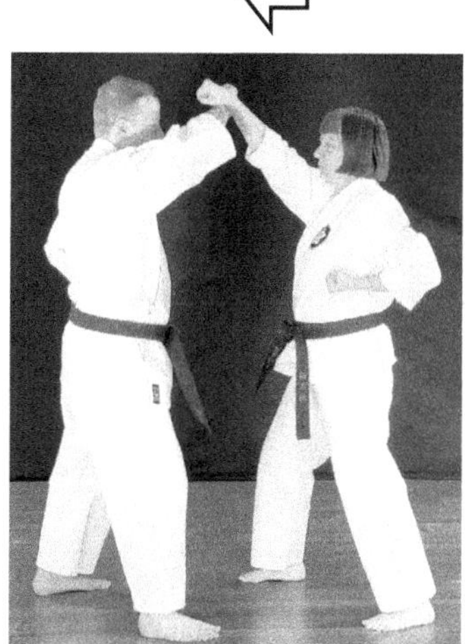

6. Left: Step Forward, Jodan Zuki / Right: Step Back, Jodan Age Uke

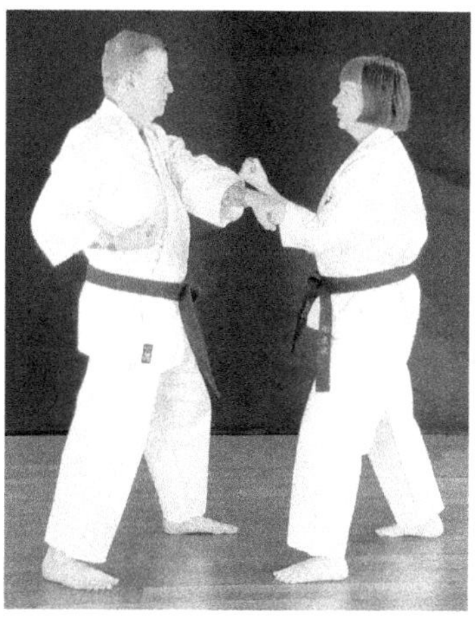

7. Left: Step Forward, Chudan Zuki / Right: Step Back, Chudan Uke

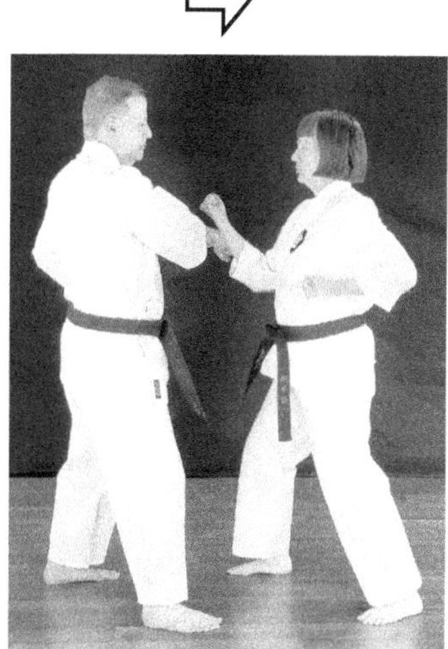

8. Left: Step Forward, Chudan Zuki / Right: Step Back, Chudan Uke

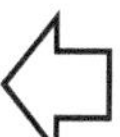
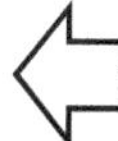

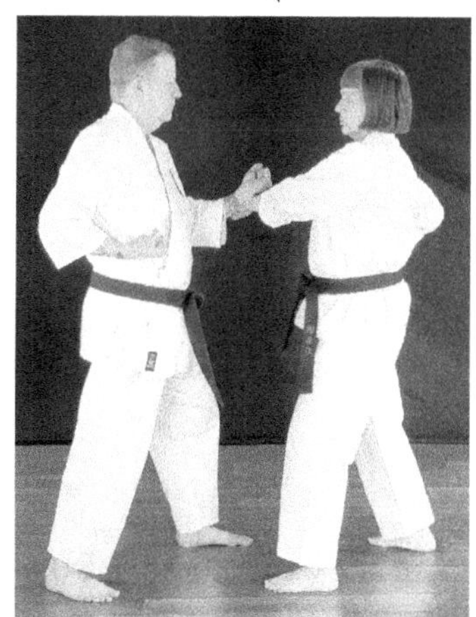

9. Left: Step Back, Chudan Uke / Right: Step Forward, Chudan Zuki

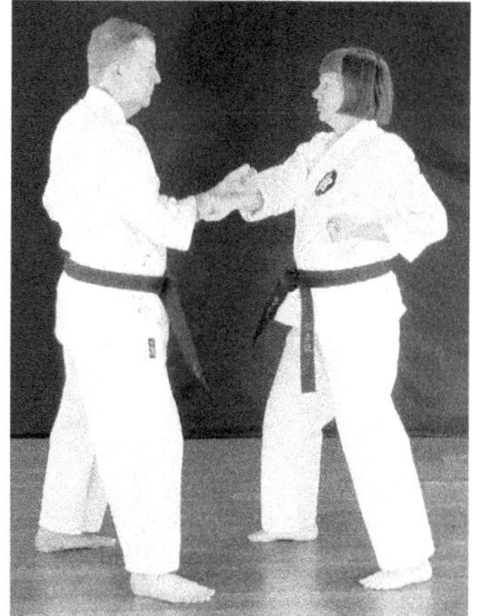

10. Left: Step Back, Chudan Uke / Right: Step Forward, Chudan Zuki

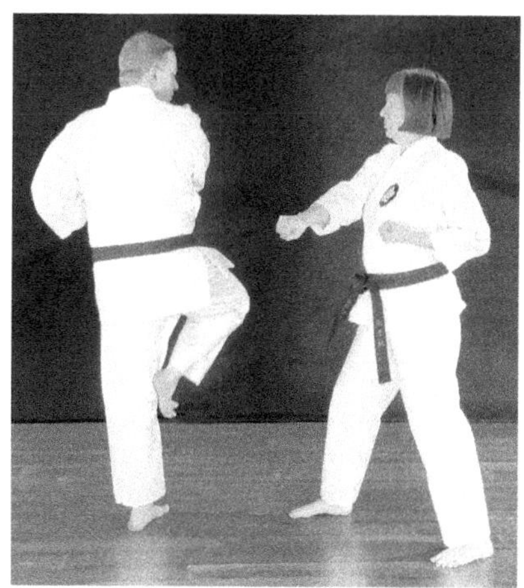

11. Left: Pivot Left, Chamber Foot and Hand for Shuto Uchi

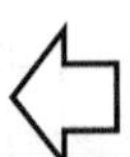

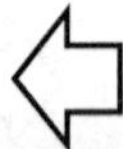

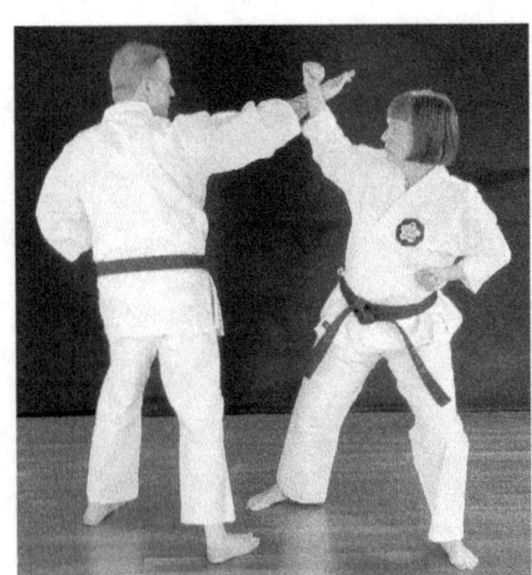

12. Left: Yoko Shuto Uchi and Fumikomi Geri / Right: Pivot Left, Jodan Yoko Age Uke

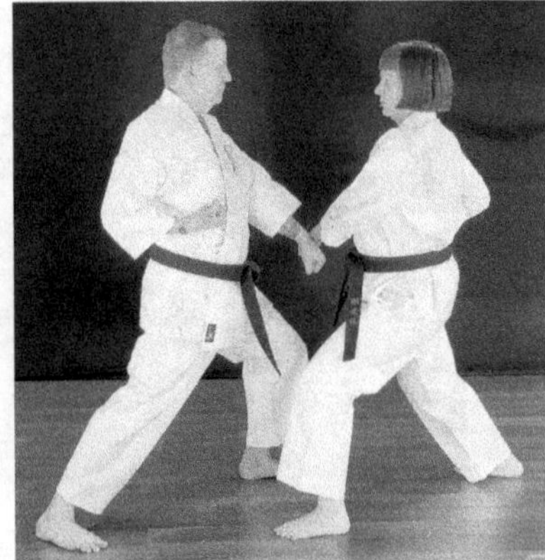

13. Left: Step Back in Zenkutsu Dachi, Gedan Barai / Right: Step Forward in Zenkutsu Dachi, Gedan Zuki

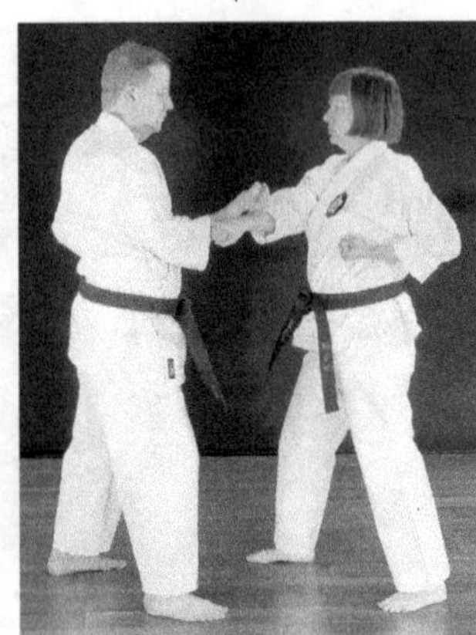

14. Left: Step Back, Chudan Uke / Right: Step Forward, Chudan Zuki

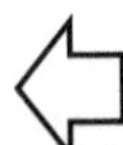

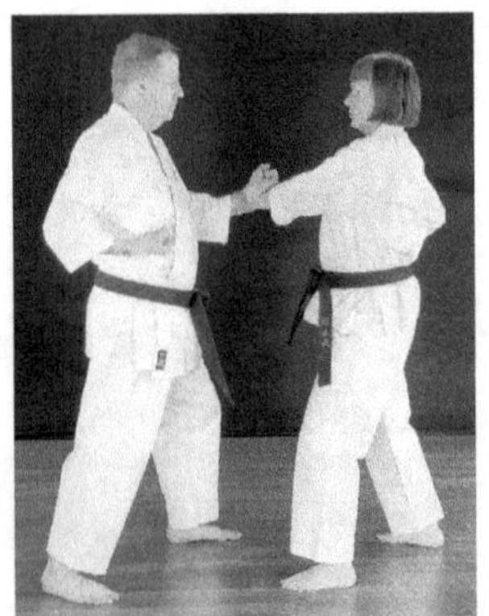

15. Left: Step Back, Chudan Uke / Right: Step Forward, Chudan Zuki

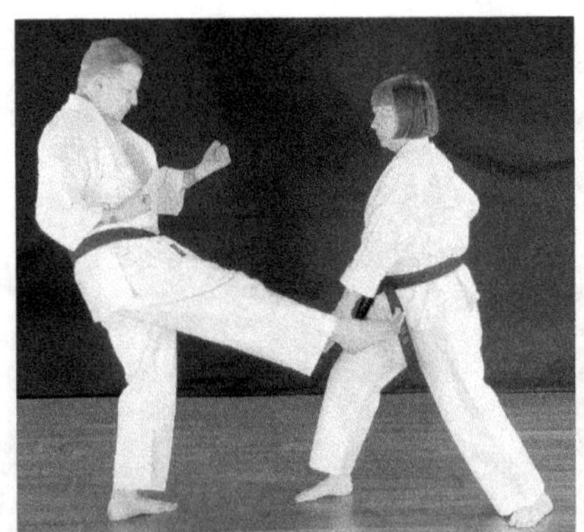

16. Left: Gedan Mae Geri / Right: Step Back into Zenkutsu Dachi, Gedan Shotei Barai

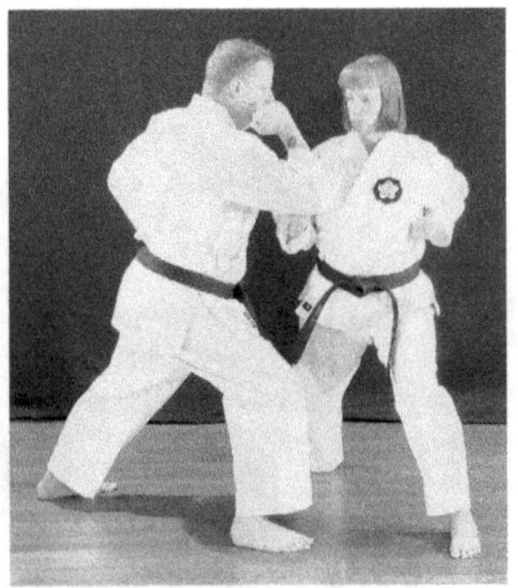

17. Left: Land in Zenkutsu Dachi, Empi Age Uchi / Right: Pivot Left, Shotei Oshi

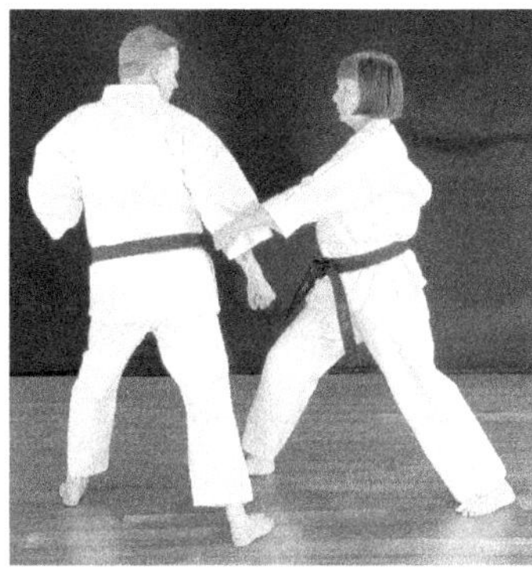

18. Left: Pivot Right, Yoko Gedan Barai / Right: Pivot Left, Gyaku Zuki

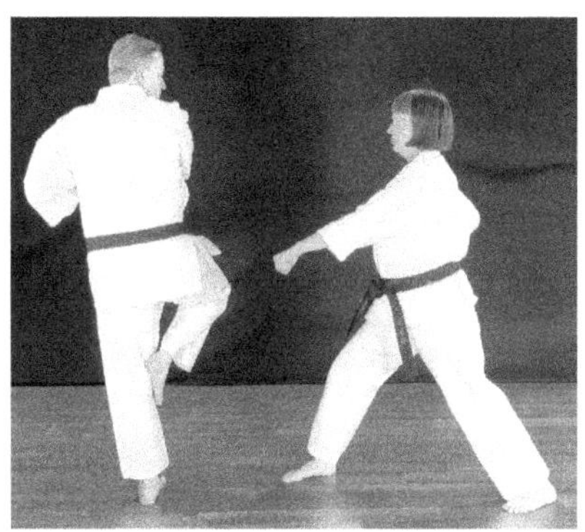

19. Left: Chamber Foot and Hand for Shuto Uchi

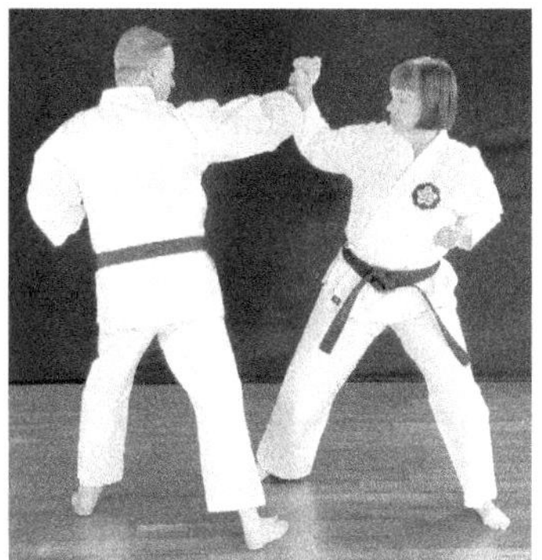

20. Left: Yoko Shuto Uchi and Fumikomi Geri / Right: Pivot Left, Jodan Yoko Age Uke

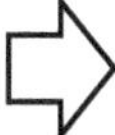

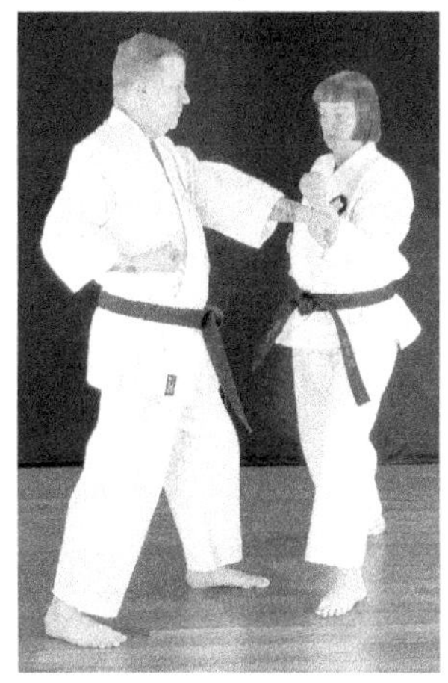

21. Left: Step Forward, Chudan Zuki / Right: Step Back on a 225° Angle into Neko Ashi Dachi with Chudan Uke, Turn Right Fist Over - Palm Down

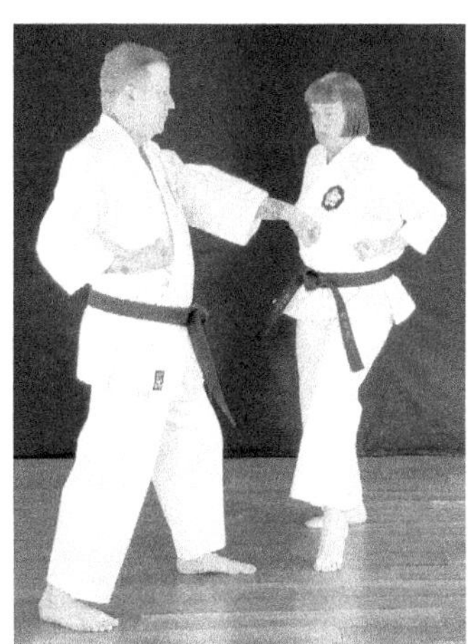

22. Right: Left Awase Zuki (Kiai)

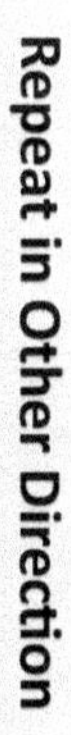

Kata Comparison to Bunkai Kumite

Gekisai Kumite Ichi and Gekisai Kumite Ni contain elements of the Gekisai Ichi and Gekisai Ni katas, namely in the following areas:

- Gedan Mae Geri (Step 9 - Gekisai Kumite Ichi, Step 16 - Gekisai Kumite Ni)
- Empi Age Uchi (Step 10 - Ichi, Step 17 - Ni)
- Gedan Barai (forward facing in kata) (Step 11 - Ichi, Step 18 - Ni)
- Gyaku Zuki (Step 11 - Ichi, Step 18 - Ni)
- Yoko Shuto Uchi (Step 13 - Ichi, Step 20 - Ni)
- Awase Zuki (Step 15 - Ichi, Step 22 - Ni)

3. Gekisai Kumite San

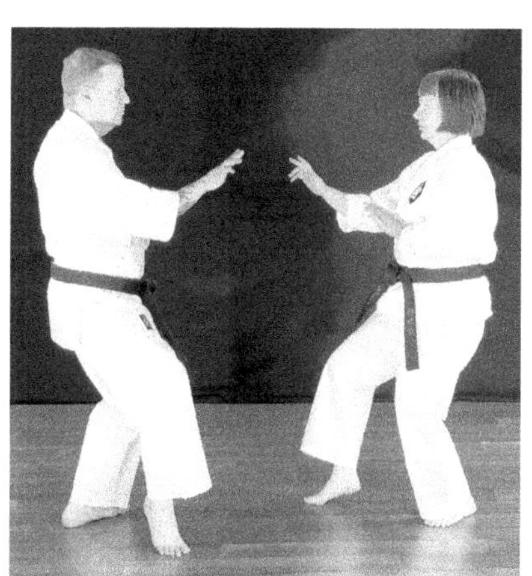

Neko Ashi Dachi Kamae Chamber Hand at Chest, Hands Open, Flat, Palms Down

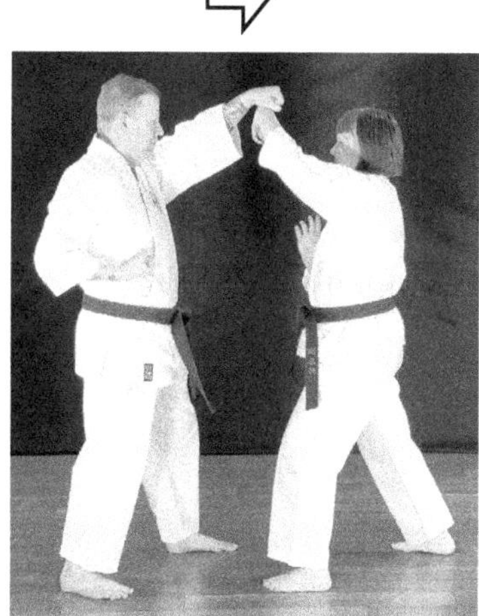

1. Left: Step Forward, Jodan Zuki / Right: Step Back, Jodan Age Ko Uke

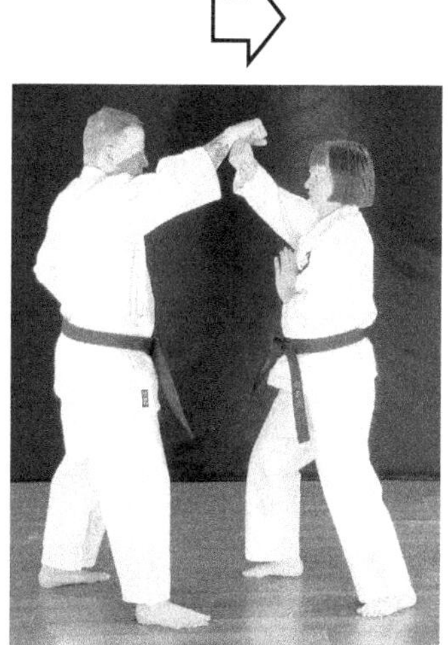

2. Left: Step Forward, Jodan Zuki / Right: Step Back, Jodan Age Ko Uke

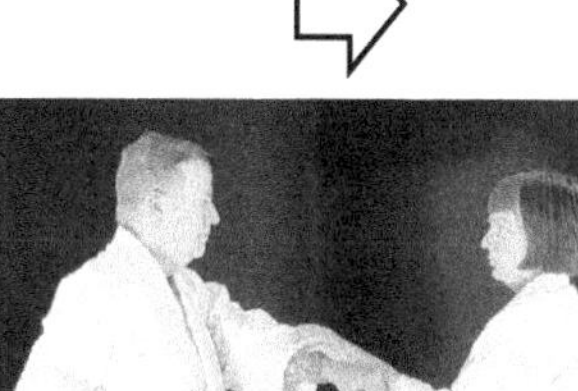

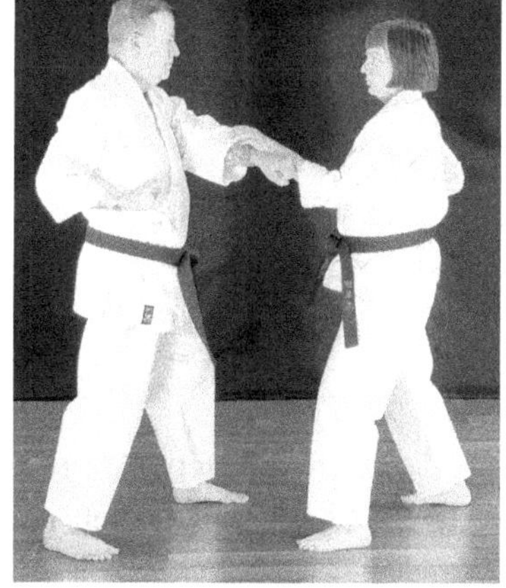

3. Left: Step Forward, Chudan Zuki / Right: Step Back, Chudan Hari to Hiki Uke

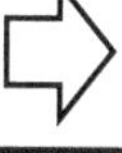

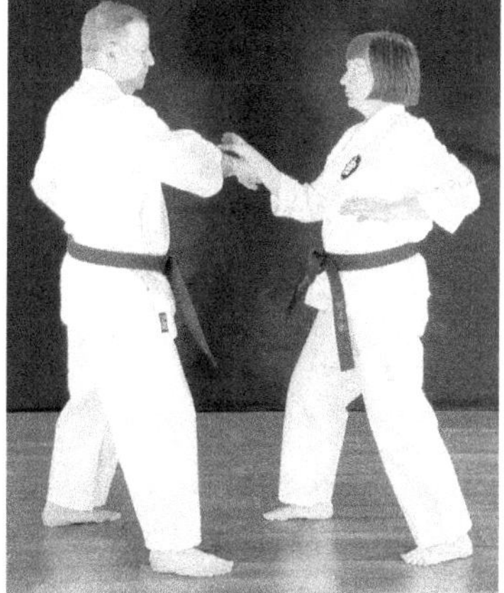

4. Left: Step Forward, Chudan Zuki / Right: Step Back, Chudan Hari to Hiki Uke

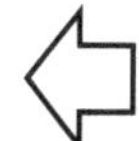

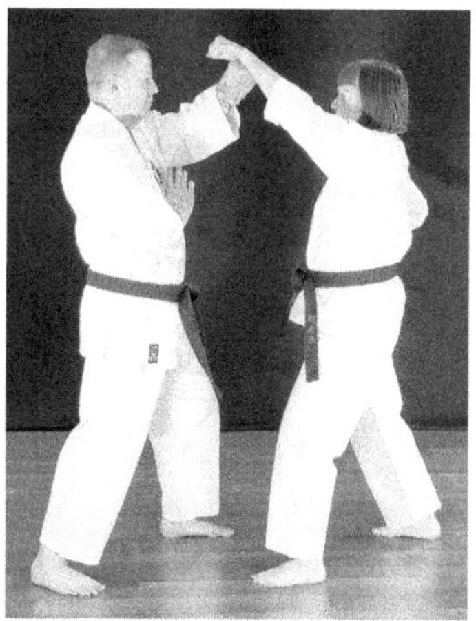

5. Left: Step Back, Jodan Age Ko Uke / Right: Step Forward, Jodan Zuki

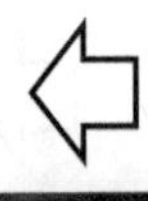
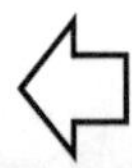

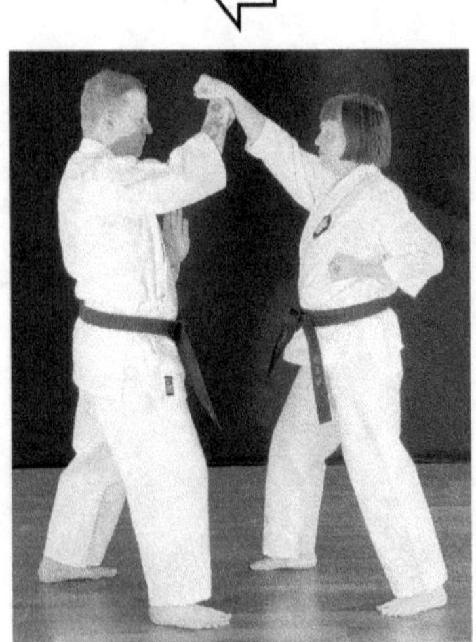

6. Left: Step Back, Jodan Age Ko Uke / Right: Step Forward, Jodan Zuki

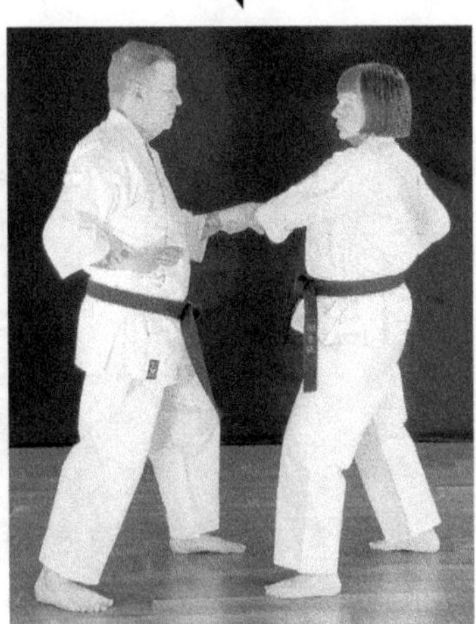

7. Left: Step Back, Chudan Hari to Hiki Uke / Right: Step Forward, Chudan Zuki

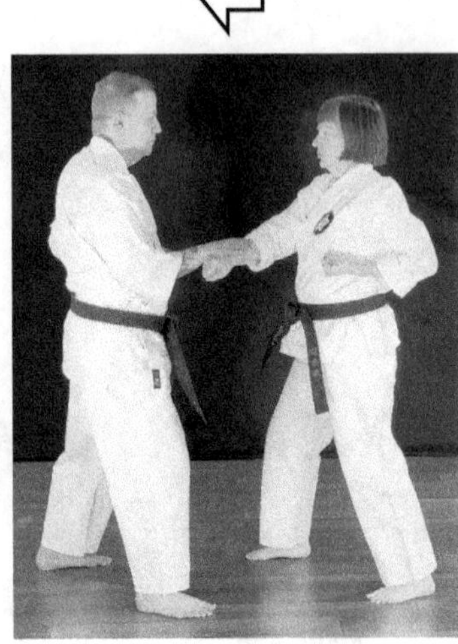

8. Left: Step Back, Chudan Hari to Hiki Uke / Right: Step Forward, Chudan Zuki

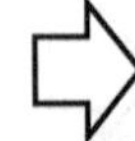
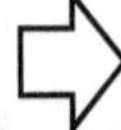
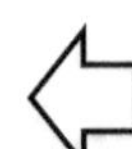

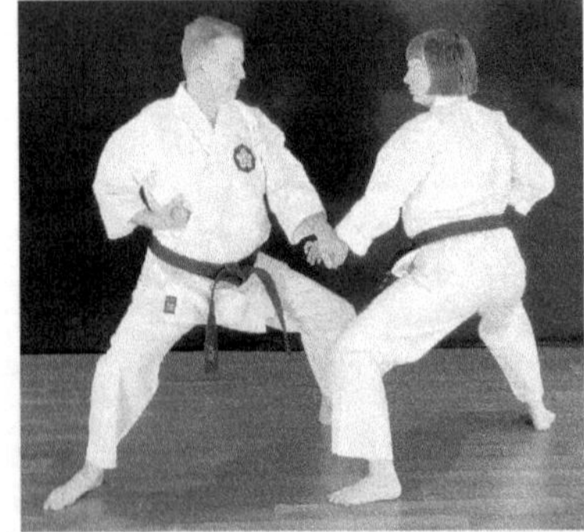

9. Left: Step Forward into Shiko Dachi, Gedan Zuki / Right: Step Back into Shiko Dachi, Gedan Shotei Barai

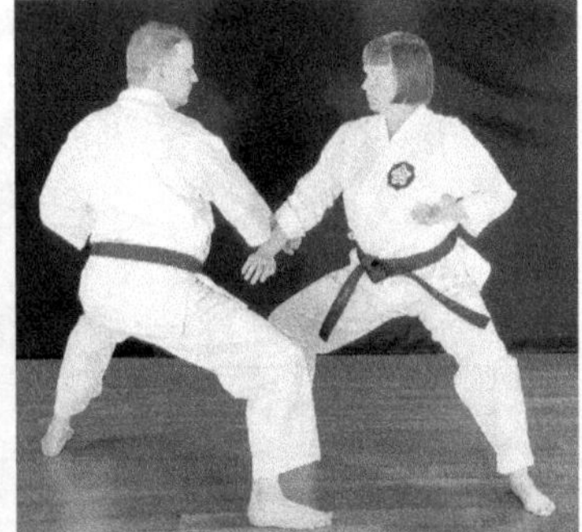

10. Left: Step Forward into Shiko Dachi, Gedan Zuki / Right: Step Back into Shiko Dachi, Gedan Shotei Barai

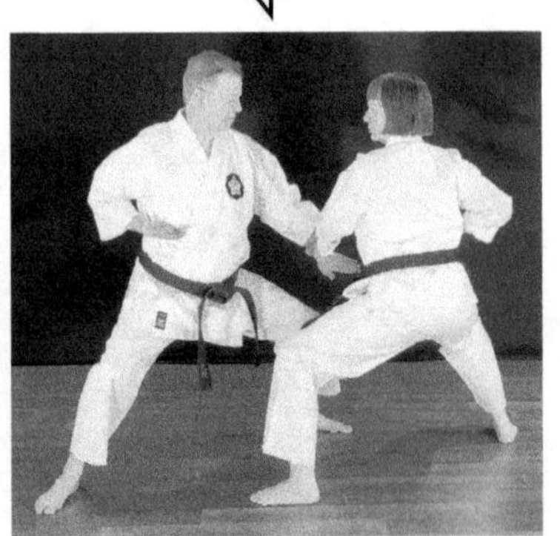

11. Left: Step Back into Shiko Dachi, Gedan Shotei Barai / Right: Step Forward into Shiko Dachi, Gedan Zuki

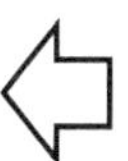

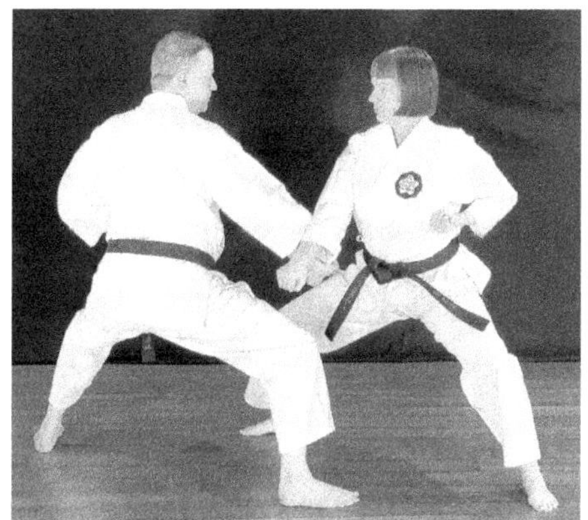

12. Left: Step Back into Shiko Dachi, Gedan Shotei Barai / Right: Step Forward into Shiko Dachi, Gedan Zuki

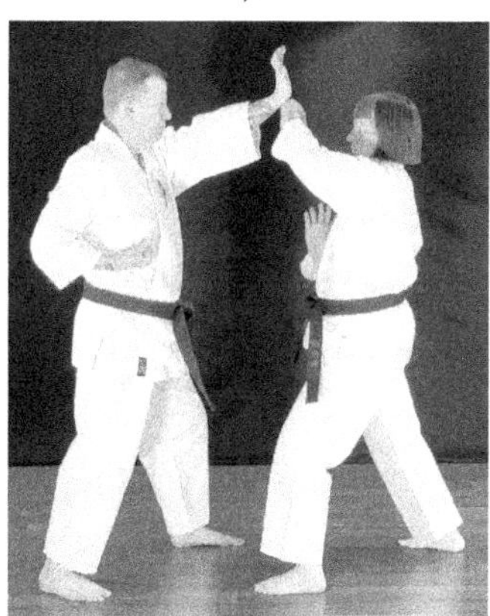

13. Left: Step Forward, Jodan Shotei Uchi / Right: Step Back, Jodan Age Ko Uke

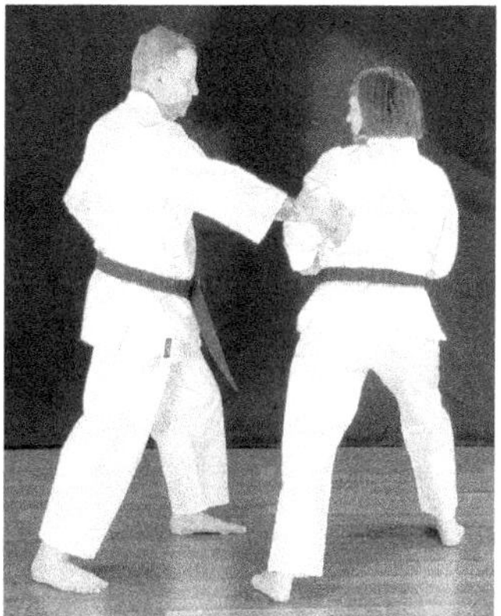

14. Left: Chudan Zuki / Right: Pivot Right, Ushiro Empi Uchi

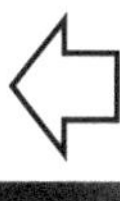

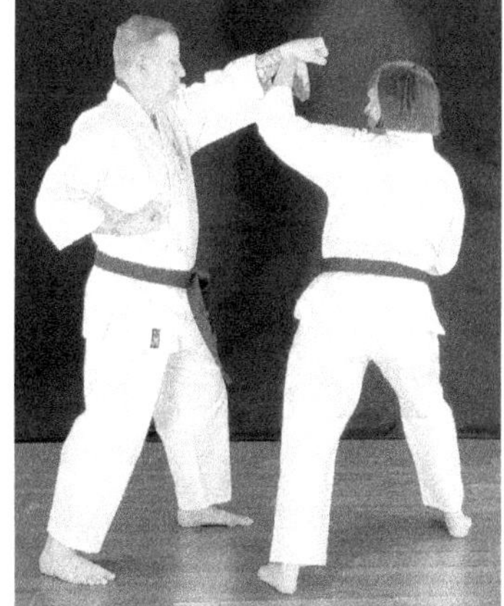

15. Left: Jodan Zuki / Right: Jodan Yoko Age Ko Uke

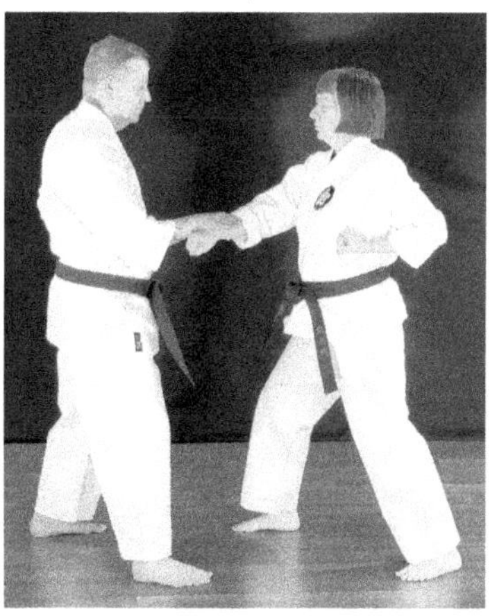

16. Left: Step Back, Chudan Hari to Hiki Uke / Right: Step Forward, Chudan Zuki

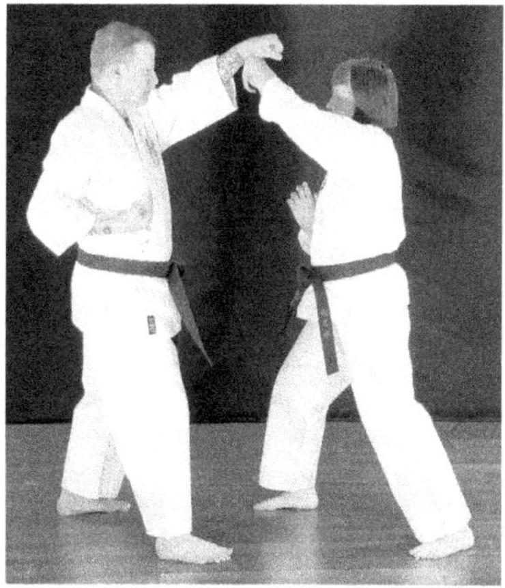

17. Left: Jodan Zuki / Right: Jodan Yoko Age Ko Uke

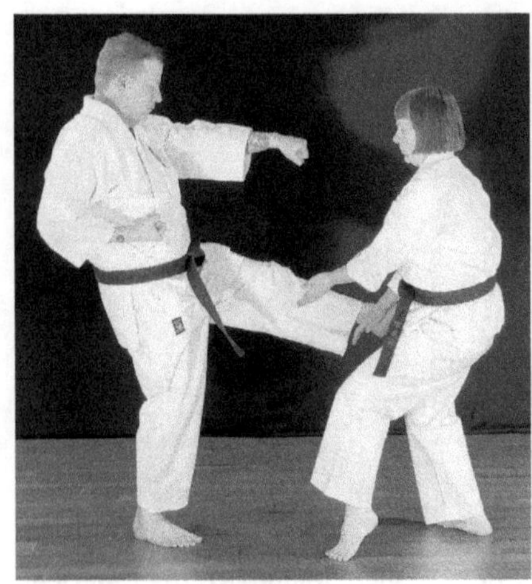

18. Left: Gedan Mae Geri / Right: Step Back into Neko Ashi Dachi, Morote Shuto Uke

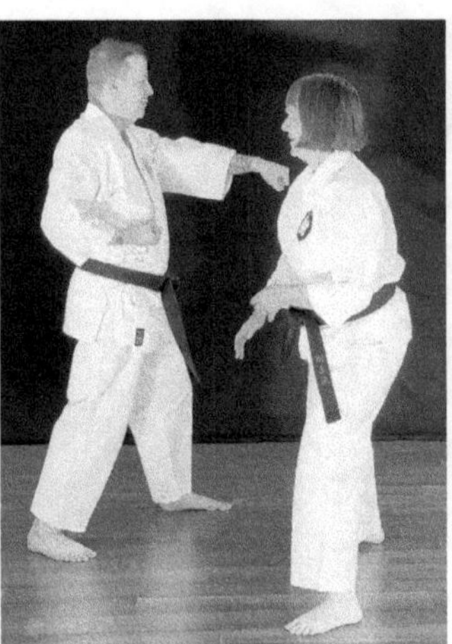

19. Right: Step to Left, Jodan Yoko Geri

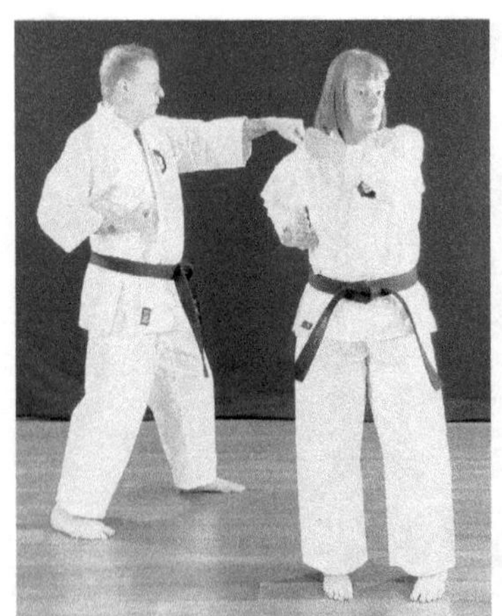

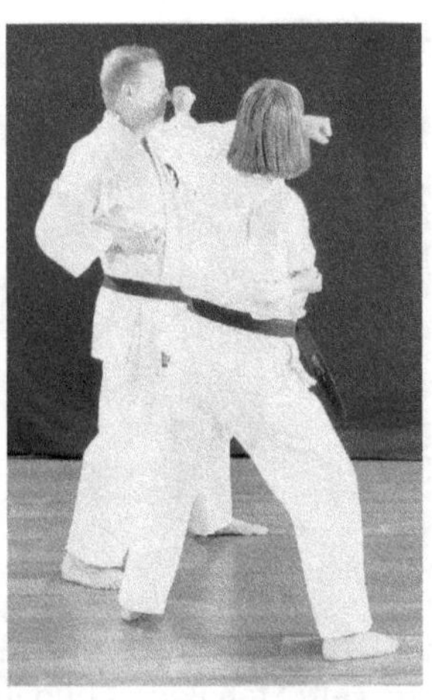

20. Right: After Kick, Bring Right Foot Back to Left Foot, Step in with Left Foot, Jodan Yoko Uraken Uchi

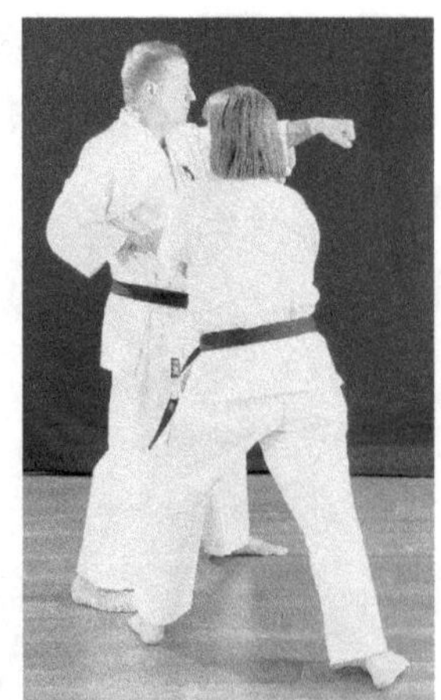

21. Right: Pivot Left, Shuto Uchi no Kamae, Ura Zuki

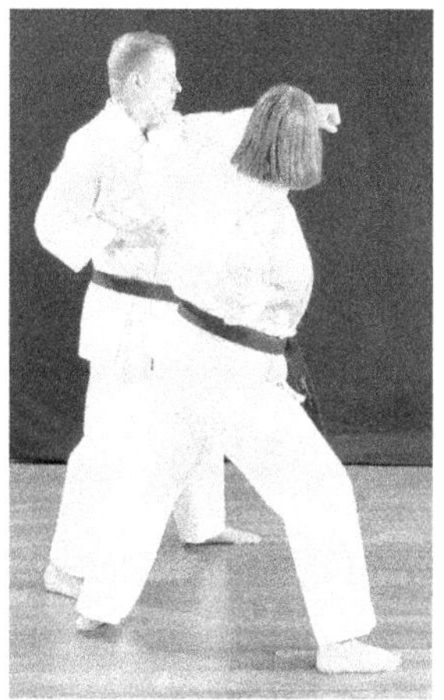

Repeat in Other Direction

22. Right: Pivot Right,
Kubi Shuto Uchi (Kiai)

Kata Comparison to Bunkai Kumite

Gekisai Kumite San does not necessarily correspond to the kata Gekisai San. For the bunkai kumite Shodai created (Gekisai Kumite San through Jokyu Kumite Ichi), he maintained the spirit of showing offensive and defensive moves together, but not necessarily from one kata. However, there are elements from Gekisai San in the following areas:

- The opening blocking sequence, Jodan Yoko Age Ko Uke is taken from an early version of Isshoni San kata (Steps 1-2, 5-6)

4. Chukyu Kumite Ichi

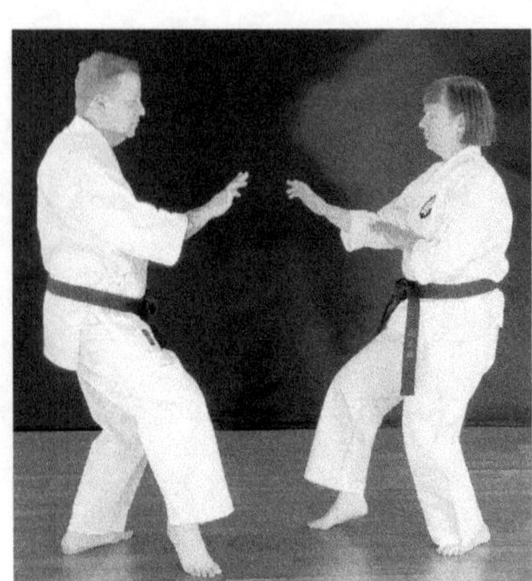

Neko Ashi Dachi Kamae Chamber Hand at Chest, Hands Open, Flat, Palms Down

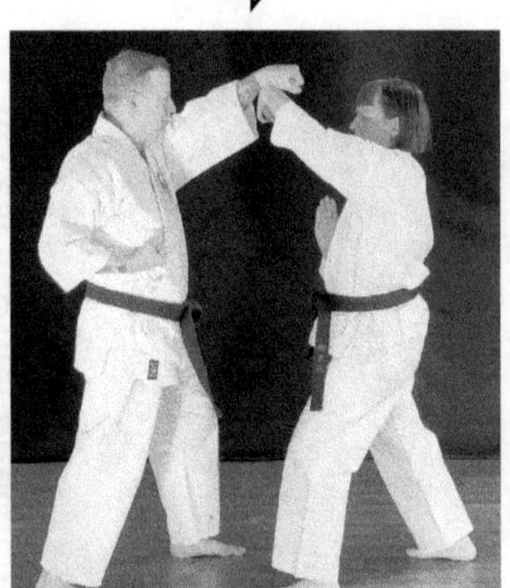

1. Left: Step Forward, Jodan Zuki / Right: Step Back, Jodan Age Ko Uke

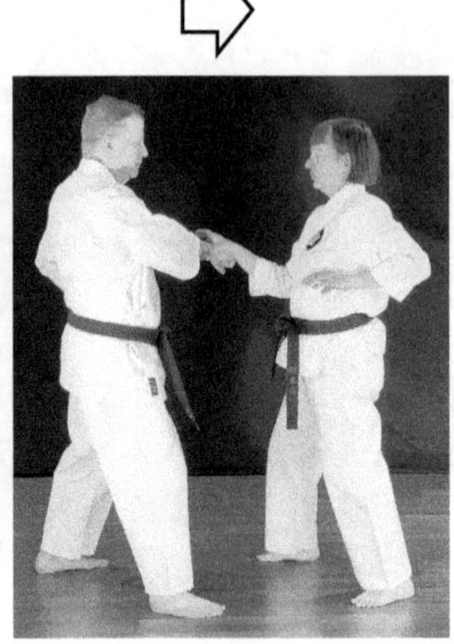

2. Left: Step Forward, Chudan Zuki / Right: Step Back, Chudan Hari to Hiki Uke

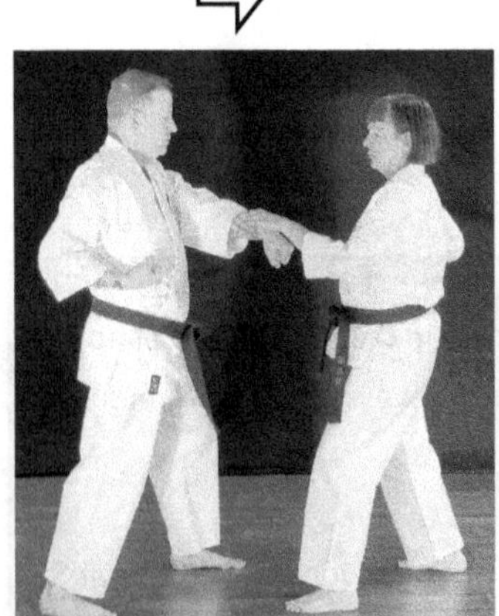

3. Left: Step Forward, Chudan Zuki / Right: Step Back, Chudan Hari to Hiki Uke

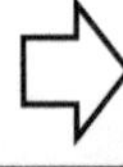

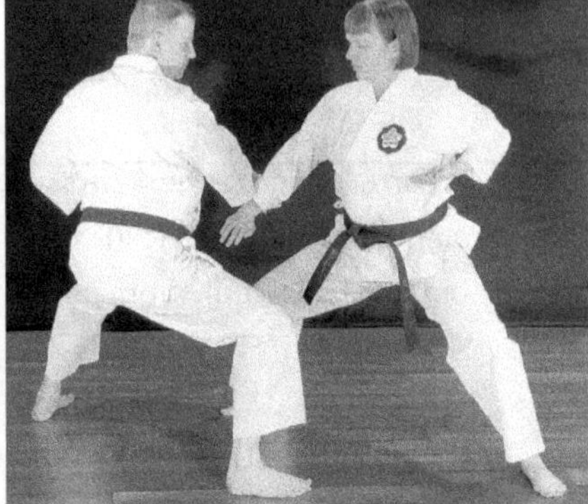

4. Left: Step Forward into Shiko Dachi, Gedan Zuki / Right: Step Back into Shiko Dachi, Gedan Shotei Barai

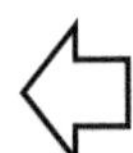

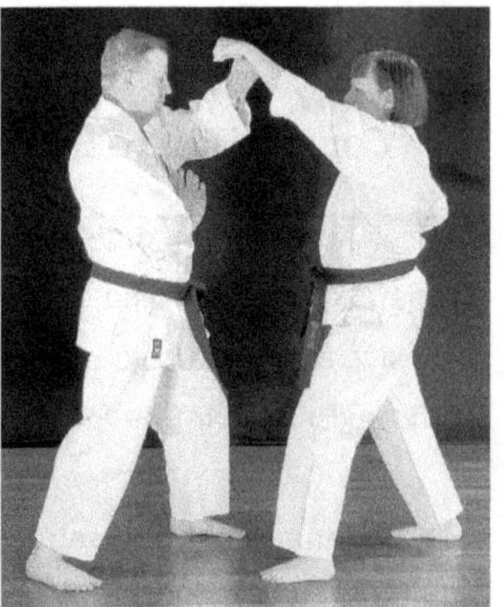

5. Left: Step Back, Jodan Age Ko Uke / Right: Step Forward, Jodan Zuki

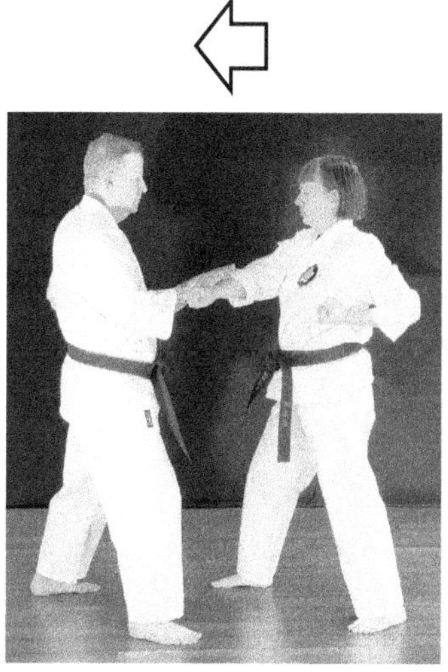

6. Left: Step Back, Chudan Hari to Hiki Uke / Right: Step Forward, Chudan Zuki

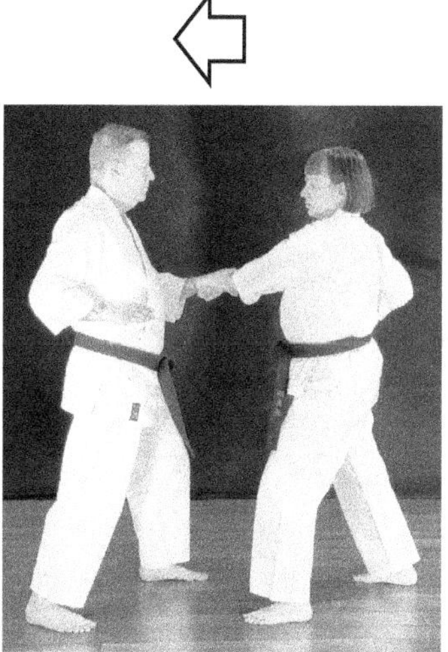

7. Left: Step Back, Chudan Hari to Hiki uke / Right: Step Forward, Chudan Zuki

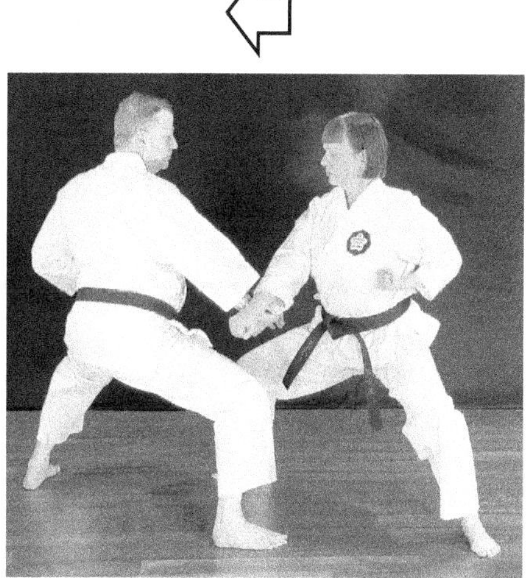

8. Left: Step Back into Shiko Dachi, Gedan Shotei Barai / Right: Step Forward into Shiko Dachi, Gedan Zuki

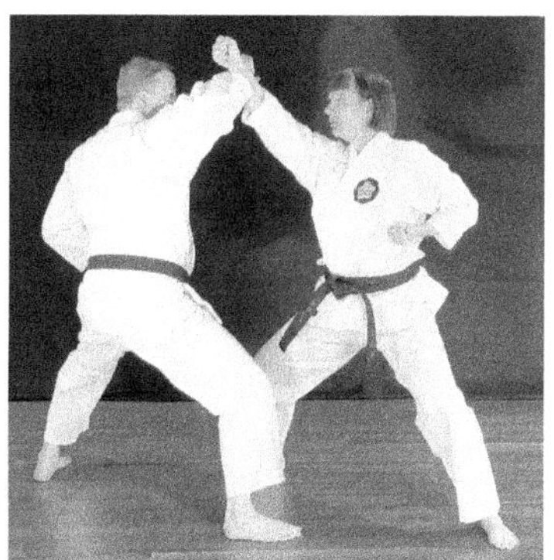

9. Left: Jodan Age Uke / Right: Jodan Yoko Uraken Uchi

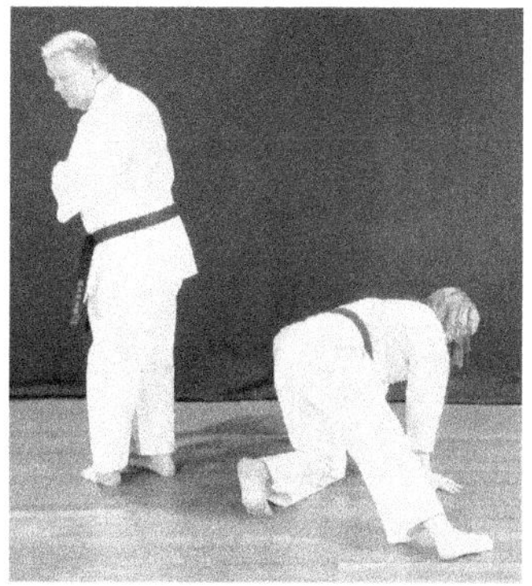

10. Left: Bring Right Leg to Left, Kake Geri / Right: Drop Down to Left Knee, Ura Mawashi Ashi Barai

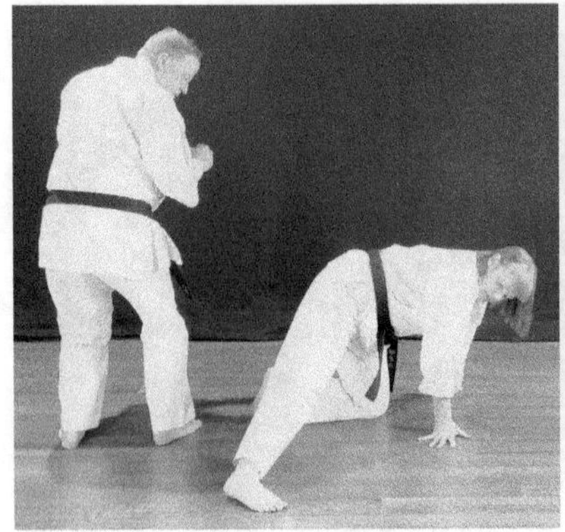
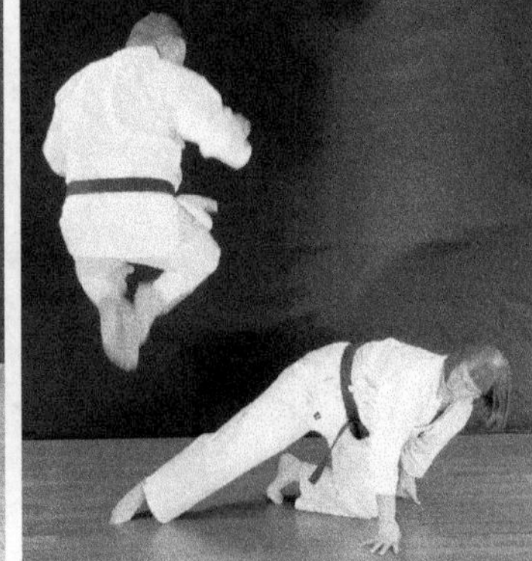
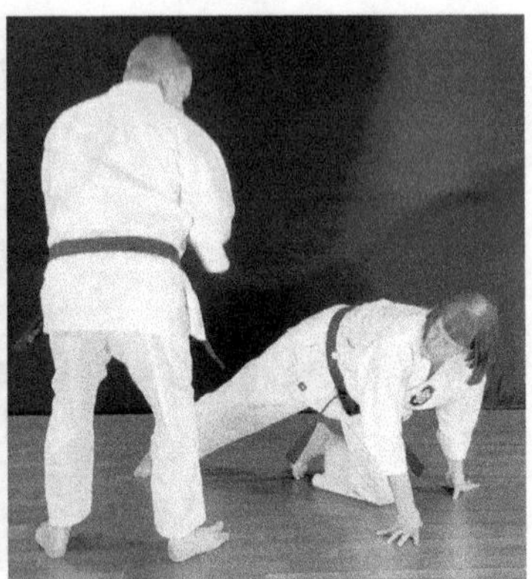

Right: Ura Mawashi Ashi Barai (cont.)

11. Left: Jump over Leg Sweep

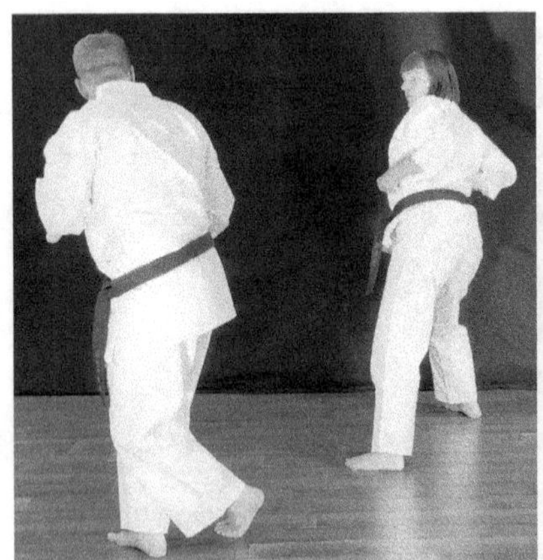
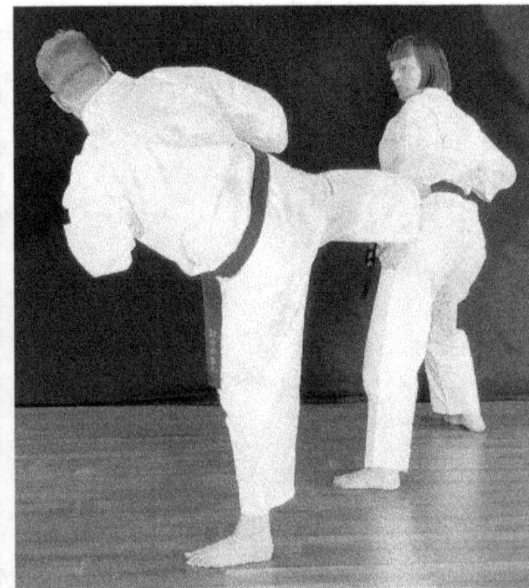

12. Left: Step Behind Yoko Geri / Right: Come Up, Yoko Otoshi Zuki on 225° Angle

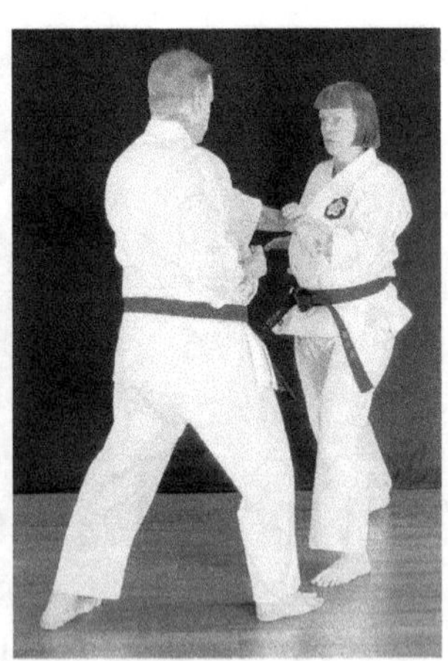

13. Left: Square Up on Opponent, Gyaku Zuki / Right: Chudan Hari to Hiki Uke

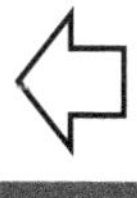

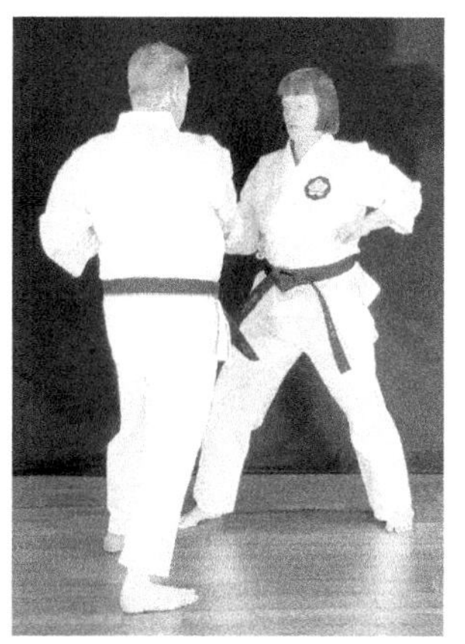

14. Left: Step Forward, Gyaku Zuki / Right: Step Back, Chudan Hari to Hiki Uke

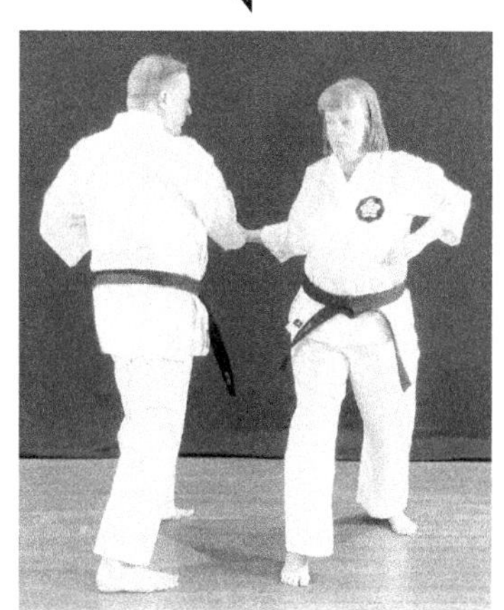

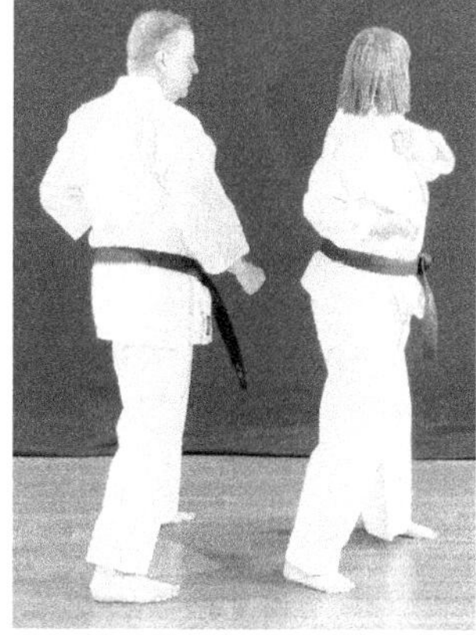

15. Right: Ushiro Mawashi Uraken Uchi

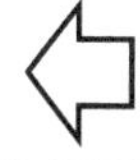

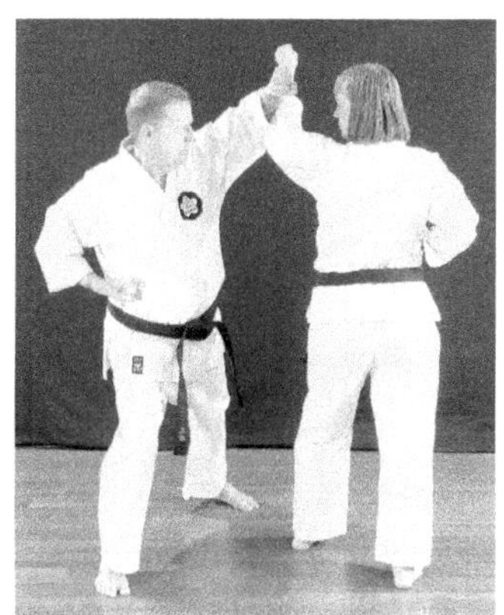

16. Left: Lean to Right, Jodan Yoko Age Uke / Right: Ushiro Mawashi Uraken Uchi (cont.)

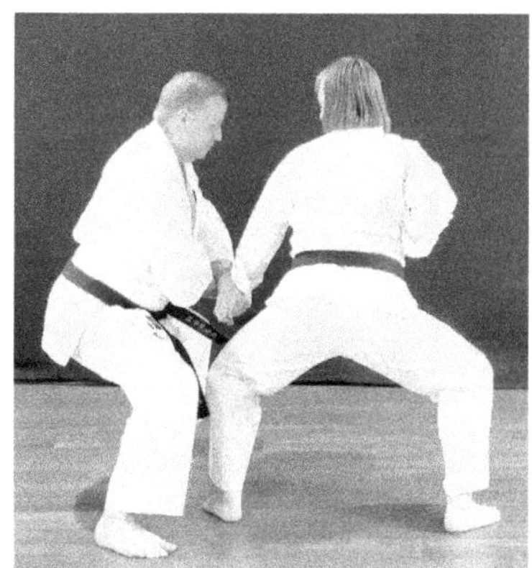

17. Left: Bring Right Foot Forward into Shiko Dachi, Juji Otoshi Uke / Right: Left Foot Step into Shiko Dachi, Yoko Tettsui Uchi

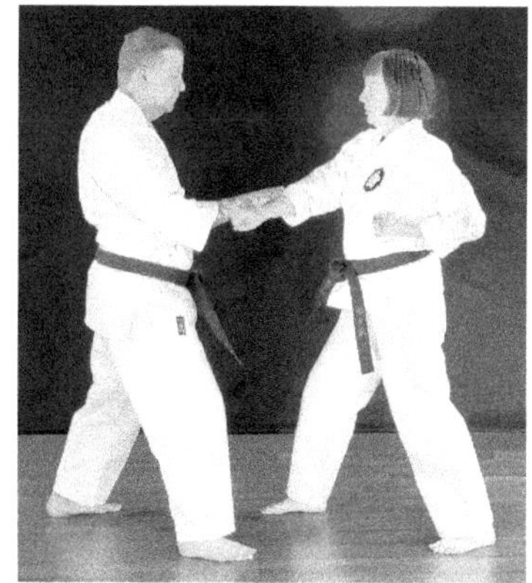

18. Left: Step Back, Chudan Hari to Hiki Uke / Right: Step Forward, Chudan Zuki

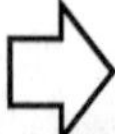

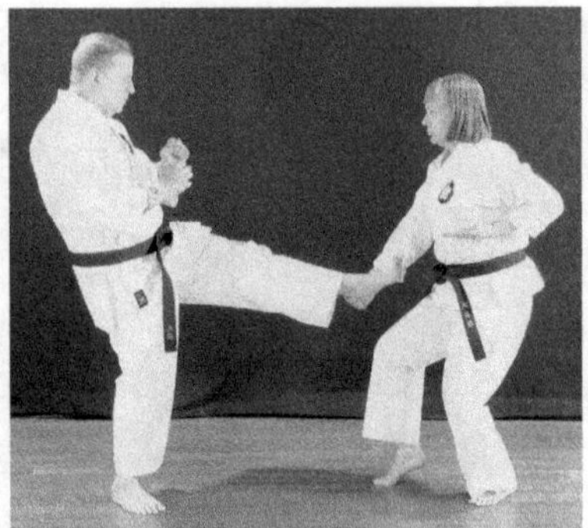

19. Left: Gedan Mae Geri / Right: Step Back with Left Foot, Drag Right Foot into Neko Ashi Dachi, Sukui Uke

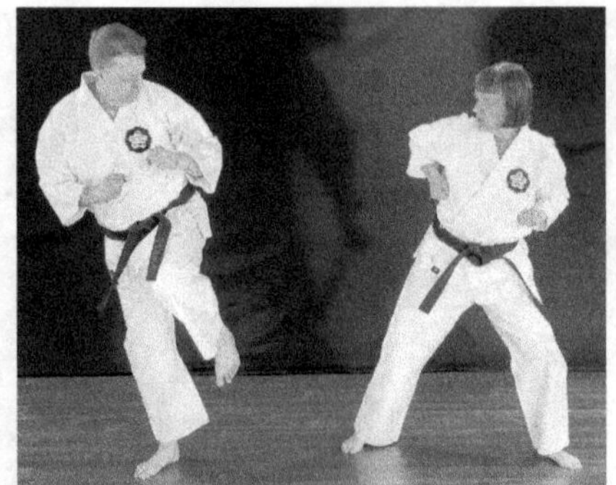

20. Left: Pivot Left (Without Putting Foot Down, Chamber Yoko Geri) / Right: Lean Away, Prepare Yoko Otoshi Zuki

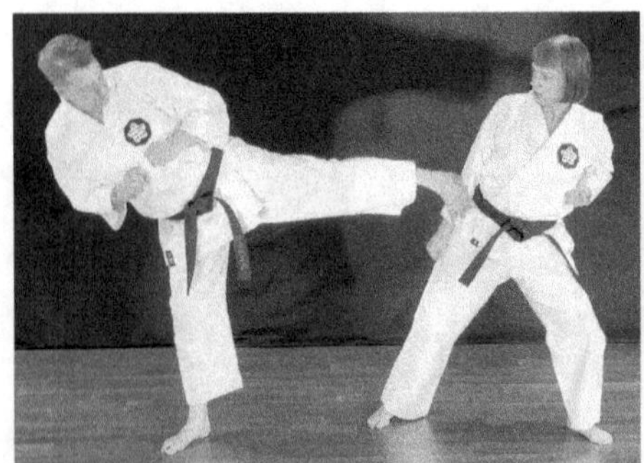

21. Left: Yoko Geri / Right: Yoko Otoshi Zuki

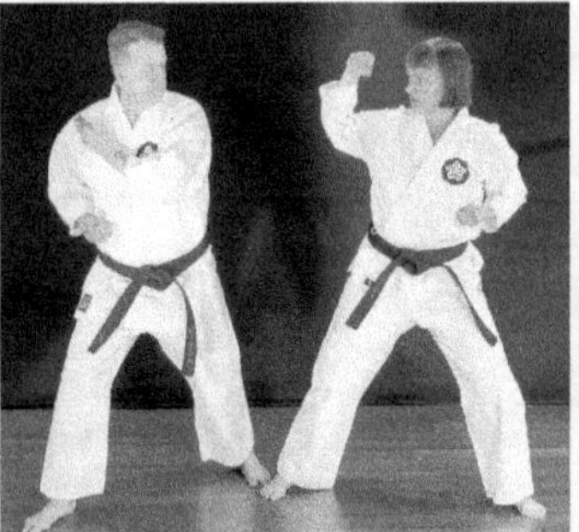

22. Left: Land Kick Just Behind Opponent, Jodan Yoko Shuto Uchi / Right: Soto Uke

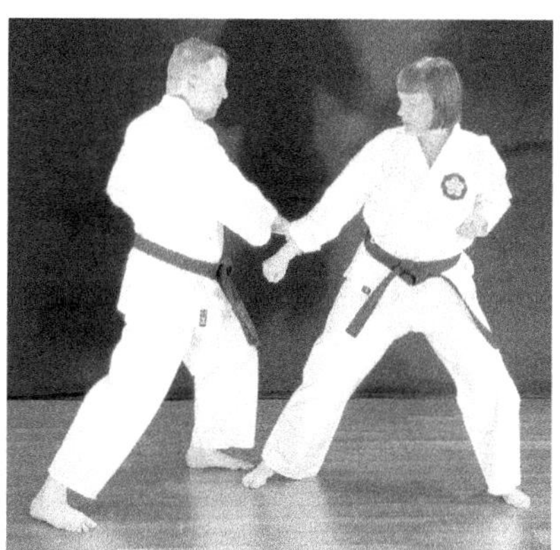

23. Left: Pivot Right, Gyaku Zuki / Right: Yoko Gedan Barai

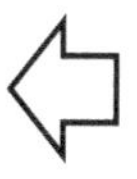

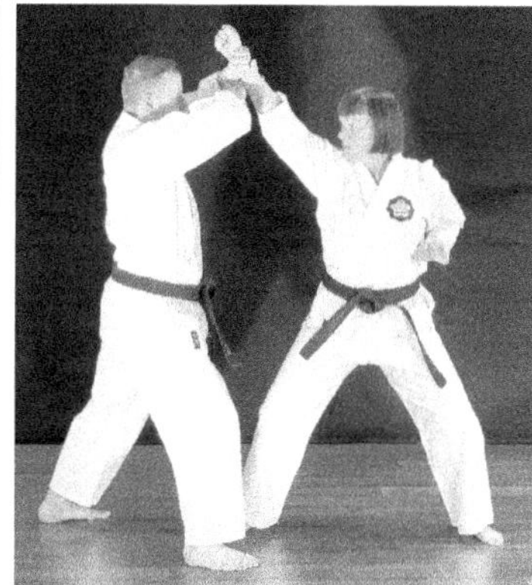

24. Left: Step Back, Juji Age Uke / Right: Step Behind Yoko Tettsui Otoshi Uchi

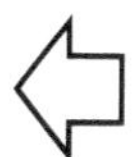

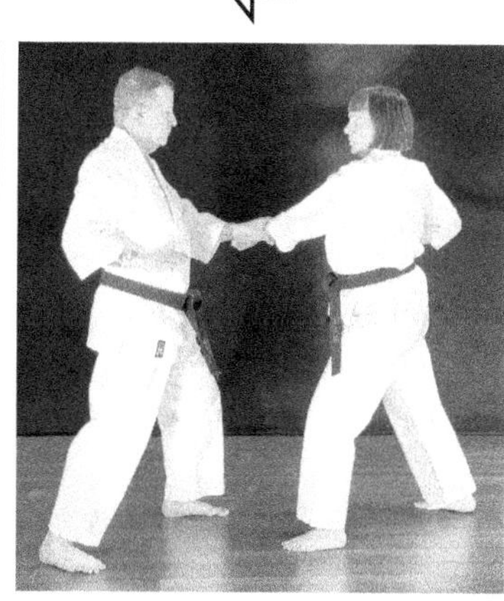

25. Left: Step Back, Chudan Hari to Hiki Uke / Right: Step Forward, Chudan Zuki

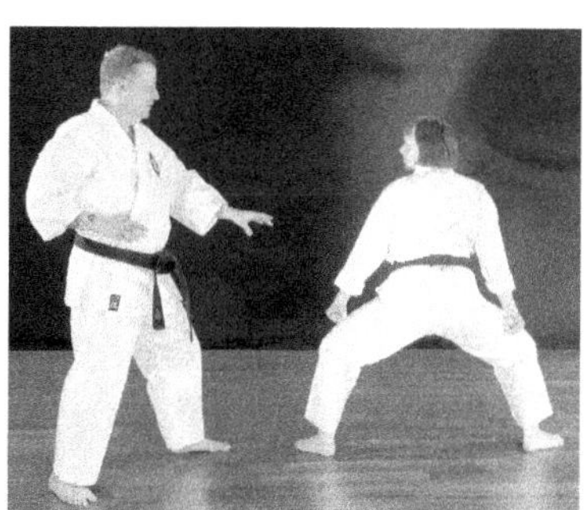

26. Left: Slide Lead Leg to Right / Right: Bring Right Leg Back into Shiko Dachi, Drop Hands

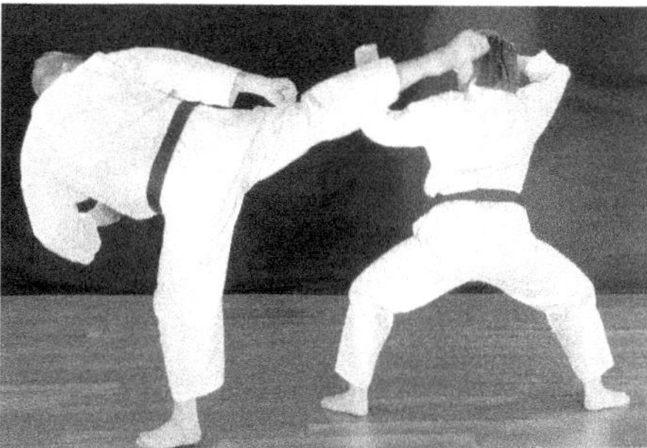

27. Left: Mawashi Geri / Right: Haiwan Uke

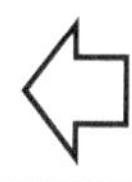

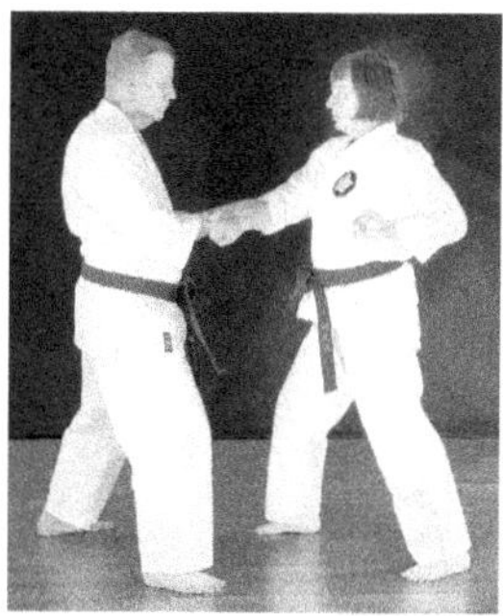

28. Left: Step Back, Chudan Hari to Hiki Uke / Right: Step Forward, Chudan Zuki

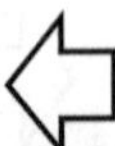

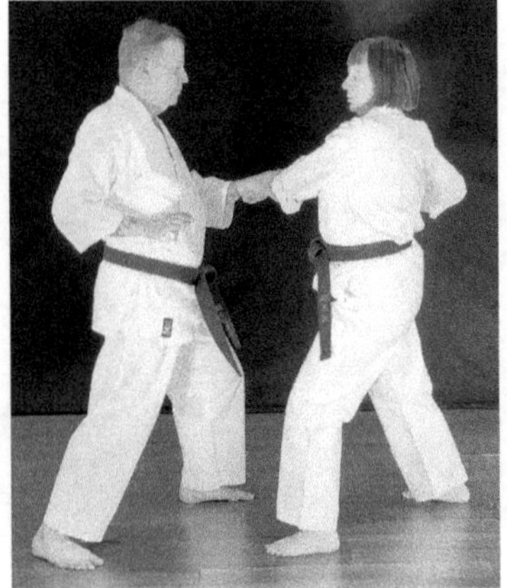

29. Left: Step Back, Chudan Hari to Hiki Uke / Right: Step Forward, Chudan Zuki

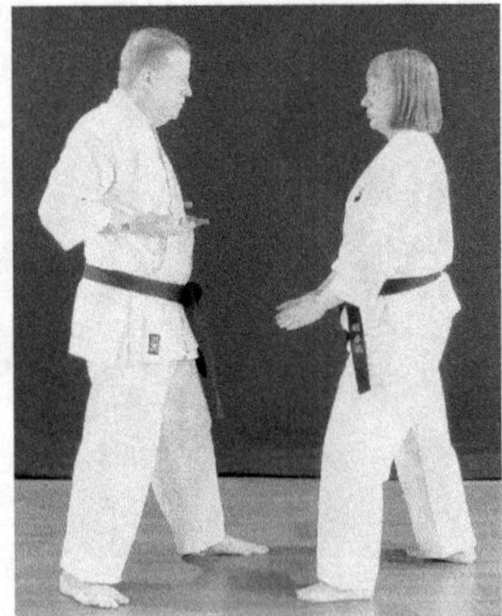

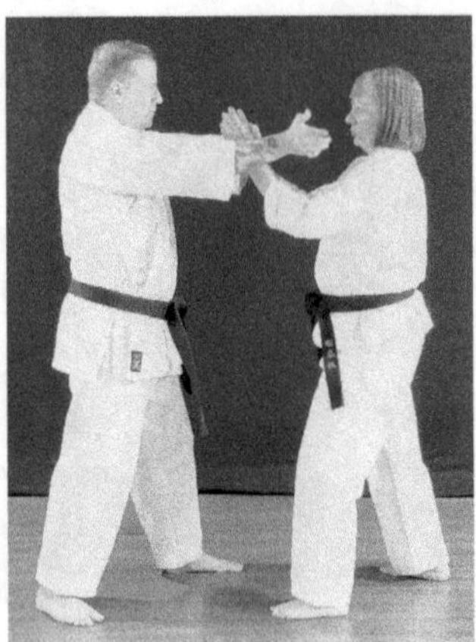

30. Left: Jodan Morote Shotei Tate Uchi / Right: Bring Hands Up Through Opponent's Hands, Separating Them

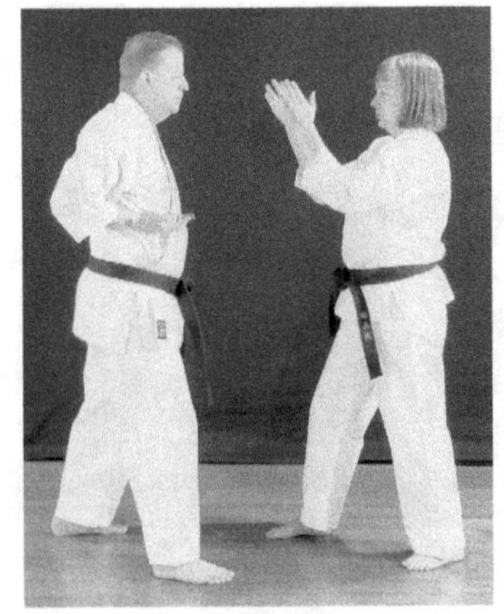

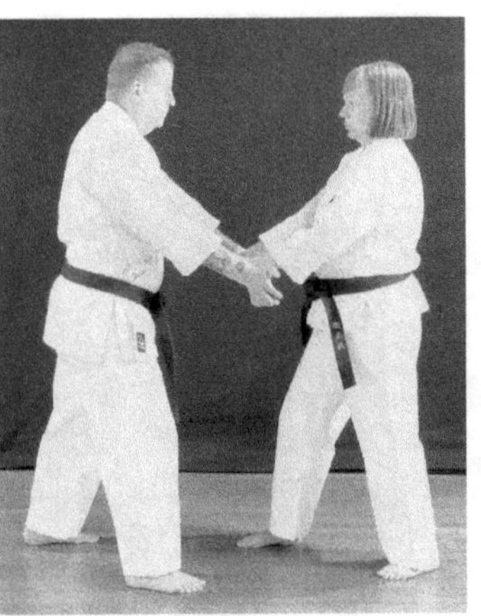

31. Left: Step Forward, Gedan Morote Tate Shotei Uchi / Right: Step Back, Bring Hands Down, Separating Opponent's Hands

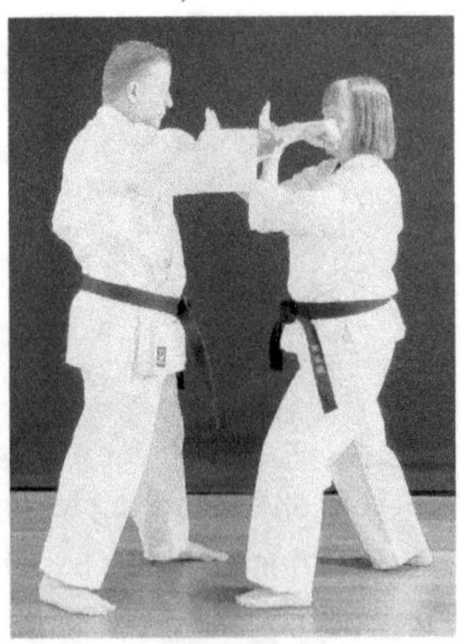

32. Left: Step Forward, Jodan Zuki / Right: Step Back, Yoko Morote Shuto Uke

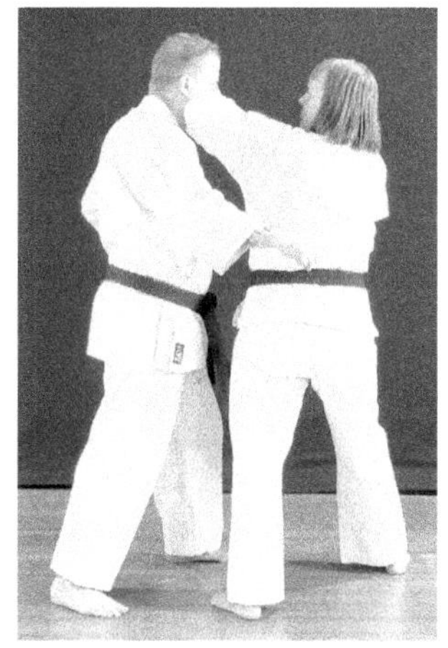

33. Right: Jodan Mawashi Empi Uchi

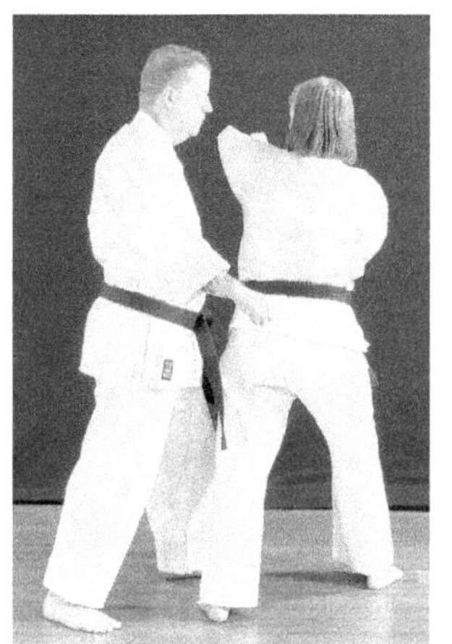

34. Right: Bring Elbow Back to Jaw (Ushiro Empi Uchi)

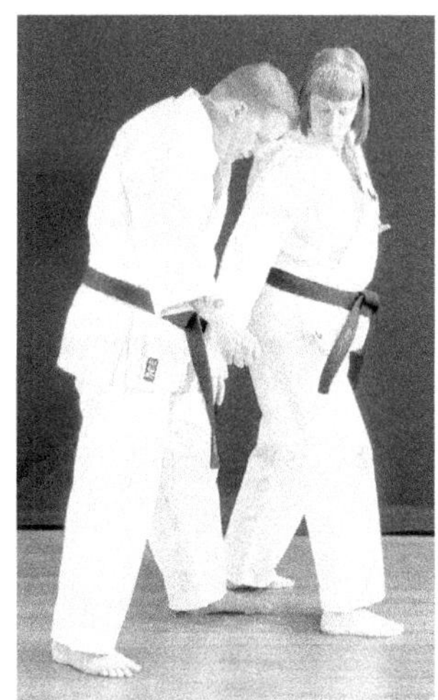

35. Right: Mawatte, Ushiro Shuto Uchi (Gedan)

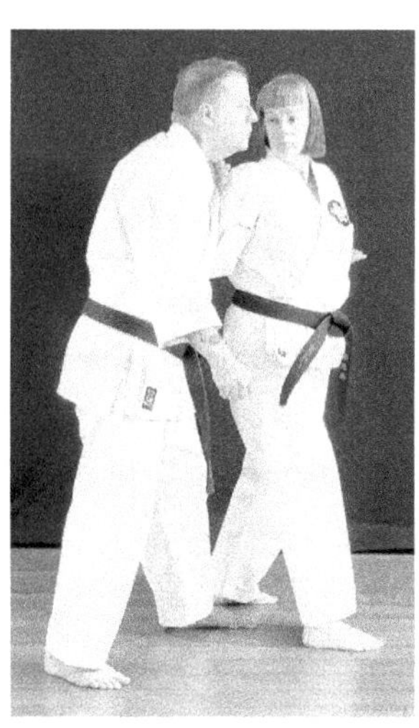

36. Right: Bring Hand Up for Haito Uchi to Opponent's Throat

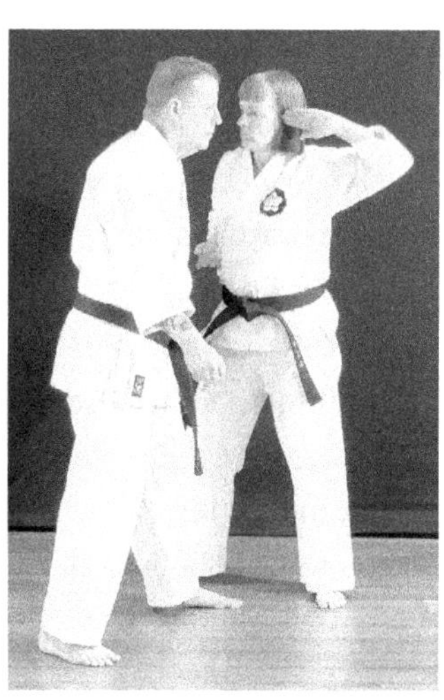

37. Right: Mawatte, Shuto Otoshi Uchi (Kokyubu) (Kiai)

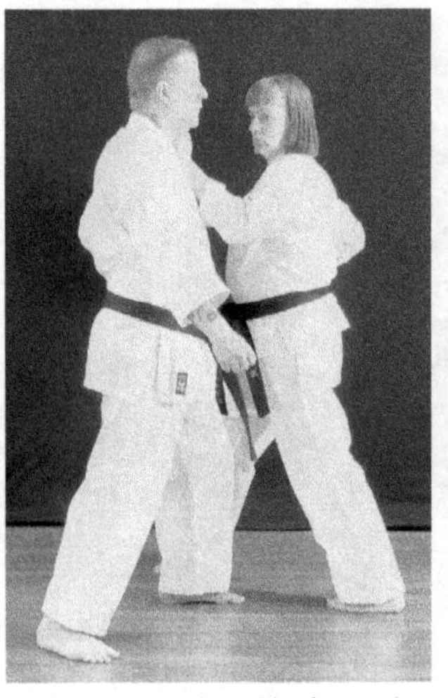

Shuto Otoshi Uchi (cont.)

Kata Comparison to Bunkai Kumite

Note: this is not an exhaustive list, but a list of observations.

Chukyu Kumite Ichi contains elements from several kata in the following areas:

- Ura Mawashi Ashi Barai (Step 10 - Kyouryoku Do)
- Yoko Tettsui Otoshi Uchi (Step 14 - Gekisai San, Genshin)
- The Ushiro Mawashi Uraken Uchi to Yoko Tettsui Uchi sequence is reminiscent of a similar move in Juhito (Uraken Uchi to Gedan Shotei Uchi) (Steps 16-17)
- The Gedan Mae Geri to Yoko Geri to Jodan Yoko Shuto Uchi sequence (Steps 19-22 - Isshoni San)
- Haiwan Uke (Step 27 - Juhito)
- Morote Tate Shotei Uchi (Steps 30-31 - Hente Do)
- Morote Shuto Uke (Step 32 - Hente Do (variation), Kyouryoku Do)

5. Chukyu Kumite Ni

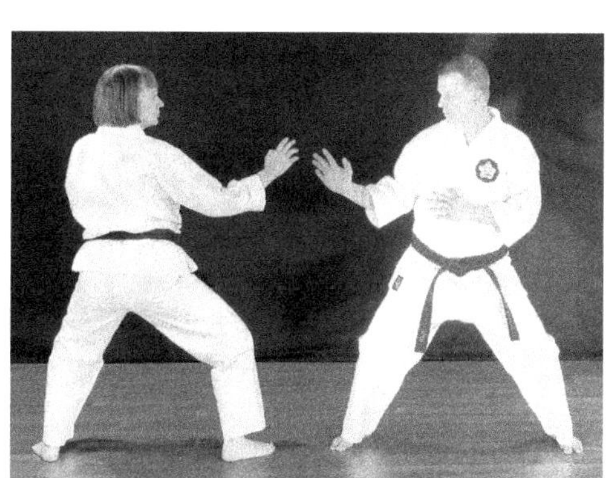

Yoko Kumite Dachi Kamae
Open Hands

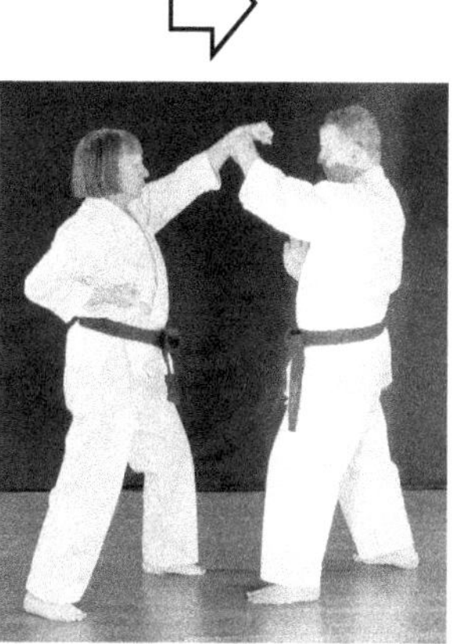

1. Left: Step Forward, Jodan Zuki / Right: Step Back, Jodan Age Ko Uke

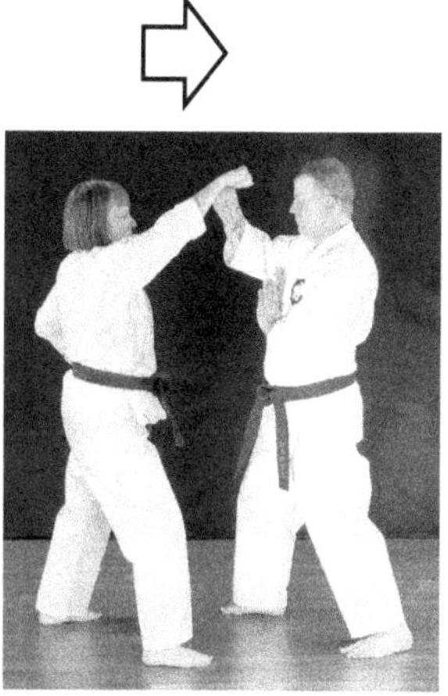

2. Left: Step Forward, Jodan Zuki / Right: Step Back, Jodan Age Ko Uke

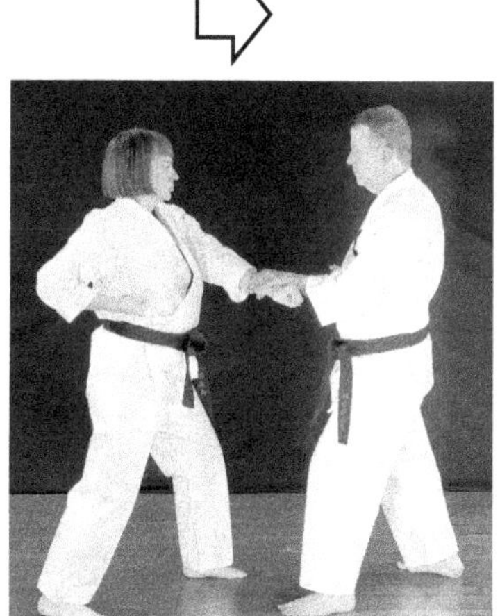

3. Left: Step Forward, Chudan Zuki / Right: Step Back, Chudan Hari to Hiki Uke

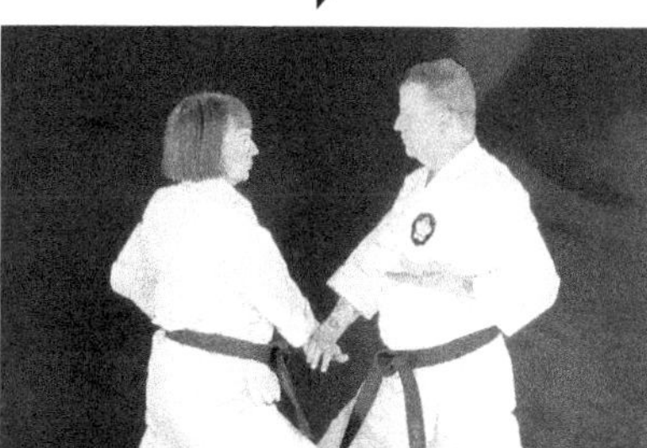

4. Left: Step Forward, Gedan Zuki in Zenkutsu Dachi / Right: Step Back, Gedan Shotei Barai in Zenkutsu Dachi

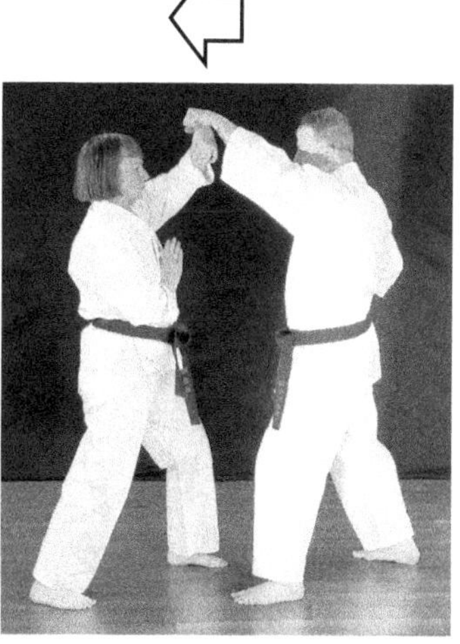

5. Left: Step Back, Jodan Age Ko Uke / Right: Step Forward, Jodan Zuki

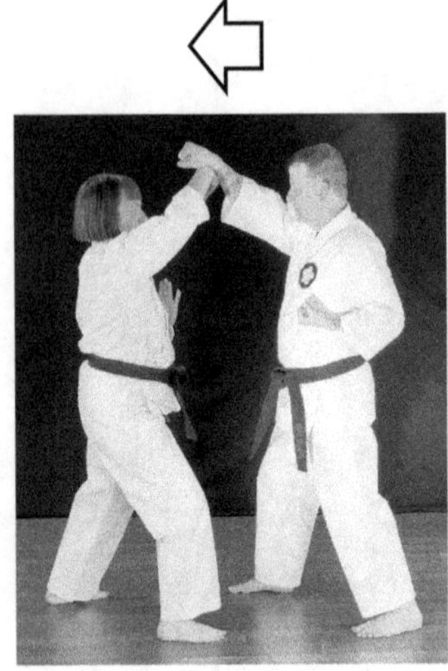

6. Left: Step Back, Jodan Age Ko Uke / Right: Step Forward, Jodan Zuki

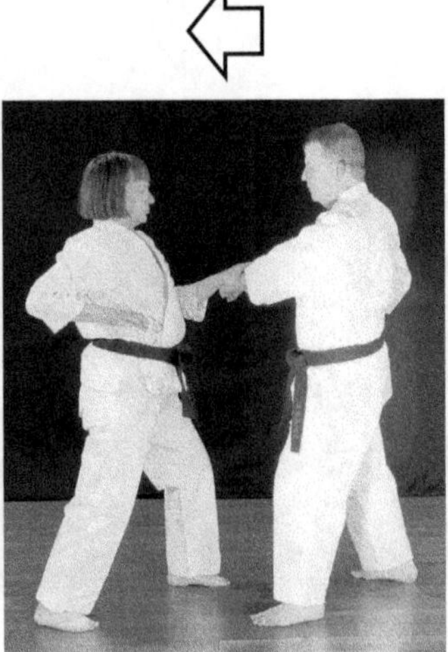

7. Left: Step Back, Chudan Hari to Hiki Uke / Right: Step Forward, Chudan Zuki

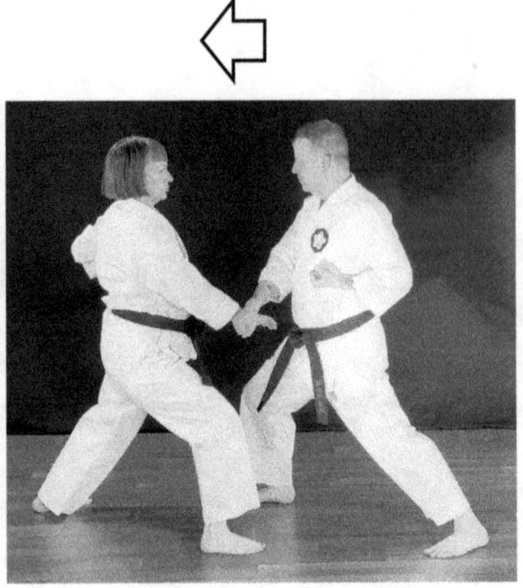

8. Left: Step Back, Gedan Shotei Barai in Zenkutsu Dachi / Right: Step Forward, Gedan Zuki in Zenkutsu Dachi

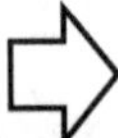

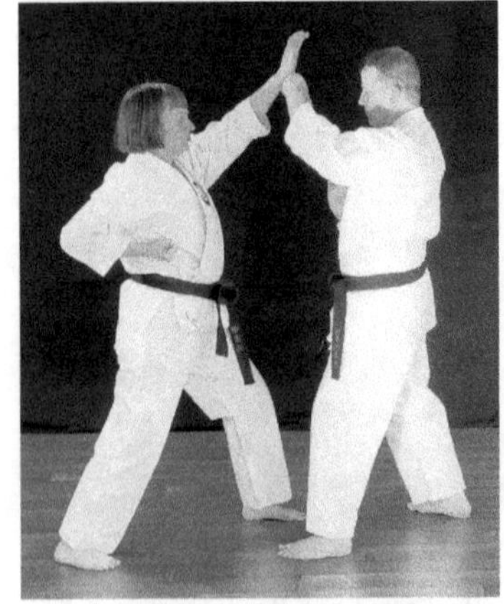

9. Left: Step Forward, Jodan Shotei Uchi / Right: Step Back, Jodan Age Ko Uke

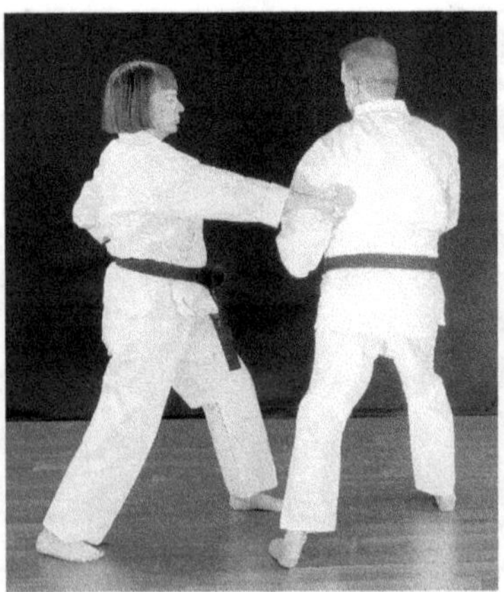

10. Left: Chudan Zuki / Right: Pivot Right, Ushiro Empi Uke

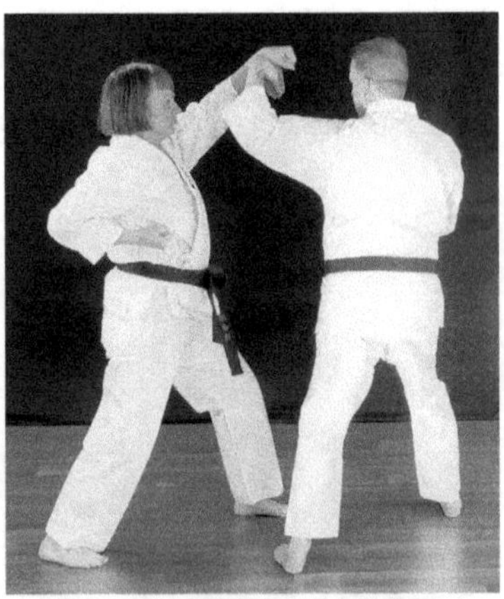

11. Left: Jodan Zuki / Right: Jodan Yoko Age Ko Uke

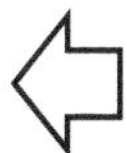

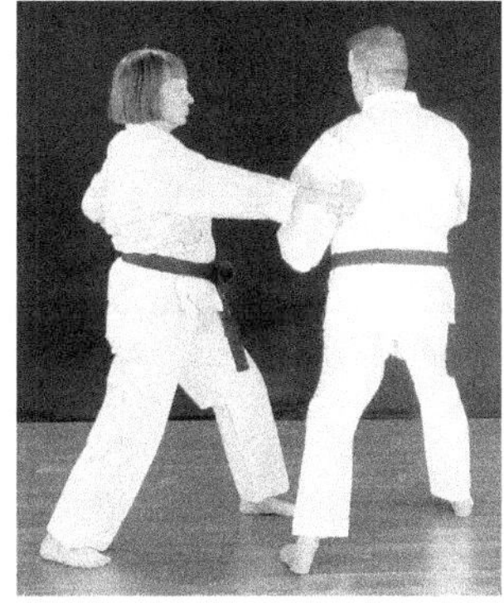

12. Left: Chudan Zuki / Right: Ushiro Empi Uke

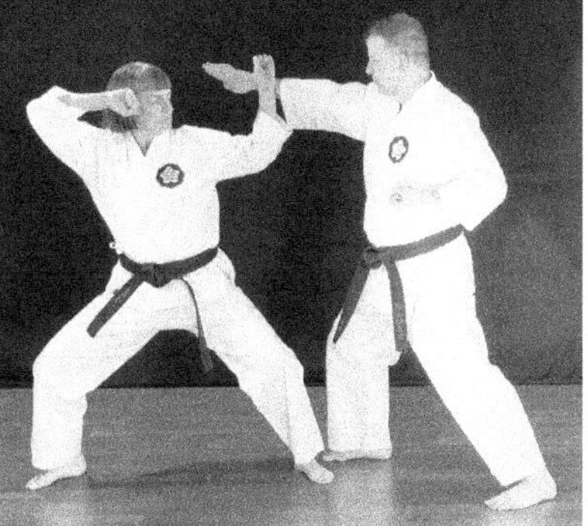

13. Left: Step Back into Yoko Shiko Dachi, Haiwan Uke / Right: Step Forward, Jodan Haito Uchi

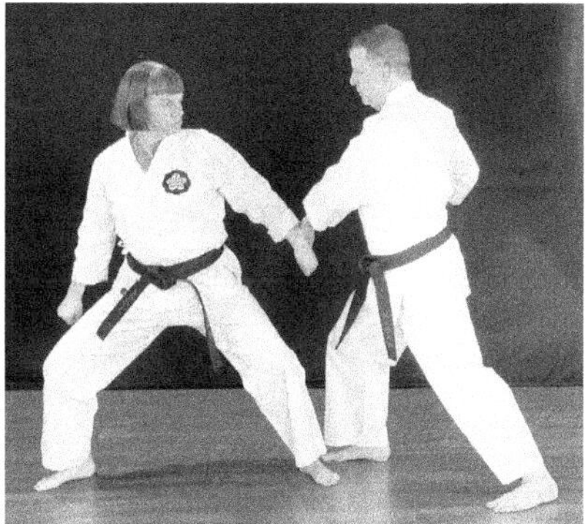

14. Left: Drop Hands, Yoko Gedan Barai / Right: Gedan Zuki

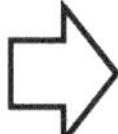

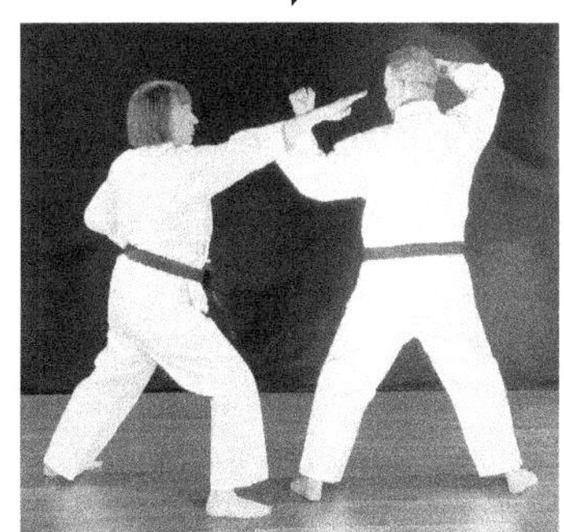

15. Left: Step Forward, Jodan Haito Uchi / Right: Step Back into Yoko Shiko Dachi, Haiwan Uke

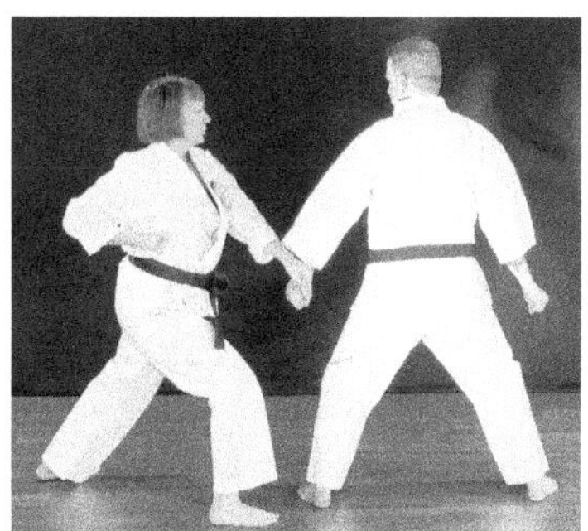

16. Left: Gedan Zuki / Right: Drop Hands, Yoko Gedan Barai

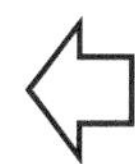

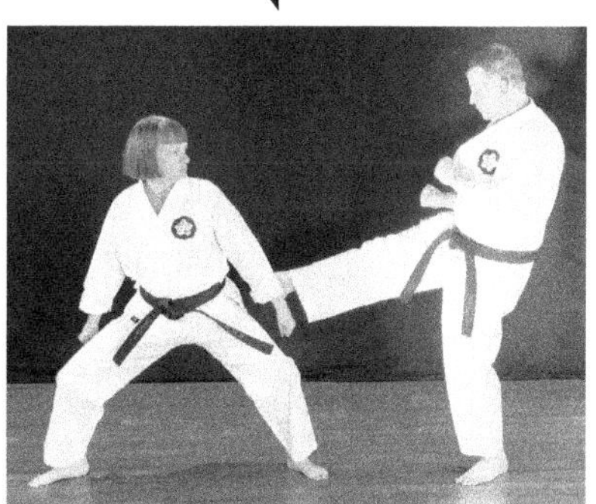

17. Left: Step Back into Yoko Shiko Dachi, Drop Hands, Yoko Gedan Barai / Right: Mae Geri

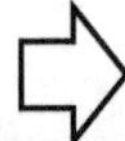

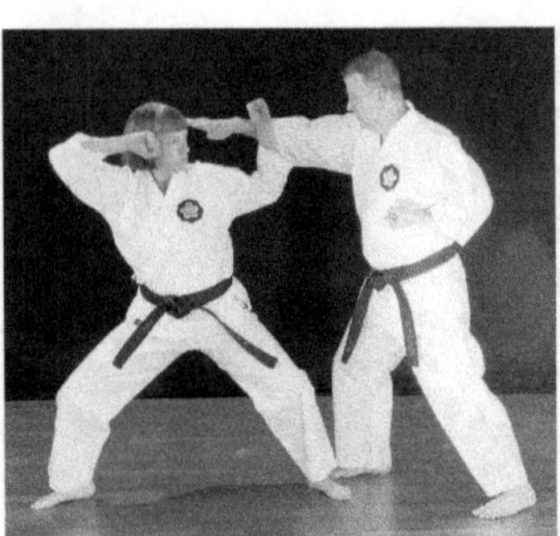

18. Left: Haiwan Uke / Right: Jodan Haito Uchi

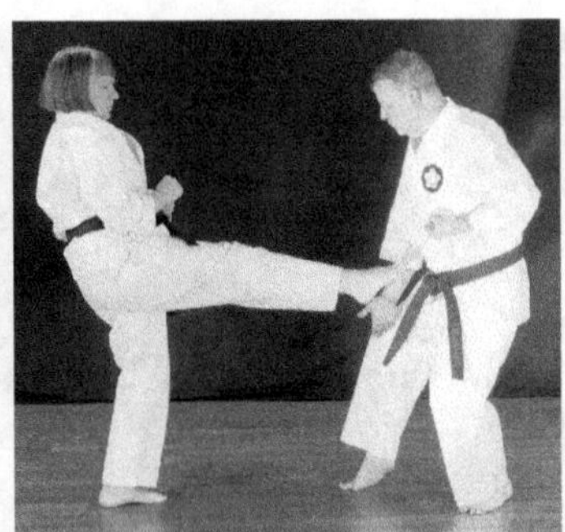

19. Left: Mae Geri / Right: Step Back with Left Foot, Sukui Uke

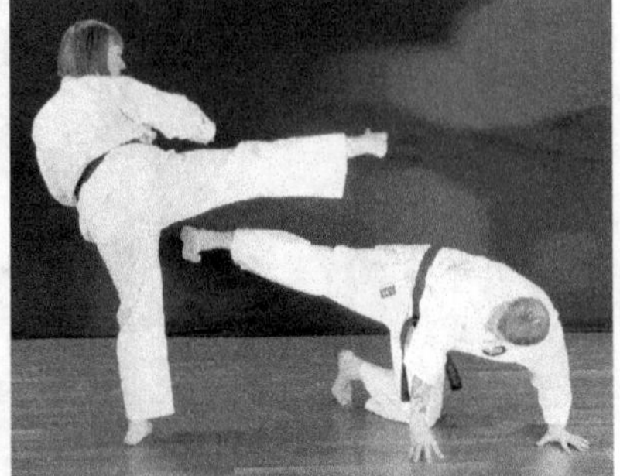

20. Left: Step Behind Yoko Geri / Right: Drop Down to Left Knee, Gedan (Age) Yoko Geri

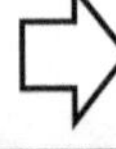

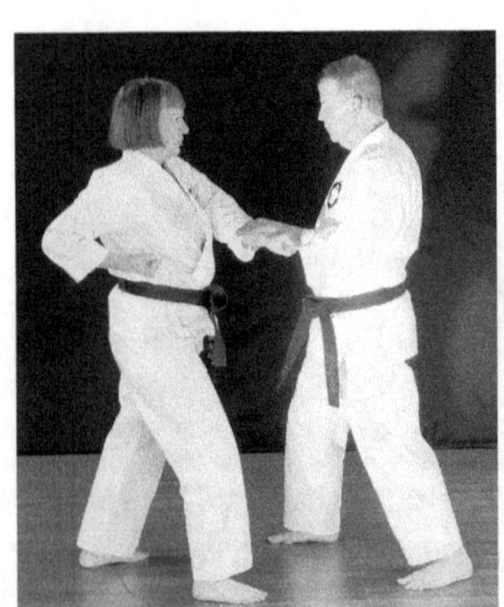

21. Left: Square Up, Gyaku Zuki / Right: Chudan Hari to Hiki Uke

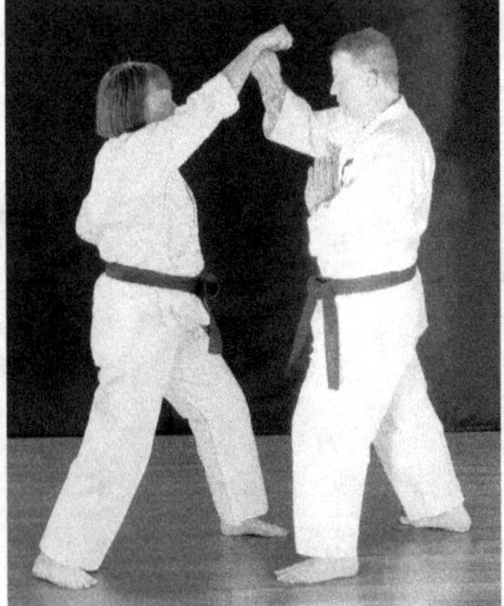

22. Left: Step Forward, Jodan Zuki / Right: Step Back, Jodan Age Ko Uke

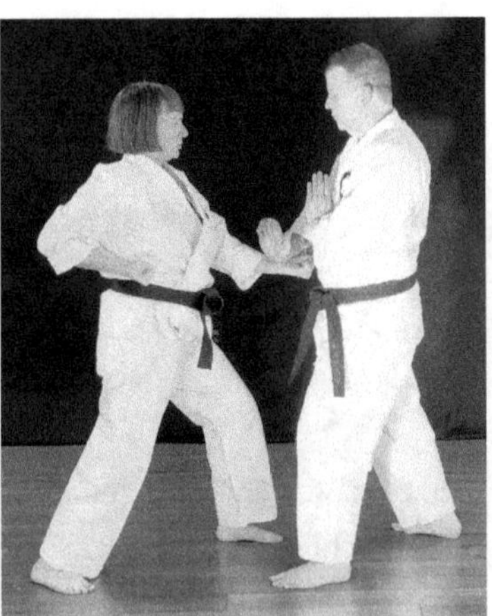

23. Left: Ura Zuki / Right: Shotei Otoshi Uke

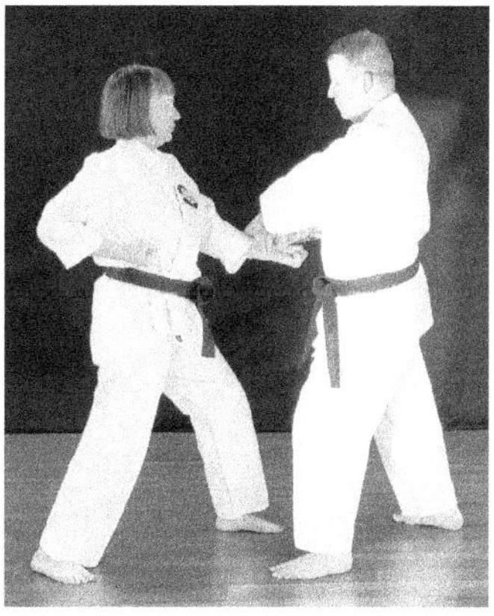

24. Right: Cross Left Hand over Opponent's Hand

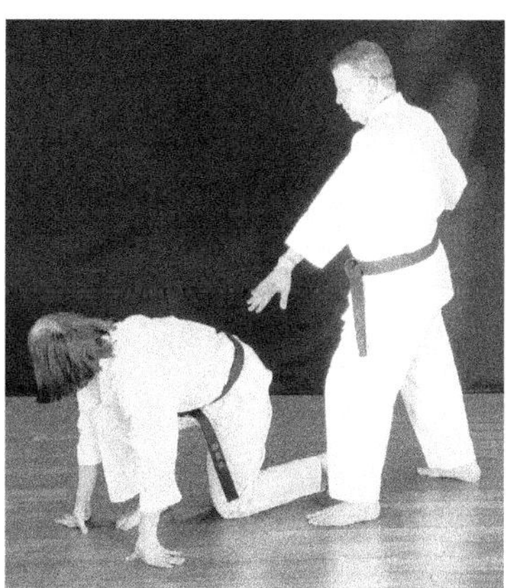

25. Left: Turn 45°, Drop to Left Knee / Right: Push Opponent's Hand Away to Left

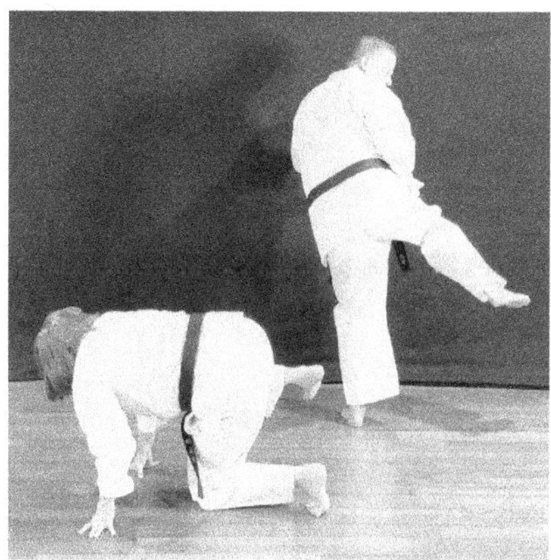

26. Right: Ushiro Ura Mawashi Geri

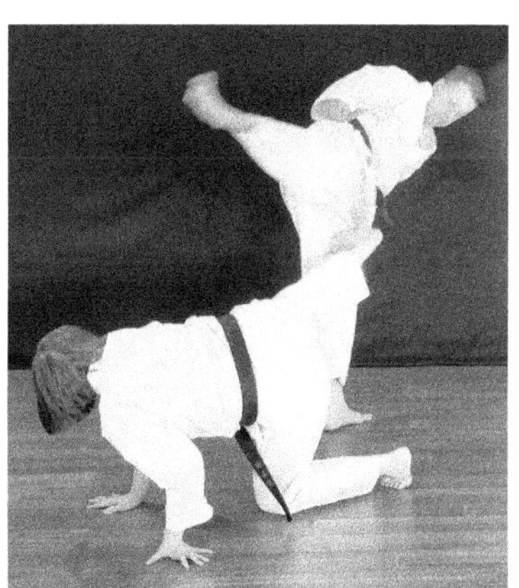

27. Left: Gedan (Age) Yoko Geri / Right: Ushiro Ura Mawashi Geri (cont.)

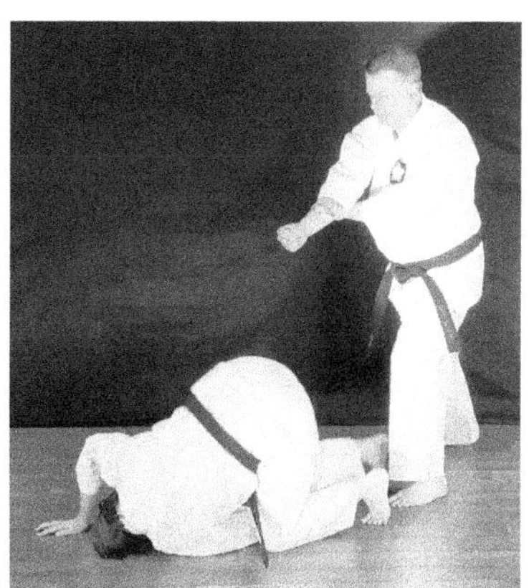

28. Left: Mae Mawari Ukemi at 45° / Right: Tettsui Otoshi Uchi

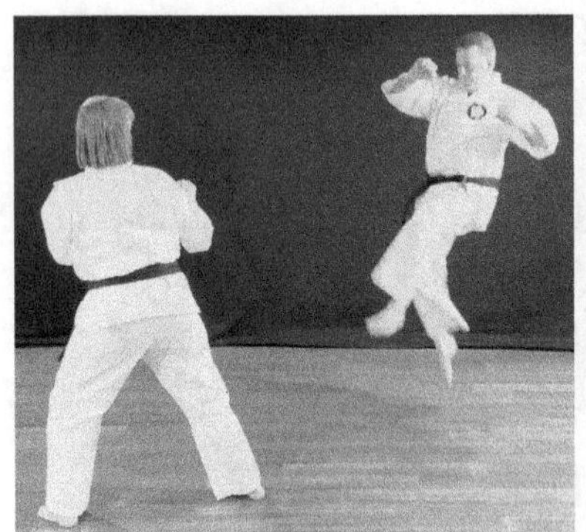
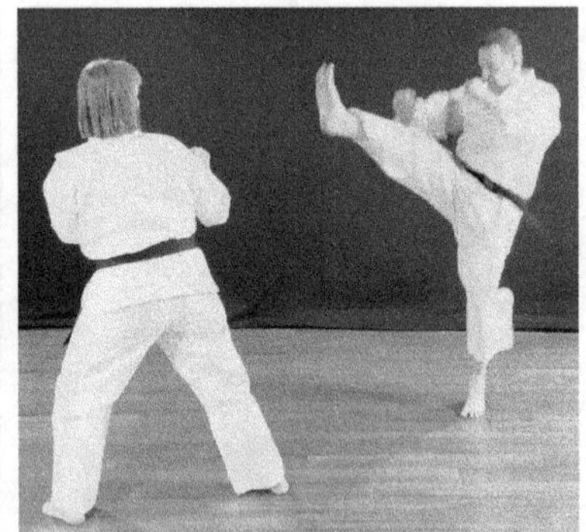
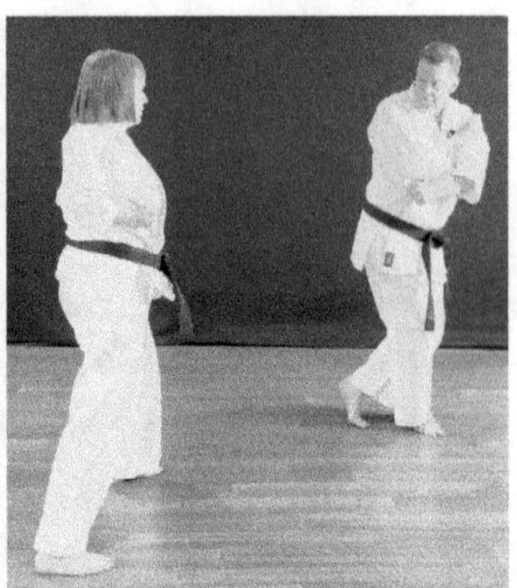

29. Left: Come Up from Roll, Lean Away from Kick / Right: Jodan Tobi Mae Geri at 45°

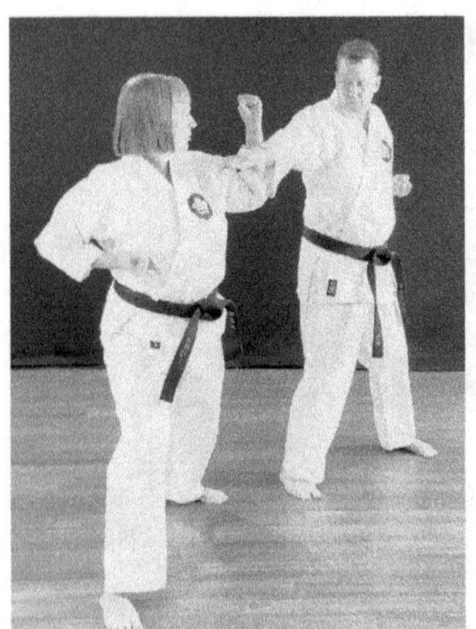

30. Left: Soto Uke at 45° / Right: Step Behind Yoko Shuto Uchi

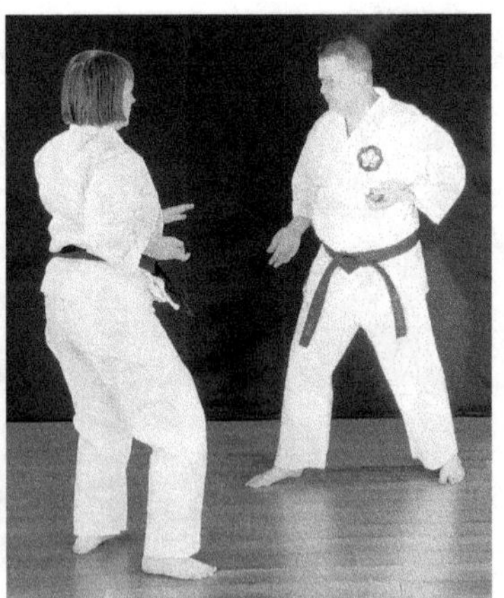

31. Right: Continue Momentum of Shuto Uchi, Clear Out Opponent in Circular Motion

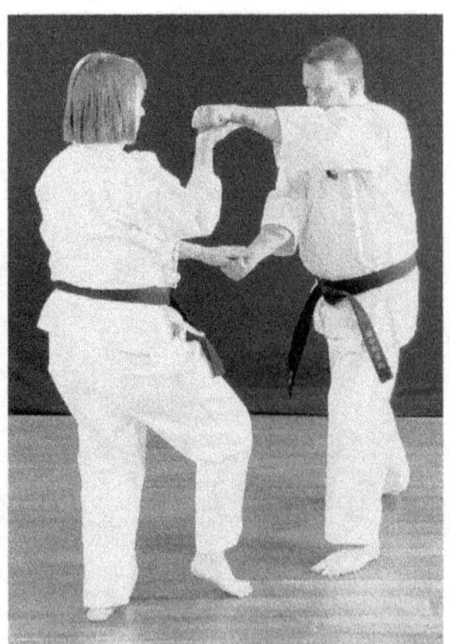

32. Left: Step Back into Neko Ashi Dachi, Left Gedan Shotei Barai and Right Chudan Sukui Uke / Right: Step Forward, Awase Zuki

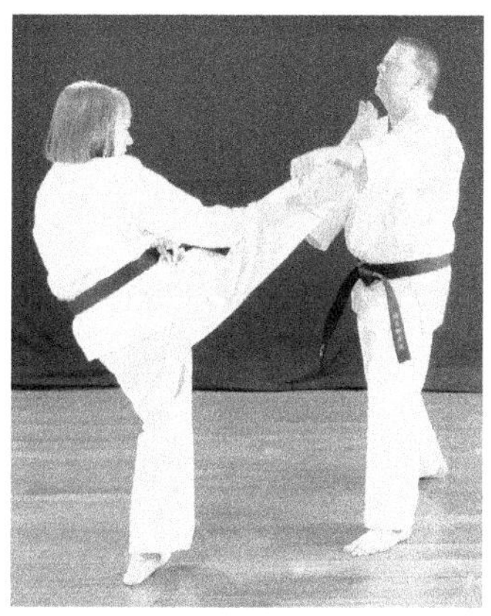

33. Left: Jodan Mae Geri on same angle (225°)

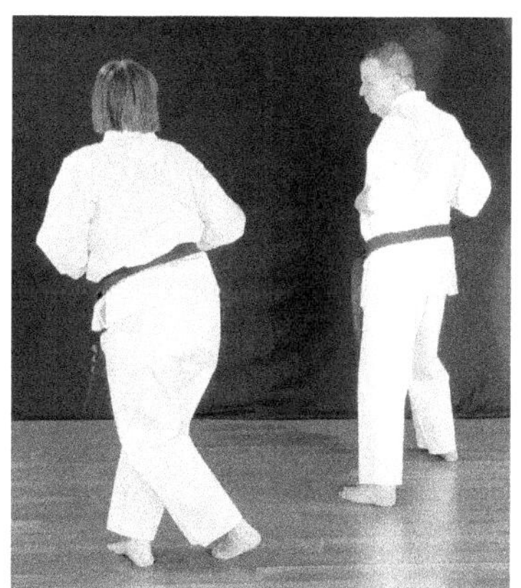

34. Left: Step Behind Yoko Geri / Right: Step Back with Right Foot, Lean Away, Yoko Otoshi Zuki (225°)

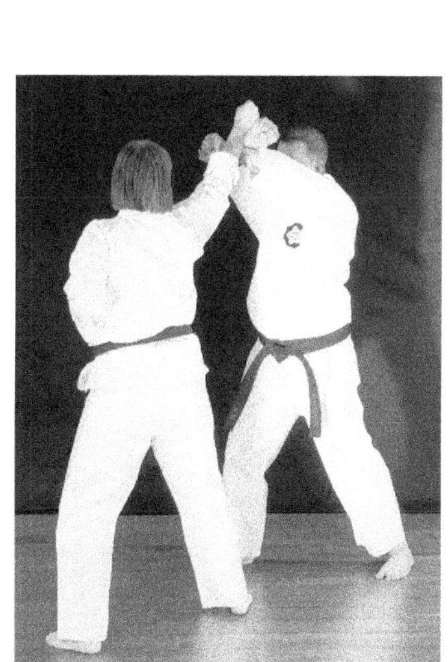

35. Left: Step Behind Yoko Tettsui Otoshi Uchi / Right: Left Step Back, Jodan Juji Age Uke (225°)

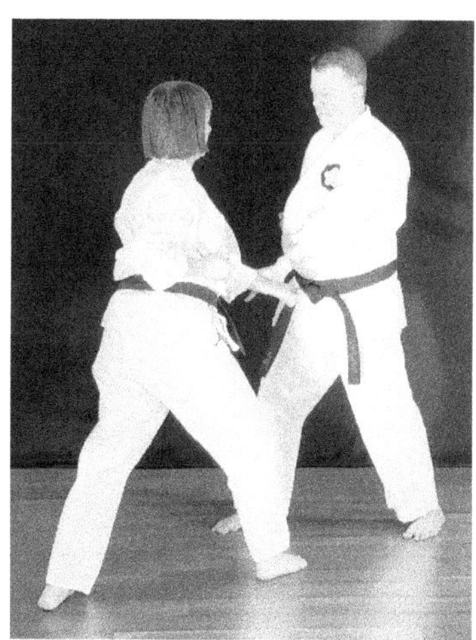

36. Left: Ura Zuki / Right: Shotei Otoshi Uke

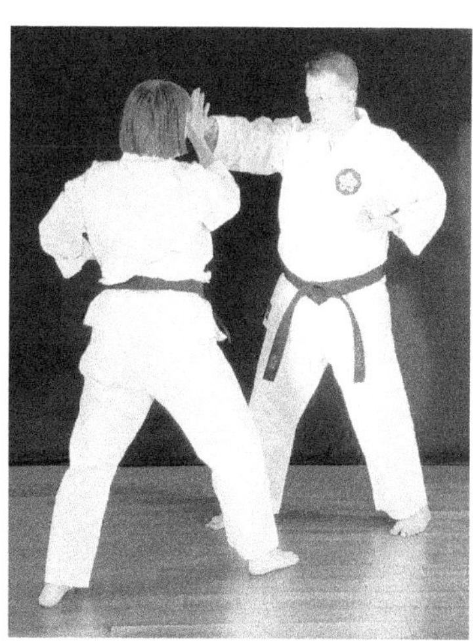

37. Left: Shotei Oshi / Right: Jodan Zuki

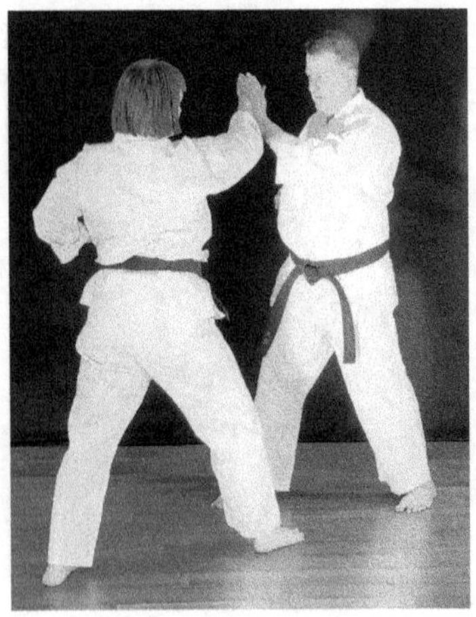
38. Left: Jodan Yoko Uraken Uchi / Right: Shotei Otoshi Uke

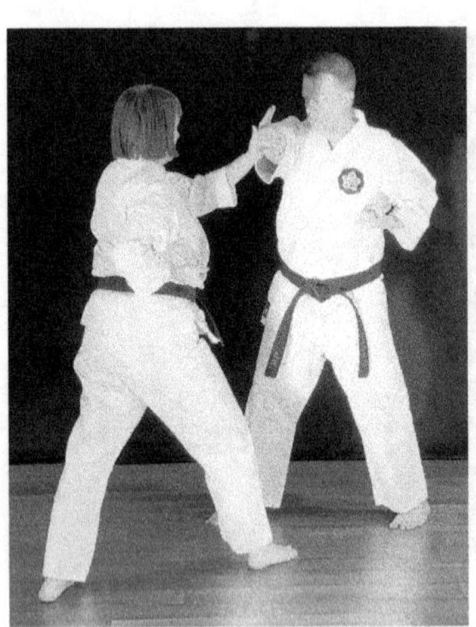
39. Left: Shotei Otoshi Uke / Right: Jodan Zuki

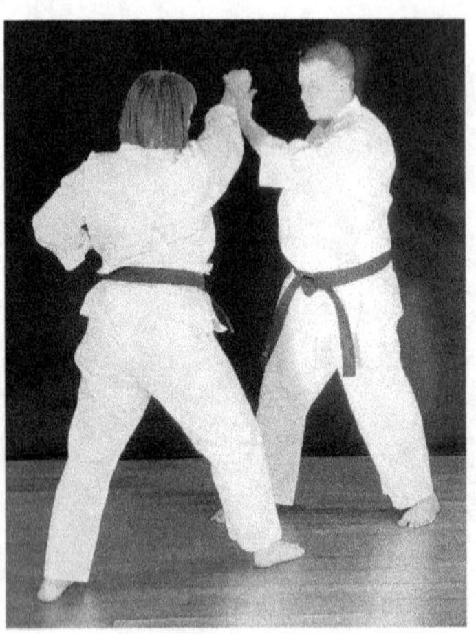
40. Left: Jodan Zuki / Right: Shotei Otoshi Uke

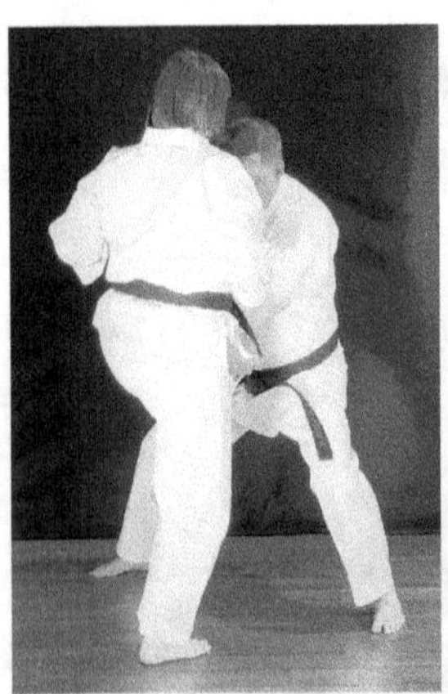
41. Left: Gedan Hiza Uchi / Right: Right Step Back into Shiko Dachi, Juji Otoshi Uke to Opponent's Leg

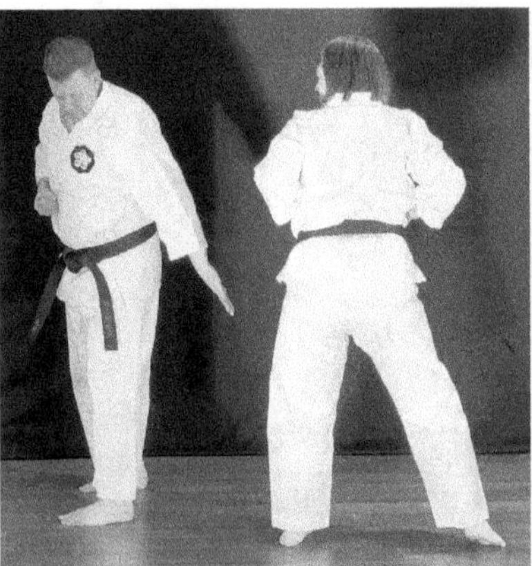
42. Left: After Juji Uke, Use Left Hand to Push Opponent to Left

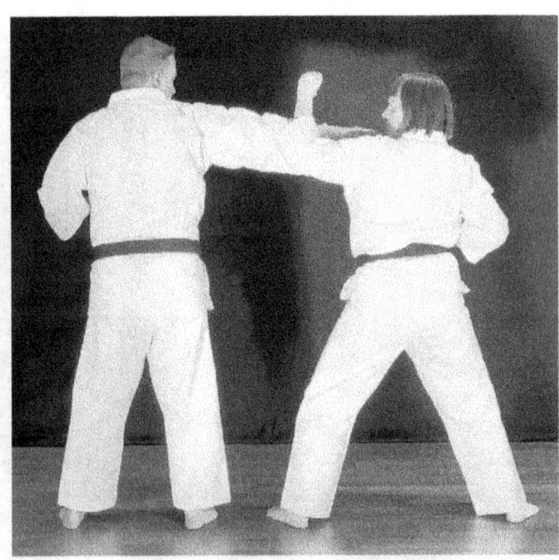
43. Left: Ushiro Mawashi Shuto Uchi / Right: Soto Uke (facing 270°)

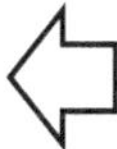

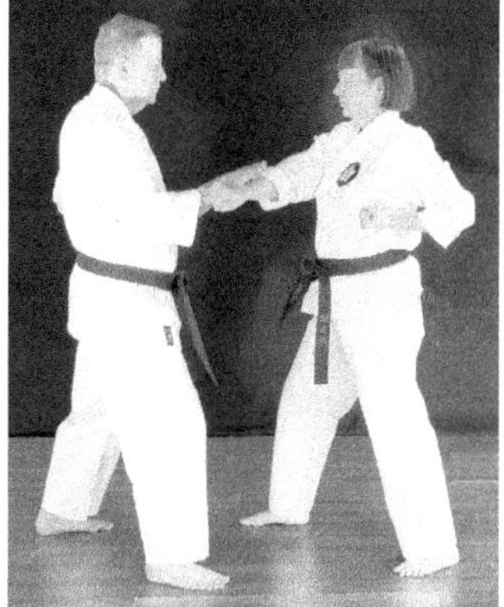

44. Left: Stutter Step Back, Chudan Hira to Hiki Uke / Right: Step Forward, Chudan Zuki

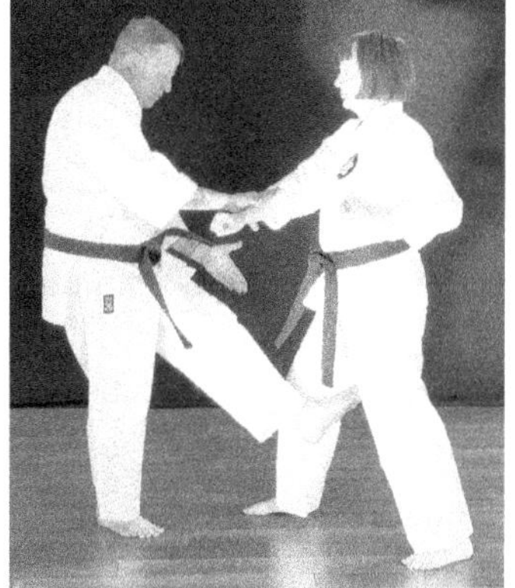

45. Left: Yoko Ukemi, Hook Opponent's Lead Leg (315°)

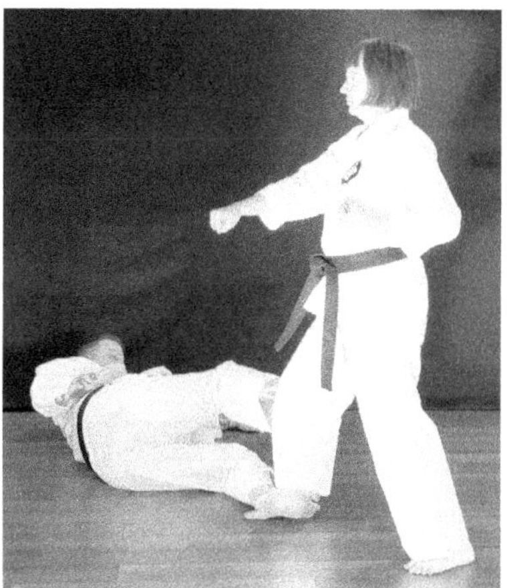

46. Left: Hiza Uchi (Kiai)

Repeat with Participants Changing Sides

Kata Comparison to Bunkai Kumite

Note: this is not an exhaustive list, but a list of observations.

Chukyu Kumite Ni contains elements from several kata in the following areas:

- Haiwan Uke (Step 18 - Juhito)
- Jodan Zuki followed by Ura Uchi is one interpretation of Awase Zuki at the end of Gekisai Ichi and Gekisai Ni (Steps 22-23)
- Ushiro Ura Mawashi Geri (Steps 26-27 - Genshin)
- Tettsui Otoshi Uchi (Step 28 - Juhito, Kyouryoku Do)
- Tobi Mae Geri (Step 29 - Juhito)
- Awase Zuki (Step 32 - Gekisai Ichi, Gekisai Ni)
- Shotei Barai and Chudan Sukui Uke defense is one interpretation of the same move in Saifa (Step 32)
- Tettsui Otoshi Uchi (Step 35 - Gekisai Ni, Genshin)
- Jodan Juji Age Uke (Step 35 - Juhito, Hente Do)
- Juji Otoshi Uke (Step 41 - Juhito, Sanseiru)
- Yoko Ukemi is similar to a sequence in Bushido Rei and Kyouroku Do (Step 45)

6. Jokyu Kumite Ichi

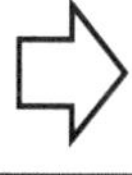

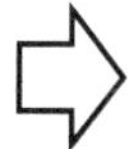

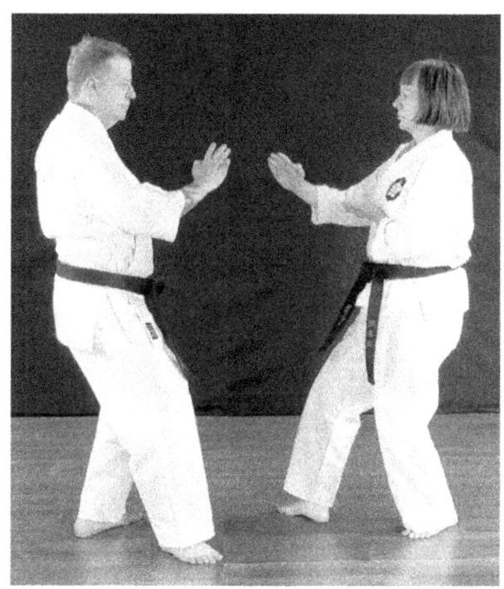

Renoji Dachi Kamae
Open Hands, Chamber Hand at Chest, Palm Up

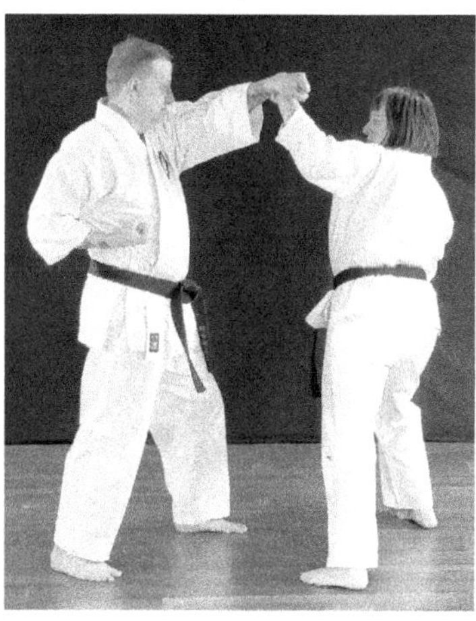

1. Left: Step Forward, Jodan Zuki / Right: Step Back to Side, Jodan Yoko Ko Uke

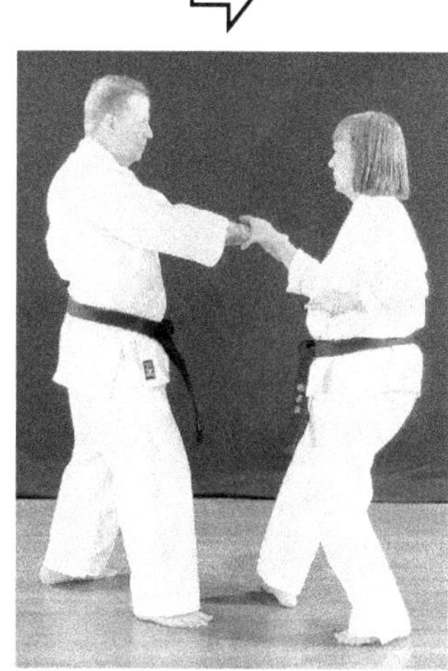

2. Left: Step Forward, Chudan Zuki / Right: Step Back, Off Center, Chudan Hari to Hiki Uke

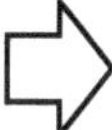

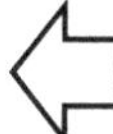

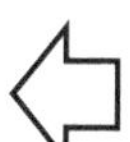

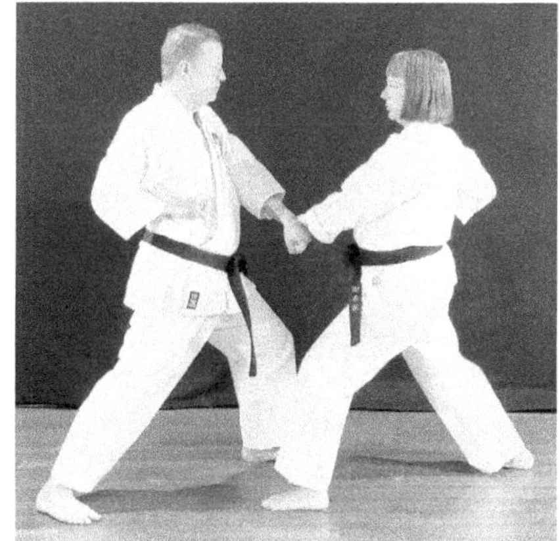

3. Left: Step Forward, Gedan Zuki in Zenkutsu Dachi / Right: Step Back, Gedan Shotei Barai in Zenkutsu Dachi

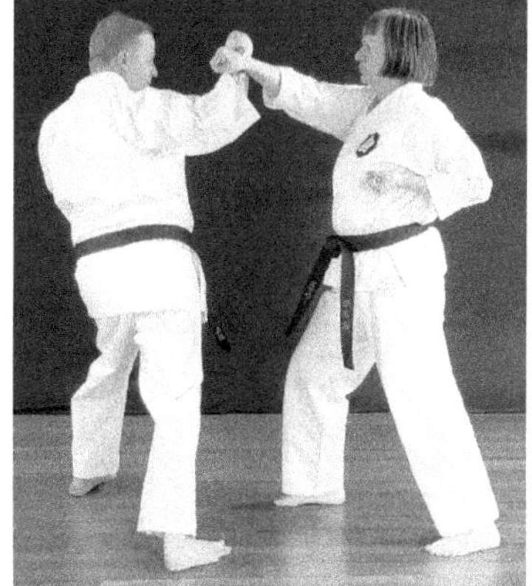

4. Left: Step Back to Side, Jodan Yoko Ko Uke / Right: Step Forward, Jodan Zuki

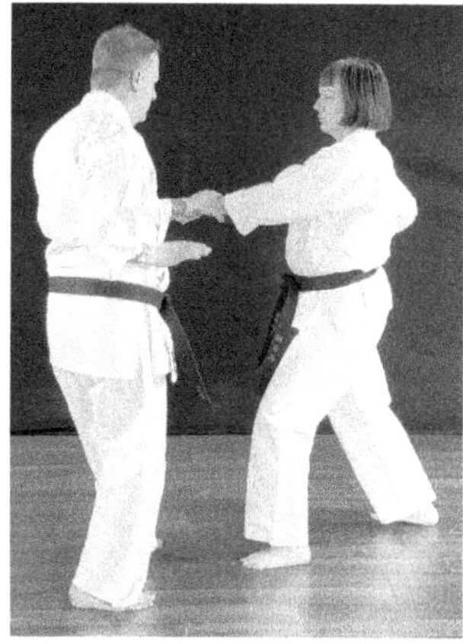

5. Left: Step Back, Off Center, Chudan Hari to Hiki Uke / Right: Step Forward, Chudan Zuki

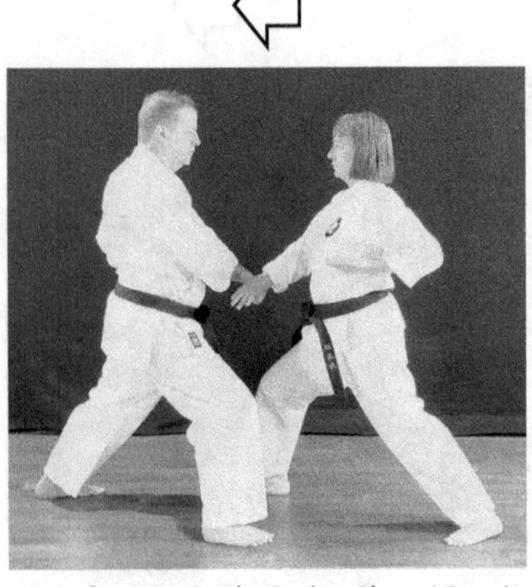

6. Left: Step Back, Gedan Shotei Barai in Zenkutsu Dachi / Right: Step Forward, Gedan Zuki in Zenkutsu Dachi

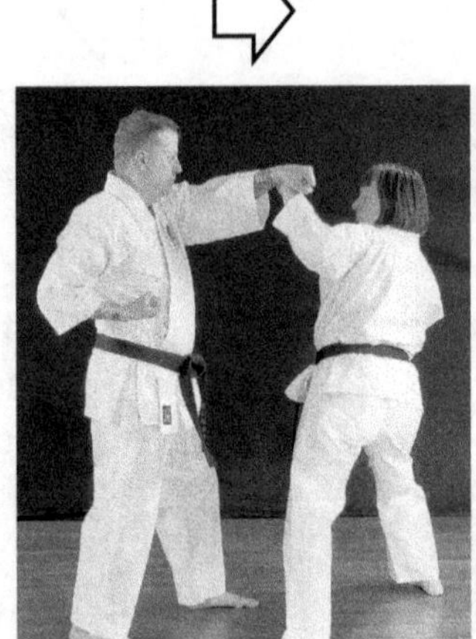

7. Left: Step Forward, Jodan Zuki / Right: Step Back to Side, Jodan Yoko Ko Uke

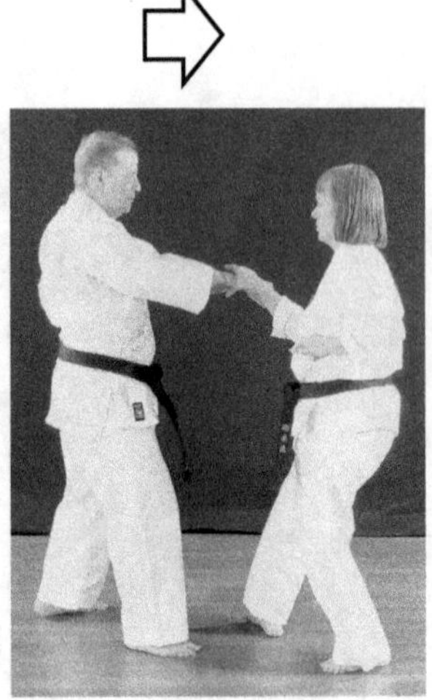

8. Left: Step Forward, Chudan Zuki / Right: Step Back, Off Center, Chudan Hari to Hiki Uke

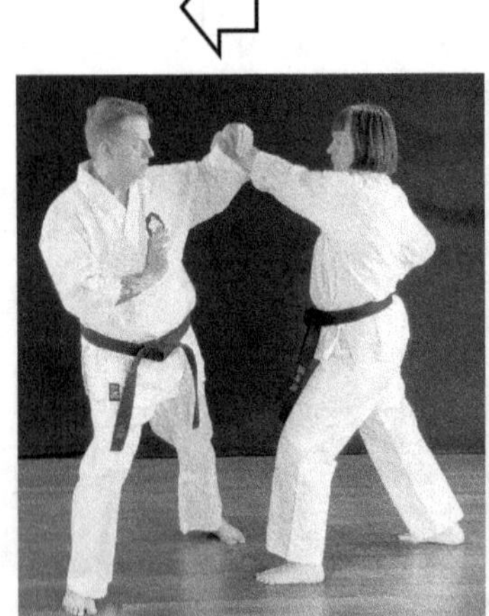

9. Left: Step Back to Side, Jodan Yoko Ko Uke / Right: Step Forward, Jodan Zuki

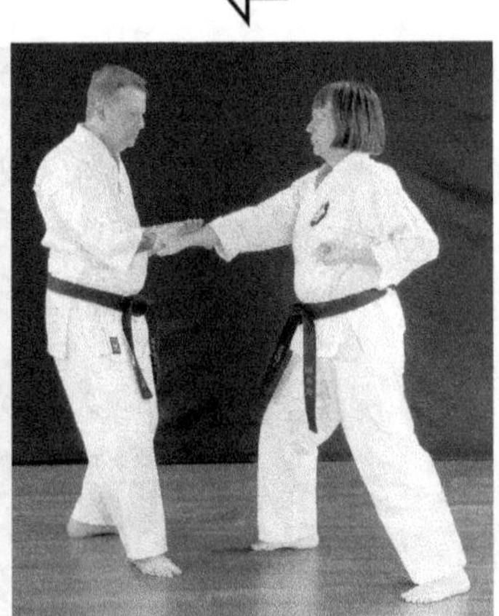

10. Left: Step Back, Off Center, Chudan Hari to Hiki Uke / Right: Step Forward, Chudan Zuki

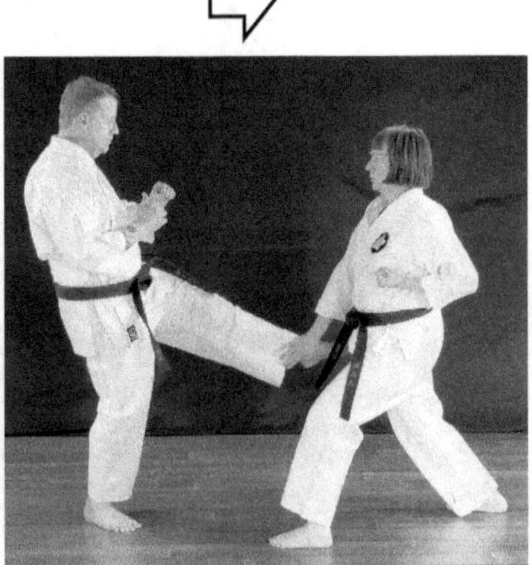

11. Left: Gedan Mae Geri / Right: Step Back in Zenkutsu Dachi, Gedan Shotei Barai

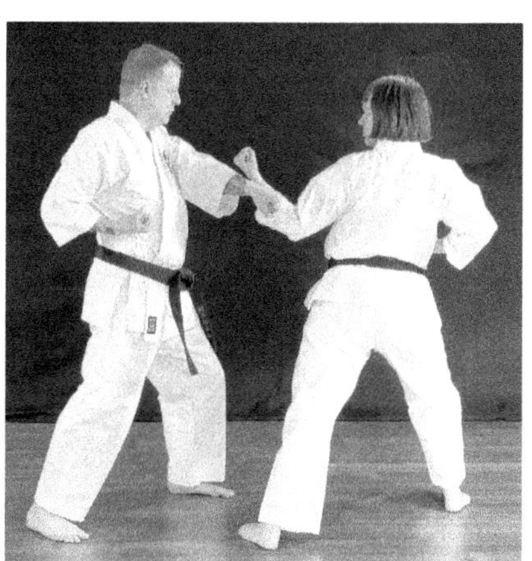

12. Left: Step Forward, Chudan Zuki / Right: Step Back to Side, Uchi Uke

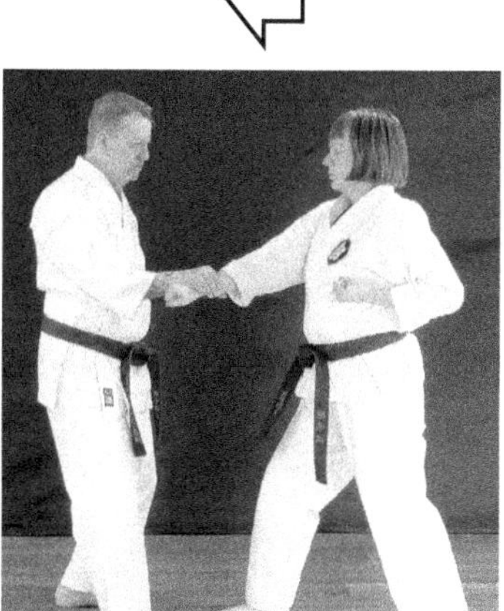

13. Left: Step Back, Off Center, Chudan Hari to Hiki Uke / Right: Step Forward, Chudan Zuki

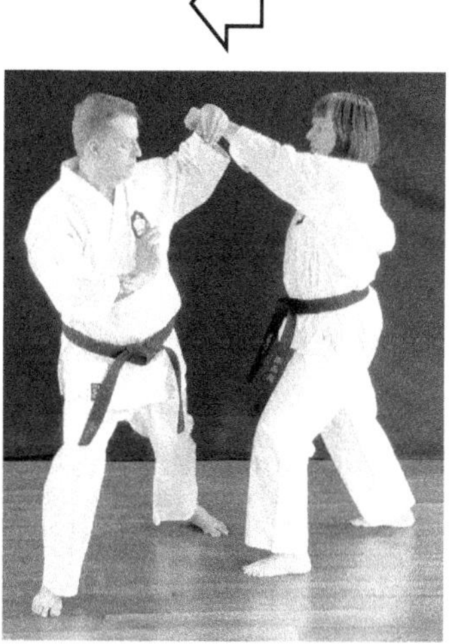

14. Left: Step Back to Side, Jodan Yoko Ko Uke / Right: Step Forward, Jodan Zuki

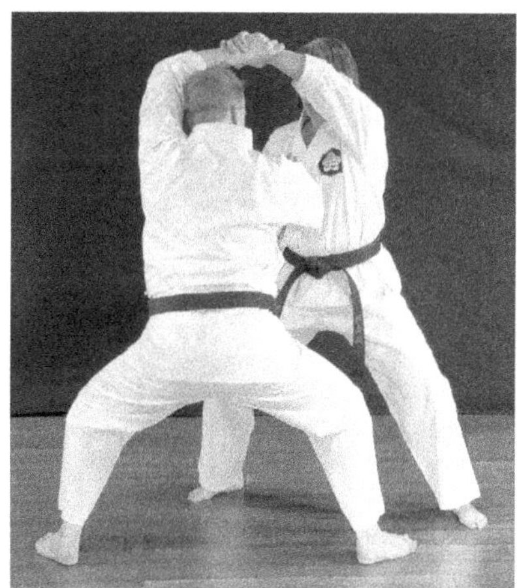

15. Left: Grab Opponent's Wrist, Right Step in, Chudan Empi Uchi in Shiko Dachi / Right: Grab Opponent's Wrist, Left Step Back with Left Hand on Opponent's Elbow

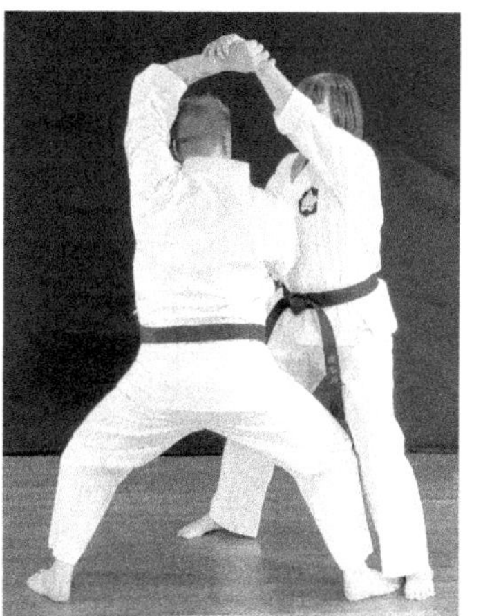

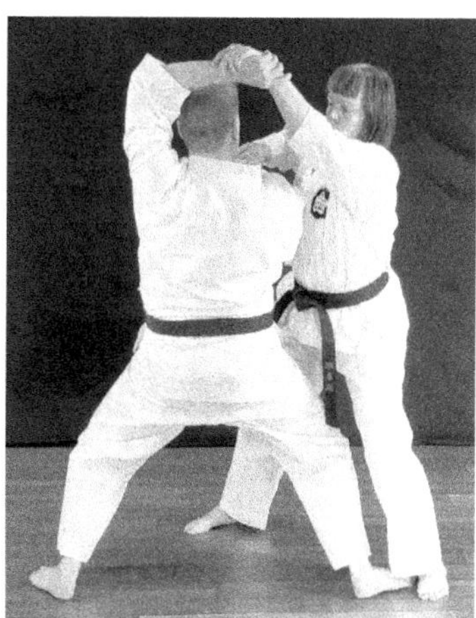

16. Right: Step Towards Opponent, Pushing Opponent's Arm Down Overhead, Keeping Pressure on Elbow, Forcing Opponent Back to Ground (45°)

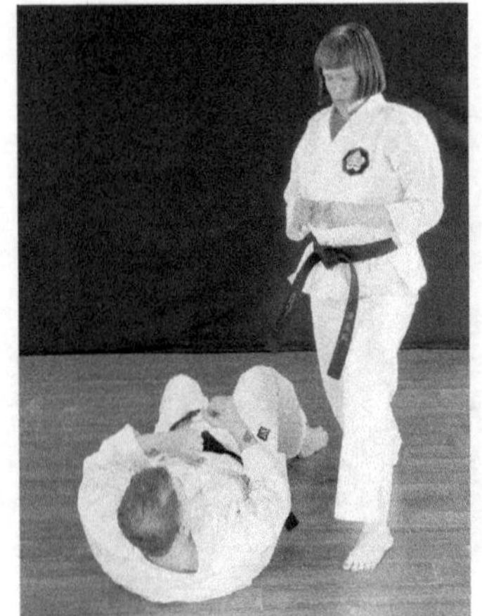
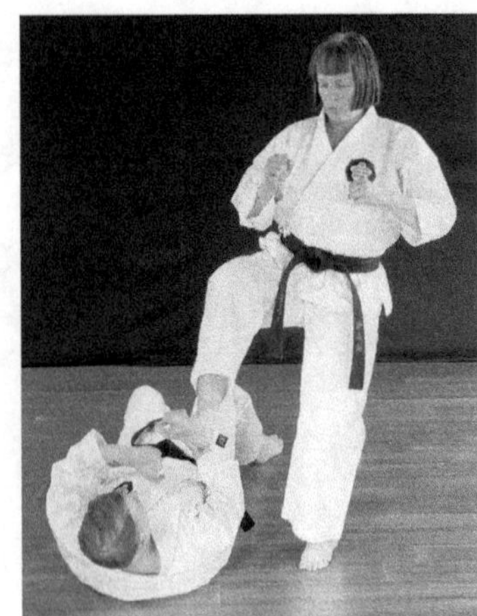
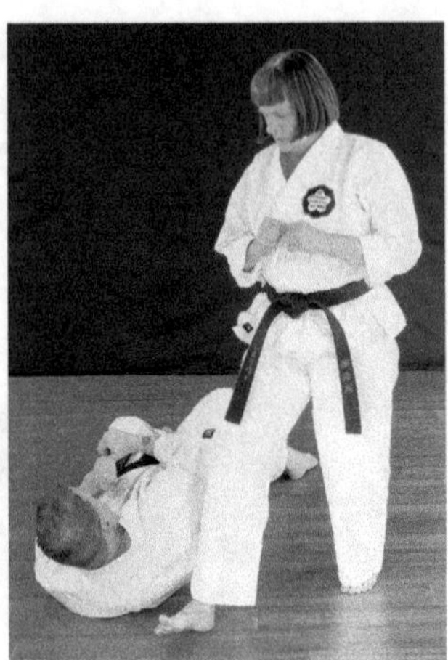

17. Left: Dodge by Rolling Parallel to Left / Right: Fumikomi Geri to Jodan

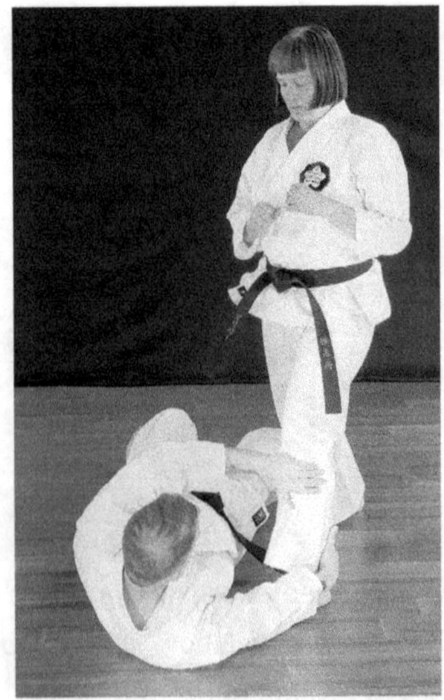
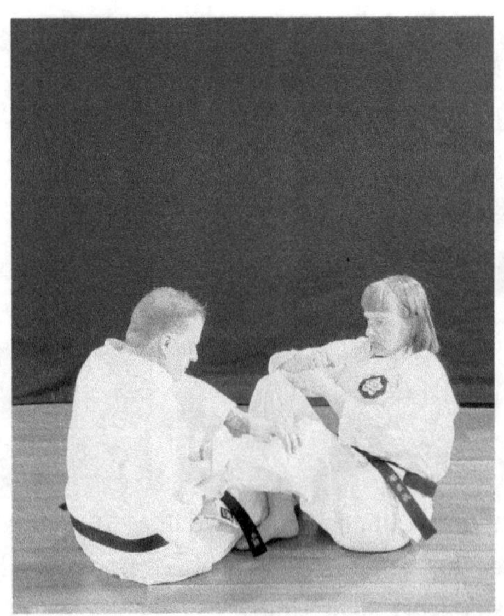

18. Left: Grab Opponent's Leg (Push with Left Hand, Pull with Right Hand), Kibisu Gaeshi (225°)

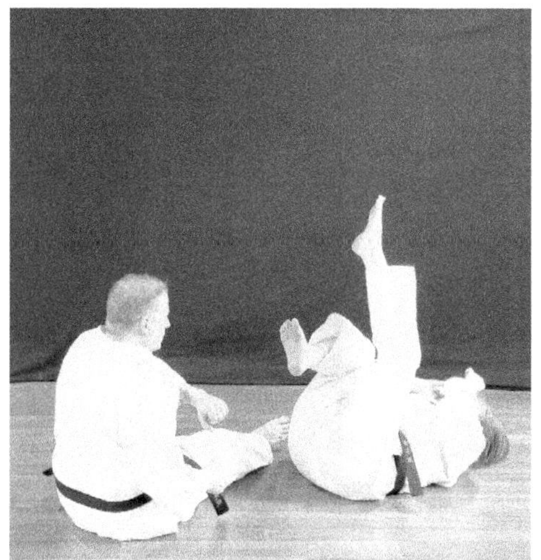
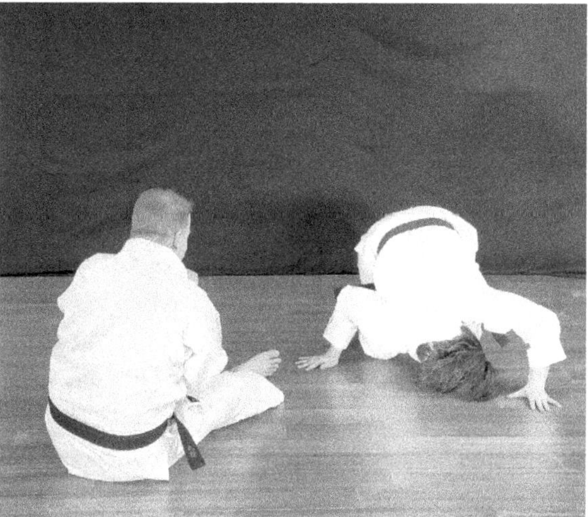

19. Right: Ushiro Mawari Ukemi

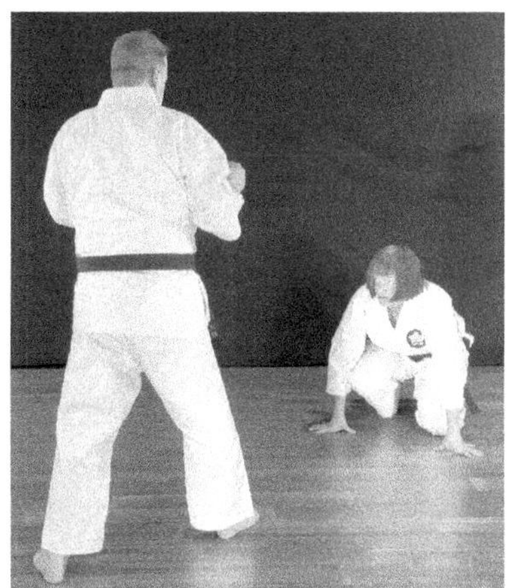
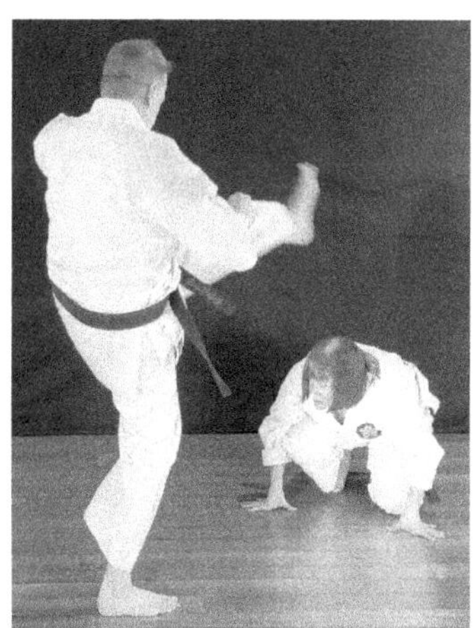
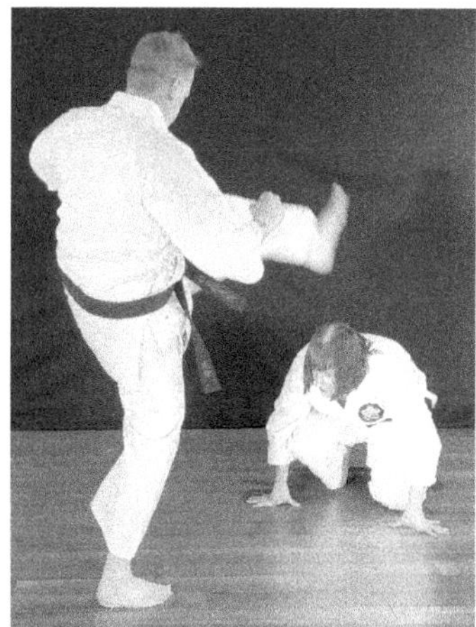

20. Left: Come Up into Left Mikazuki Geri / Right: Duck Away from Kick

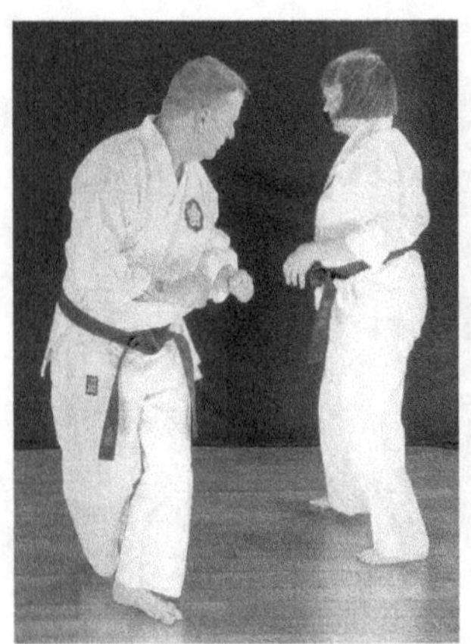

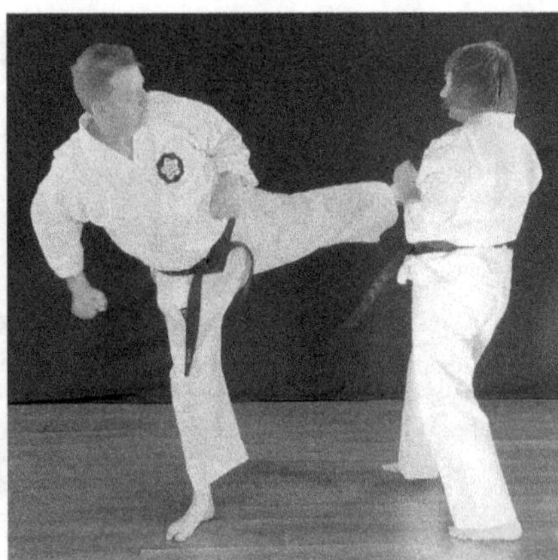

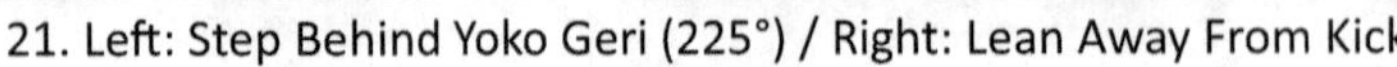

21. Left: Step Behind Yoko Geri (225°) / Right: Lean Away From Kick

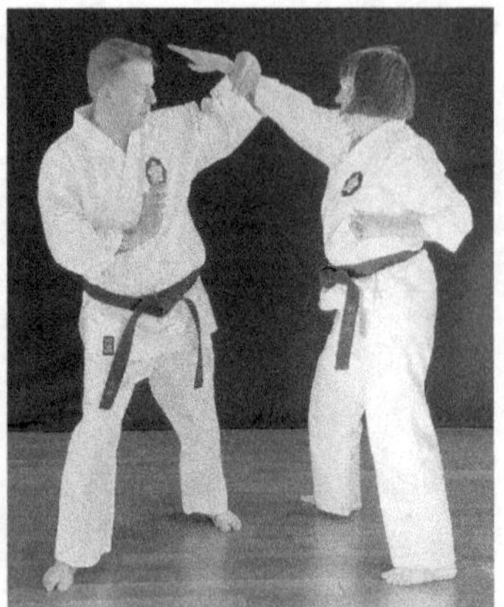

22. Left: Jodan Yoko Ko Uke / Right: Jodan Haito Uchi (315°)

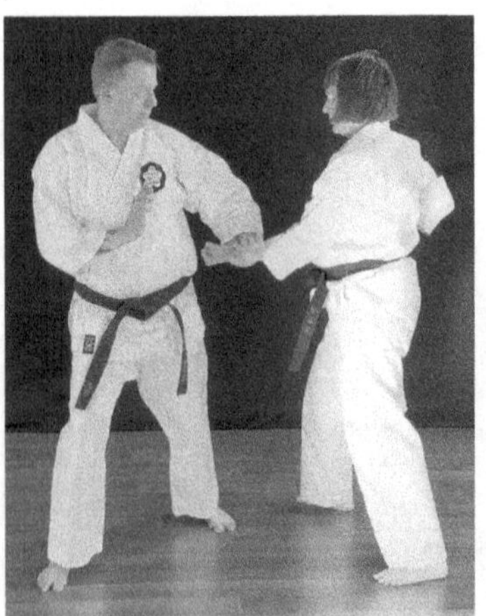

23. Left: Shotei Otoshi Uke / Right: Ura Zuki

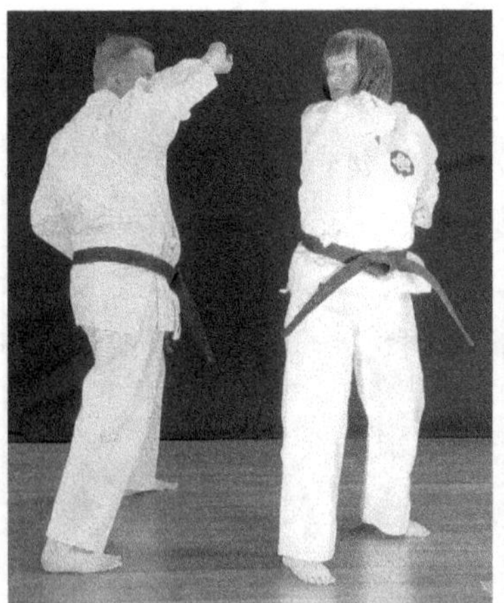

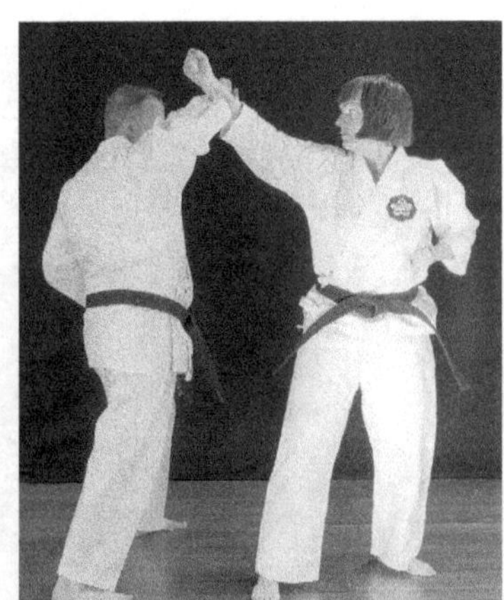

24. Left: Jodan Yoko Ko Uke / Right: Ushiro Mawashi Uraken Uchi

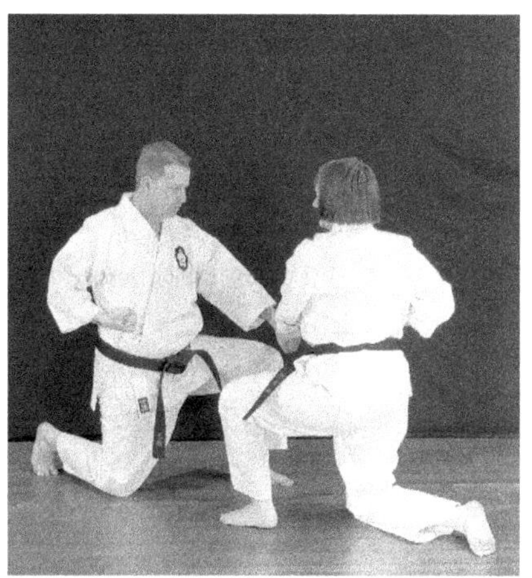

25. Left: Step Back, Drop to Right Knee, Gedan Barai / Right: Step Forward, Drop to Right Knee, Gedan Zuki (315°)

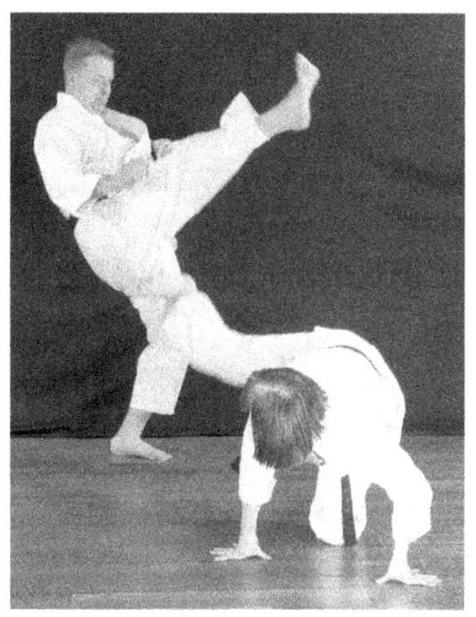

26. Left: Jodan Mae Geri / Right: Switch to Left Knee, Gedan Yoko Geri

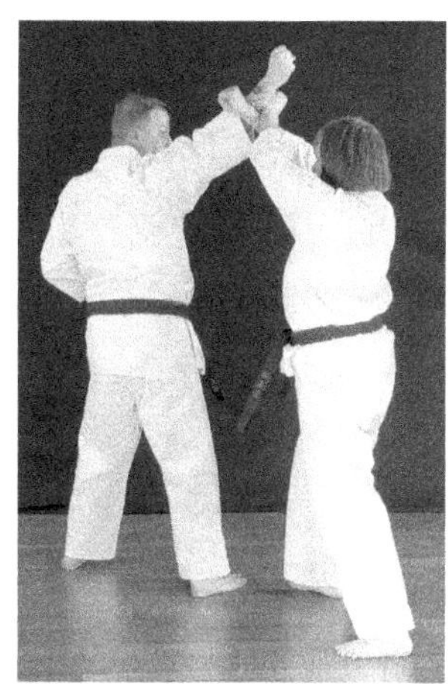

27. Left: Step Behind Tettsui Otoshi Uchi / Right: Step Back, Juji Age Uke (135°)

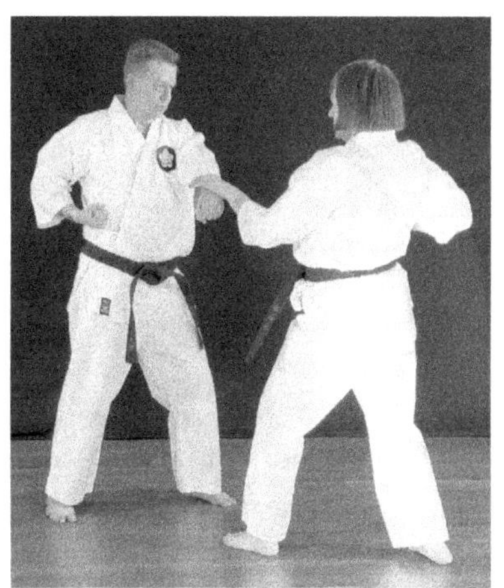

28. Left: Step Forward, Chudan Zuki / Right: Step Back, Chudan Hari to Hiki Uke

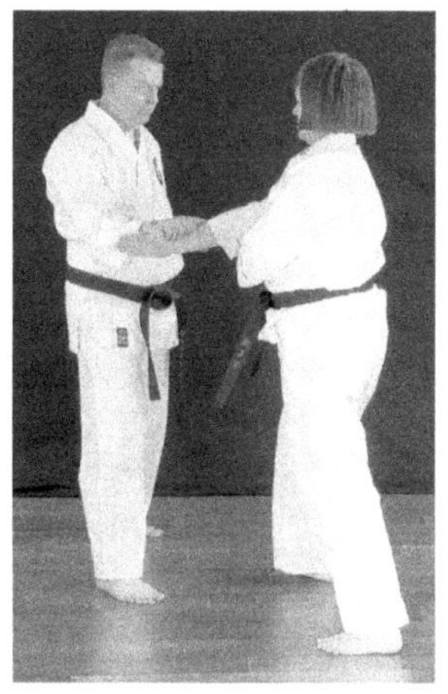

29. Left: Step Back, Chudan Hari to Hiki Uke / Right: Step Forward, Supported Chudan Nukite Uchi (315°)

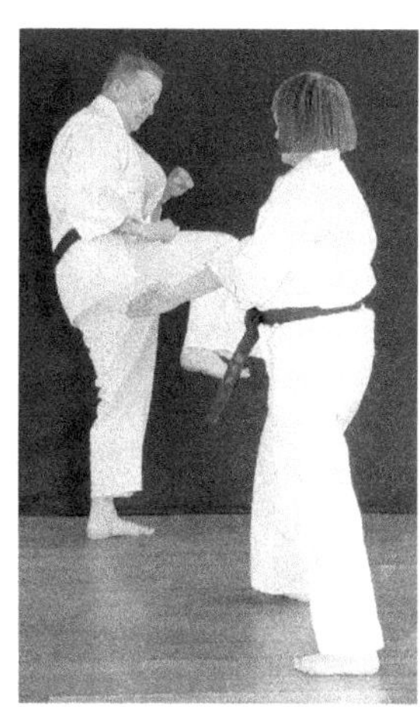

30. Left: Step to Left Side, Hiza Geri no Kamae

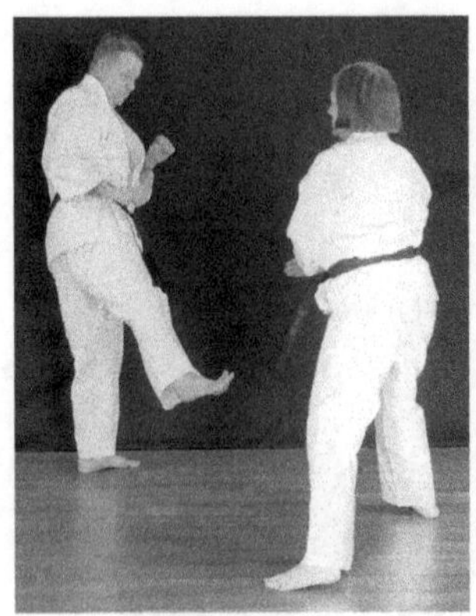
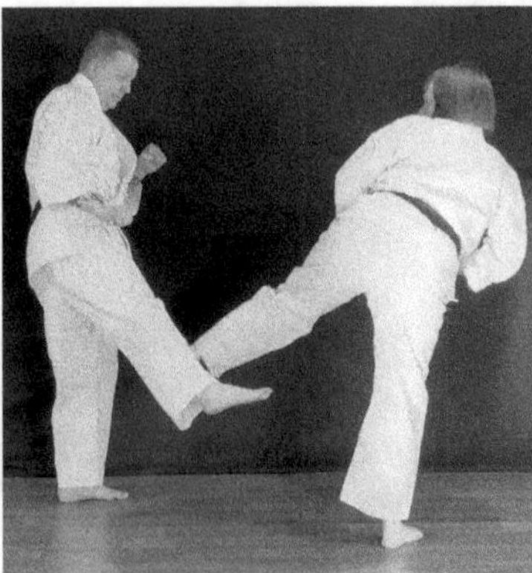

31. Left: Hiza Geri / Right: Step to Right Side, Left Hiza Geri

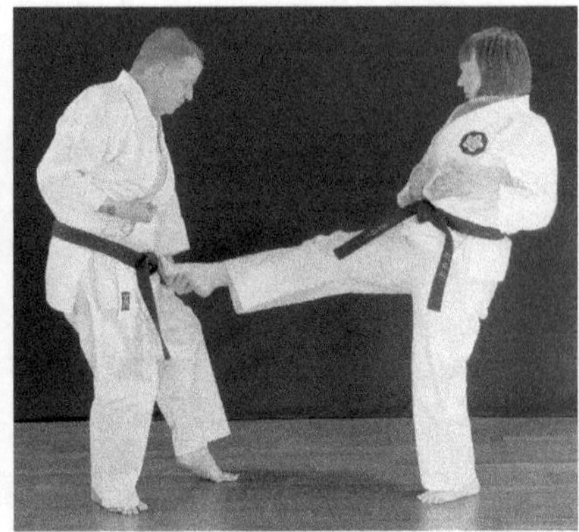

32. Left: Left Sukui Uke / Right: Gedan Mae Geri

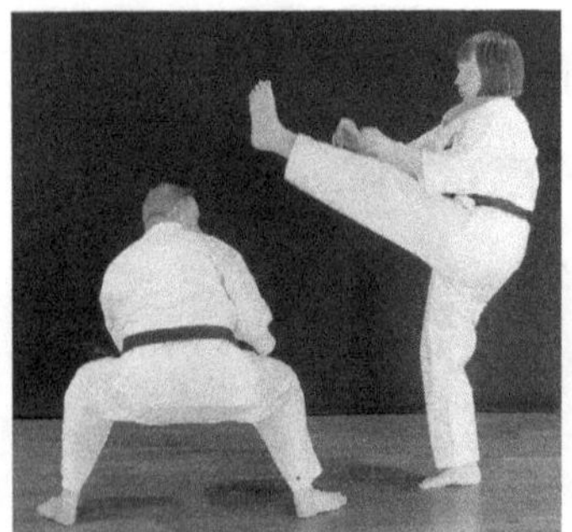
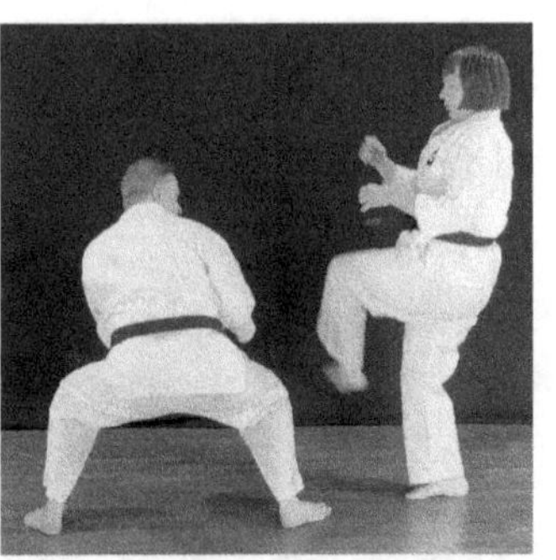

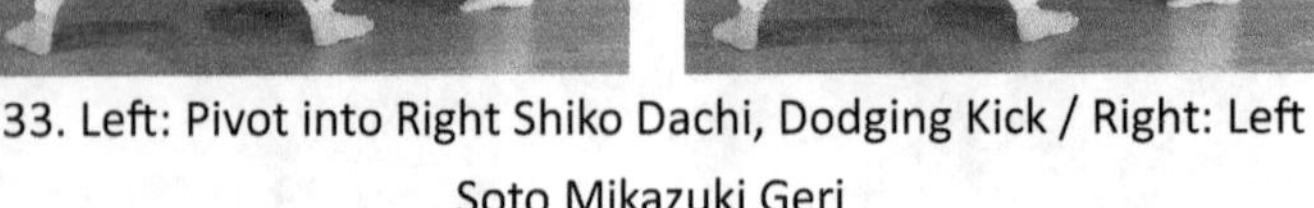

33. Left: Pivot into Right Shiko Dachi, Dodging Kick / Right: Left Soto Mikazuki Geri

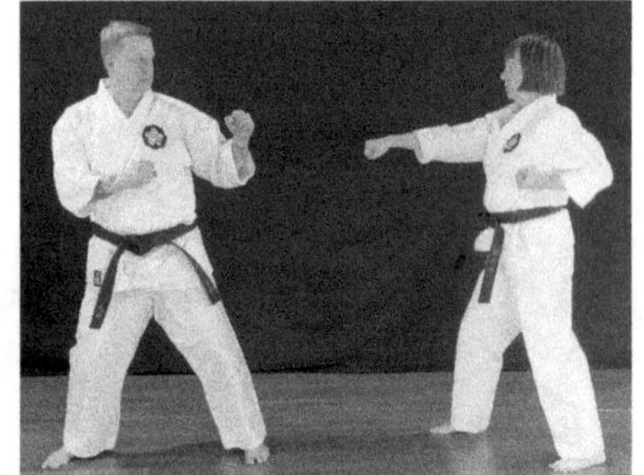

34. Left: Pivot into Left Heiko Dachi / Right: Step Forward, Chudan Zuki

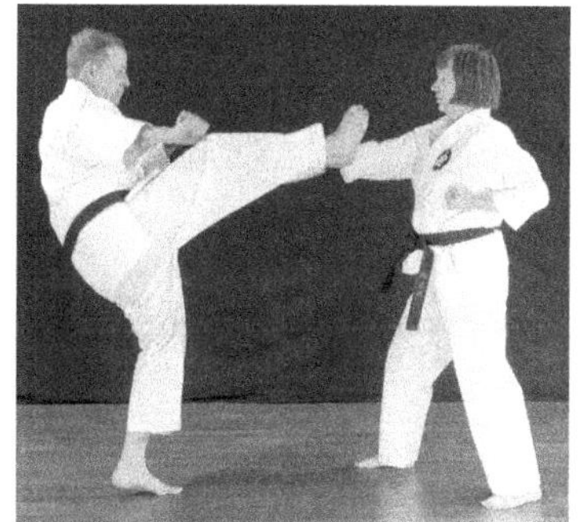
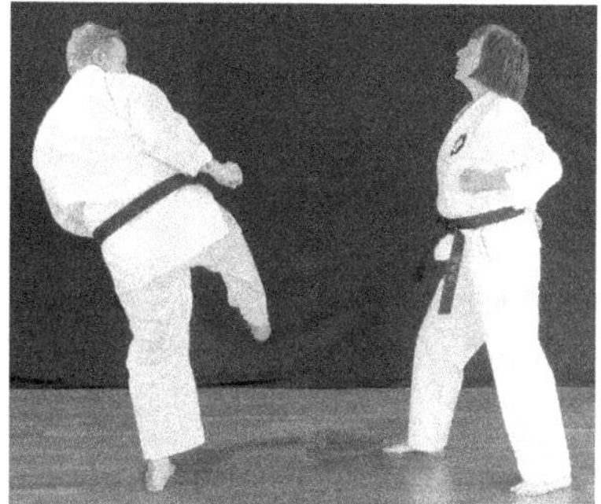
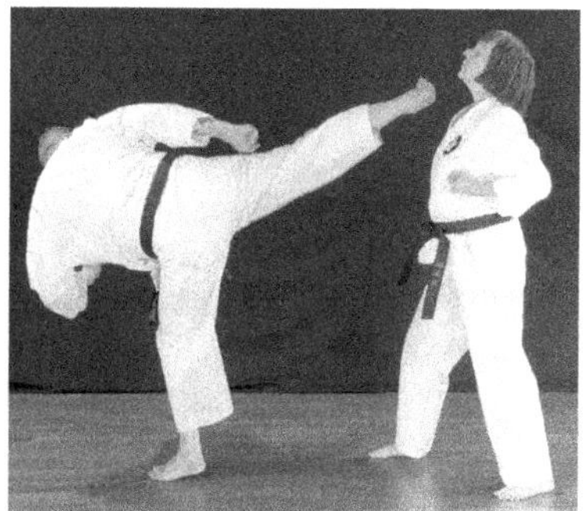

35. Left: Right Soto Mikazuki Geri into Opponent's Arm, Pivot Immediately into Jodan Yoko Geri

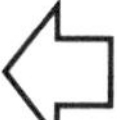
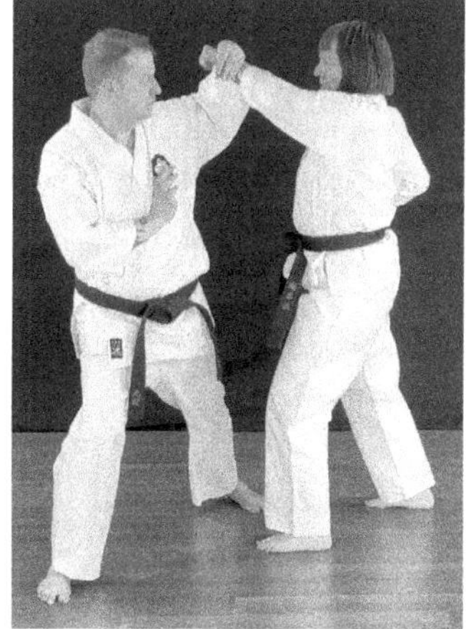

36. Left: Step Back to Side, Jodan Yoko Ko Uke / Right: Step Forward, Jodan Zuki

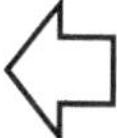
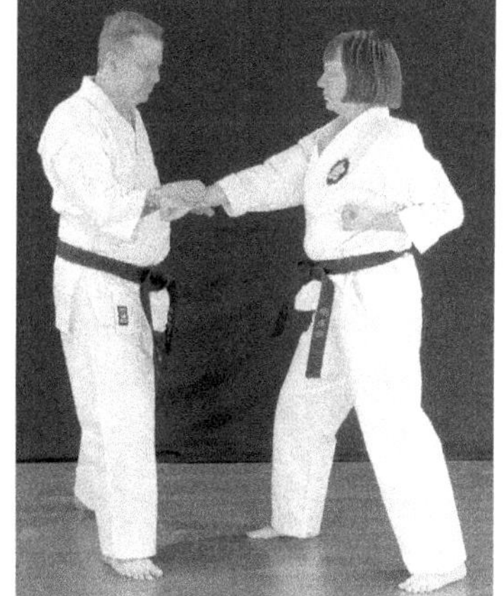

37. Left: Step Back, Off Center, Chudan Hari to Hiki Uke / Right: Step Forward, Chudan Zuki

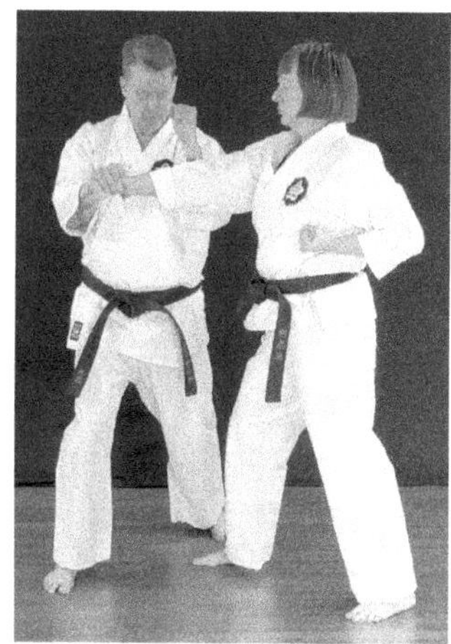

38. Left: Grab Arm, Step Around to Side, Kote Uchi on Opponent's Arm, Just Above the Elbow

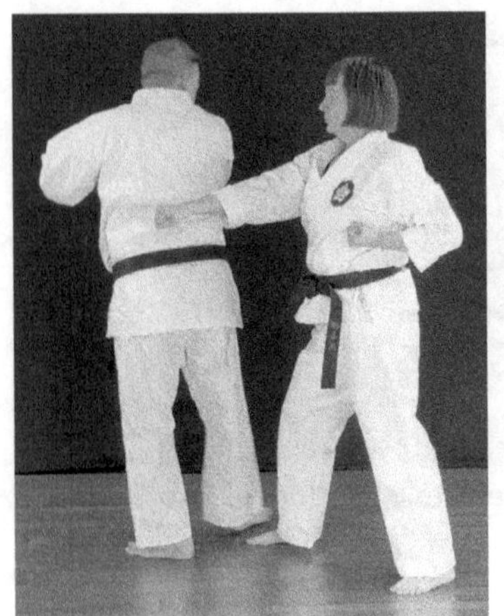

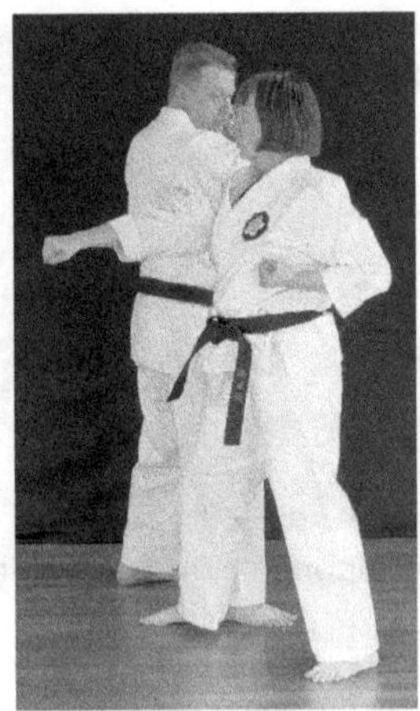

39. Left: Mawatte, Empi Uchi to Opponent's Kidney

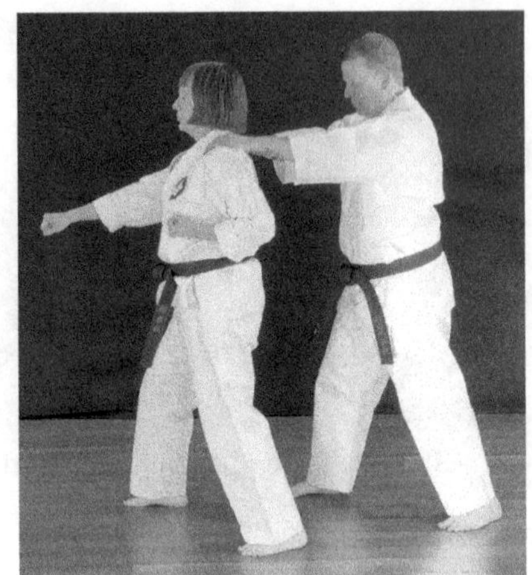

40. Left: Pull Opponent From the Shoulders

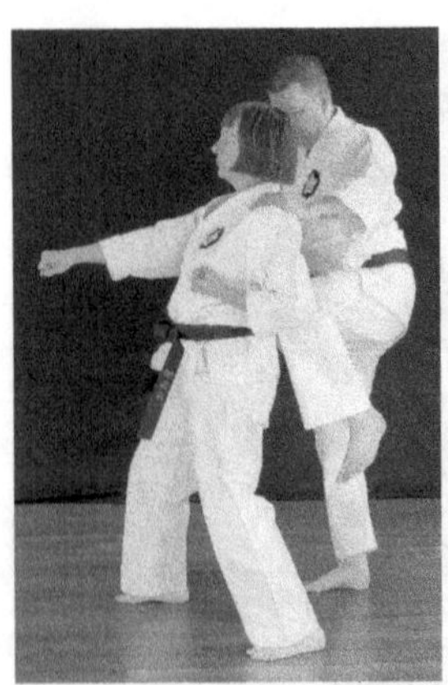

41. Left: Age Hiza Uchi to Opponent's Back

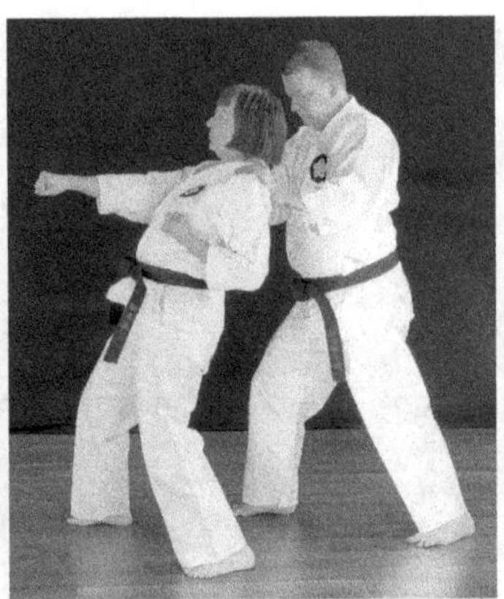

42. Left: Continue Pulling Opponent Down to Ground

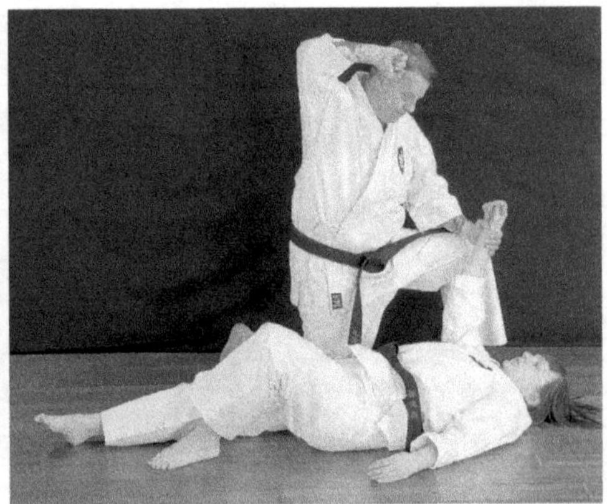

43. Left: Tettsui Otoshi Uchi to Chest

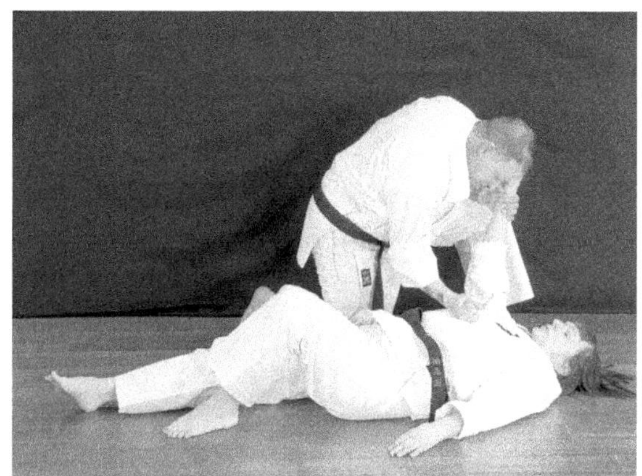
Tettsui Otoshi Uchi to Chest (cont.)

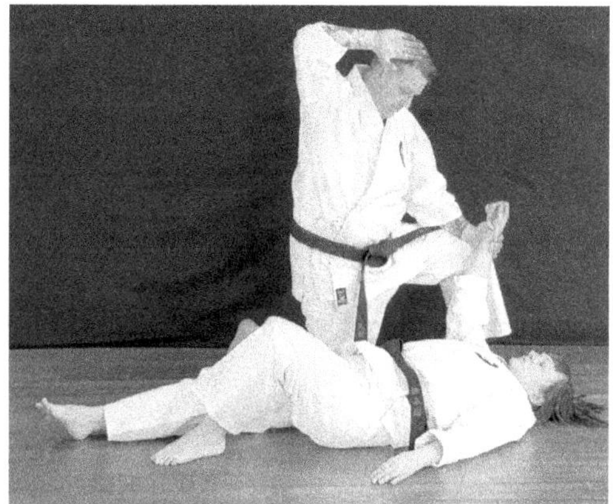
44. Left: Nodo Kaki (Kiai)

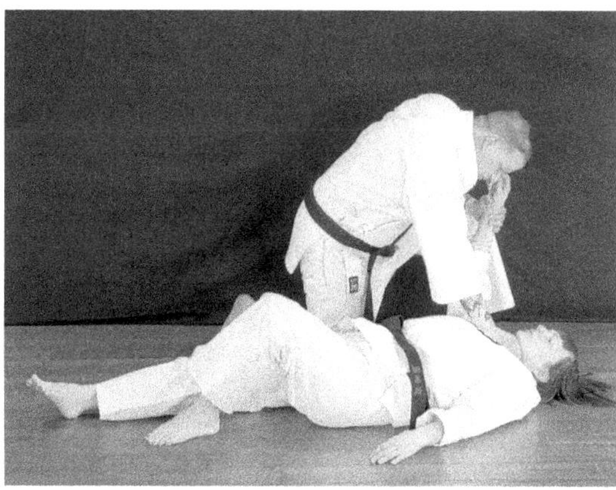
Nodo Kaki (cont.)

Repeat in Other Direction

Kata Comparison to Bunkai Kumite

Note: this is not an exhaustive list, but a list of observations.

Jokyu Kumite Ichi contains elements from several kata in the following areas:

- Gedan Mae Geri & Gedan Shotei Barai (Step 11 - Gekisai Ichi, Gekisai Ni)
- Chudan Empi Uke in Shiko Dachi (Step 15 - Sanseiru)
- Fumikomi Geri (Step 17 - Hon'nogeki, Juhito)
- Juji Age Uke (Step 27 - Genshin, Juhito)
- Mikazuki Geri into Yoko Geri (Step 35 - Hon'nogeki)
- Age Hiza Uchi (Step 41 - Juhito)

Kiso Kumite

Kiso Kumite, much like Bunkai Kumite, is a two-person exercise in which two people move together, punching and blocking at the same time. The main difference is that, after the opening punching and blocking sequence, the person on offense completes a final strike while the defensive person executes a counter. This exercise has many of the same benefits as Bunkai Kumite, but the principal benefit is the concept of countering after a block and refining the countering techniques themselves.

Like Bunkai Kumite, the participants begin by punching and blocking at the same time in one direction, then after a final strike, the defensive partner completes a counterstrike or sequence of strikes. After each counterstrike, the two people line up and go in the other direction so that each person is on offense and defense for each counter.

Kiso Kumite drills are an important training exercise for learning and practicing counterstriking. In the beginning, Kiso Kumite counters are simple, helping the student become accustomed to countering immediately after a block. Eventually, the counters become more complex and must be practiced repeatedly until the technique is sound.

However, once the techniques are learned, it is important to practice them first at greater speed, and then in an unstructured environment, such as sparring, where the defender does not allow the student to simply practice the move. Takedowns, for example, are far more difficult to accomplish without a willing partner. While Kumite drills do not, in and of themselves, resemble a real fight, the techniques should be refined enough to be used whenever applicable and adapted to nearly any situation.

Note: For space considerations, the bow-ins and bow-outs have been omitted; also under each image, the steps have been numbered.

For example:

The offensive attacking side, has been shortened to "Off" with a direction of whatever side the offensive is on (L for Left Side, R for Right Side)

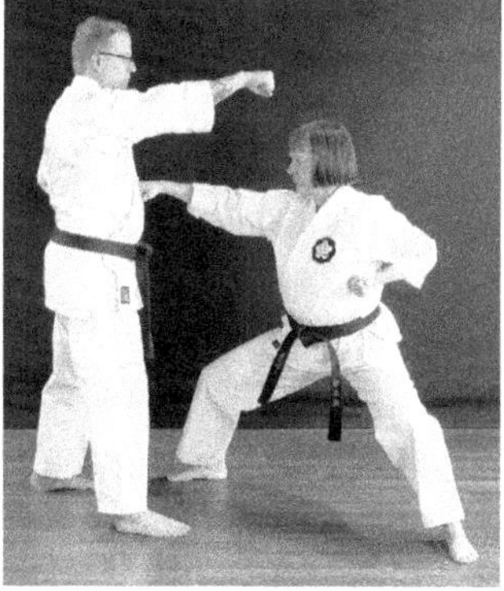

4. **(Off - L)**: Step Forward, Jodan Zuki / **(Def - R)**: Step Back, Chudan Zuki (Kiai) in Shiko Dachi

The defensive or countering side has been shorted to "Def" with a direction for whatever side that person is on, (L for Left Side, R for Right Side)

7. Kumite Ichi (1)

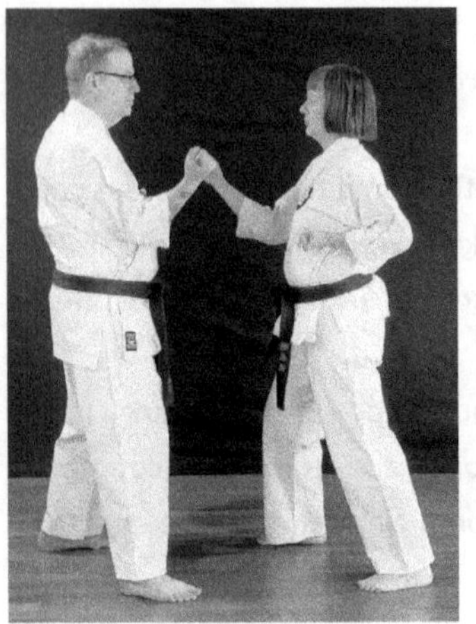

Basic Front Facing Closed Hand Kamae

Begin Counter 1

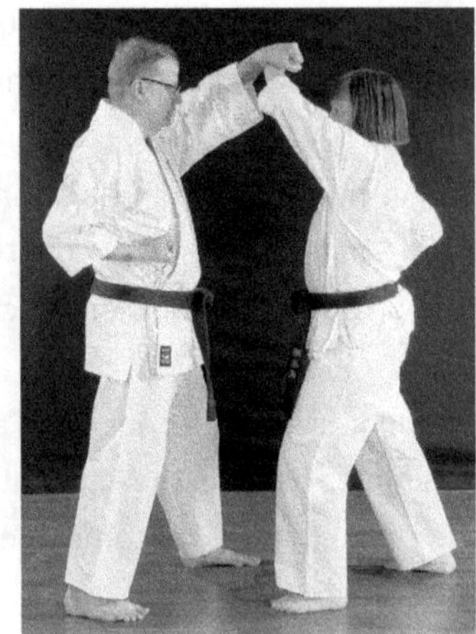

1. (Off - L): Step Forward, Jodan Zuki / (Def - R): Step Back, Jodan Age Uke

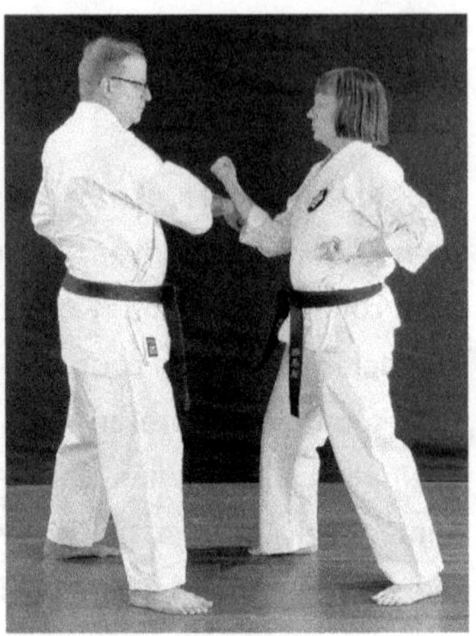

2. (Off - L): Step Forward, Chudan Zuki / (Def - R): Step Back, Chudan Uke

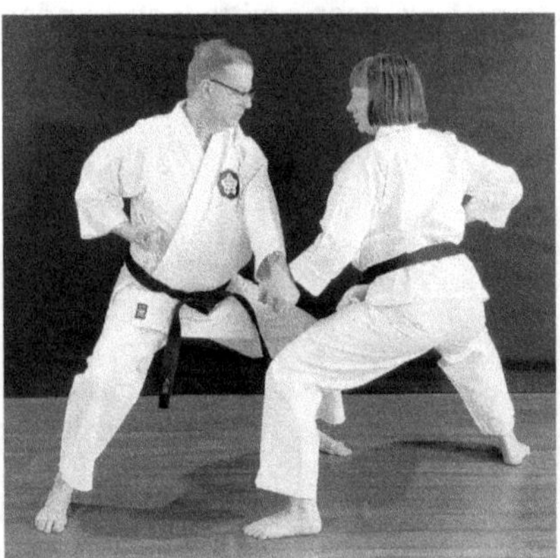

3. (Off - L): Step Forward, Gedan Zuki in Shiko Dachi / (Def - R): Step Back, Gedan Barai in Shiko Dachi

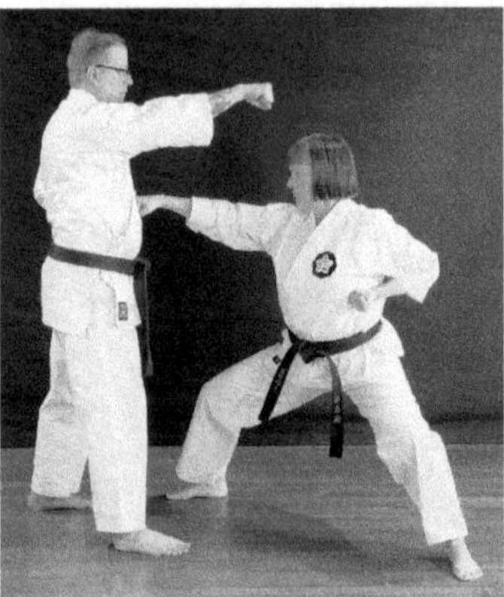

4. (Off - L): Step Forward, Jodan Zuki / (Def - R): Step Back, Chudan Zuki (Kiai) in Shiko Dachi

Repeat in Other Direction

Begin Counter 2

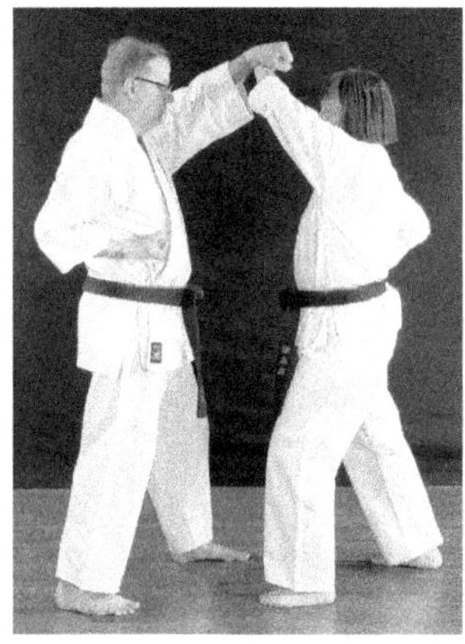

1. (Off - L): Step Forward, Jodan Zuki / (Def - R): Step Back, Jodan Age Uke

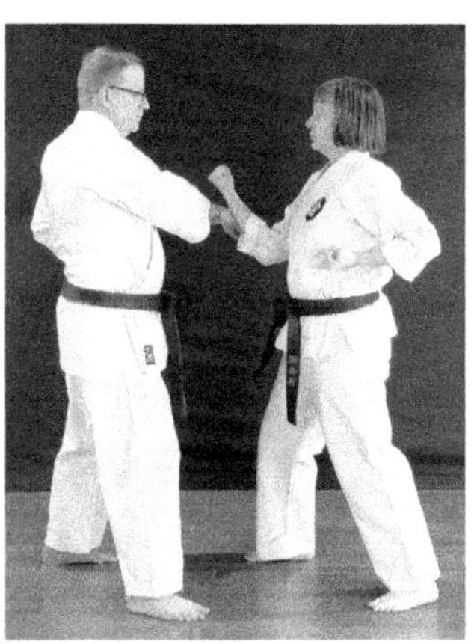

2. (Off - L): Step Forward, Chudan Zuki / (Def - R): Step Back, Chudan Uke

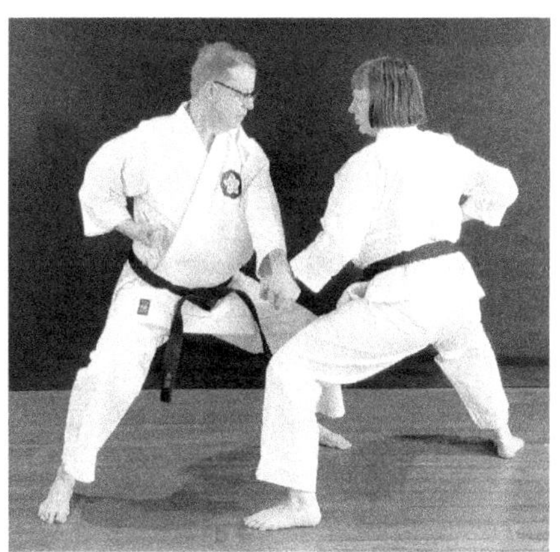

3. (Off - L): Step Forward, Gedan Zuki in Shiko Dachi / (Def - R): Step Back, Gedan Barai in Shiko Dachi

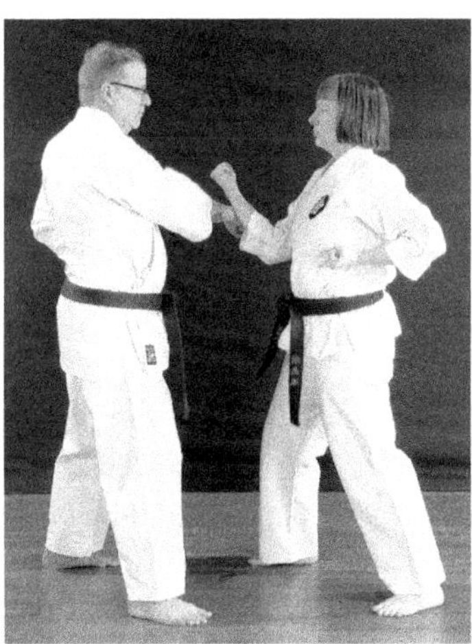

4. (Off - L): Step Forward, Chudan Zuki / (Def - R): Step Back, Chudan Uke

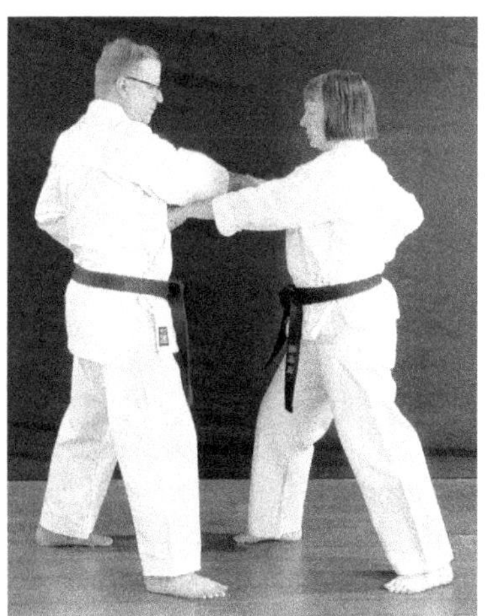

5. (Def - R): Chudan Zuki (Kiai)

Repeat in Other Direction

Begin Counter 3

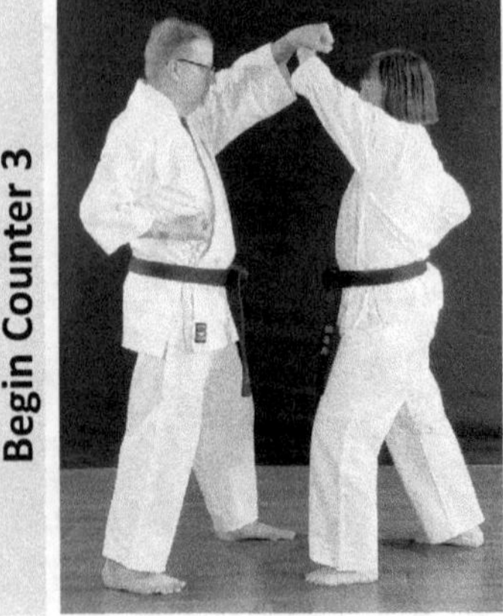

1. (Off - L): Step Forward, Jodan Zuki / (Def - R): Step Back, Jodan Age Uke

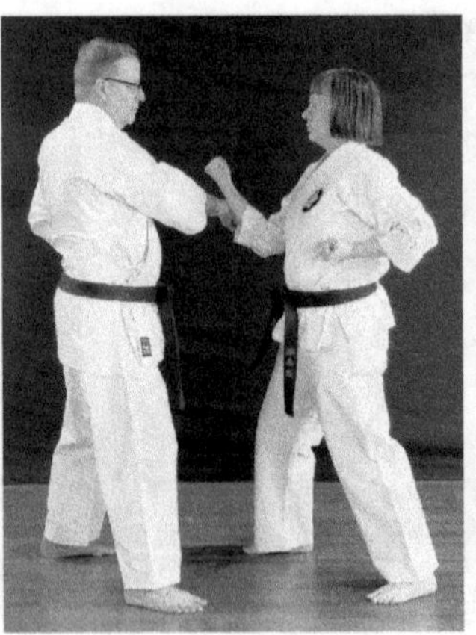

2. (Off - L): Step Forward, Chudan Zuki / (Def - R): Step Back, Chudan Uke

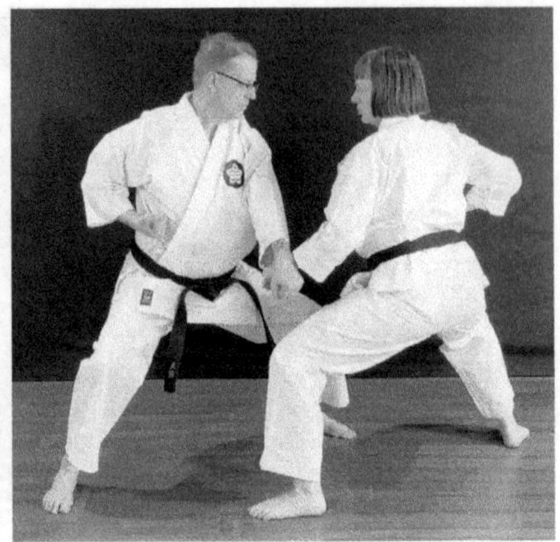

3. (Off - L): Step Forward, Gedan Zuki in Shiko Dachi / (Def - R): Step Back, Gedan Barai in Shiko Dachi

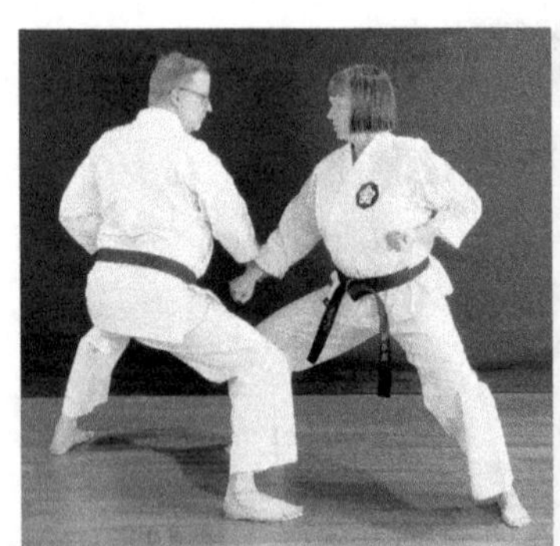

4. (Off - L): Step Forward, Gedan Zuki in Shiko Dachi / (Def - R): Step Back, Gedan Barai in Shiko Dachi

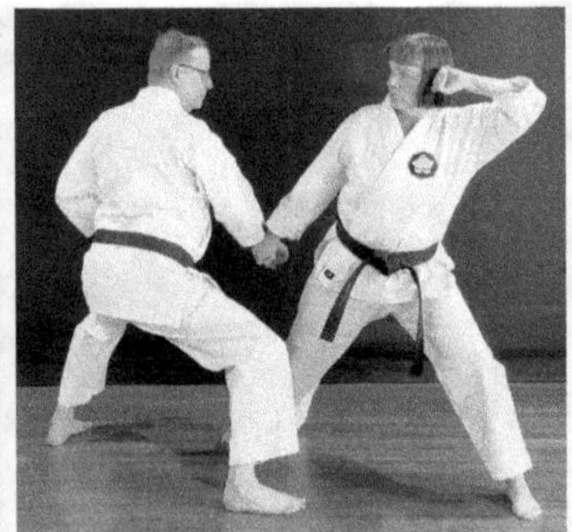

5. (Def - R): Pivot Back, Chamber Right Hand

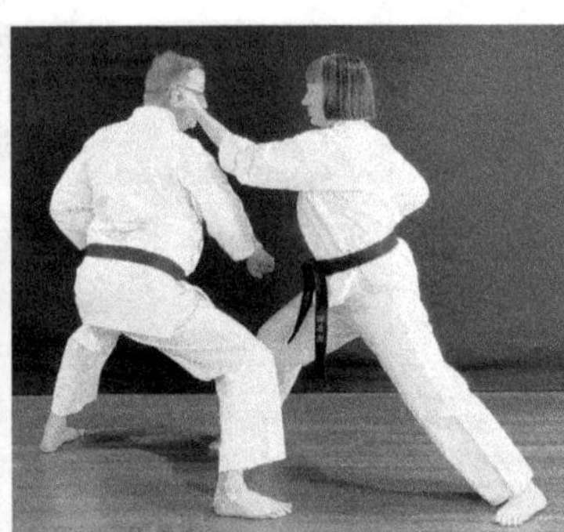

6. (Def - R): Pivot Right, Jodan Tettsui Uchi (Kiai)

Repeat in Other Direction

Begin Counter 4

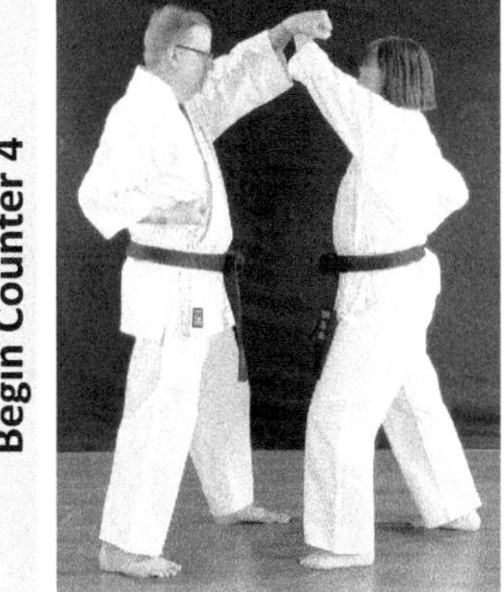

1. (Off - L): Step Forward, Jodan Zuki / (Def - R): Step Back, Jodan Age Uke

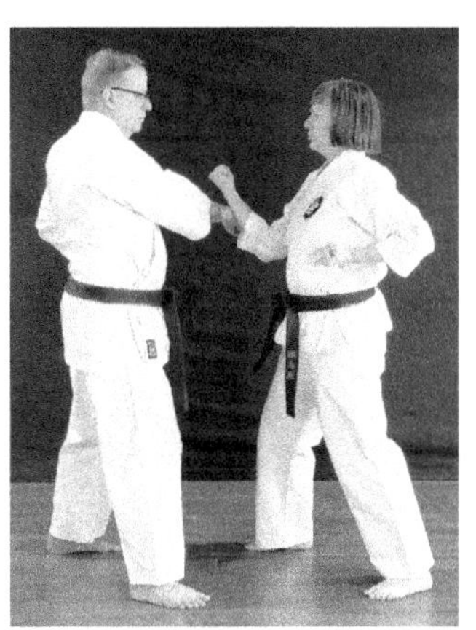

2. (Off - L) Step Forward, Chudan Zuki / (Def - R): Step Back, Chudan Uke

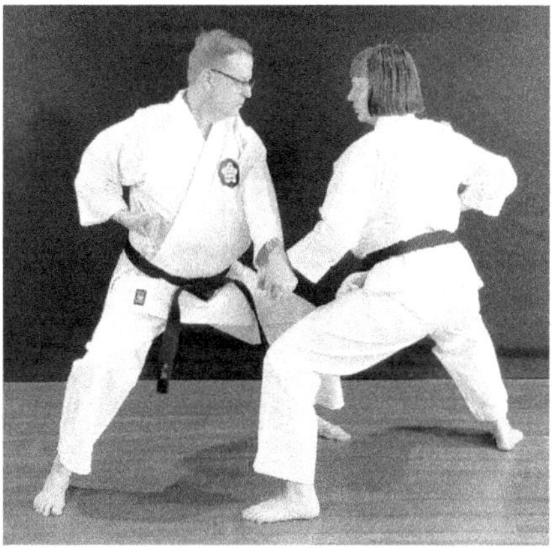

3. (Off - L): Step Forward, Gedan Zuki in Shiko Dachi / (Def - R): Step Back, Gedan Barai in Shiko Dachi

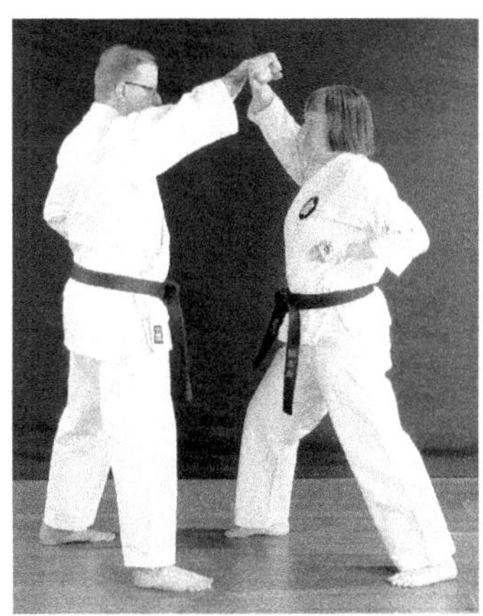

4. (Off - L): Step Forward, Jodan Zuki / (Def - R): Step Back, Jodan Age Uke

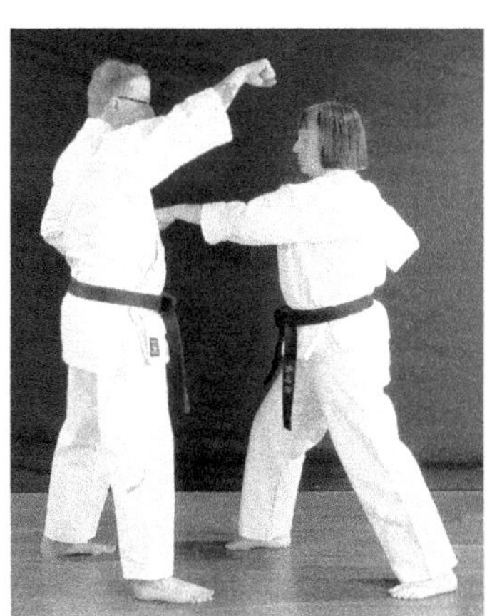

5. (Def - R): Left Chudan Zuki

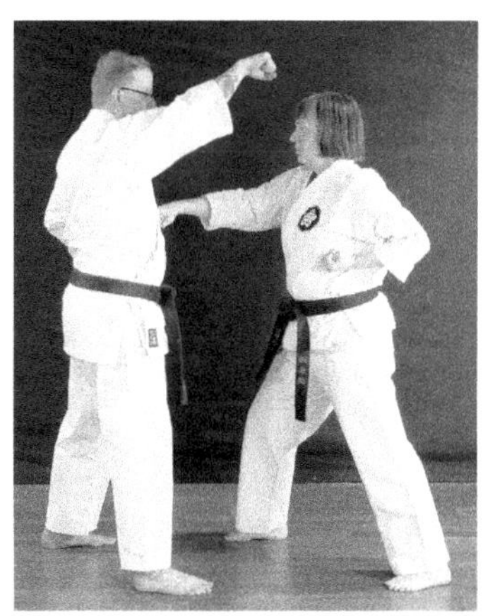

6. (Def - R): Right Chudan Zuki (Kiai)

Repeat in Other Direction

Begin Counter 5

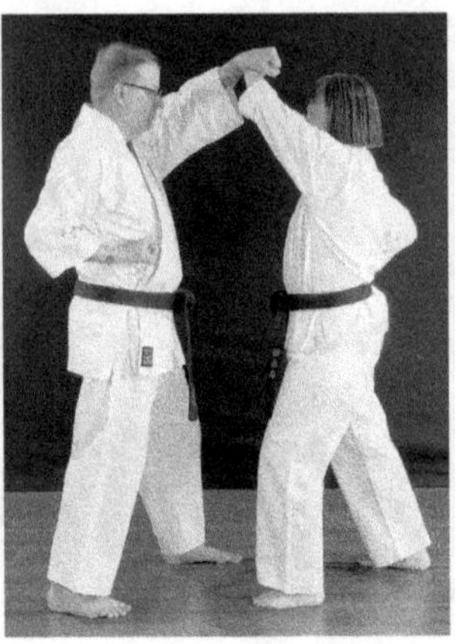

1. (Off - L): Step Forward, Jodan Zuki / (Def - R): Step Back, Jodan Age Uke

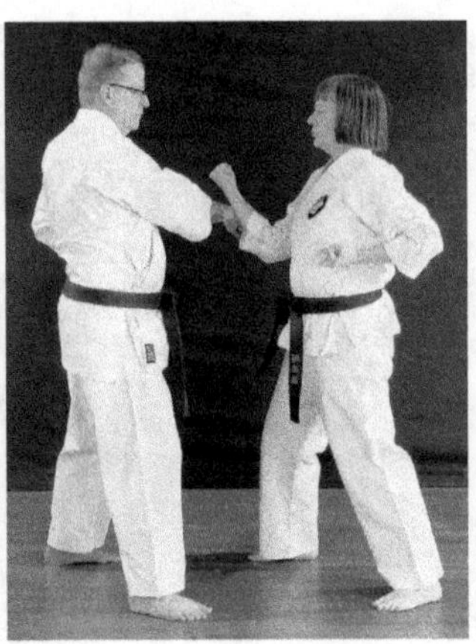

2. (Off - L) Step Forward, Chudan Zuki / (Def - R): Step Back, Chudan Uke

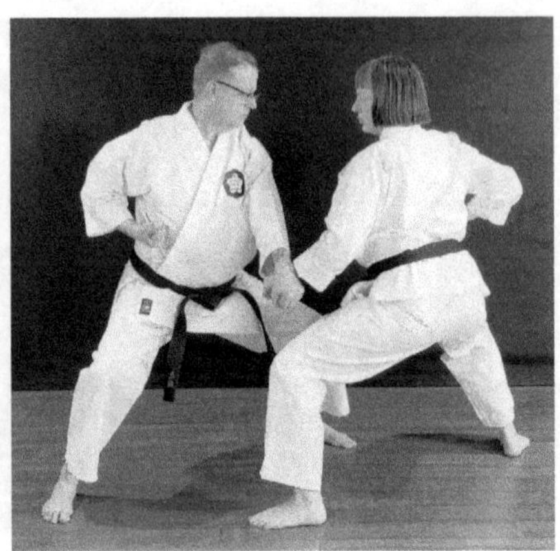

3. (Off - L): Step Forward, Gedan Zuki in Shiko Dachi / (Def - R): Step Back, Gedan Barai in Shiko Dachi

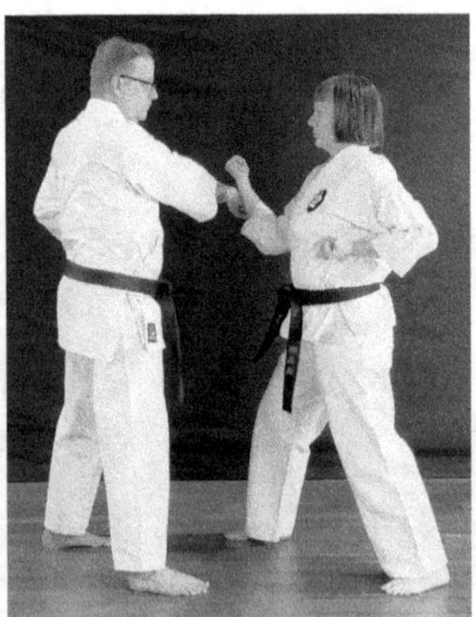

4. (Off - L): Step Forward, Chudan Zuki / (Def - R): Step Back, Chudan Uke

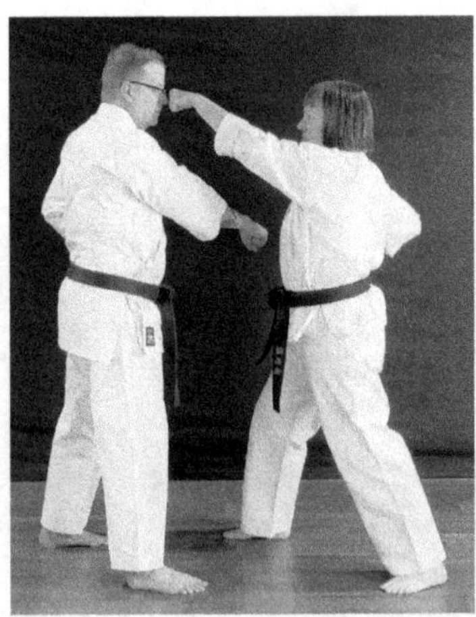

5. (Def - R): Jodan Zuki (Kiai)

Repeat in Other Direction

Begin Counter 6

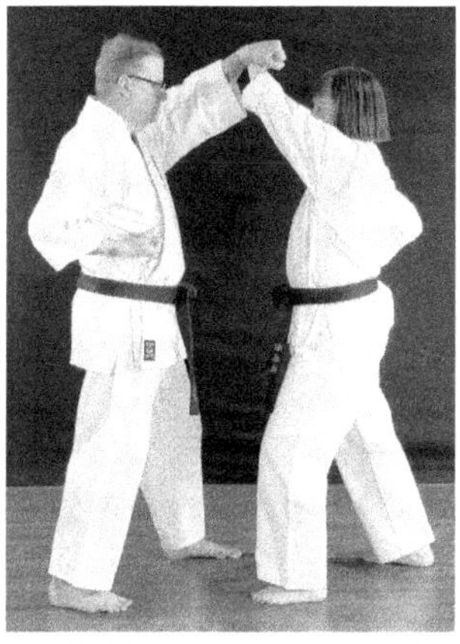
1. (Off - L): Step Forward, Jodan Zuki / (Def - R): Step Back, Jodan Age Uke

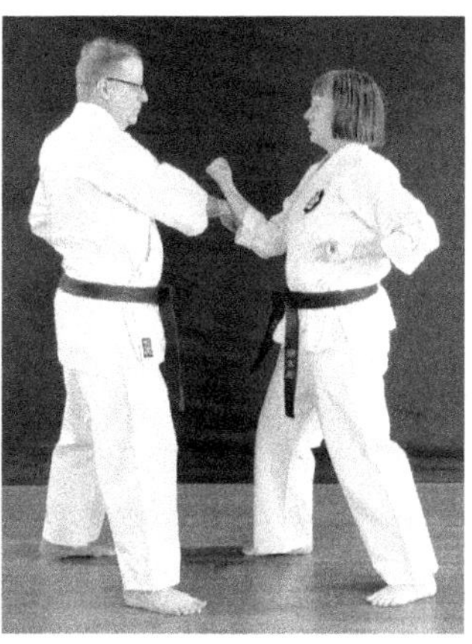
2. (Off - L) Step Forward, Chudan Zuki / (Def - R): Step Back, Chudan Uke

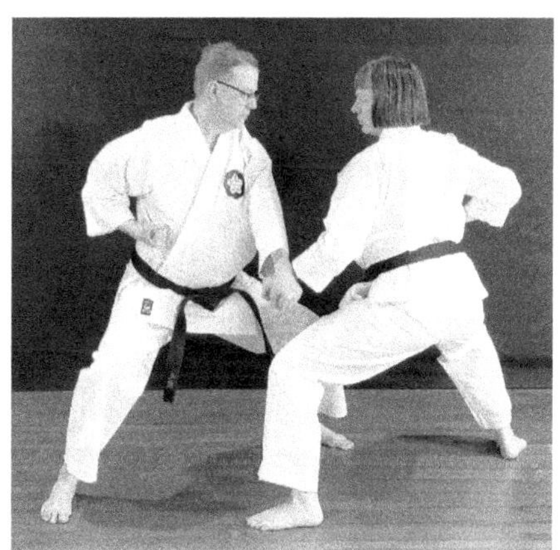
3. (Off - L): Step Forward, Gedan Zuki in Shiko Dachi / (Def - R): Step Back, Gedan Barai in Shiko Dachi

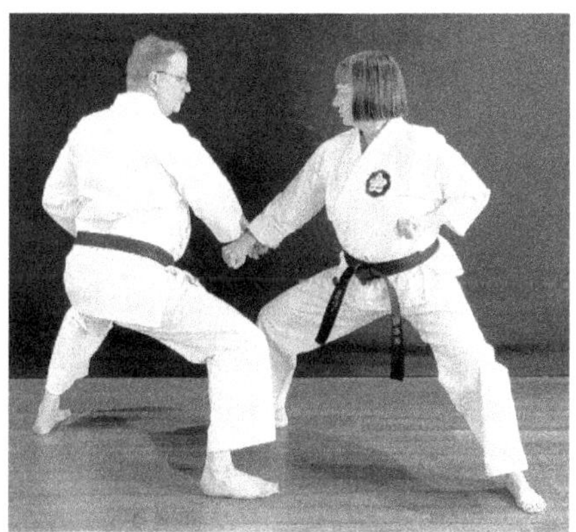
4. (Off - L): Step Forward, Gedan Zuki in Shiko Dachi / (Def - R): Step Back, Gedan Barai in Shiko Dachi

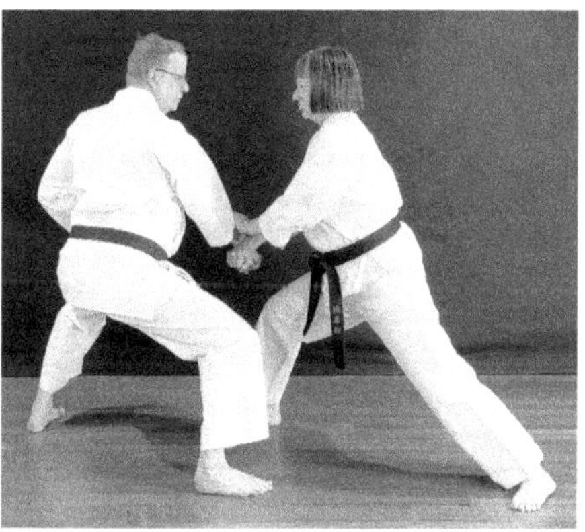
5. (Def - R): Pivot Right, Left Shotei Otoshi Uke

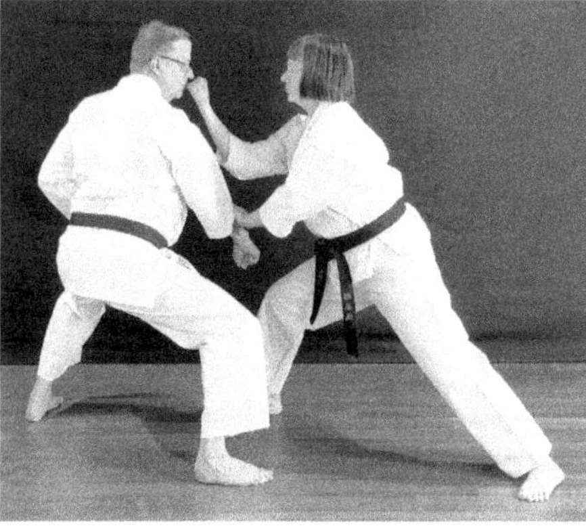
6. (Def - R): Right Uraken Uchi (Kiai)

Repeat in Other Direction

Kumite Ichi - Bag Work

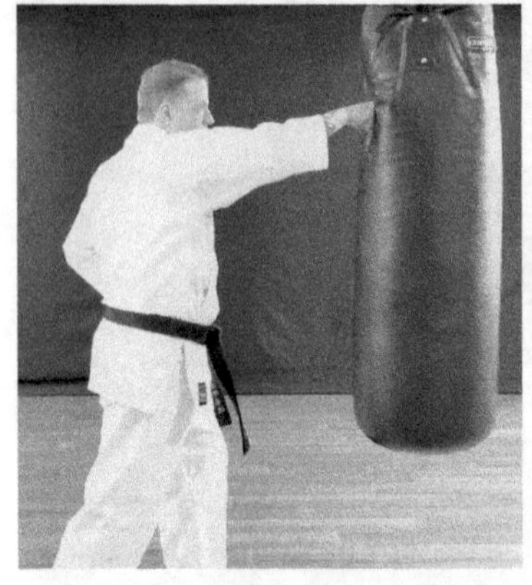

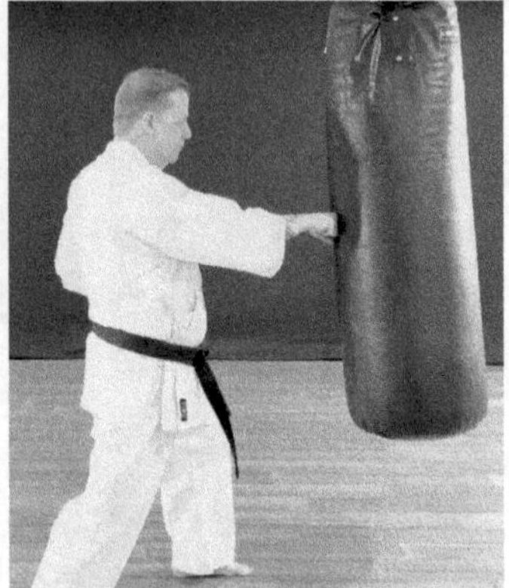

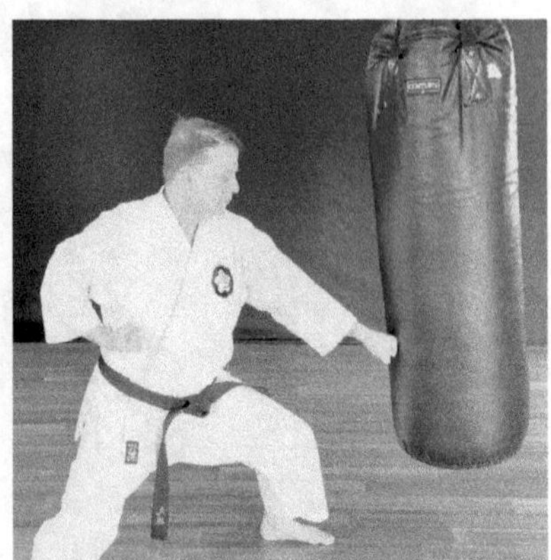

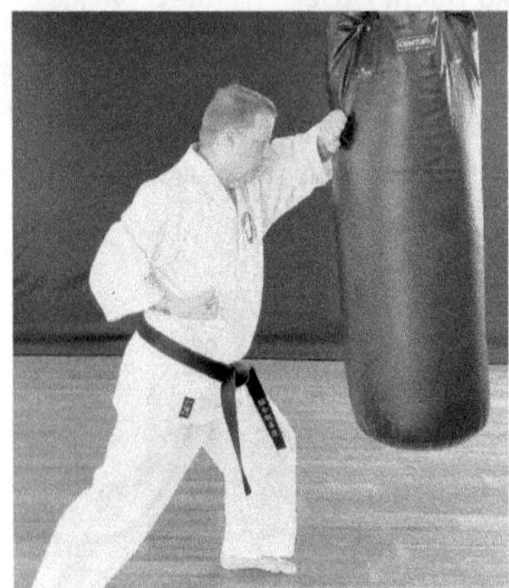

Jodan Zuki (Top) & Jodan Age Uke (Bottom)

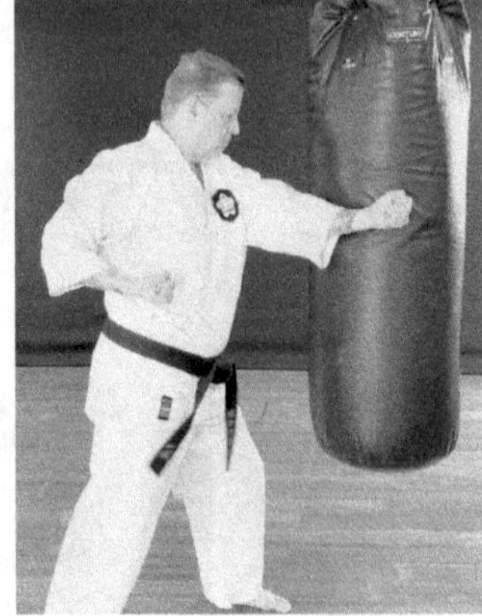

Chudan Zuki (top) & Uchi Uke (bottom)

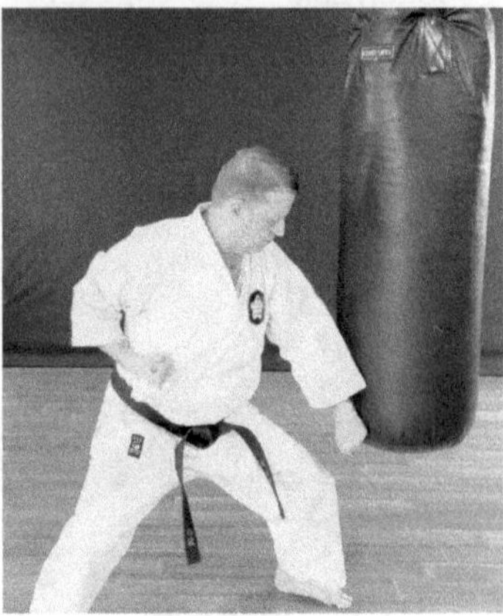

Gedan Zuki in Shiko Dachi (Top) & Gedan Barai (Bottom)

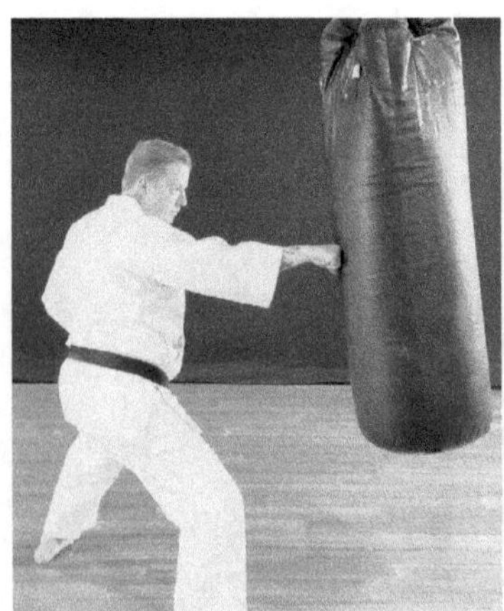

Counter 1: Chudan Zuki in Shiko Dachi

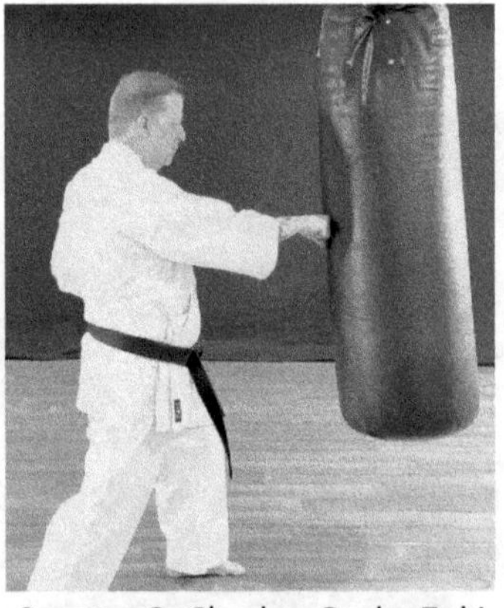

Counter 2: Chudan Gyaku Zuki

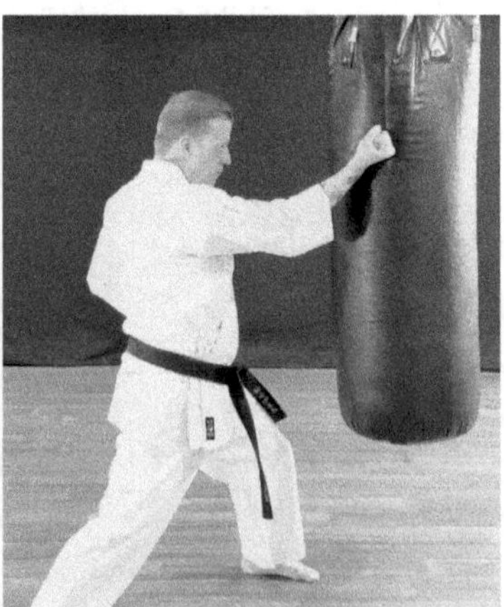

Counter 3: Jodan Tettsui Uchi in Shiko Dachi

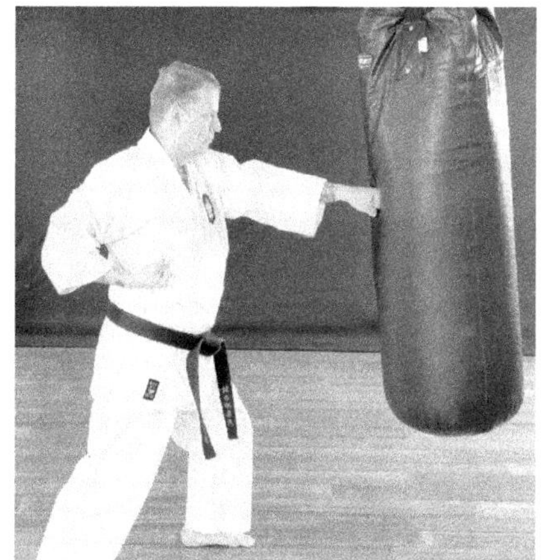

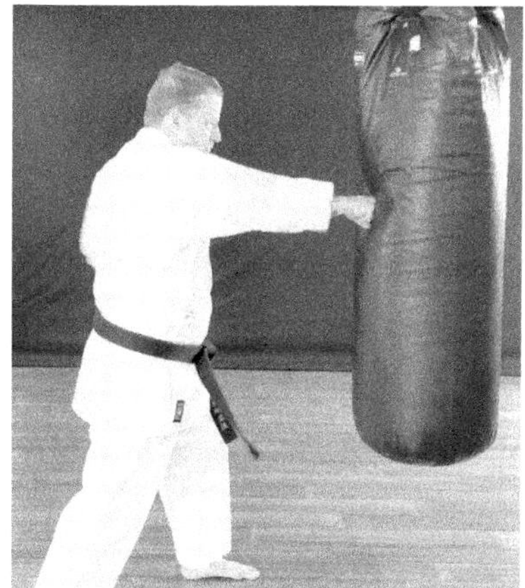

Counter 4: Left, then Right Chudan Zuki

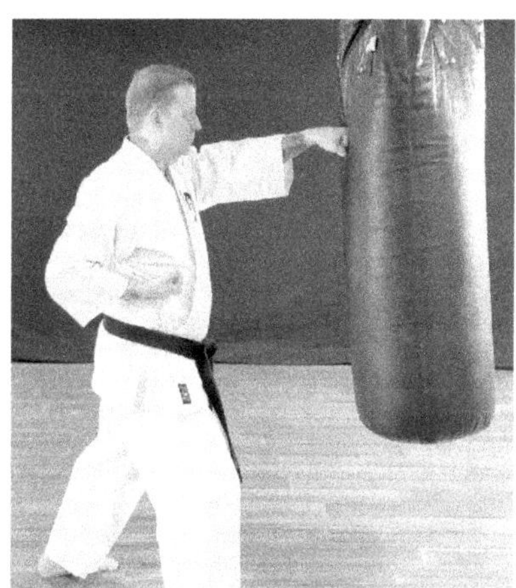

Counter 5: Jodan Gyaku Zuki

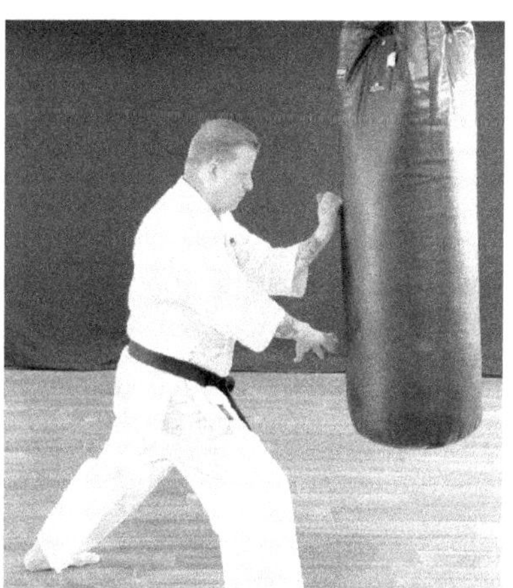

Counter 6: Uraken Uchi

8. Kumite Ni (2)

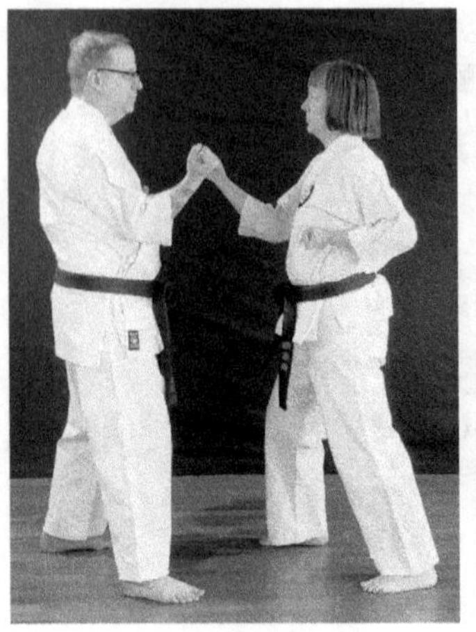

Basic Front Facing Closed Hand Kamae

Begin Counter 1

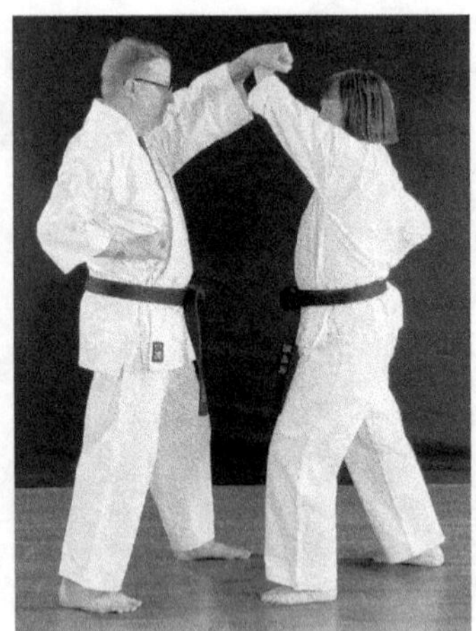

1. (Off - L): Step Forward, Jodan Zuki / (Def - R): Step Back, Jodan Age Uke

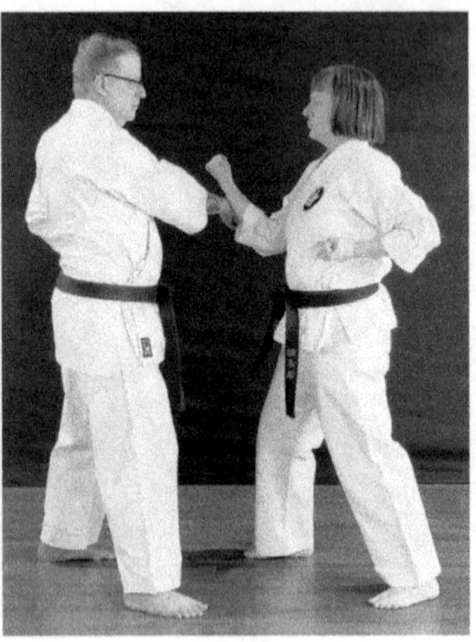

2. (Off - L): Step Forward, Chudan Zuki / (Def - R): Step Back, Chudan Uke

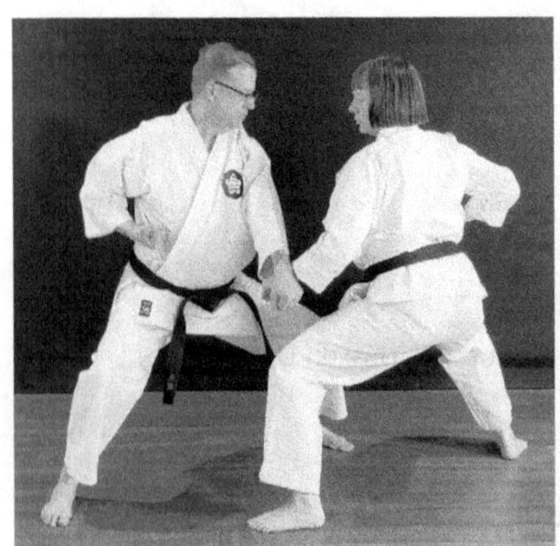

3. (Off - L): Step Forward, Gedan Zuki in Shiko Dachi / (Def - R): Step Back, Gedan Barai in Shiko Dachi

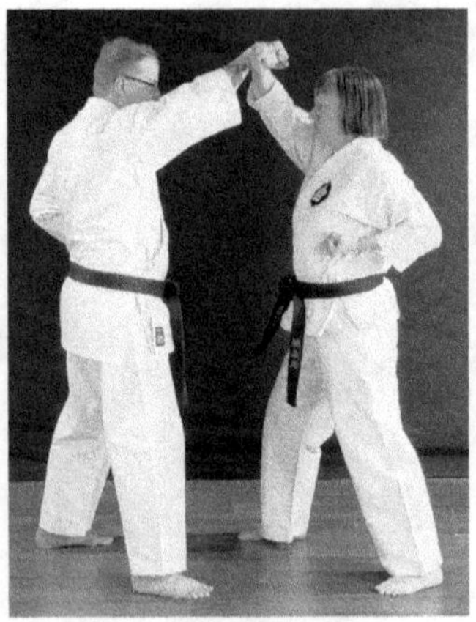

4. (Off - L): Step Forward, Jodan Zuki / (Def - R): Step Back, Jodan Age Uke

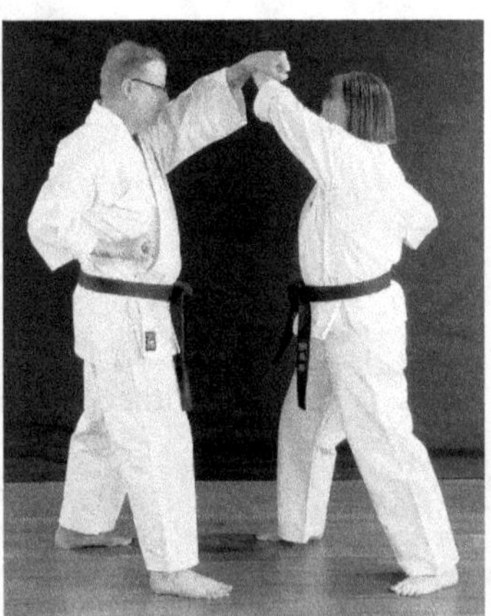

5. (Off - L): Jodan Zuki / (Def - R): Jodan Age Uke

6. (Off - L): Jodan Zuki / (Def - R): Jodan Age Uke

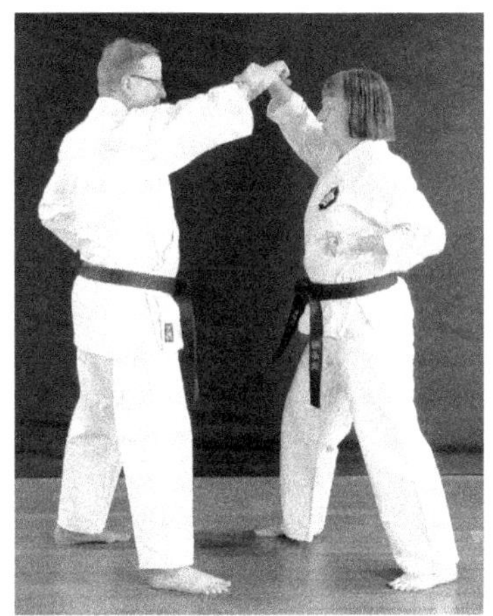

7. (Def - R): Grab Wrist

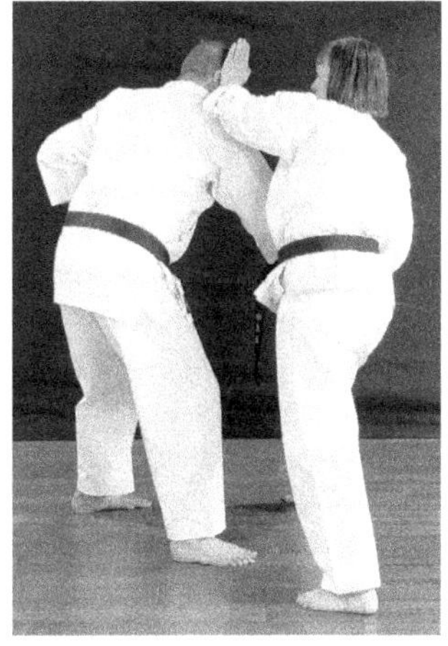

8. (Def - R): Step Out, Jodan Shotei Uchi (Kiai)

Repeat in Other Direction

Begin Counter 2

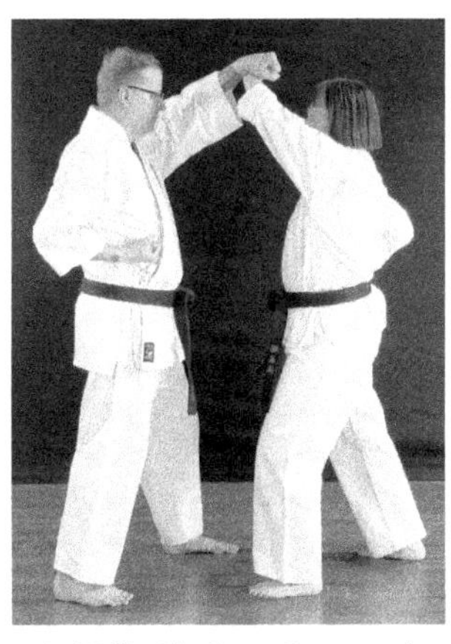

1. (Off - L): Step Forward, Jodan Zuki / (Def - R): Step Back, Jodan Age Uke

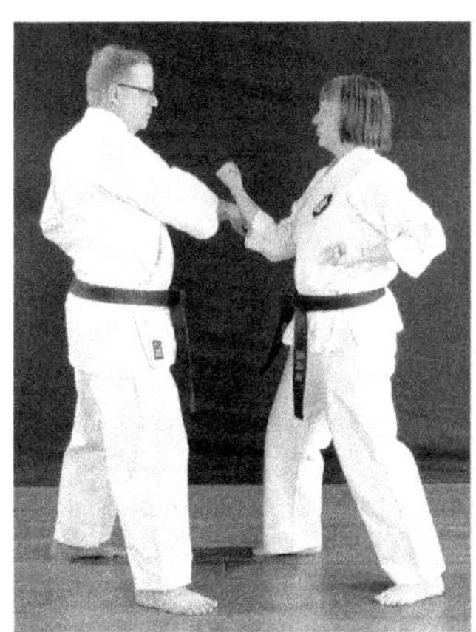

2. (Off - L): Step Forward, Chudan Zuki / (Def - R): Step Back, Chudan Uke

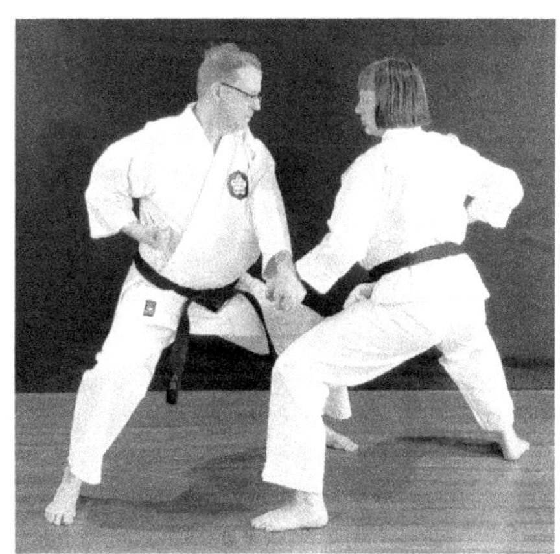

3. (Off - L): Step Forward, Gedan Zuki in Shiko Dachi / (Def - R): Step Back, Gedan Barai in Shiko Dachi

4. (Off - L): Step Forward, Chudan Zuki / (Def - R): Step Back, Chudan Uke

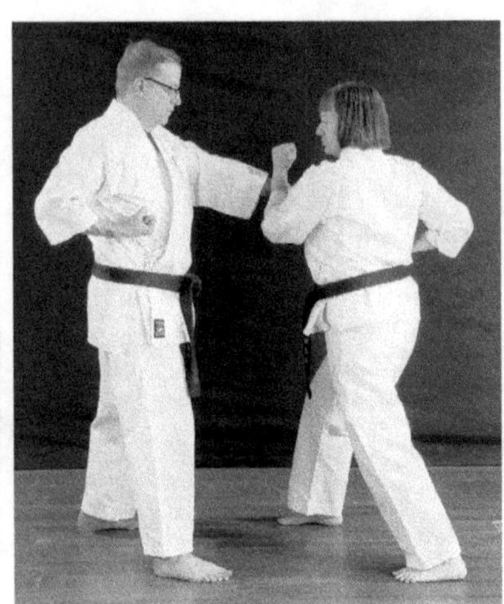

5. (Off - L): Chudan Zuki / (Def - R): Soto Uke

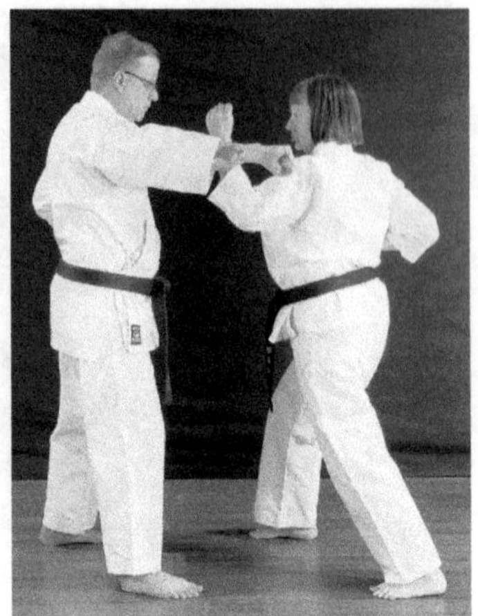

6. (Off - L): Chudan Zuki / (Def - R): Uchi Uke

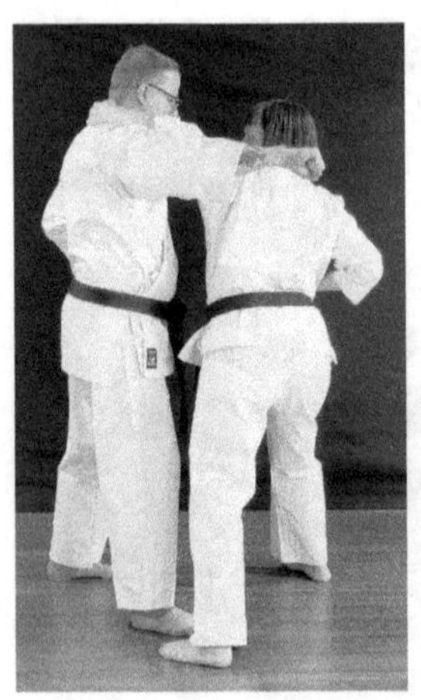

7. (Def - R): Step In, Hand Behind Opponent's Neck

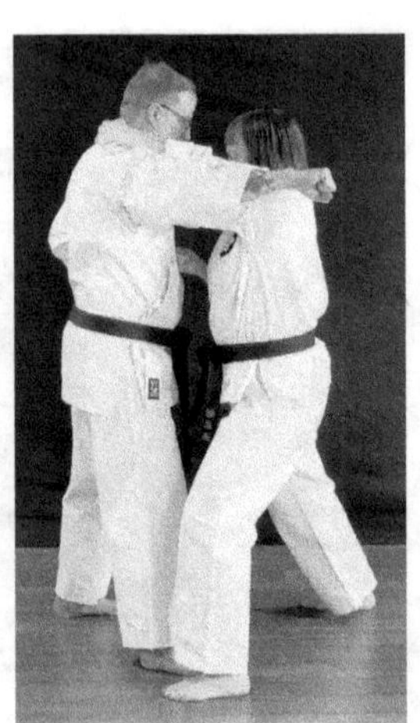

8. (Def - R): Pivot Left, Ura Uchi (Kiai)

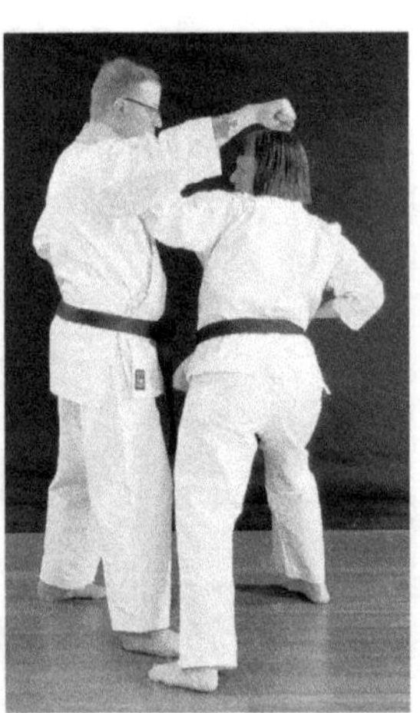

9. (Def - R): Push Away with Left Forearm on Opponent's Shoulder

Repeat in Other Direction

Begin Counter 3

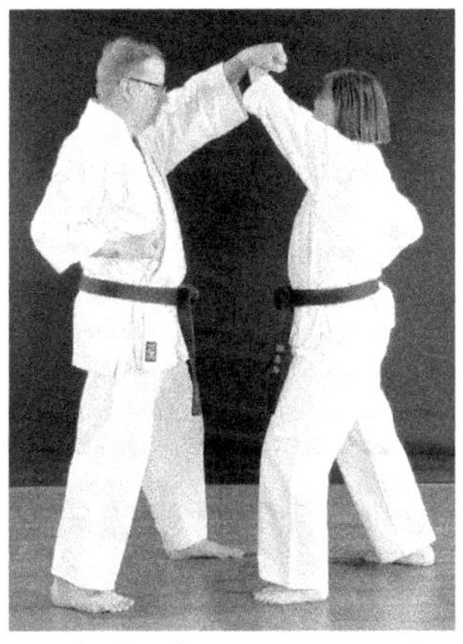

1. (Off - L): Step Forward, Jodan Zuki / (Def - R): Step Back, Jodan Age Uke

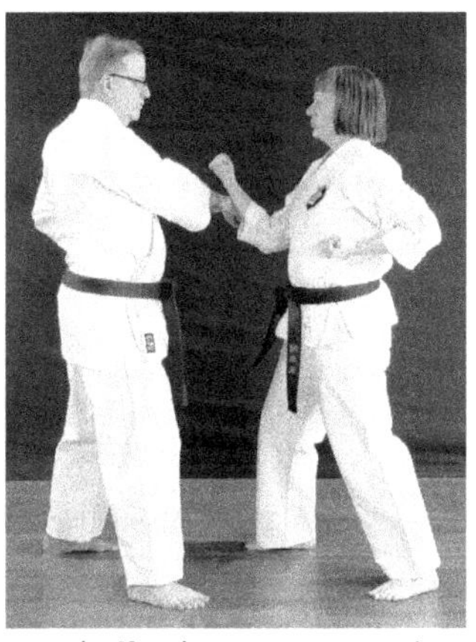

2. (Off - L): Step Forward, Chudan Zuki / (Def - R): Step Back, Chudan Uke

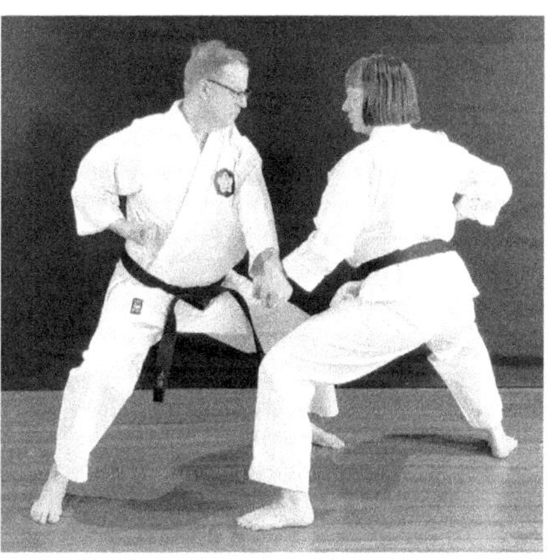

3. (Off - L): Step Forward, Gedan Zuki in Shiko Dachi / (Def - R): Step Back, Gedan Barai in Shiko Dachi

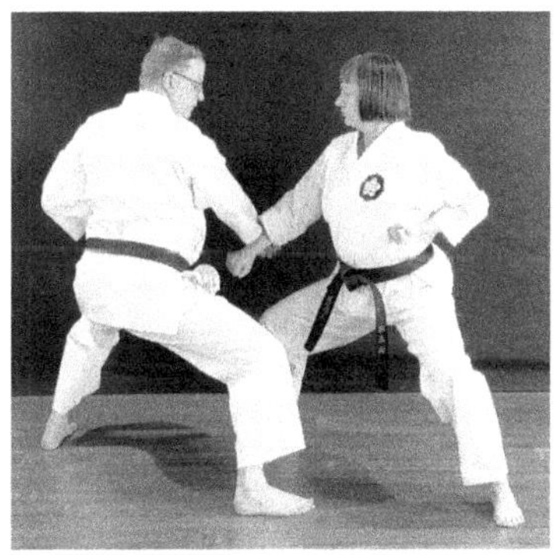

4. (Off - L): Step Forward, Gedan Zuki in Shiko Dachi / (Def - R): Step Back, Gedan Barai in Shiko Dachi

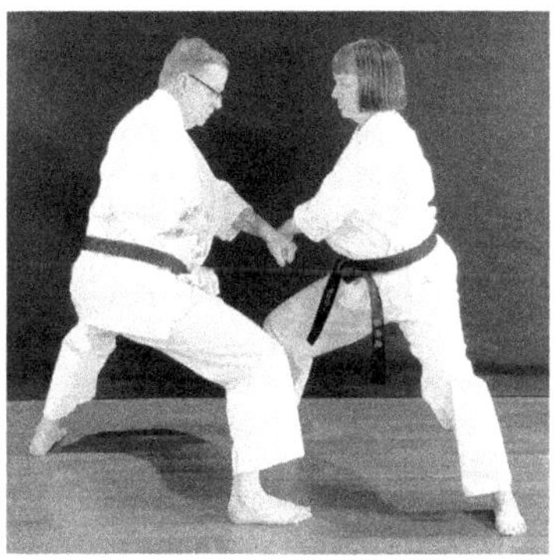

5. (Off - L): Gedan Zuki in Shiko Dachi / (Def - R): Gedan Barai in Shiko Dachi

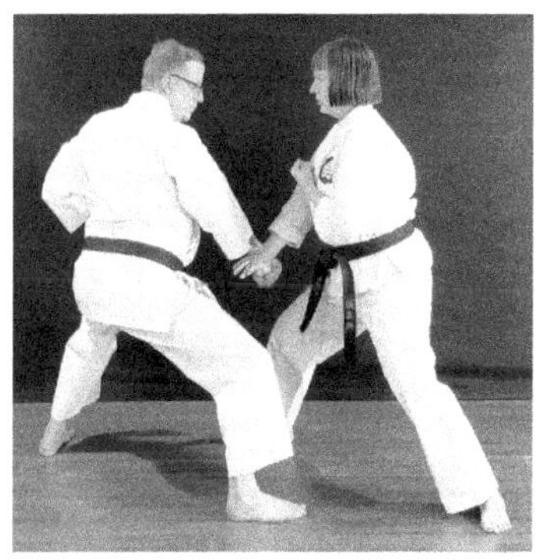

6. (Off - L): Gedan Zuki in Shiko Dachi / (Def - R): Right Shotei Otoshi Uke

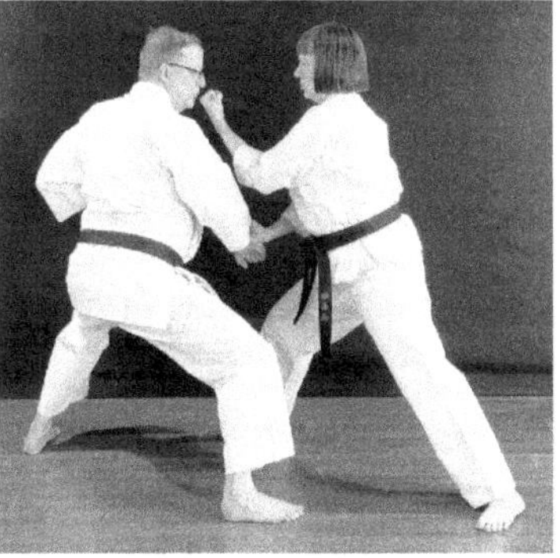

7. (Def - R): Leave Right Hand on Opponent's Arm, Uraken Uchi (Kiai)

Repeat in Other Direction

Begin Counter 4

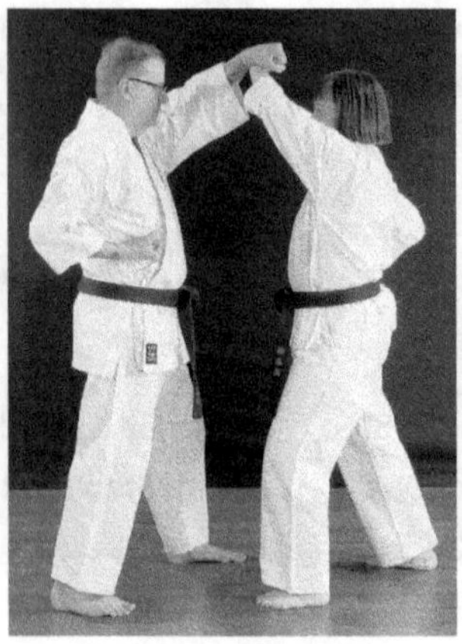

1. (Off - L): Step Forward, Jodan Zuki / (Def - R): Step Back, Jodan Age Uke

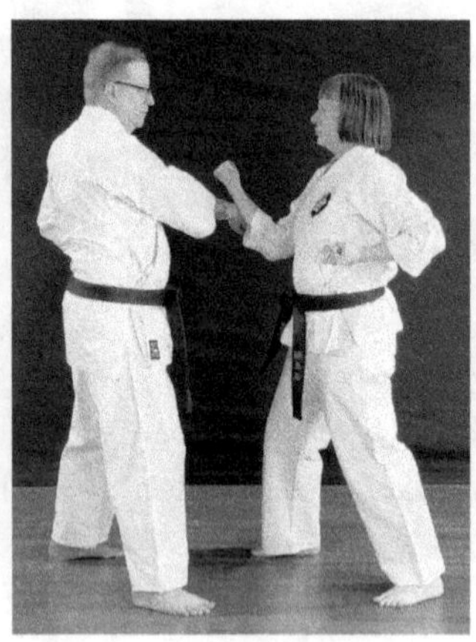

2. (Off - L): Step Forward, Chudan Zuki / (Def - R): Step Back, Chudan Uke

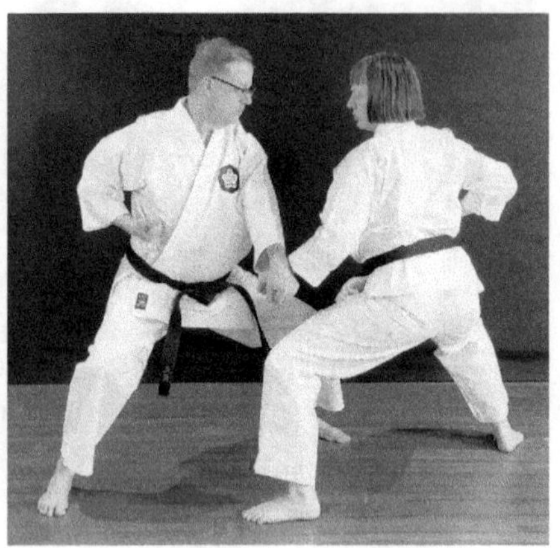

3. (Off - L): Step Forward, Gedan Zuki in Shiko Dachi / (Def - R): Step Back, Gedan Barai in Shiko Dachi

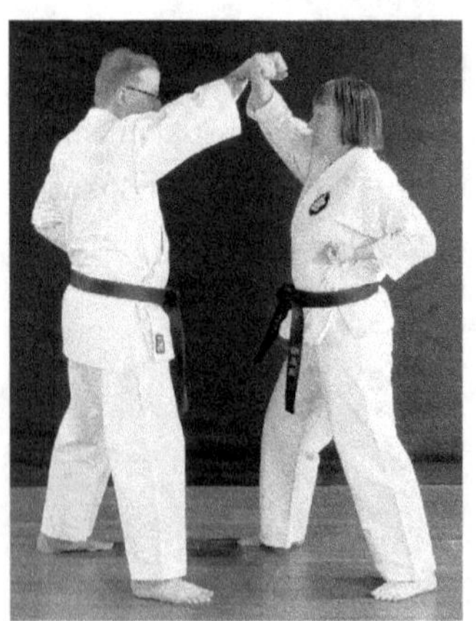

4. (Off - L): Step Forward, Jodan Zuki / (Def - R): Step Back, Jodan Age Uke

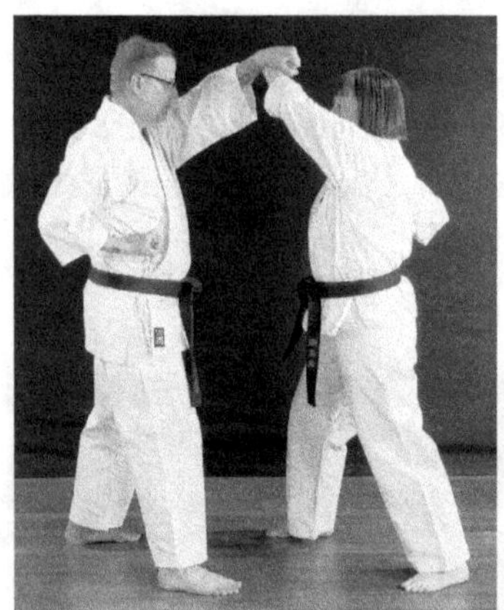

5. (Off - L): Jodan Zuki / (Def - R): Jodan Age Uke

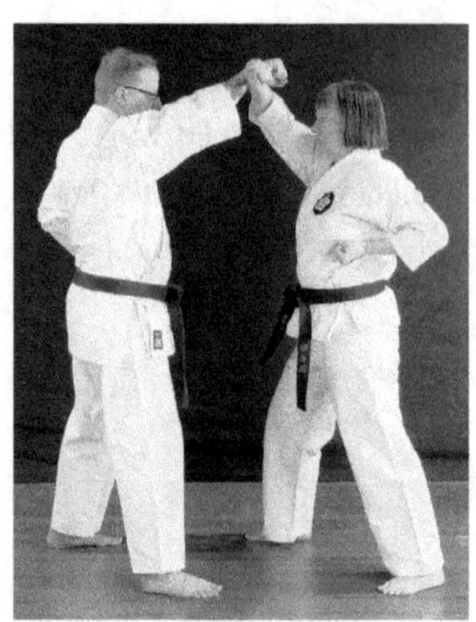

6. (Off - L): Jodan Zuki / (Def - R): Jodan Age Uke

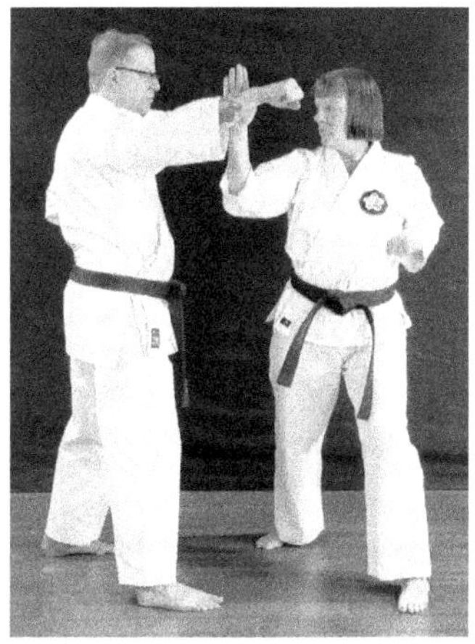

7. (Def - R): Jodan Shotei Oshi Pivoting Left

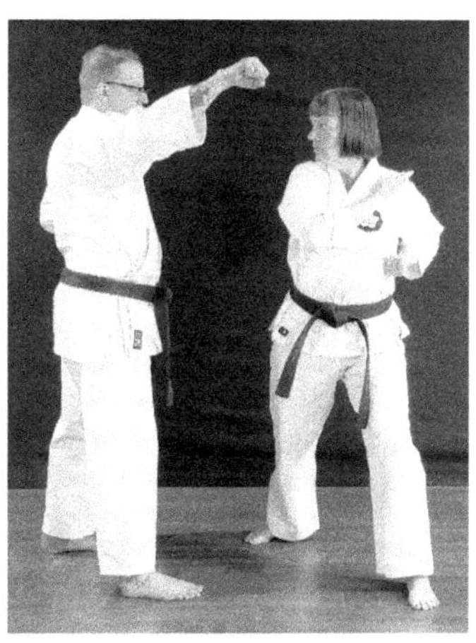

8. (Def - R): Chamber Shuto Hand to Shoulder

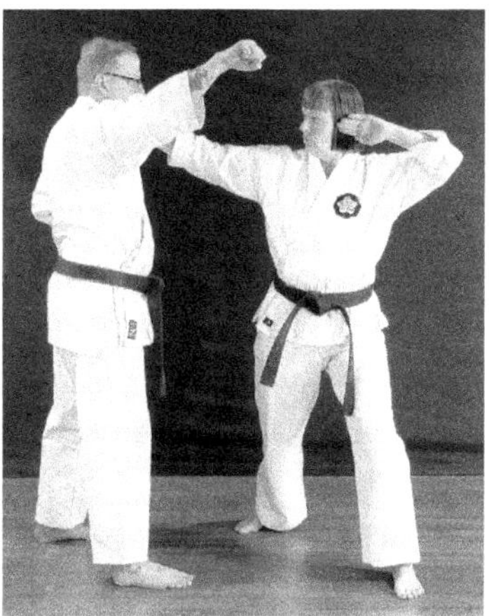

9. (Def - R): Right Jodan Yoko Shuto Uchi While Chambering Left Shuto Hand to Head

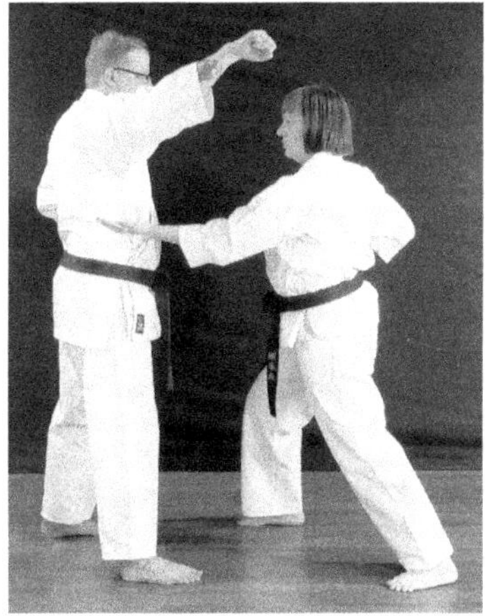

10. (Def - R): Pivot Right, Shuto Uchi to Ribs (Kiai)

Repeat in Other Direction

Begin Counter 5

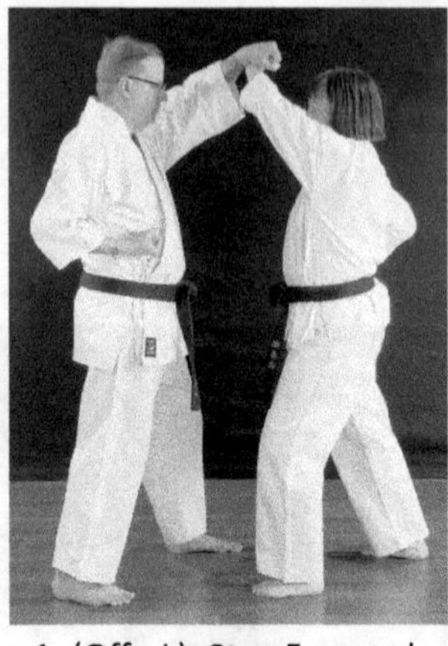

1. (Off - L): Step Forward, Jodan Zuki / (Def - R): Step Back, Jodan Age Uke

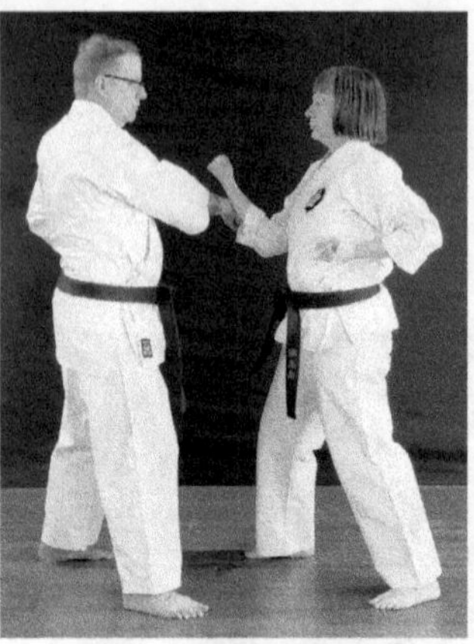

2. (Off - L): Step Forward, Chudan Zuki / (Def - R): Step Back, Chudan Uke

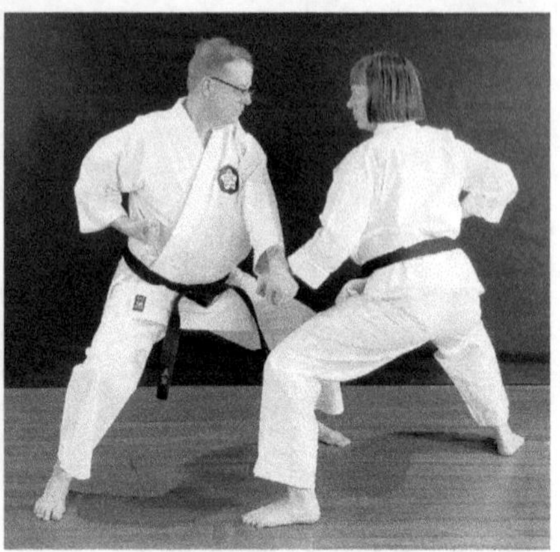

3. (Off - L): Step Forward, Gedan Zuki in Shiko Dachi / (Def - R): Step Back, Gedan Barai in Shiko Dachi

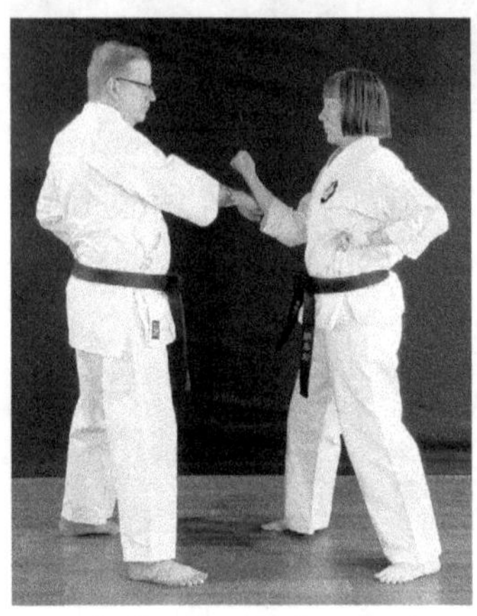

4. (Off - L): Step Forward, Chudan Zuki / (Def - R): Step Back, Chudan Uke

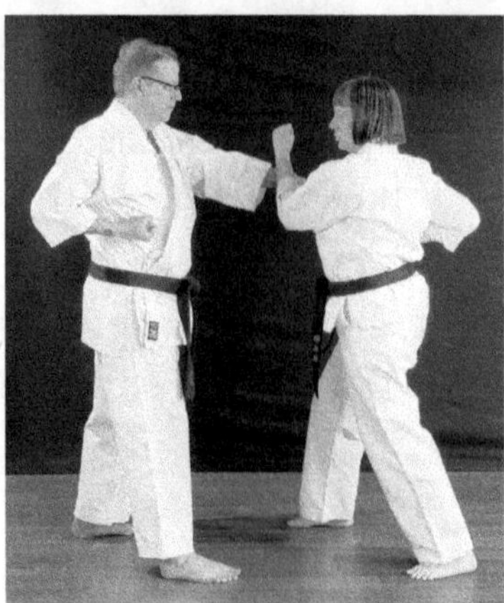

5. (Off - L): Chudan Zuki / (Def - R): Left Soto Uke

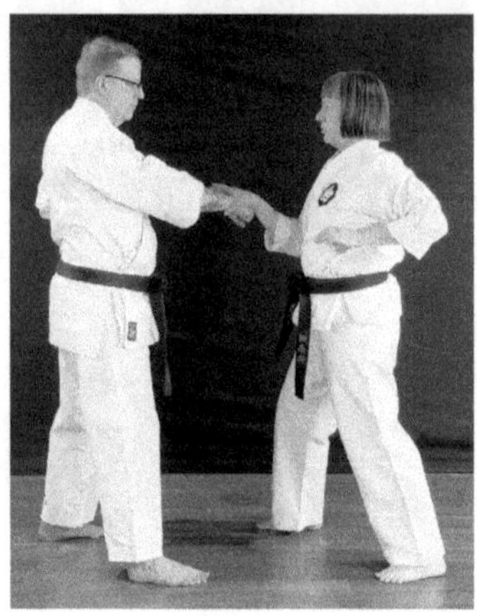

6. (Off - L): Chudan Zuki / (Def - R): Right Chudan Hari to Hiki Uke

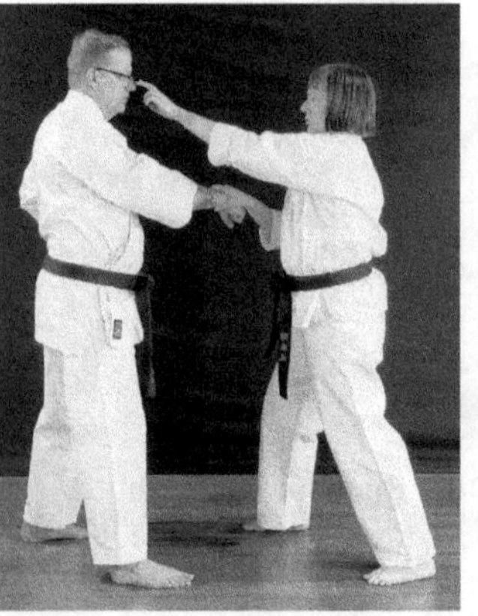

7. (Def - R): Grab Opponent's Wrist, Left Nihon Nukite to Opponent's Eyes (Kiai)

Repeat in Other Direction

Begin Counter 6

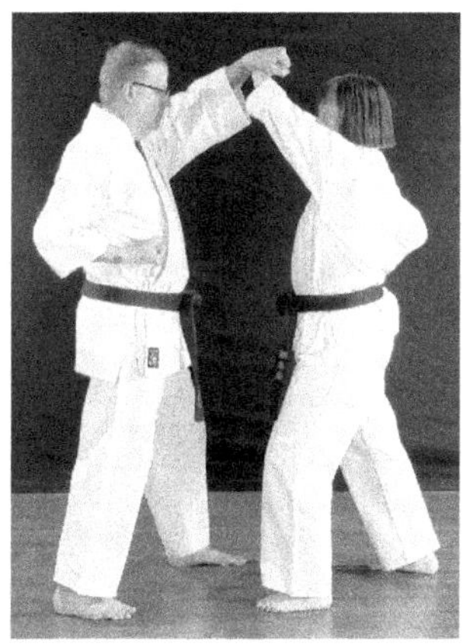

1. (Off - L): Step Forward, Jodan Zuki / (Def - R): Step Back, Jodan Age Uke

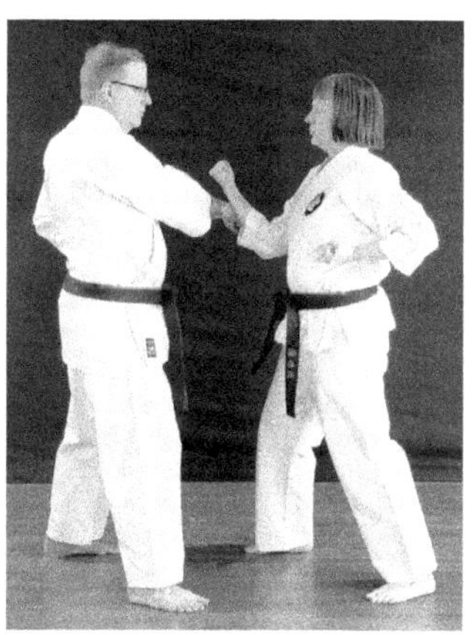

2. (Off - L): Step Forward, Chudan Zuki / (Def - R): Step Back, Chudan Uke

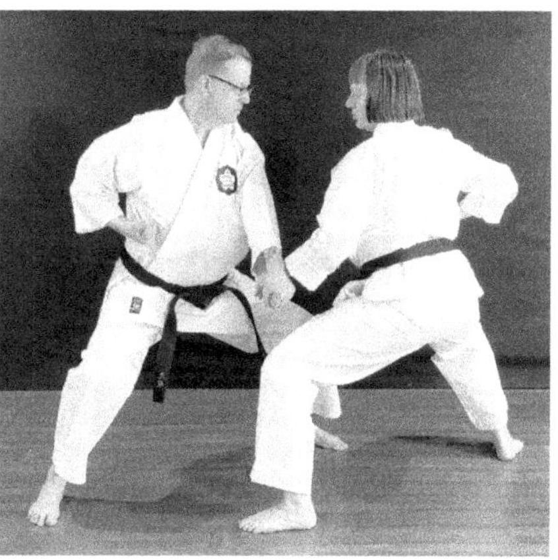

3. (Off - L): Step Forward, Gedan Zuki in Shiko Dachi / (Def - R): Step Back, Gedan Barai in Shiko Dachi

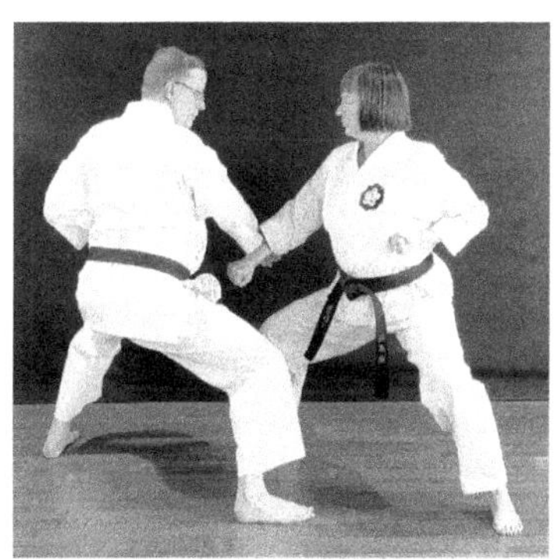

4. (Off - L): Step Forward, Gedan Zuki in Shiko Dachi / (Def - R): Step Back, Gedan Barai in Shiko Dachi

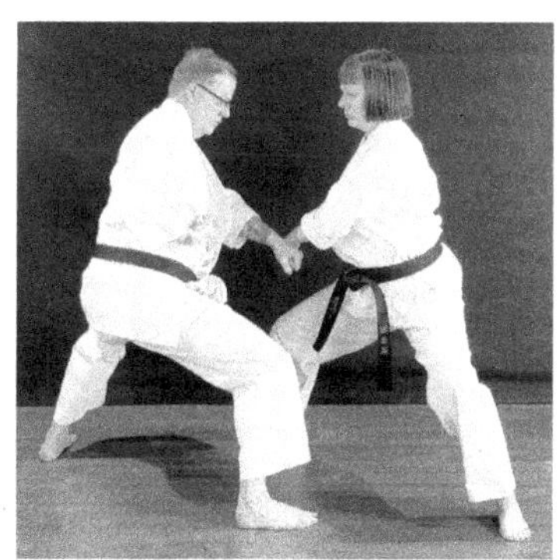

5. (Off - L): Gedan Zuki in Shiko Dachi / (Def - R): Gedan Barai in Shiko Dachi

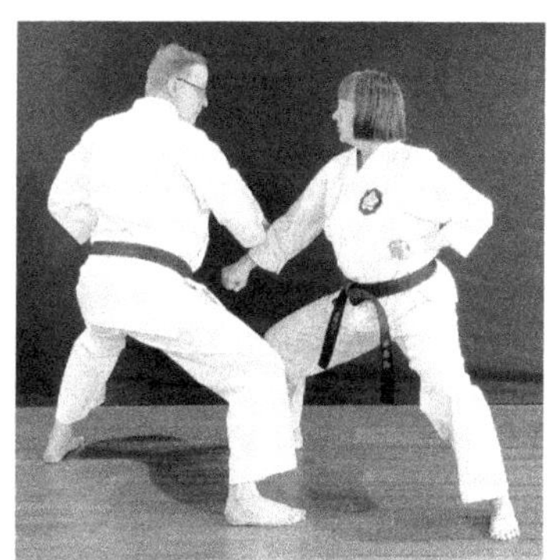

6. (Off - L): Gedan Zuki in Shiko Dachi / (Def - R): Gedan Barai in Shiko Dachi

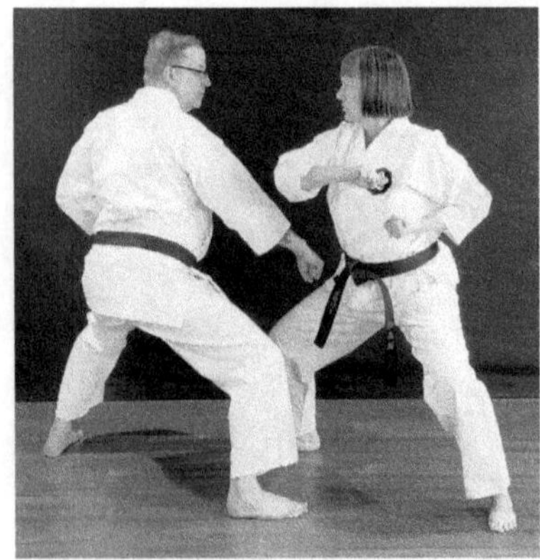
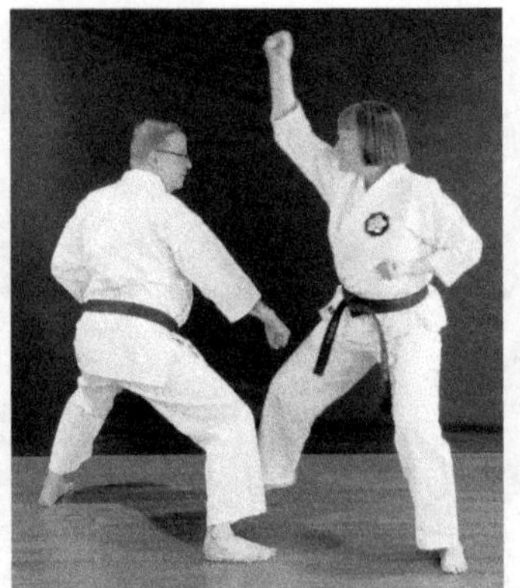
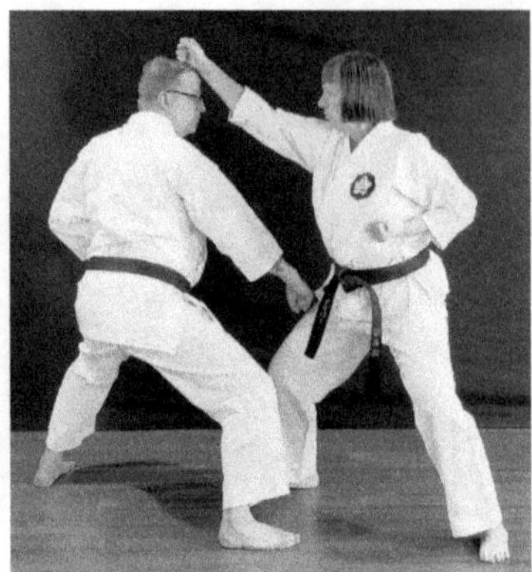

7. (Def - R): Right Tettsui Otoshi Uchi

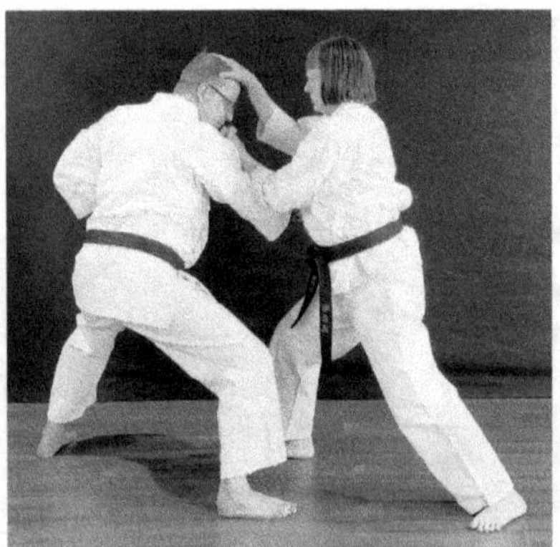

8. (Def - R): Grab Head/Hair, Pivot Right, Ura Zuki (Kiai)

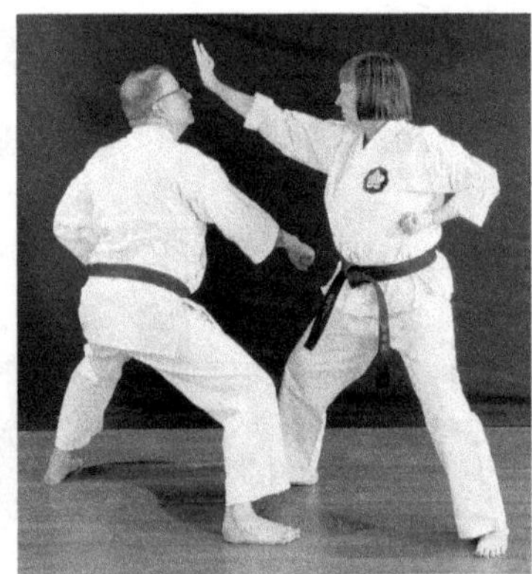

9. (Def - R): Push Away Head

Repeat in Other Direction

Kumite Ni - Bag Work

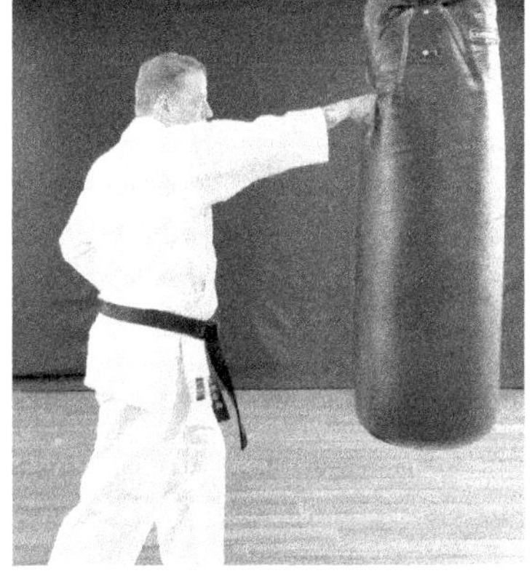
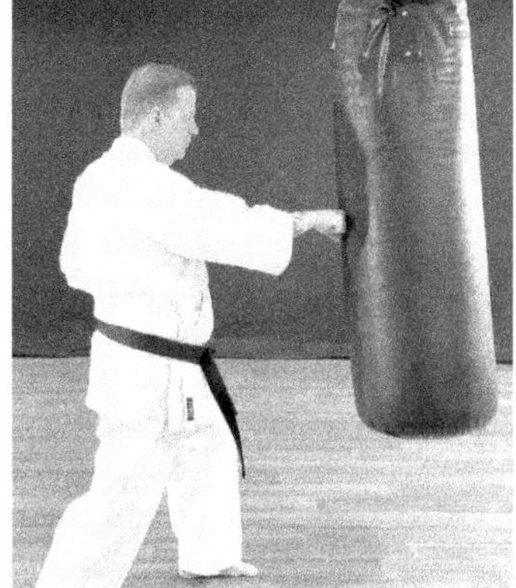
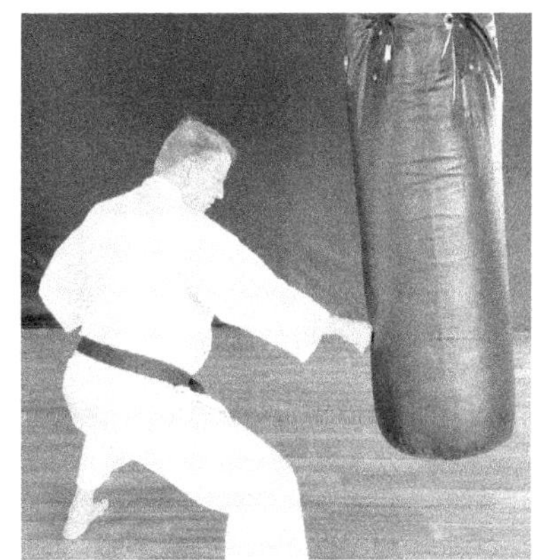

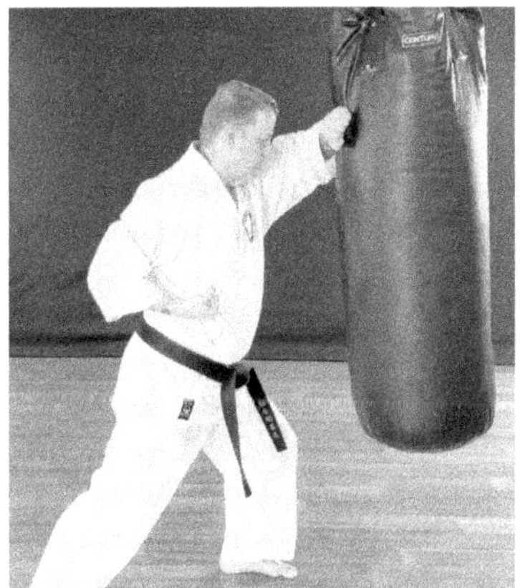

Jodan Zuki (Top) & Jodan Age Uke (Bottom)

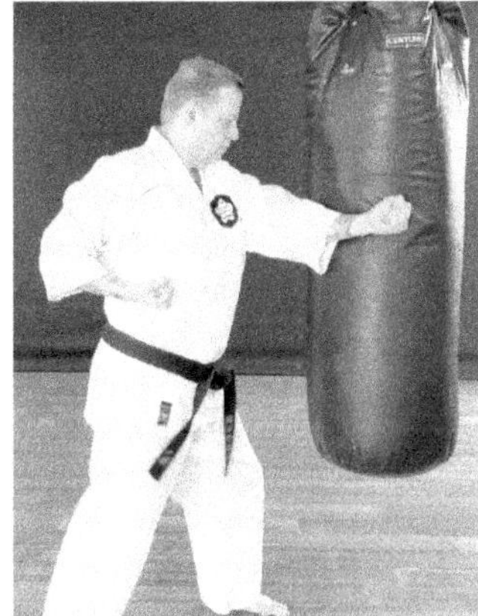

Chudan Zuki (Top) & Uchi Uke (Bottom)

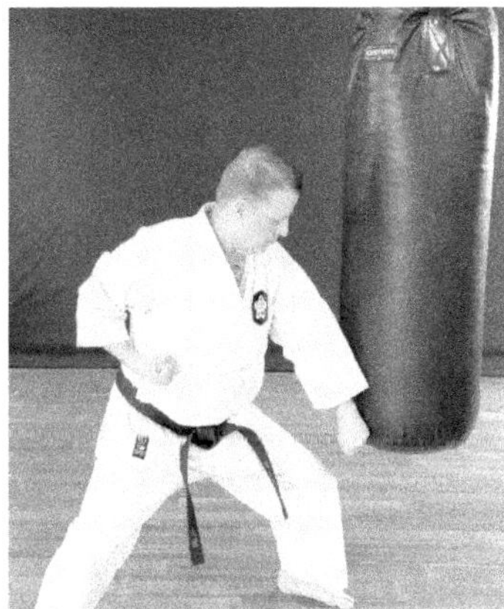

Gedan Zuki in Shiko Dachi (Top) & Gedan Barai (Bottom)

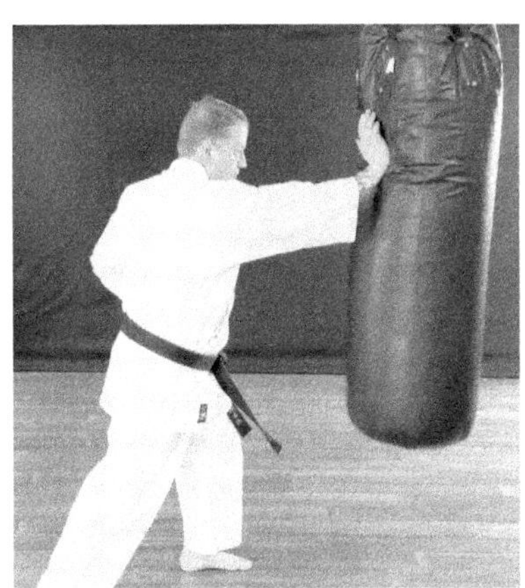

Counter 1: Jodan Shotei Uchi

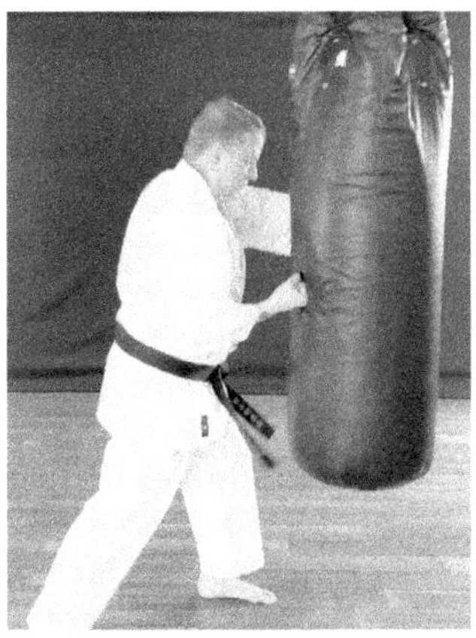

Counter 2: Ura Zuki

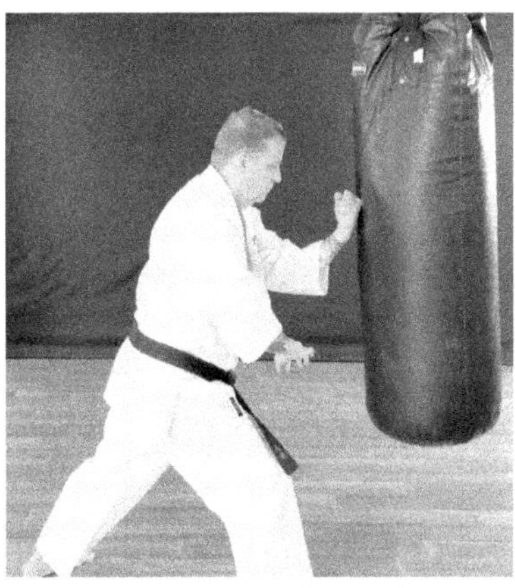

Counter 3: Uraken Uchi

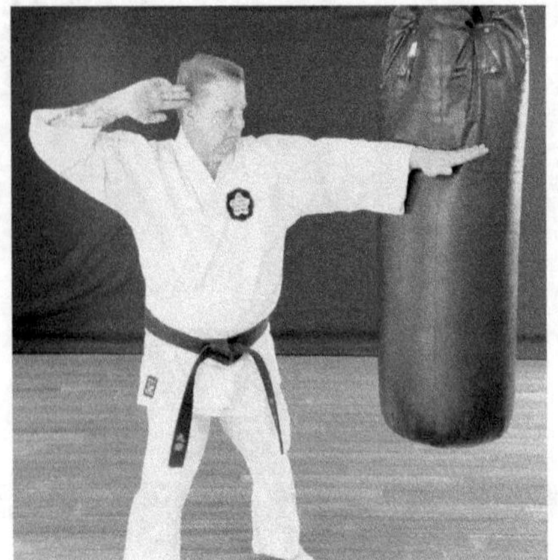
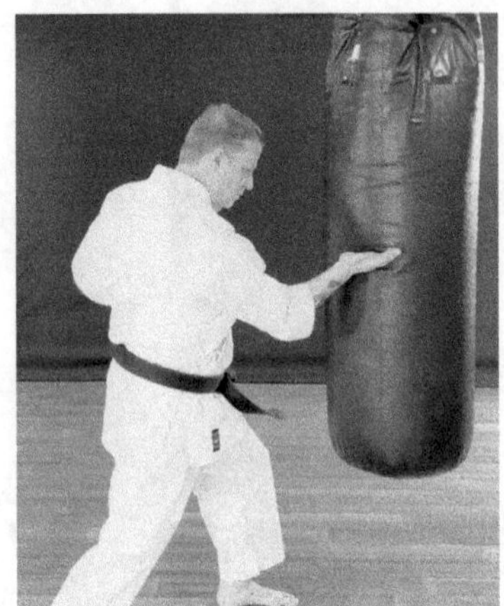

Counter 4: Yoko Shuto Uchi & Shuto Uchi

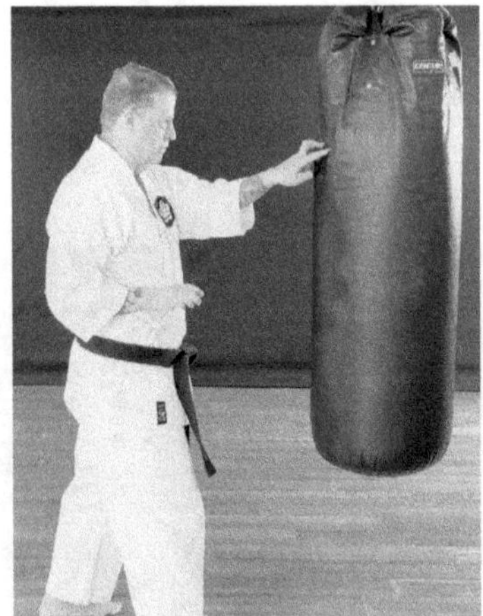

Counter 5: Nihon Nukite

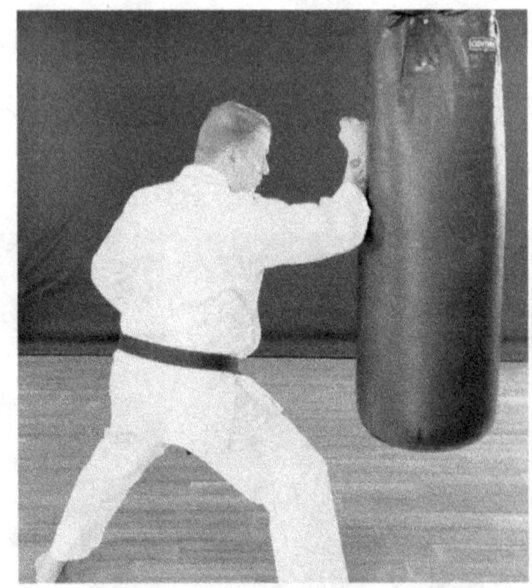

Counter 6: Tettsui Otoshi Uchi

Takedowns and Breakfalls

Takedowns are formally introduced at Kumite San, but there are other kiso kumite drills that contain takedowns, and officially, the first double lapel grab self-defense introduces the concept of doing a takedown and learning to breakfall. Starting at Kumite San, the student will learn the standing single leg takedown, the double handed breakfall, and a variation on the standing single leg takedown where a planted foot and a hard pivot is used to move the opponent.

Takedowns should be practiced carefully at first, but should always be a fully committed action. Stopping partway through a takedown can result in serious injury to one or both students and the instructor should pay close attention to students practicing takedowns.

The first takedown is a Judo move called **Osoto-gari**. Student A steps to the outside of the strike and grabs Student B at both shoulders, then while remaining outside, lifts the inside leg behind Student B, then brings the leg through the opponent's leg, calf to calf. At the same time, Student A should push the shoulders back hard. The takedown should not depend completely on the leg, nor should it completely rely on the shoulder push. Student A will hold onto the arm while Student B completes a side breakfall. Key safety point when training: don't stop halfway through the takedown, always follow through and commit fully.

For Osoto Gari, some people will train to go back of thigh to back of thigh and some go calf to calf. We train calf to calf, but this will largely be determined by the height of the participants. To practice osoto gari when sparring, it will typically work best in a clinch-type situation. For the defender, it's simple enough to just step out of a single leg takedown attempt, so speed is key.

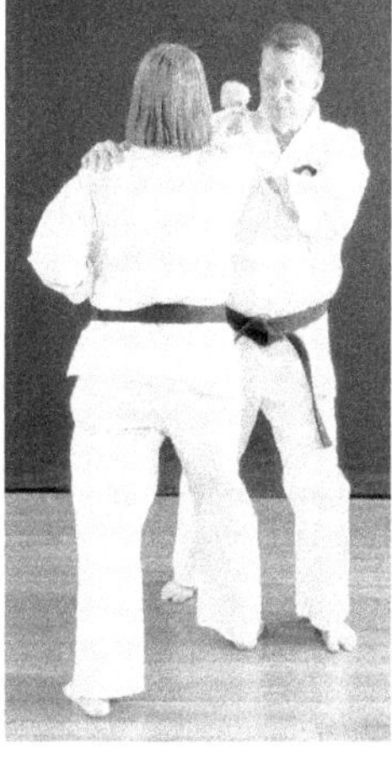

Step to the Side
Grabbing Shoulders

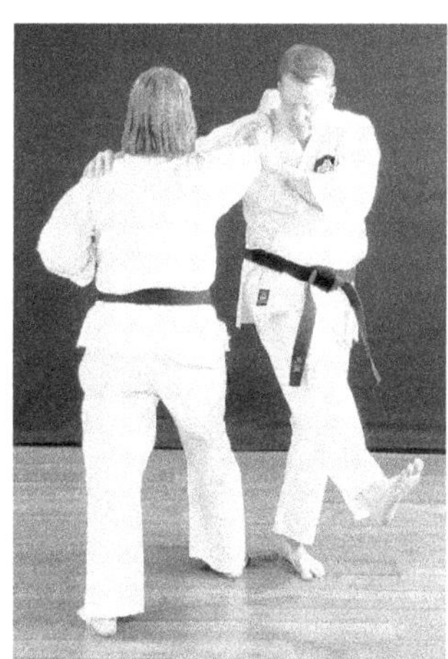

Lift Inside Leg

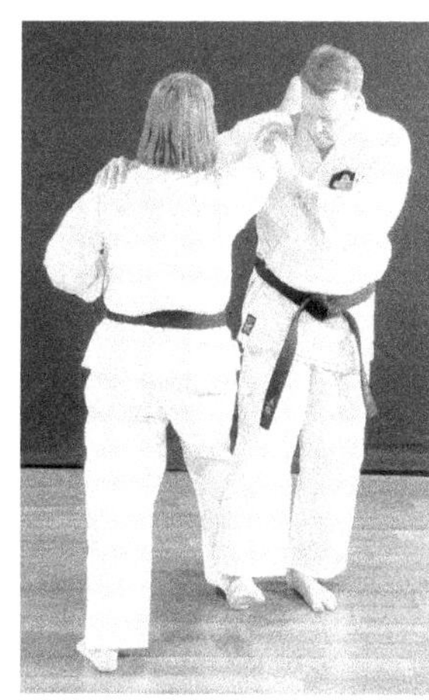

Follow Through
With Leg, Calf to Calf

The 3rd counter is a wrist lock takedown. After the block, the defender reaches around with both hands, thumbs on the back of the opponent's hand. The defender will push down with the thumbs and use the rest of the hand for support, then bringing Student B's hand to Student A's chest for leverage, with elbow on elbow, it's a matter of using the body weight to engineer the takedown. This can be done with one hand as well, but start by getting the technique down with two hands.

To practice the wrist lock takedown when sparring, the fighter should be wearing gloves with enough room in the fingers to manipulate the opponent's hand and wrist.

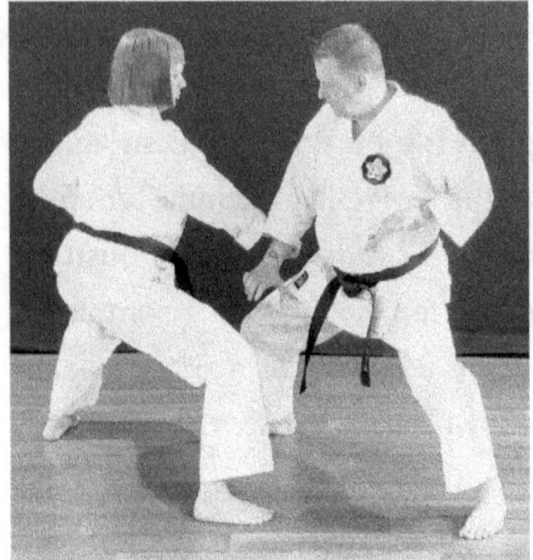

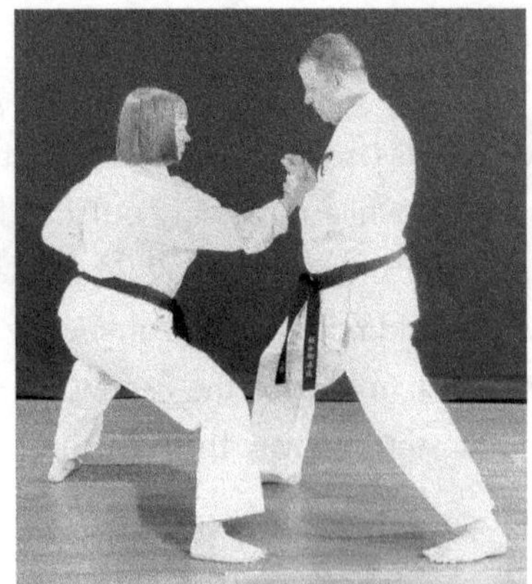

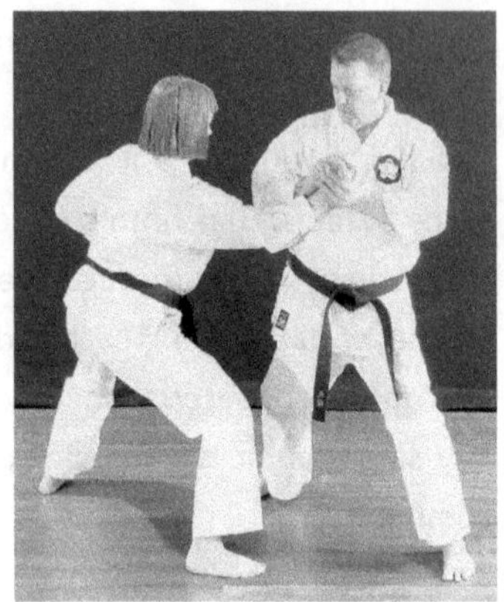

The 6th counter is a variation of **Osoto-gari**. The defender steps around the opponent, locking the back of the knee to the back of the opponent's knee with foot planted on the ground. The defender pivots hard to the outside, using the hip and leg to throw the opponent. When practicing this variation, quick commitment is extremely important so the defender doesn't collapse into the defender's knee.

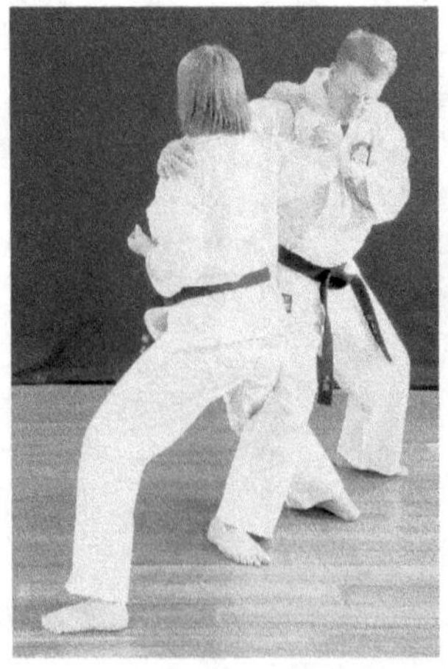

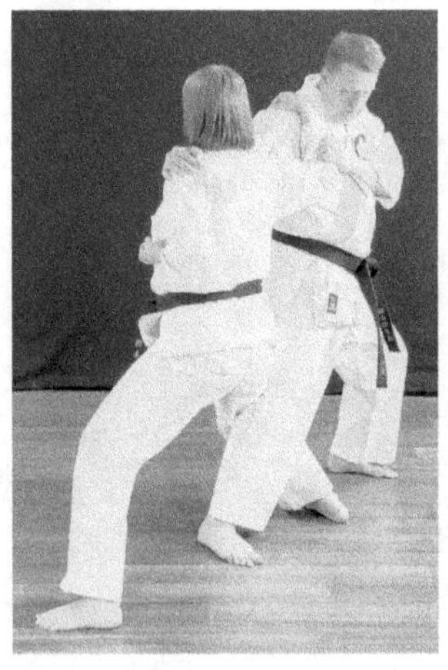

9. Kumite San (3)

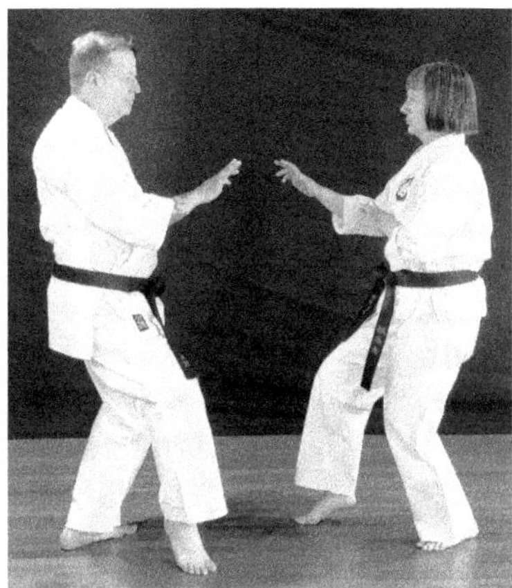

Neko Ashi Dachi Kamae Chamber Hand at Chest, Palm Down

Begin Counter 1

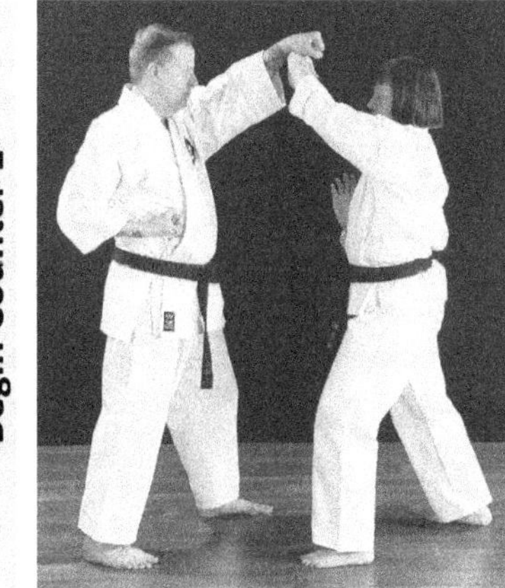

1. (Off - L): Step Forward, Jodan Zuki / (Def - R): Step Back, Jodan Age Ko Uke

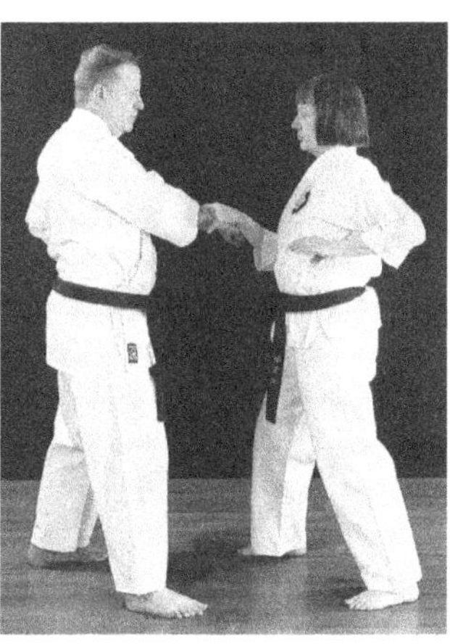

2. (Off - L): Step Forward, Chudan Zuki / (Def - R): Step Back, Chudan Hari to Hiki Uke

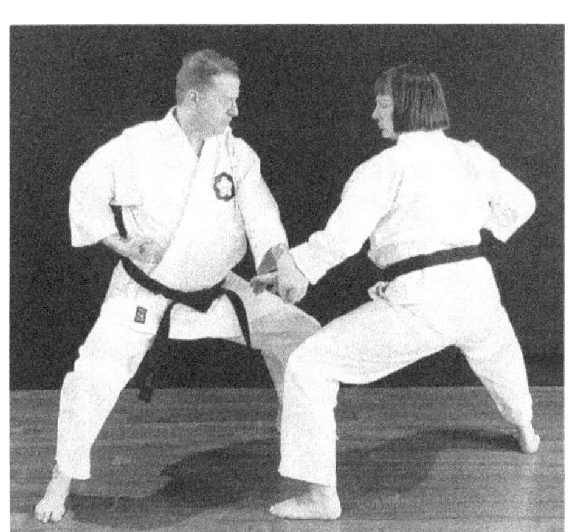

3. (Off - L): Step Forward, Gedan Zuki in Shiko Dachi / (Def - R): Step Back, Gedan Shotei Barai in Shiko Dachi

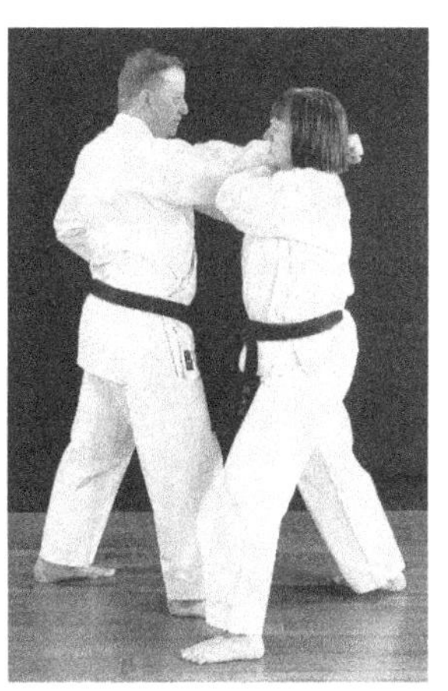

4. (Off - L): Step Forward, Jodan Zuki / (Def - R): Step to Side, Osoto-gari

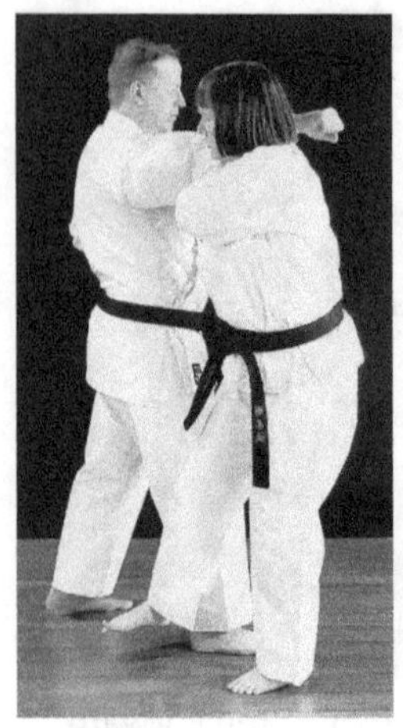

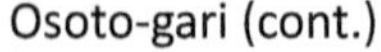

Osoto-gari (cont.)

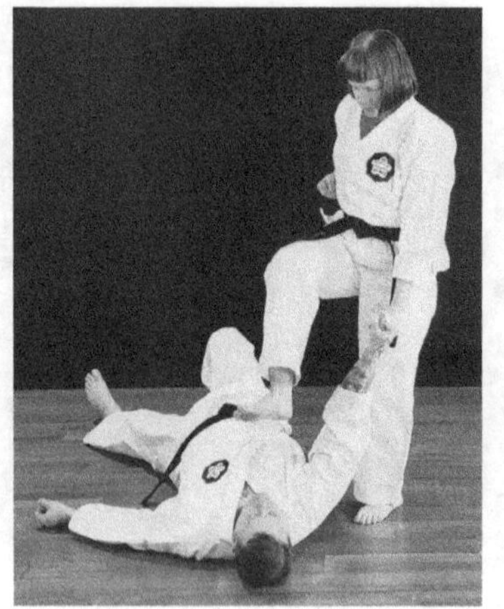

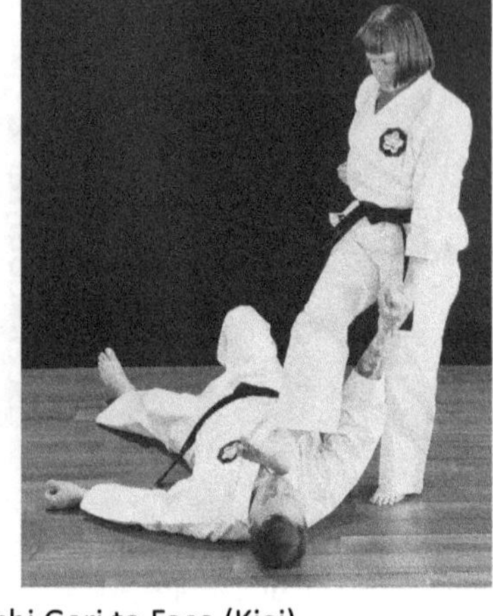

5. (Def - R): Kakato Otoshi Geri to Face (Kiai)

Repeat in Other Direction

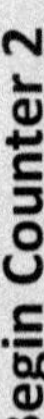

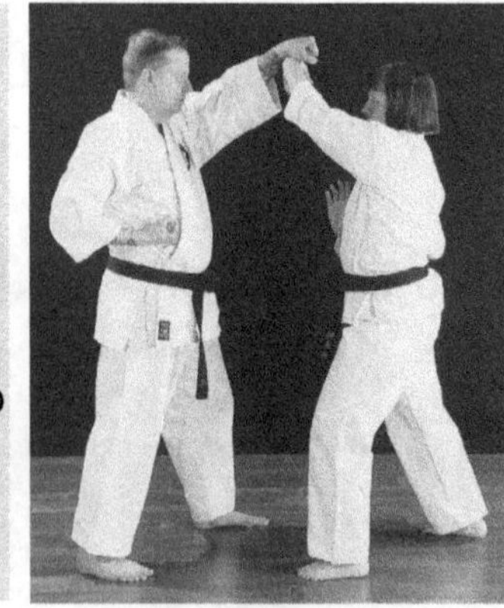

1. (Off - L): Step Forward, Jodan Zuki / (Def - R): Step Back, Jodan Age Ko Uke

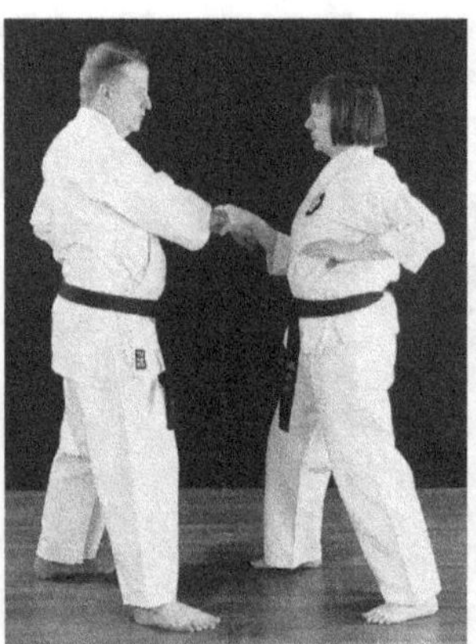

2. (Off - L): Step Forward, Chudan Zuki / (Def - R): Step Back, Chudan Hari to Hiki Uke

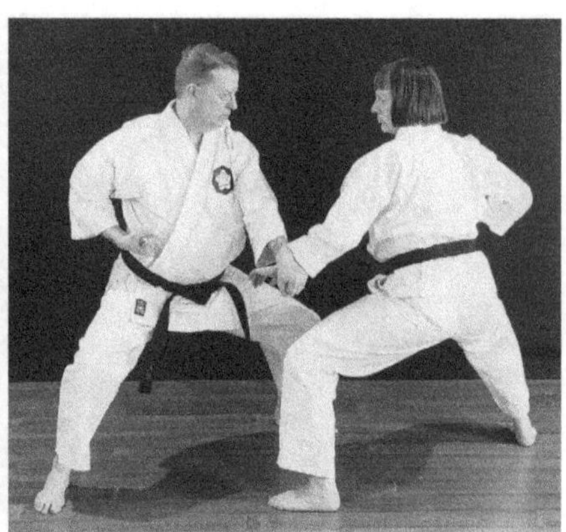

3. (Off - L): Step Forward, Gedan Zuki in Shiko Dachi / (Def - R): Step Back, Gedan Shotei Barai in Shiko Dachi

4. (Off - L): Step Forward, Chudan Zuki / (Def - R): Step Back, Chudan Hari to Hiki Uke

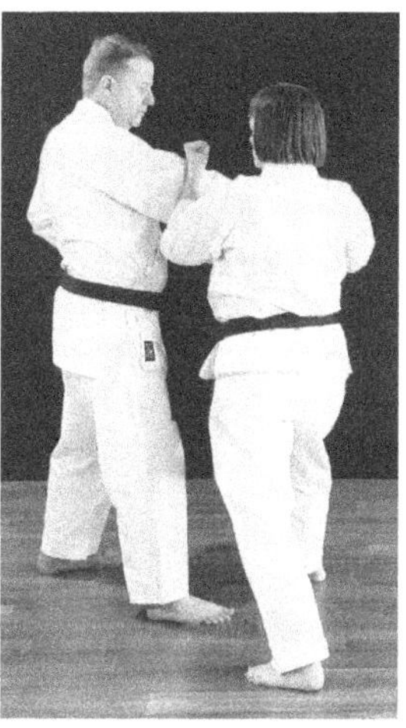

5. (Def - R): Grab Arm, Step Around to Side, Kote Uchi on Opponent's Arm, just above the elbow

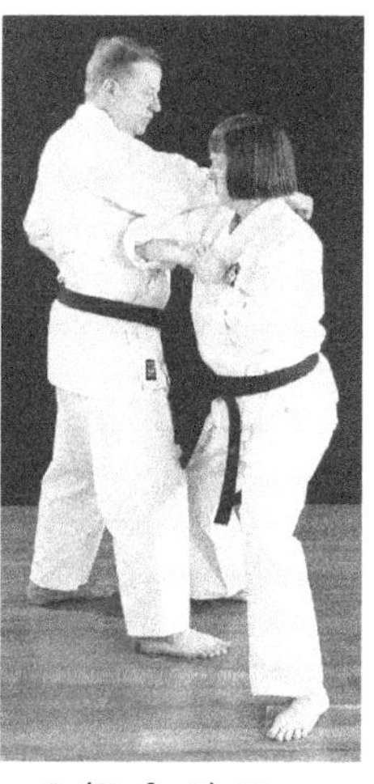

6. (Def - R): Step Inside, Yoko Empi Uchi to Opponent's Ribs

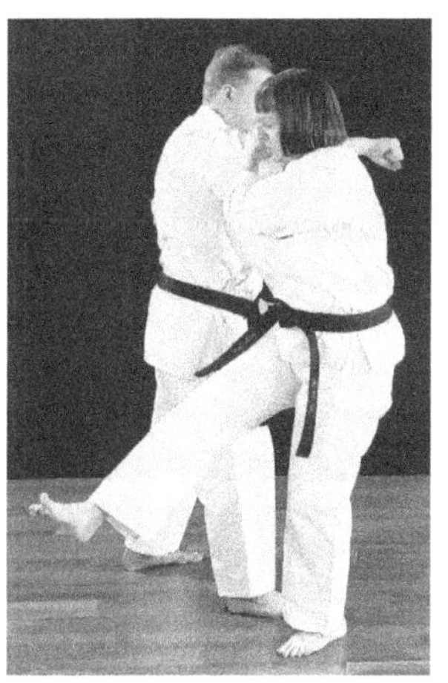

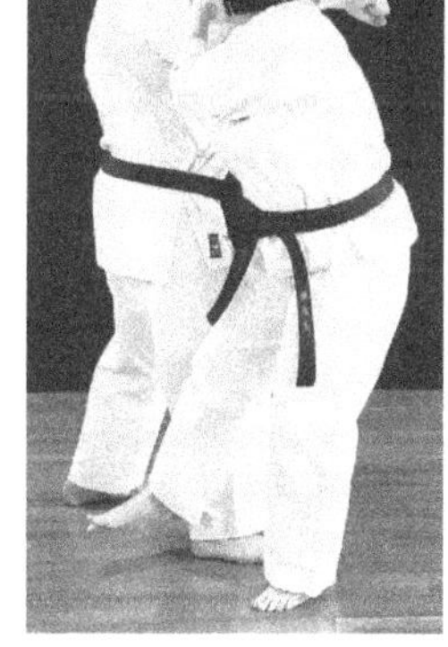

7. (Def - R): Quickly Reposition by Grabbing the Opponent's Inside or Outside Shoulder (Depending on Student's Reach), Osoto-gari

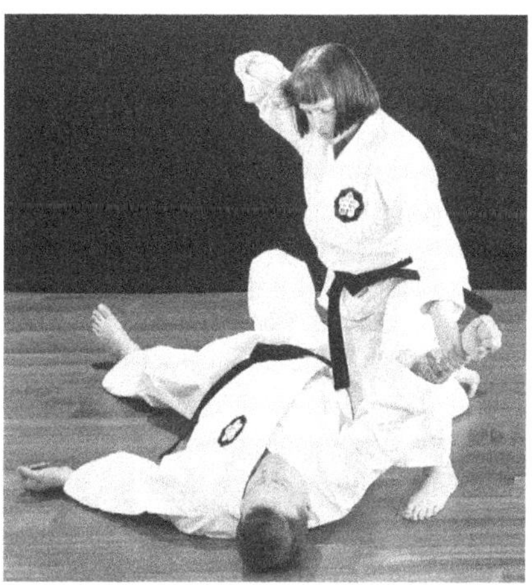

Repeat in Other Direction

8. (Def - R): Holding Opponent's Arm During Takedown, Follow Opponent Down, Jodan or Chudan Tettsui Otoshi Uchi (Kiai)

Begin Counter 3

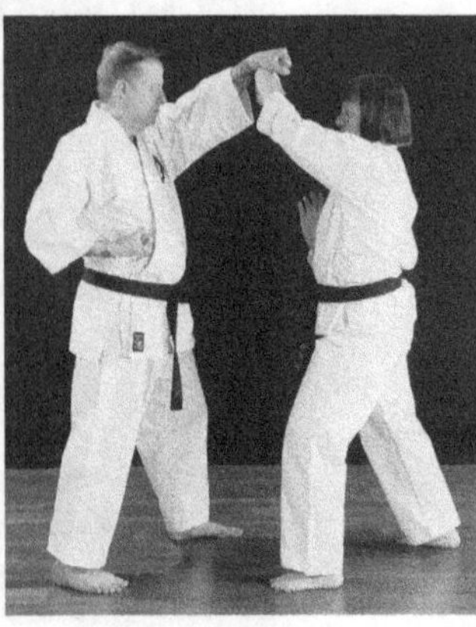

1. (Off - L): Step Forward, Jodan Zuki / (Def - R): Step Back, Jodan Age Ko Uke

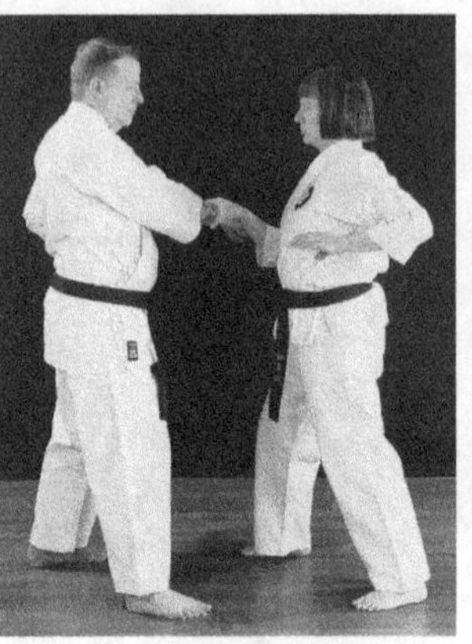

2. (Off - L): Step Forward, Chudan Zuki / (Def - R): Step Back, Chudan Hari to Hiki Uke

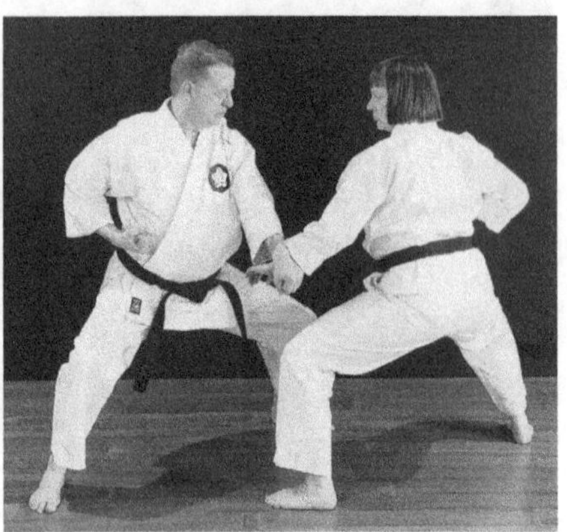

3. (Off - L): Step Forward, Gedan Zuki in Shiko Dachi / (Def - R): Step Back, Gedan Shotei Barai in Shiko Dachi

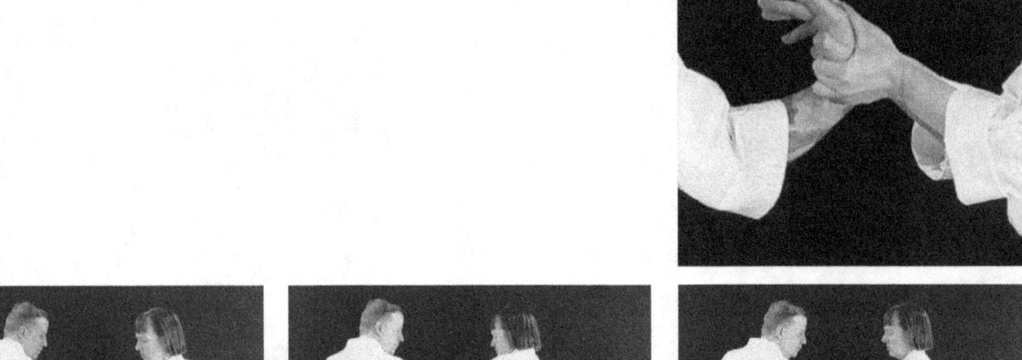

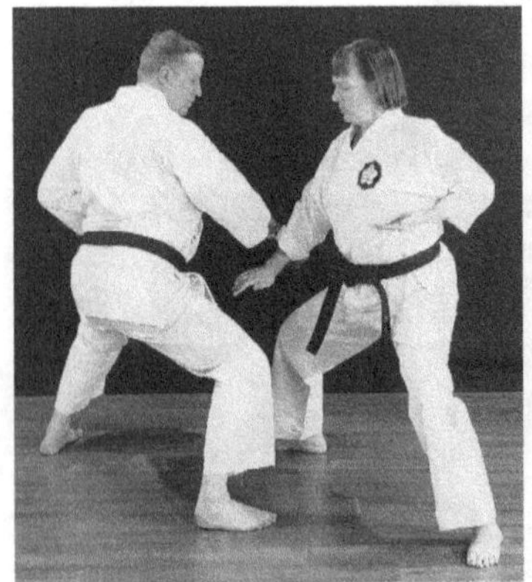

4. (Off - L): Step Forward, Gedan Zuki in Shiko Dachi / (Def - R): Step Back, Gedan Shotei Barai in Shiko Dachi

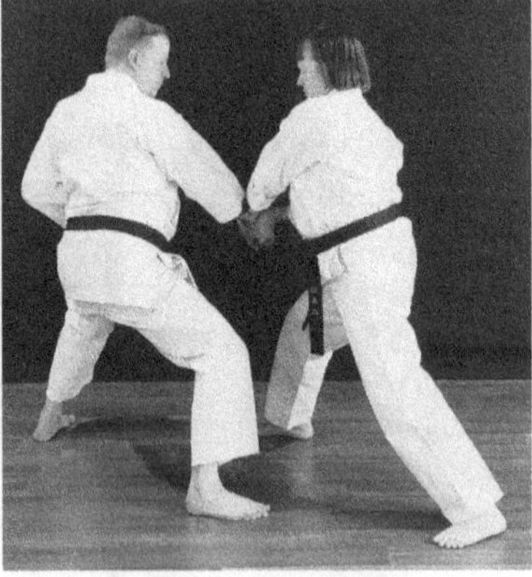

5. (Def - R): Pivot Right, Grab Opponents Wrist and Hand with Both Hands

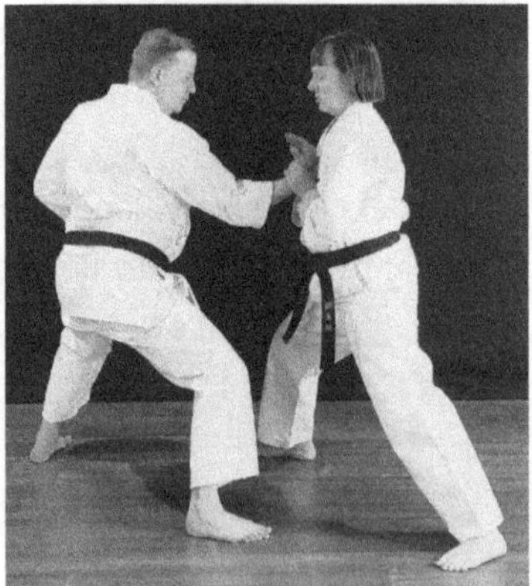

6. (Def - R): Use Thumbs to Push Opponent's Hand Down for Wrist Lock

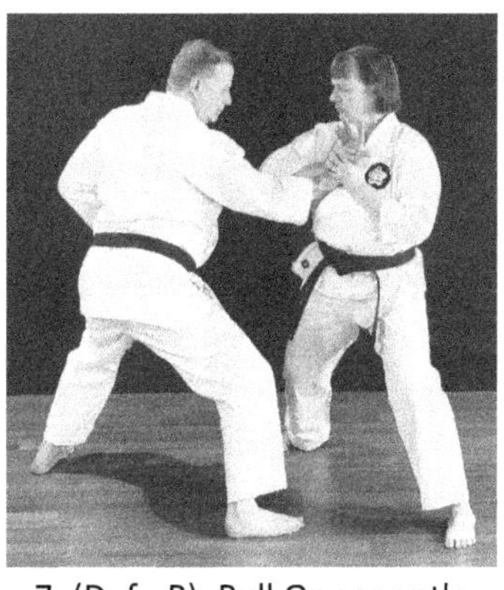

7. (Def - R): Pull Opponent's Wrist to Chest

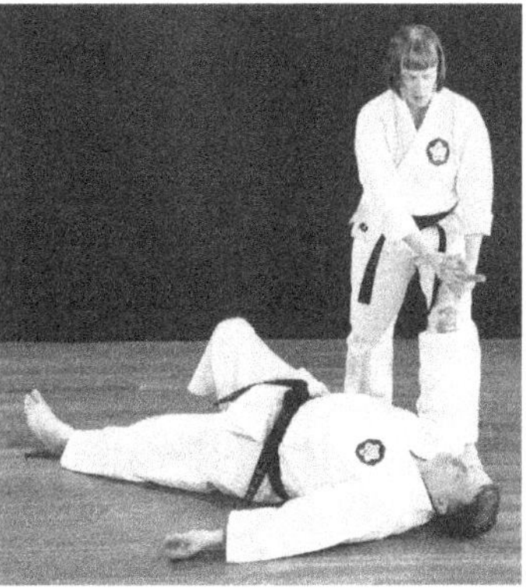

8. (Def - R): Pivot Left with Elbow on Opponent's Arm for Takedown

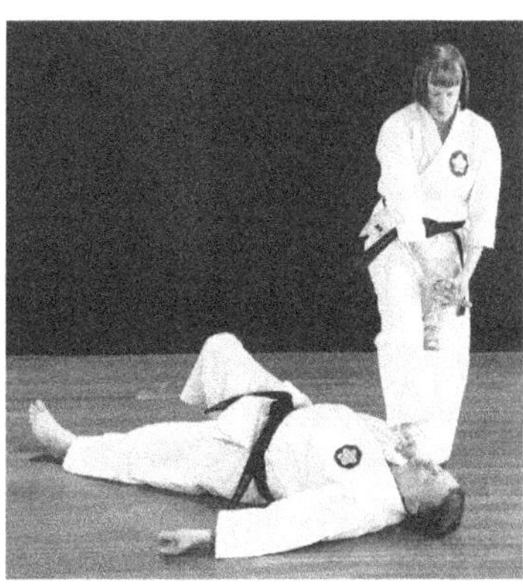

9. (Def - R): Kakato Otoshi Geri to Face (Kiai)

Repeat in Other Direction

Begin Counter 4

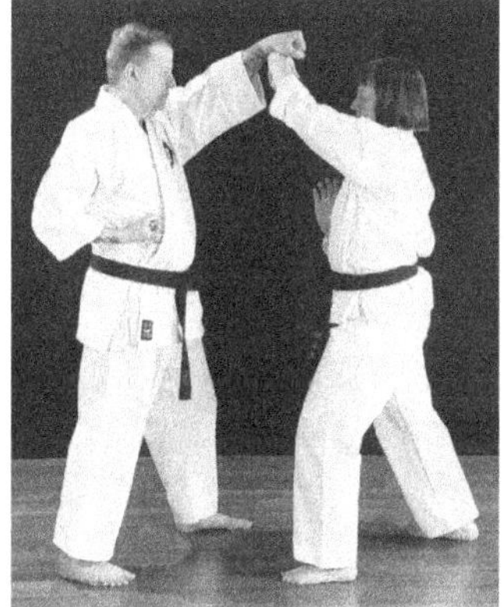

1. (Off - L): Step Forward, Jodan Zuki / (Def - R): Step Back, Jodan Age Ko Uke

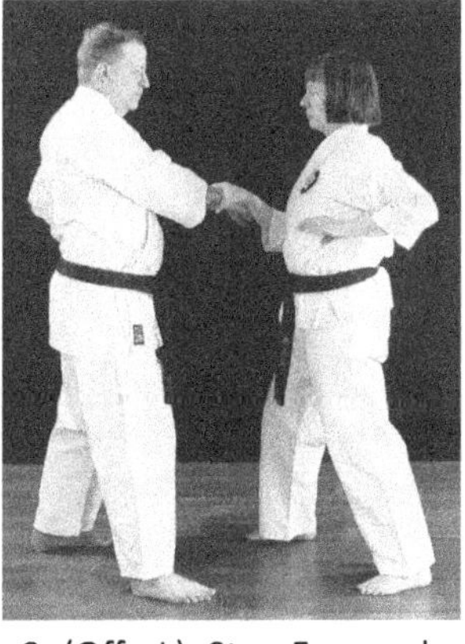

2. (Off - L): Step Forward, Chudan Zuki / (Def - R): Step Back, Chudan Hari to Hiki Uke

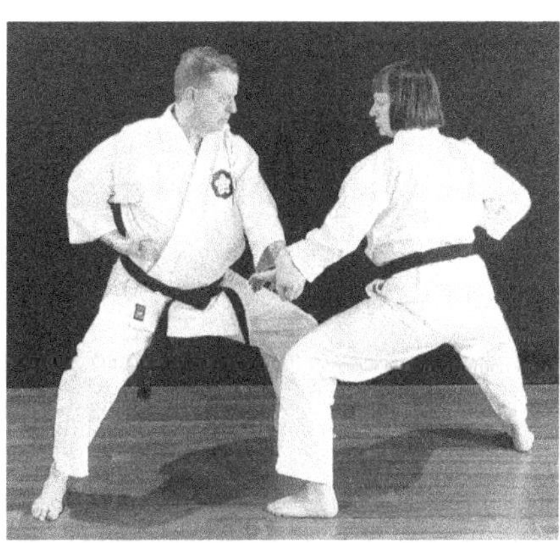

3. (Off - L): Step Forward, Gedan Zuki in Shiko Dachi / (Def - R): Step Back, Gedan Shotei Barai in Shiko Dachi

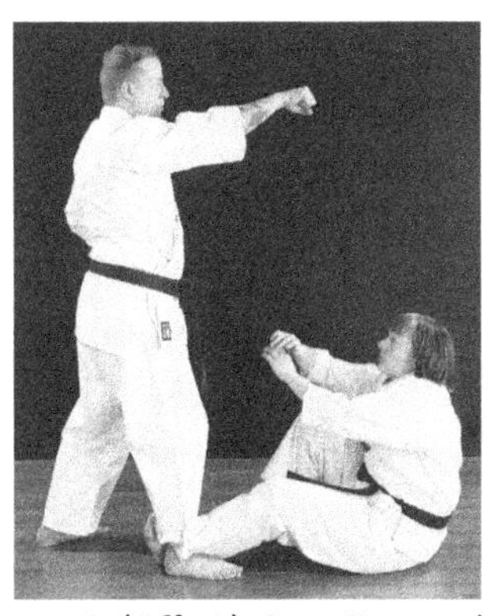

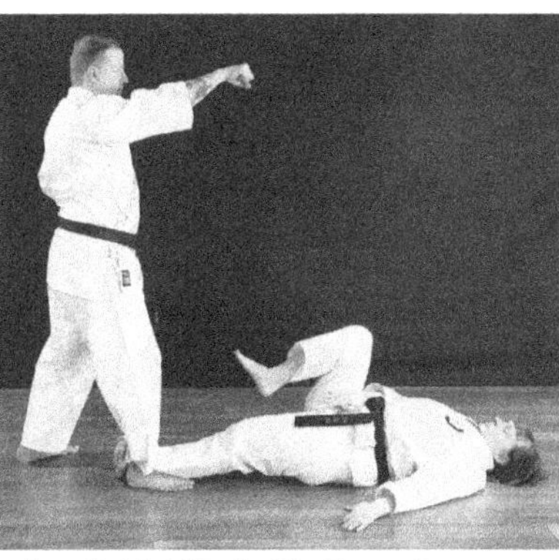

4. (Off - L): Step Forward, Jodan Zuki / (Def - R): Drop Down (Ushiro Ukemi), Hooking Left Leg on Opponent's Front Leg

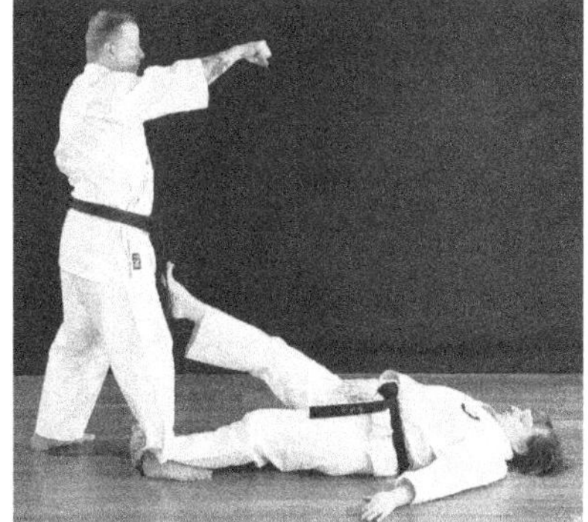

5. (Def - R): Mae Geri

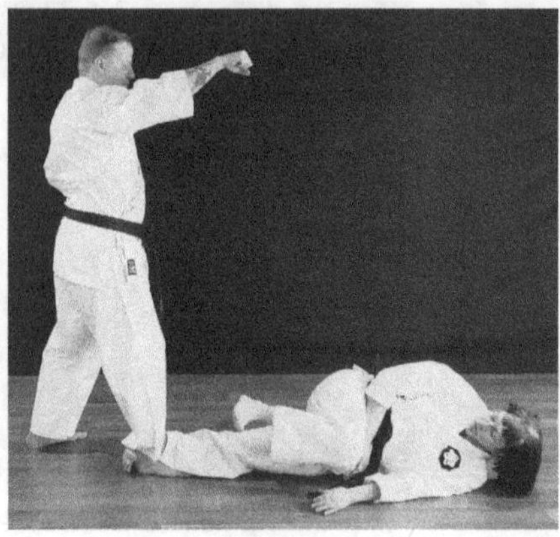

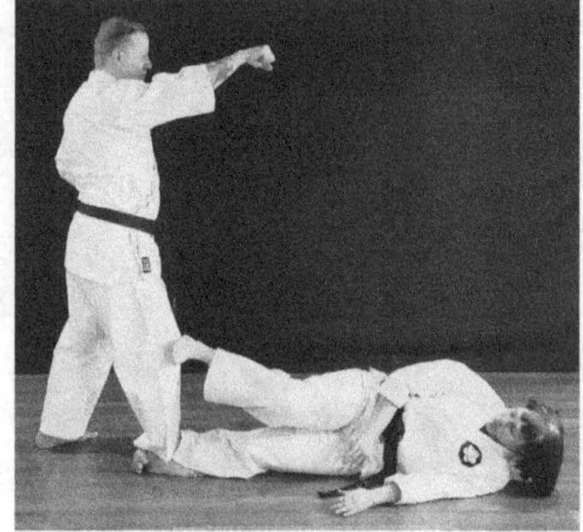

Repeat in Other Direction

6. (Def - R): Pivot on Left Hip, Yoko Geri to Knee (Kiai)

Begin Counter 5

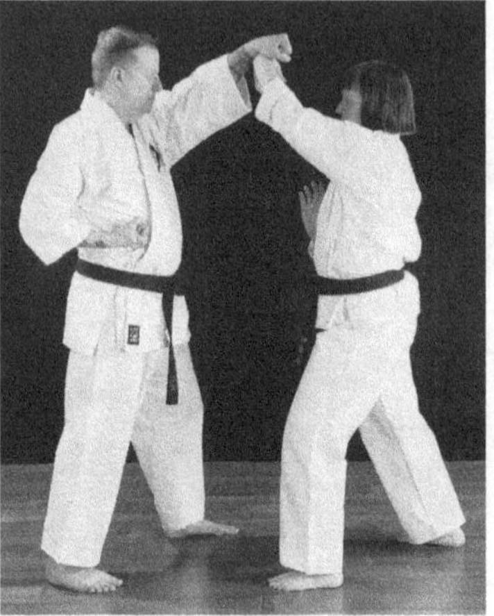

1. (Off - L): Step Forward, Jodan Zuki / (Def - R): Step Back, Jodan Age Ko Uke

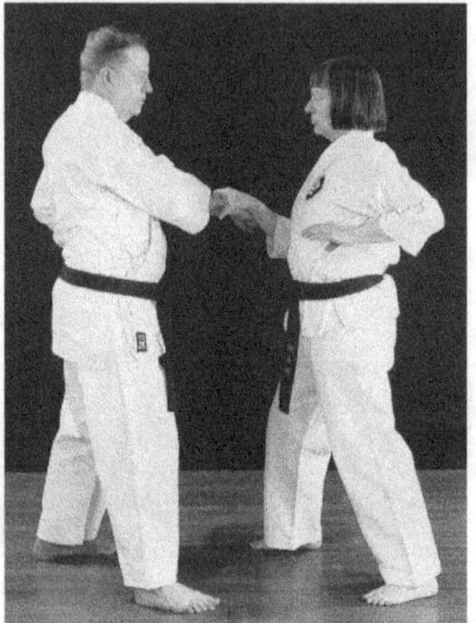

2. (Off - L): Step Forward, Chudan Zuki / (Def - R): Step Back, Chudan Hari to Hiki Uke

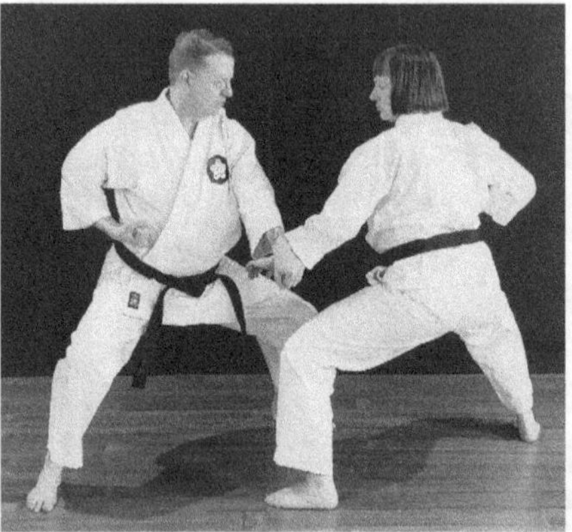

3. (Off - L): Step Forward, Gedan Zuki in Shiko Dachi / (Def - R): Step Back, Gedan Shotei Barai in Shiko Dachi

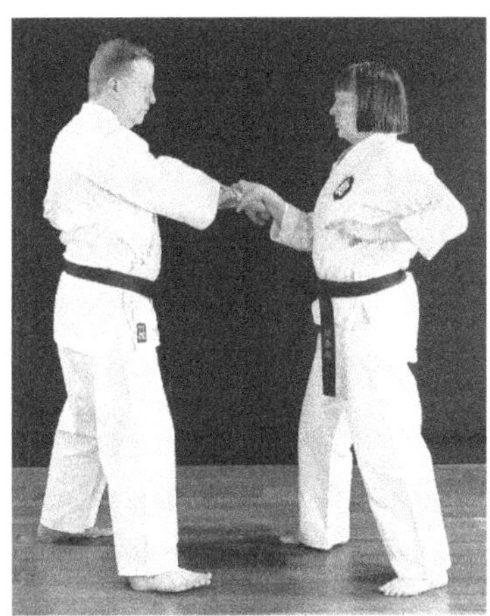

4. (Off - L): Step Forward, Chudan Zuki / (Def - R): Step Back, Chudan Hari to Hiki Uke

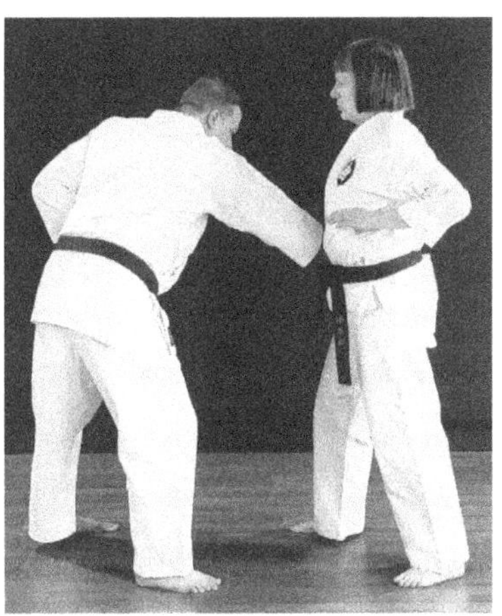

5. (Def - R): Grab Opponent's Arm, Pull Down to Right Side of Waist

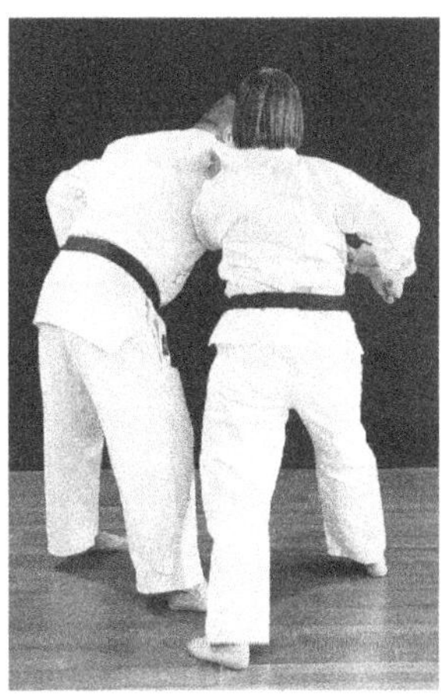

6. (Def - R) Pivot Right and Bring Left Forearm Under Base of Opponent's Arm

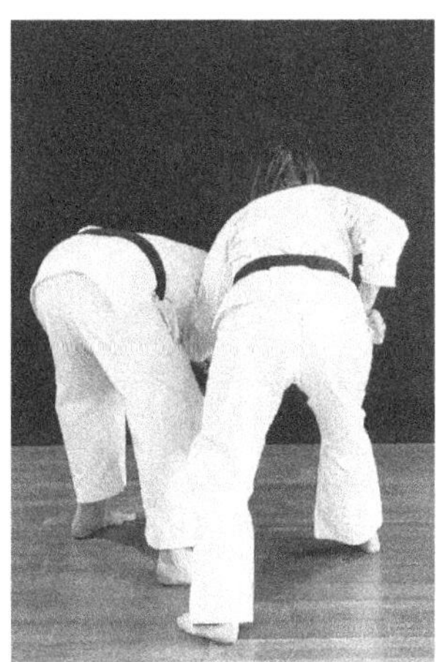

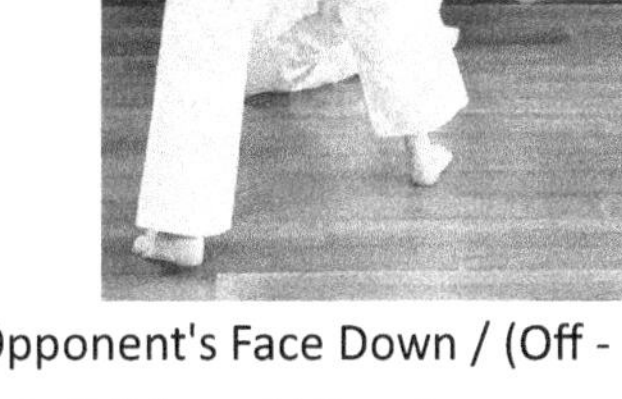

7. (Def - R): Attempt to Drive Opponent's Face Down / (Off - L): Defensive Shoulder Roll (Mawari Ukemi)

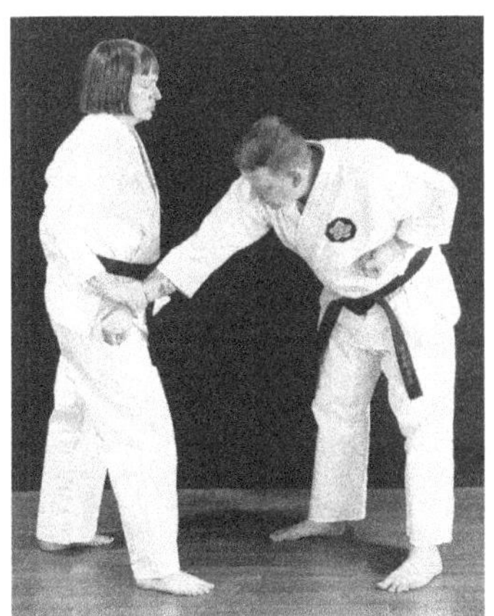

Forward POV of Step 5

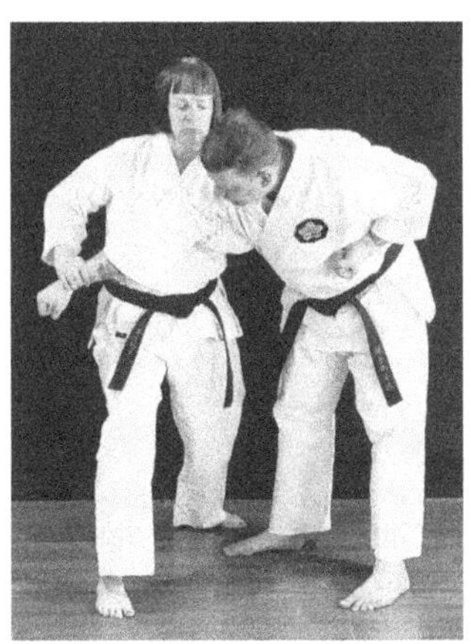

Forward POV of Step 6

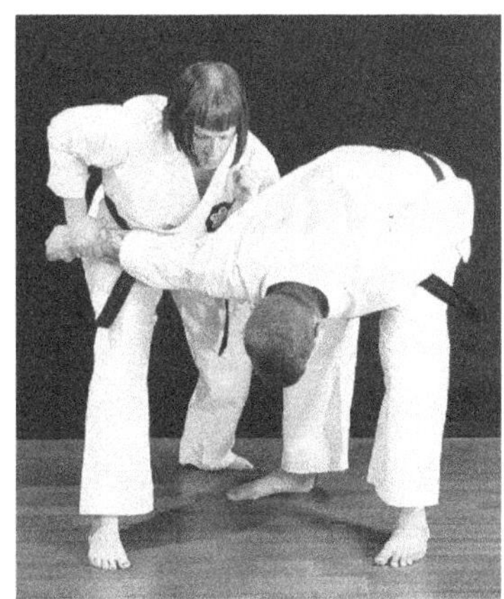

Forward POV of Step 7

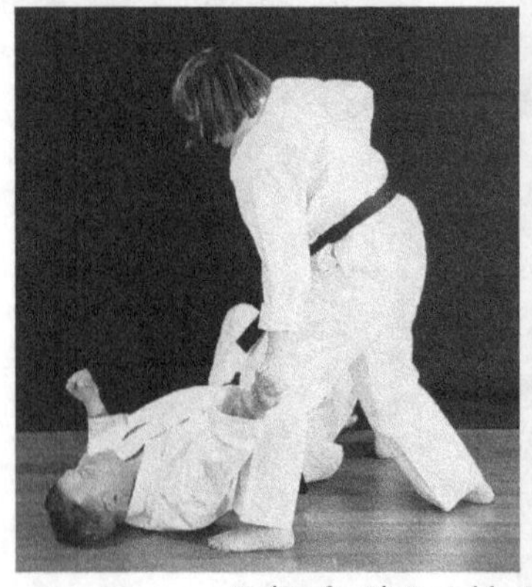
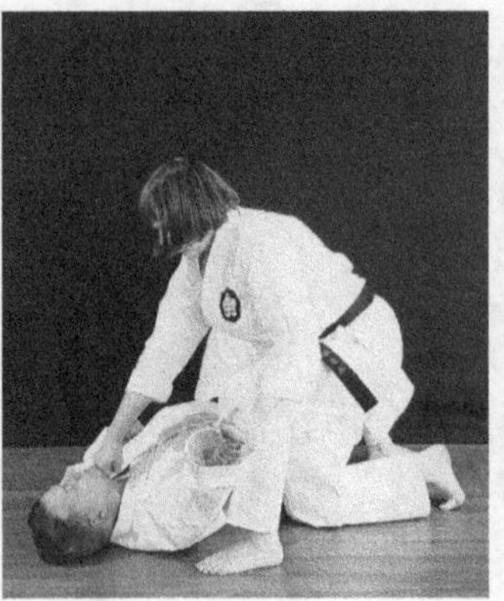
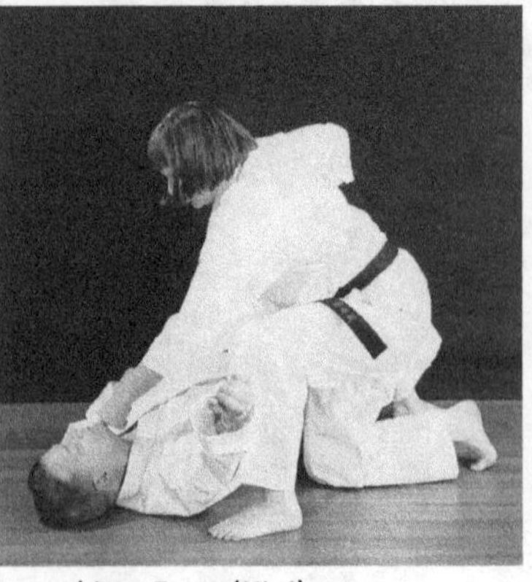

Repeat in Other Direction

8. (Def - R) Quickly Follow Opponent to Ground, Nidan-zuki to Face (Kiai)

Begin Counter 6

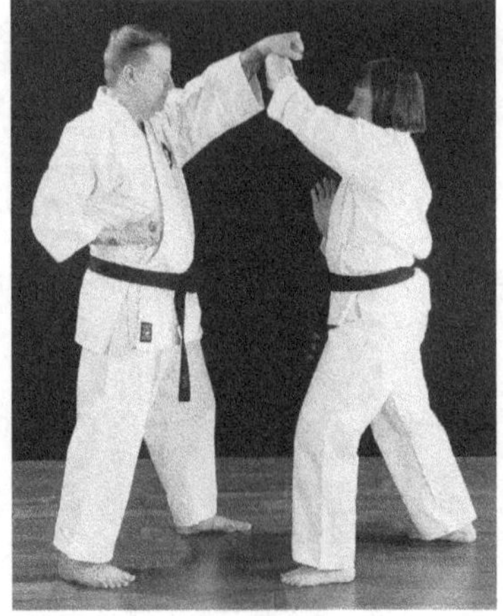

1. (Off - L): Step Forward, Jodan Zuki / (Def - R): Step Back, Jodan Age Ko Uke

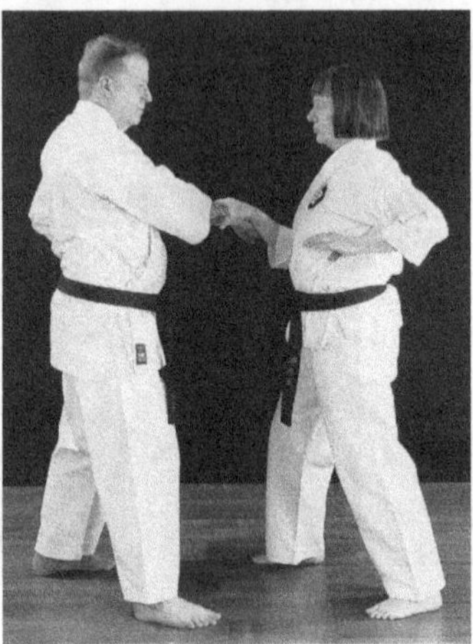

2. (Off - L): Step Forward, Chudan Zuki / (Def - R): Step Back, Chudan Hari to Hiki Uke

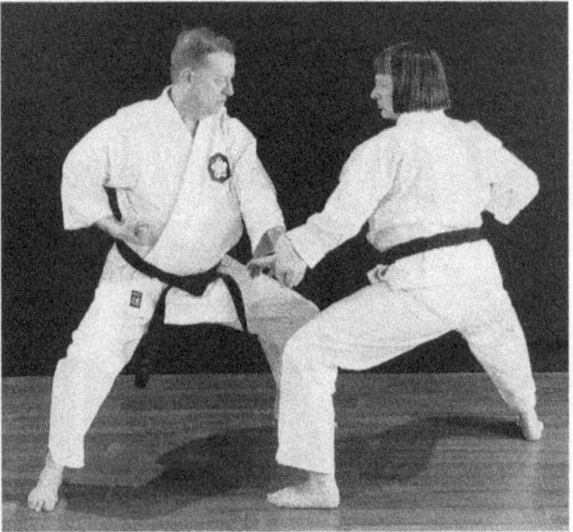

3. (Off - L): Step Forward, Gedan Zuki in Shiko Dachi / (Def - R): Step Back, Gedan Shotei Barai in Shiko Dachi

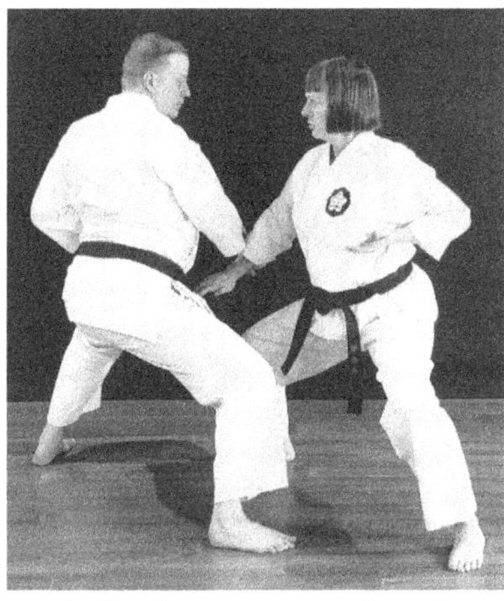

4. (Off - L): Step Forward, Gedan Zuki in Shiko Dachi / (Def - R): Step Back, Gedan Shotei Barai in Shiko Dachi

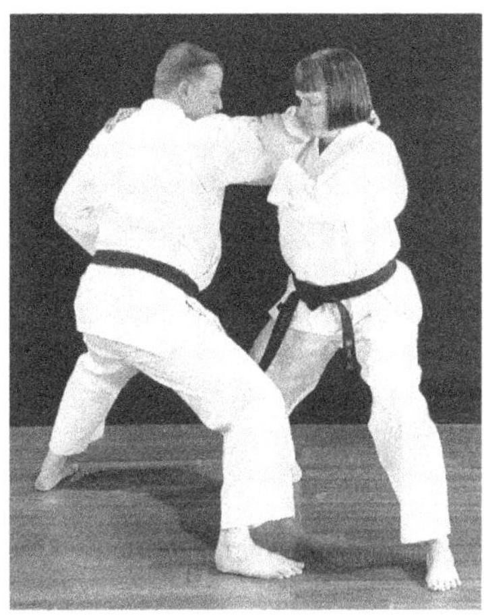

5. (Def - R) Continuing Block, Bring Right Arm Around to Opponent's Shoulder (One Fluid Movement)

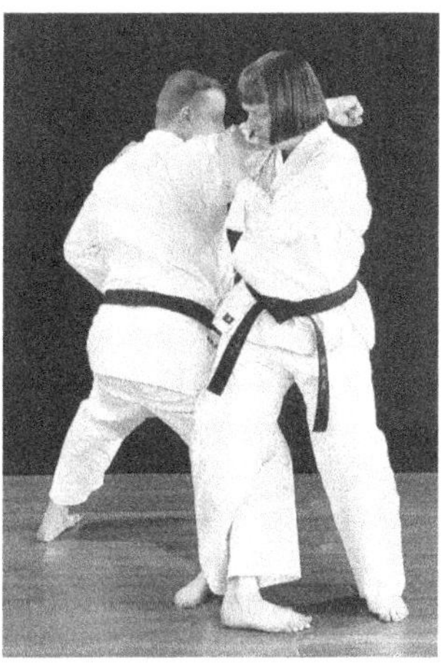

6. (Def - R): Hook Lead Leg Around Opponent's Leg (Back of Knee to Back of Knee)

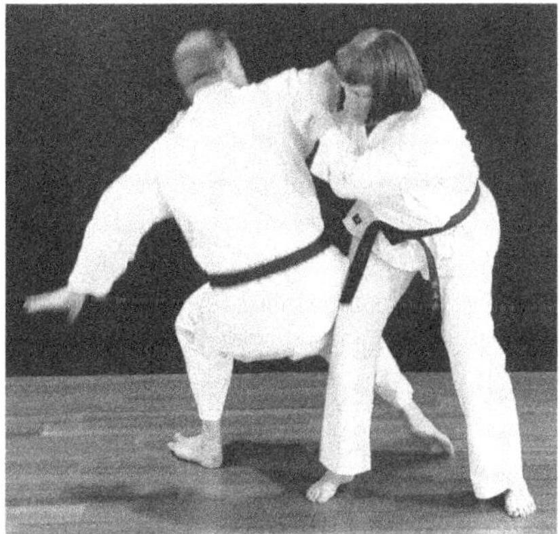

7. (Def - R) Pivot Hard Left While Pushing Opponent’s Shoulders, Throwing Opponent (Osoto-gari variation)

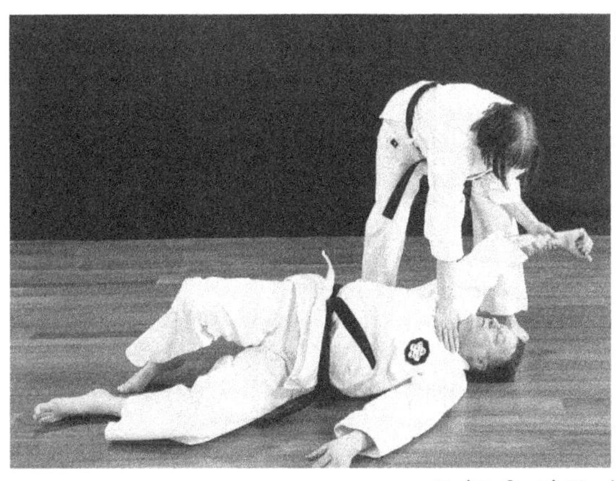

8. (Def - R) Nodo Kaki (Kiai)

Repeat in Other Direction

Kumite San - Bag Work

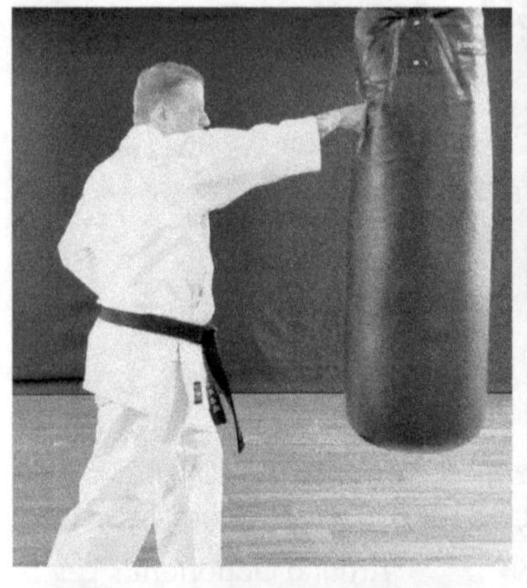

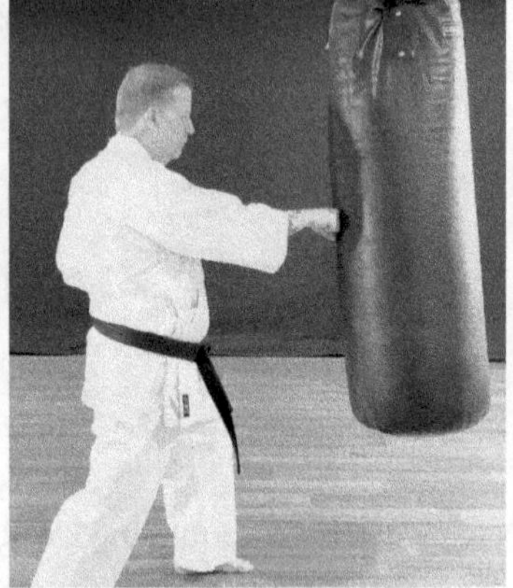

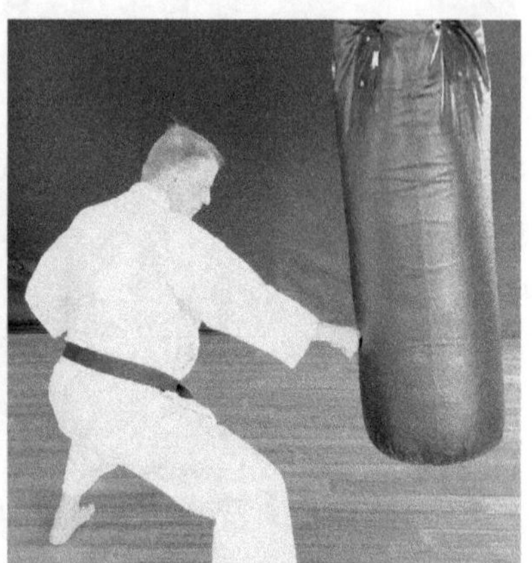

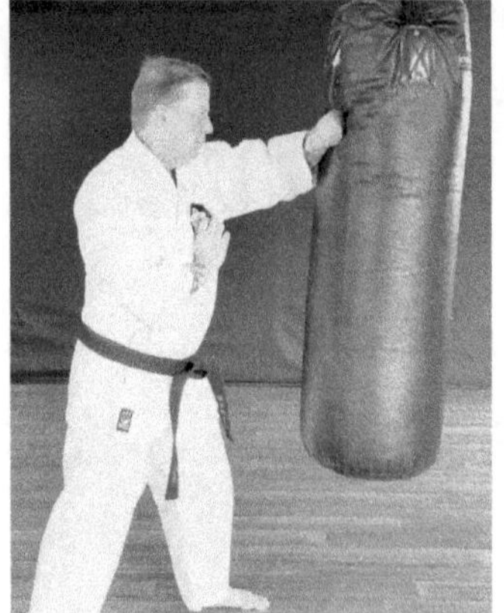

Jodan Zuki (Top) & Jodan Age Ko Uke (Bottom)

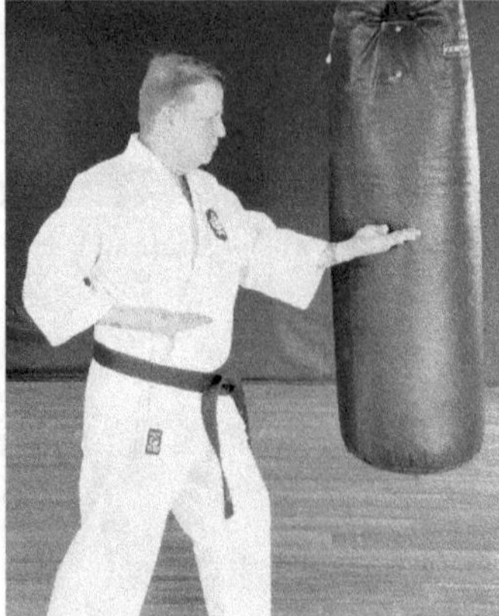

Chudan Zuki (Top) & Chudan Hari Uke (Bottom)

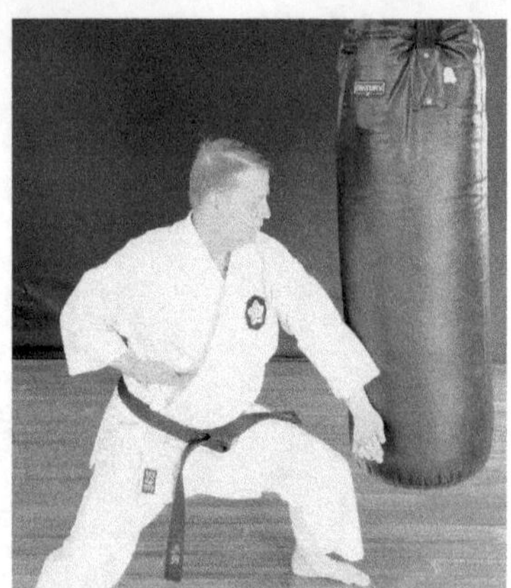

Gedan Zuki (Top) & Gedan Shotei Barai (Bottom)

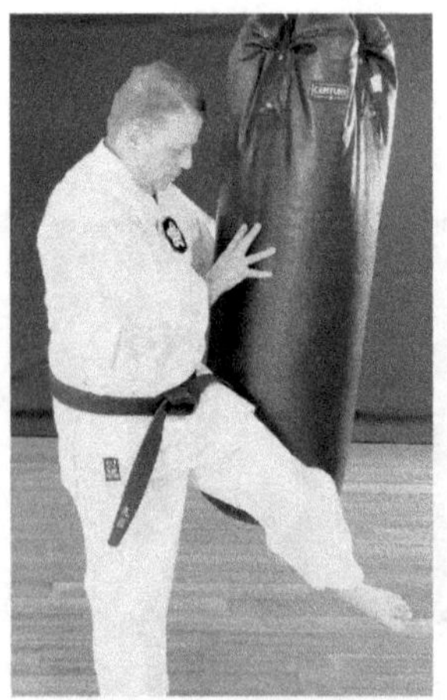

Counter 1: Osoto-gari (Calf to Calf)

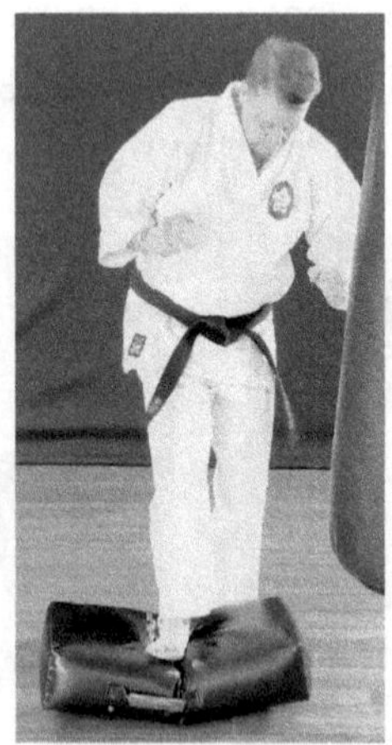

Counter 1: Kakato Otoshi Geri on Focus Pad

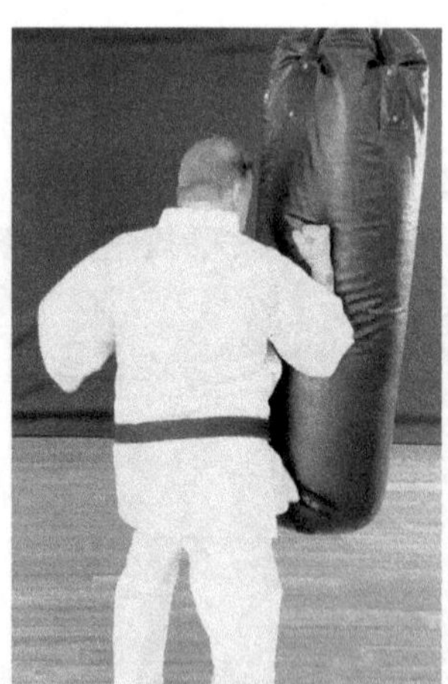

Counter 2: Kote Uchi

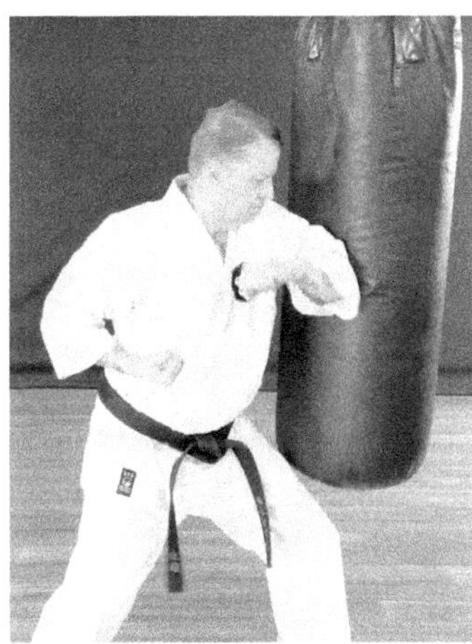

Counter 2: Yoko Empi Uchi

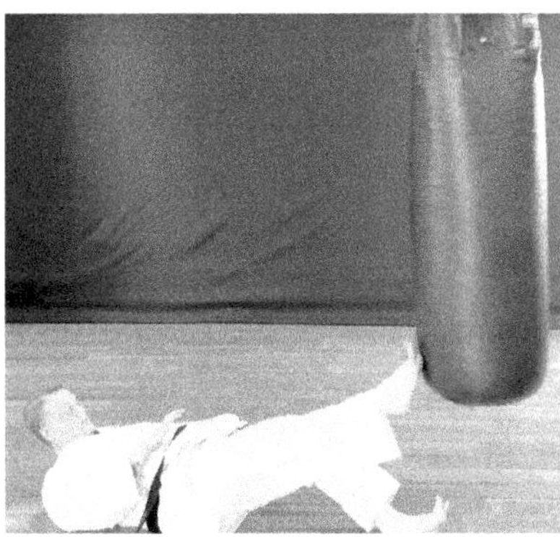

Counter 4: From Prone Position, Mae Geri

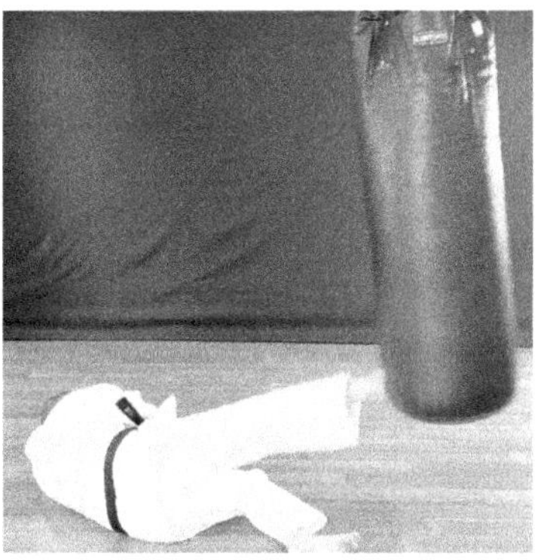

Counter 4: From Prone Position, Yoko Geri

10. Kumite Shi (4)

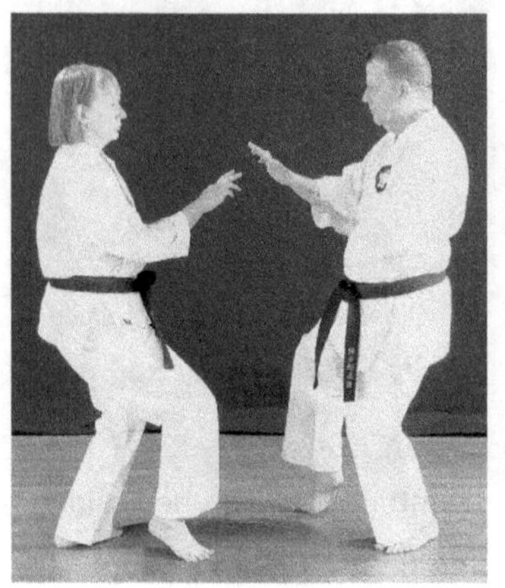

Neko Ashi Dachi Kamae Chamber Hand at Chest, Palm Down

Begin Counter 1

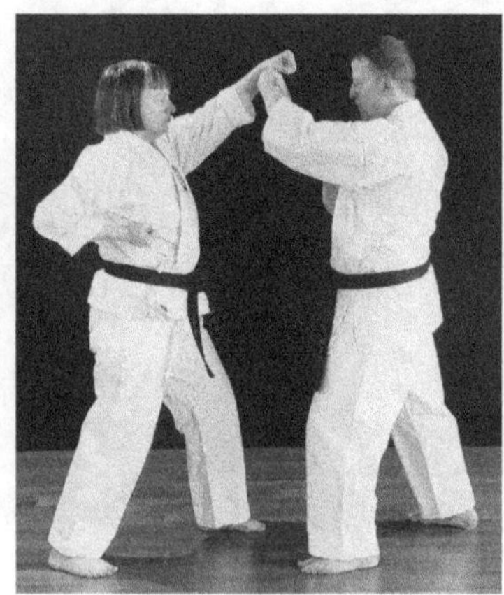

1. (Off - L): Step Forward, Jodan Zuki / (Def - R): Step Back, Jodan Age Ko Uke

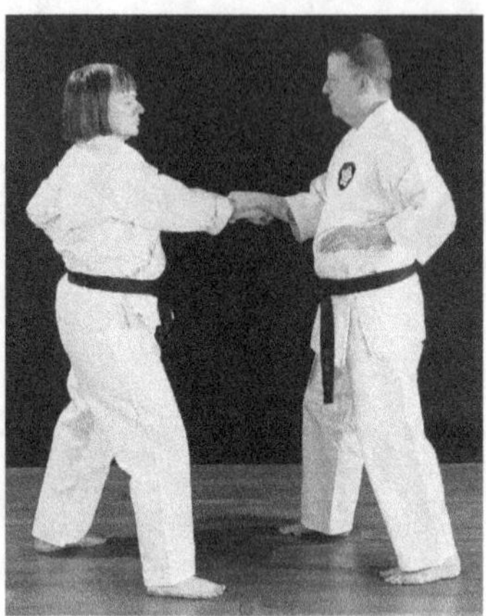

2. (Off - L): Step Forward, Chudan Zuki / (Def - R): Step Back, Chudan Hari to Hiki Uke

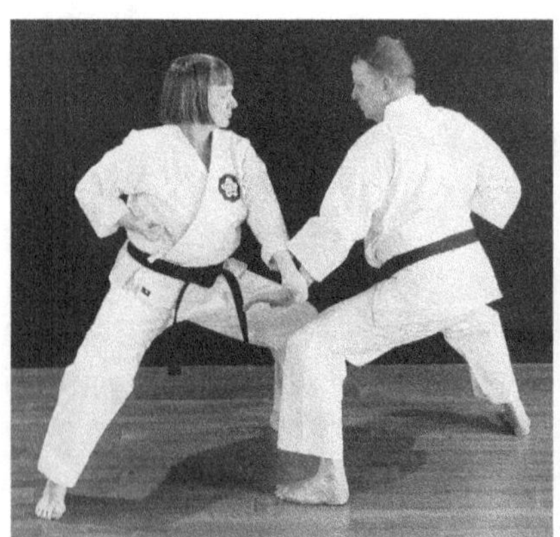

3. (Off - L): Step Forward, Gedan Zuki in Shiko Dachi / (Def - R): Step Back, Gedan Shotei Barai in Shiko Dachi

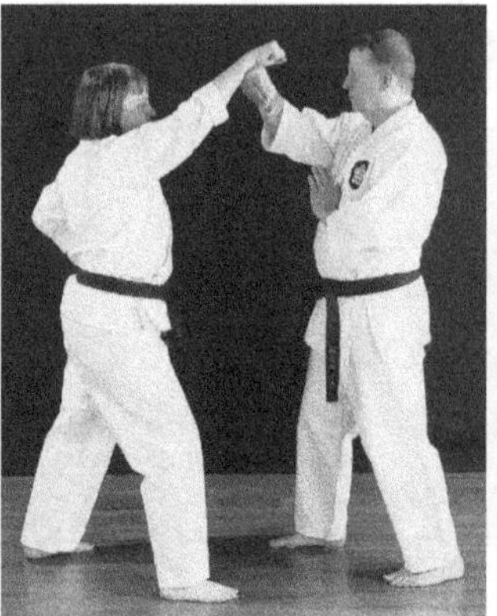

4. (Off - L): Step Forward, Jodan Zuki / (Def - R): Step Back, Jodan Age Ko Uke, Grab Wrist, Jodan Mae Geri

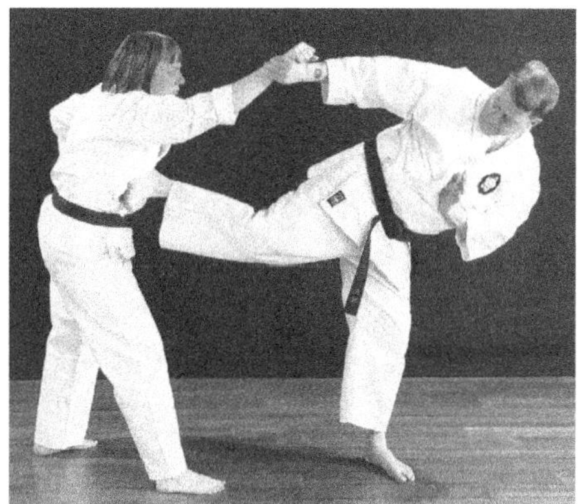

Repeat in Other Direction

5. (Def - R): Pivot Left, Chudan Yoko Geri (Kiai)

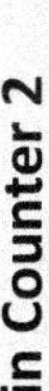

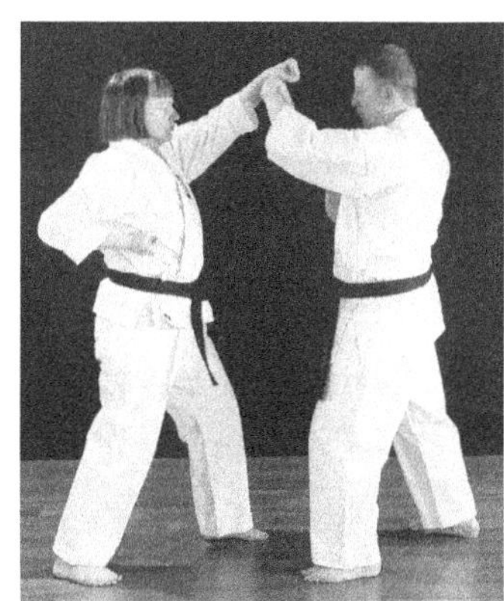

1. (Off - L): Step Forward, Jodan Zuki / (Def - R): Step Back, Jodan Age Ko Uke

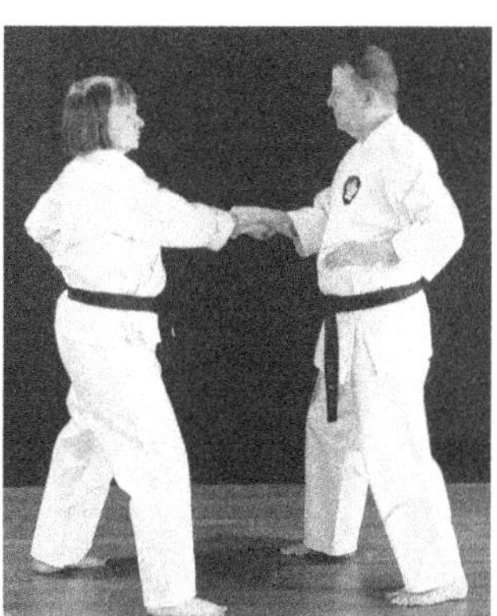

2. (Off - L): Step Forward, Chudan Zuki / (Def - R): Step Back, Chudan Hari to Hiki Uke

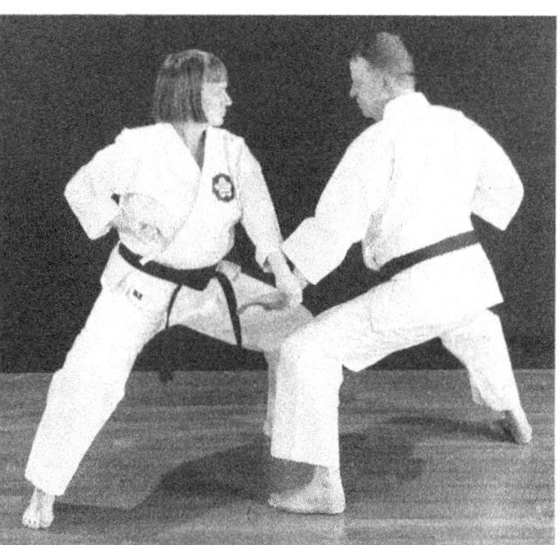

3. (Off - L): Step Forward, Gedan Zuki in Shiko Dachi / (Def - R): Step Back, Gedan Shotei Barai in Shiko Dachi

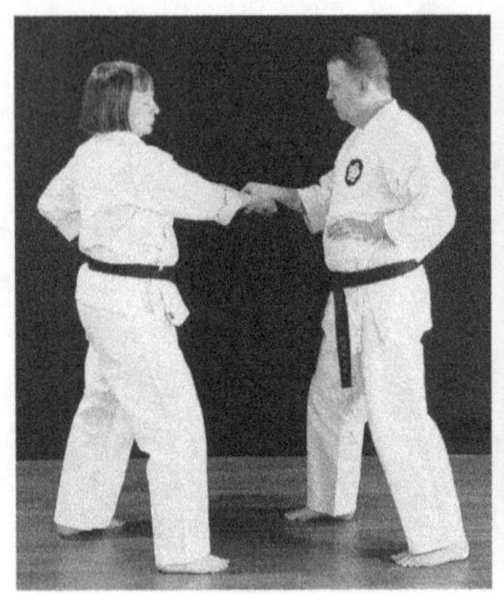

4. (Off - L): Step Forward, Chudan Zuki / (Def - R): Step Back, Chudan Hari to Hiki Uke

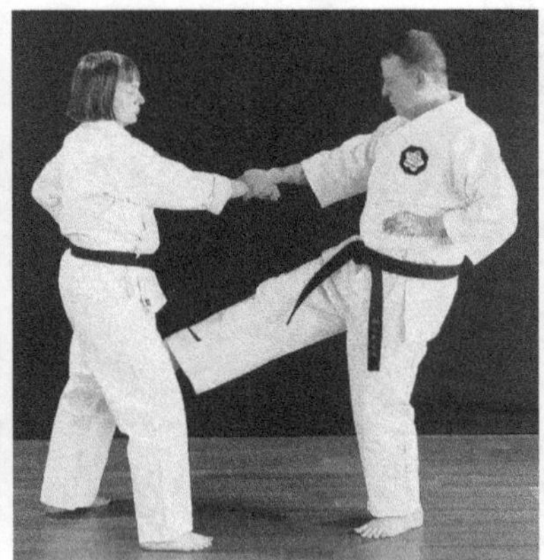

5. (Def - R): Kin Geri

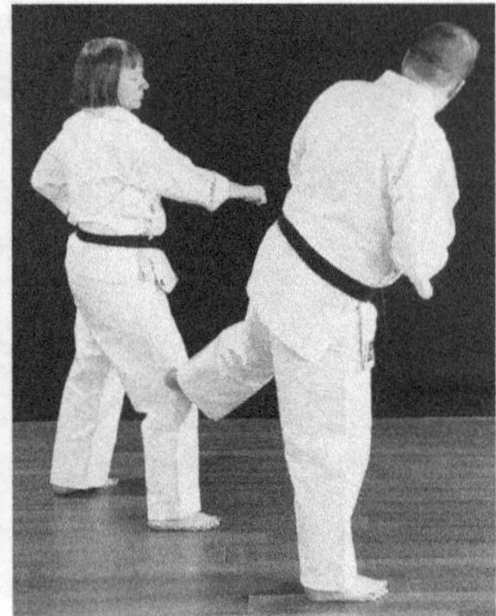

6. (Def - R): Step Out to Left, Mawatte, Hiza Geri (Kiai)

Repeat in Other Direction

Begin Counter 3

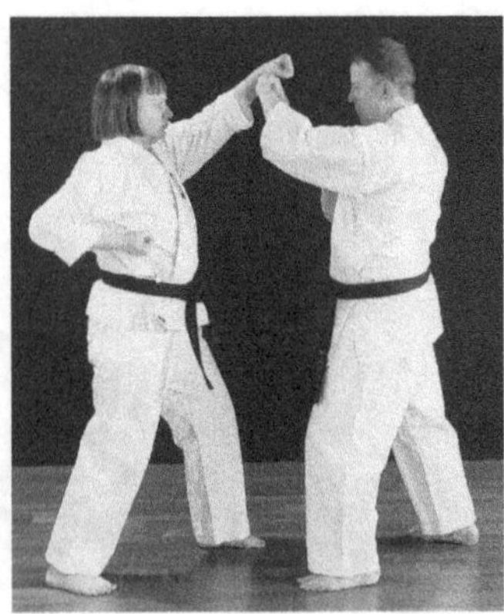

1. (Off - L): Step Forward, Jodan Zuki / (Def - R): Step Back, Jodan Age Ko Uke

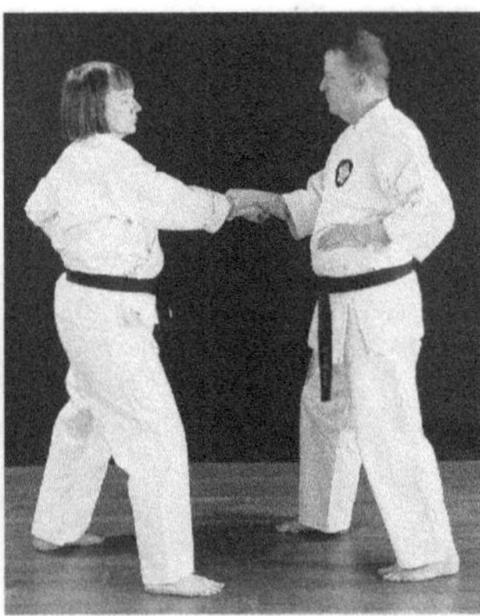

2. (Off - L): Step Forward, Chudan Zuki / (Def - R): Step Back, Chudan Hari to Hiki Uke

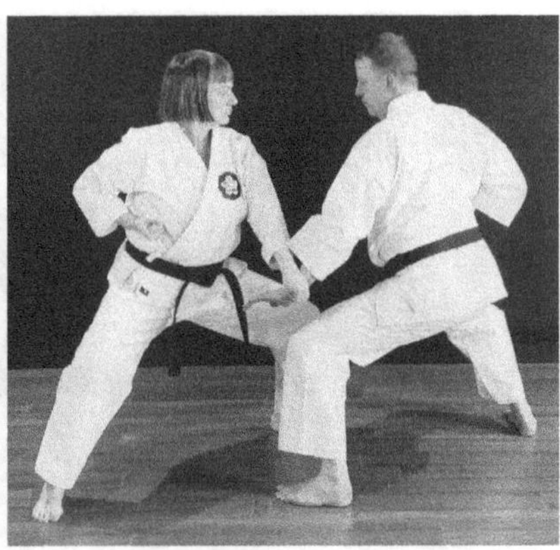

3. (Off - L): Step Forward, Gedan Zuki in Shiko Dachi / (Def - R): Step Back, Gedan Shotei Barai in Shiko Dachi

Repeat in Other Direction

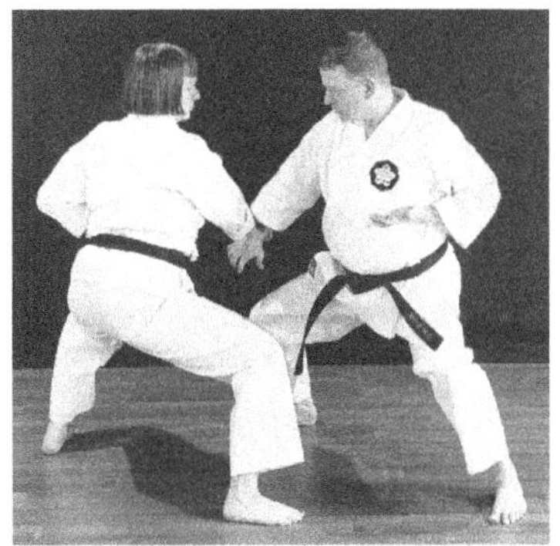
4. (Off - L): Step Forward, Gedan Zuki in Shiko Dachi / (Def - R): Step Back, Gedan Shotei Barai in Shiko Dachi

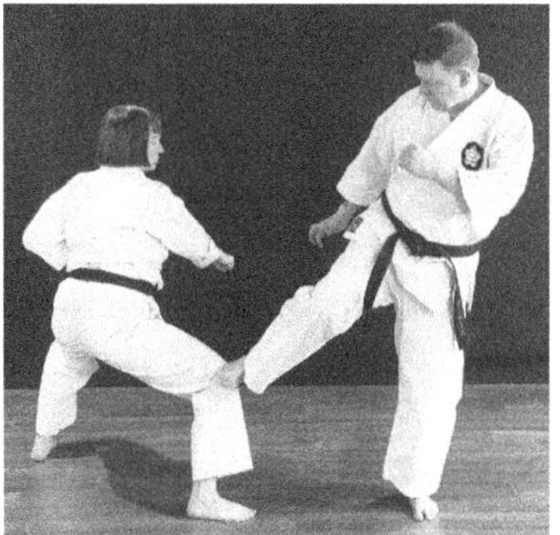
5. (Def - R): Step Out to Left, Right Hiza Geri

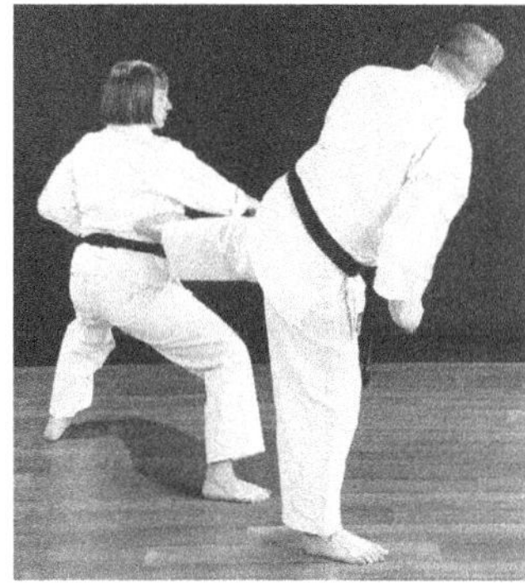
6. (Def - R): Mawatte, Left Chudan Yoko Geri (Kiai)

Begin Counter 4

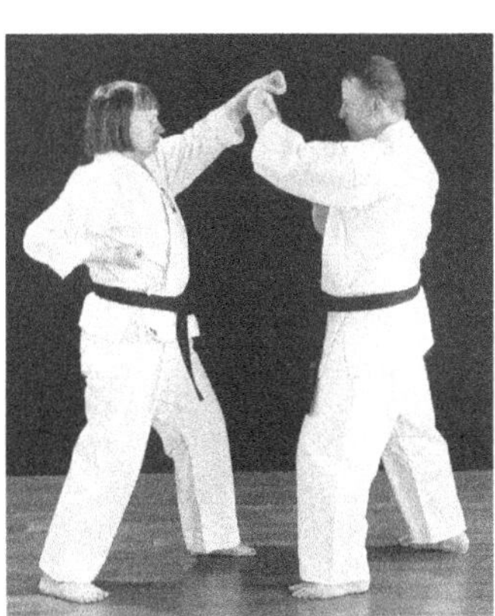
1. (Off - L): Step Forward, Jodan Zuki / (Def - R): Step Back, Jodan Age Ko Uke

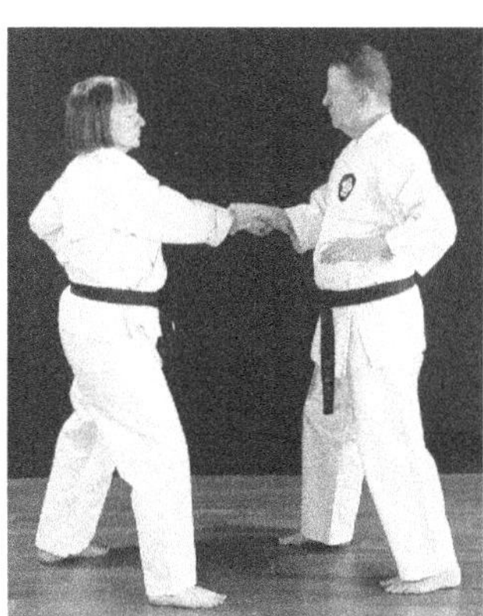
2. (Off - L): Step Forward, Chudan Zuki / (Def - R): Step Back, Chudan Hari to Hiki Uke

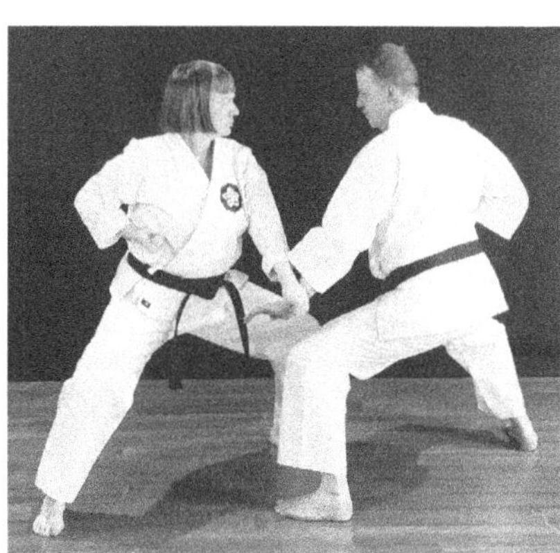
3. (Off - L): Step Forward, Gedan Zuki in Shiko Dachi / (Def - R): Step Back, Gedan Shotei Barai in Shiko Dachi

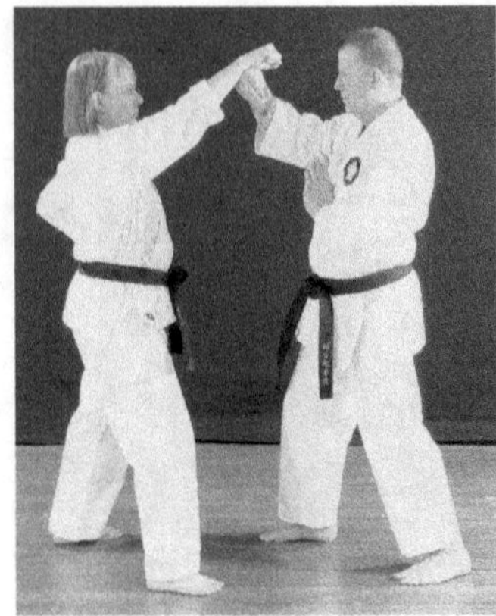

4. Off - L): Step Forward, Jodan Zuki / (Def - R): Step Back, Jodan Age Ko Uke

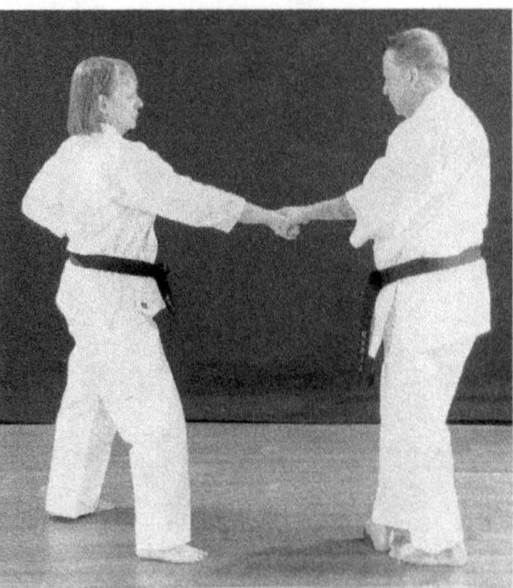

5. (Def - R): Grab Opponent's Wrist

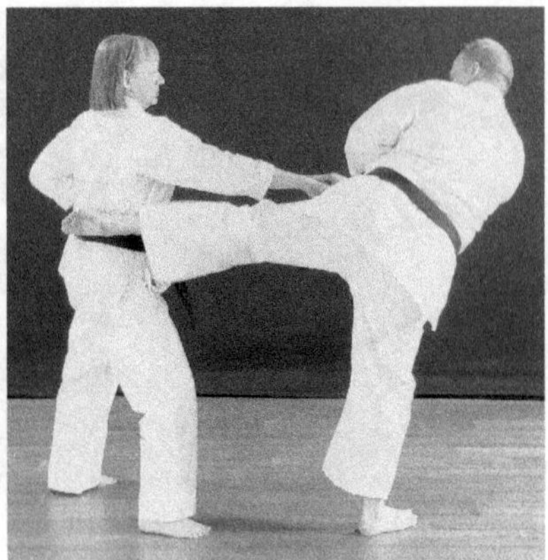

6. (Def - R): Left Chudan (or Jodan) Mawashi Geri

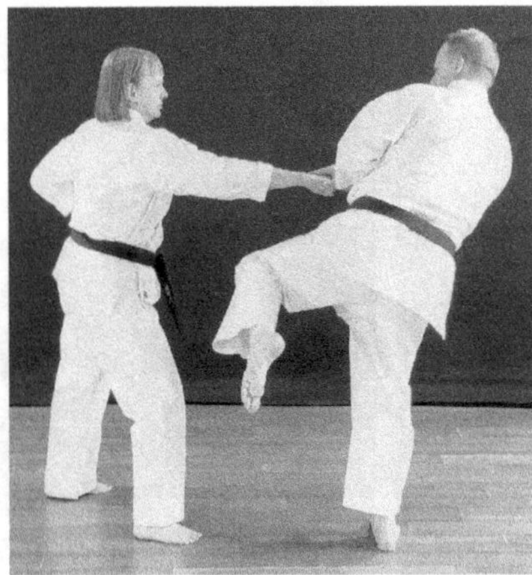

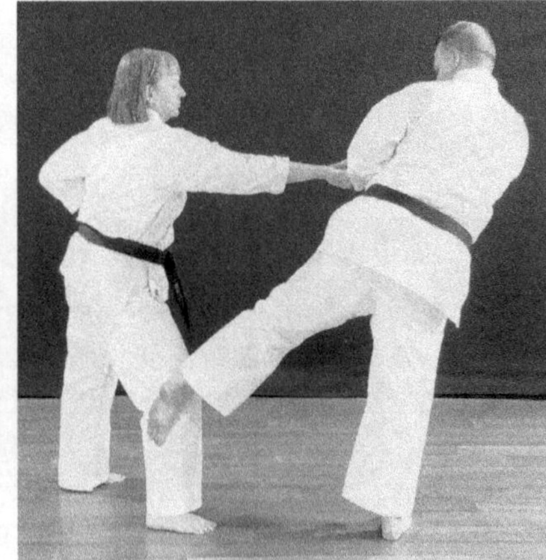

Repeat in Other Direction

7. (Def - R): Without Putting Foot Down, Complete Left Gedan (or Chudan) Mawashi Geri (Kiai)

Begin Counter 5

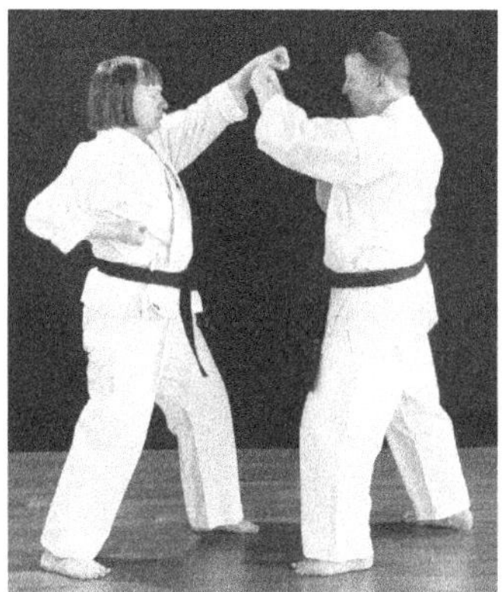

1. (Off - L): Step Forward, Jodan Zuki / (Def - R): Step Back, Jodan Age Ko Uke

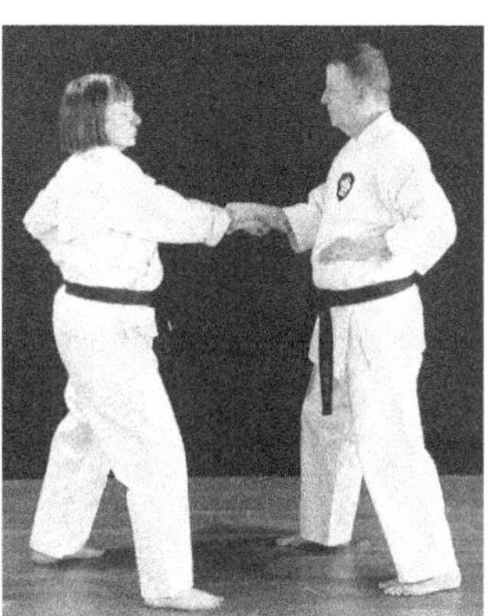

2. (Off - L): Step Forward, Chudan Zuki / (Def - R): Step Back, Chudan Hari to Hiki Uke

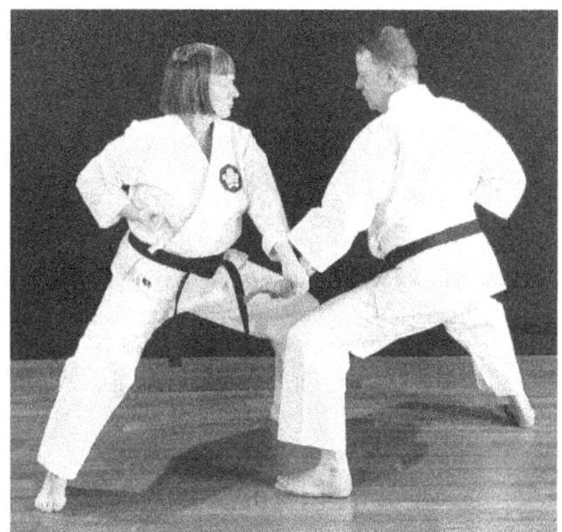

3. (Off - L): Step Forward, Gedan Zuki in Shiko Dachi / (Def - R): Step Back, Gedan Shotei Barai in Shiko Dachi

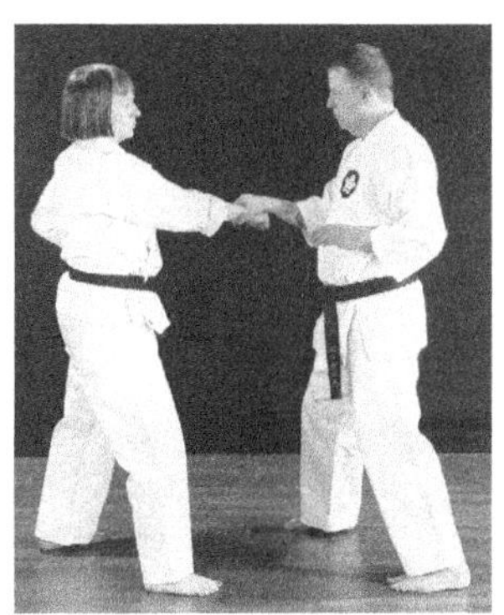

4. (Off - L): Step Forward, Chudan Zuki / (Def - R): Step Back, Chudan Hari to Hiki Uke

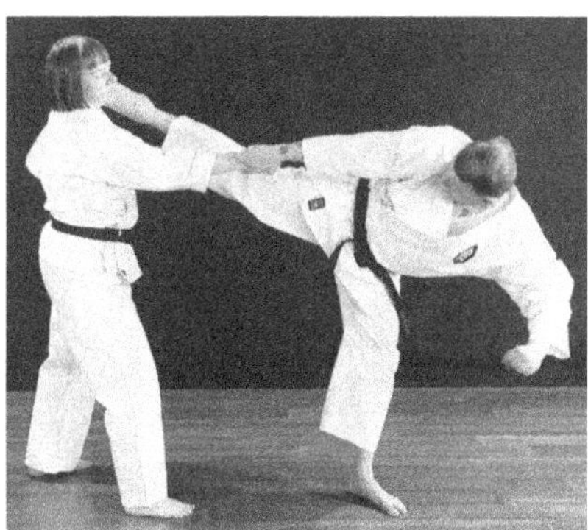

5. (Def - R): Grab Opponent's Wrist, Right Jodan Mawashi Geri

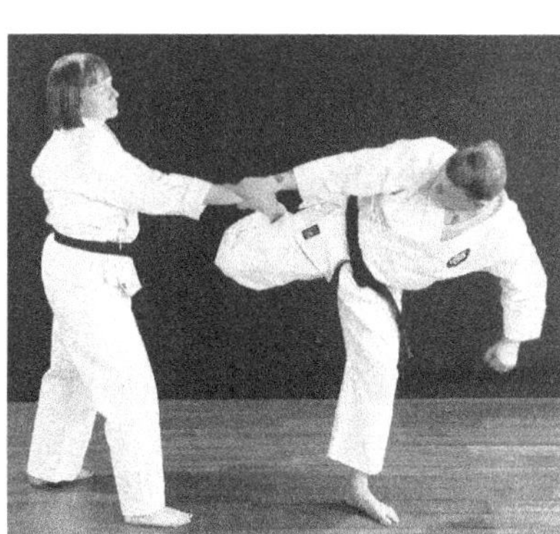

6. (Def - R): Without Putting Foot Down, Begin Right Chudan Mawashi Geri (using ball of foot)

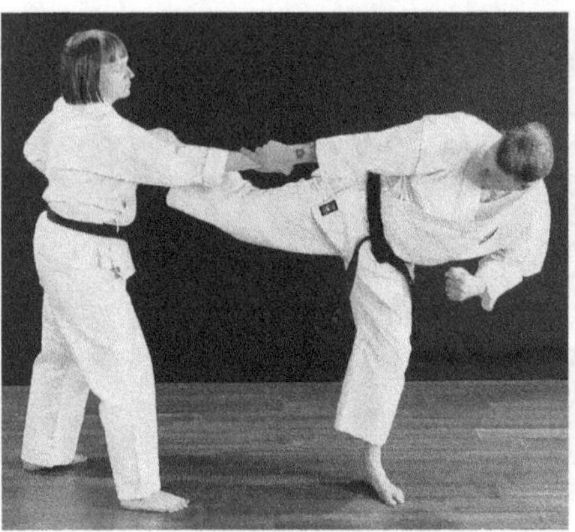

Repeat in Other Direction

7. (Def - R): Right Chudan Mawashi Geri (cont.) (Kiai)

Begin Counter 6

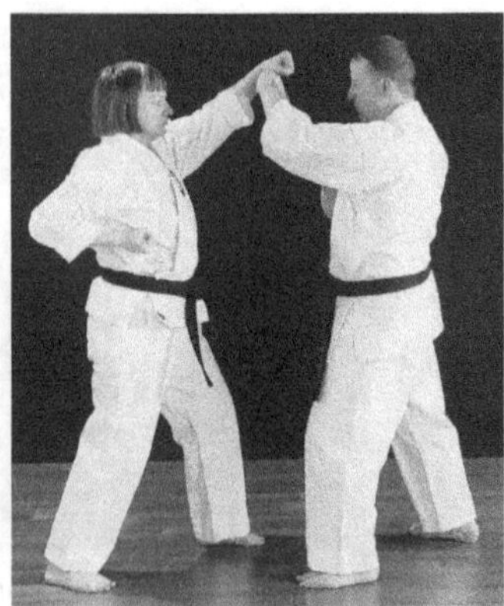

1. (Off - L): Step Forward, Jodan Zuki / (Def - R): Step Back, Jodan Age Ko Uke

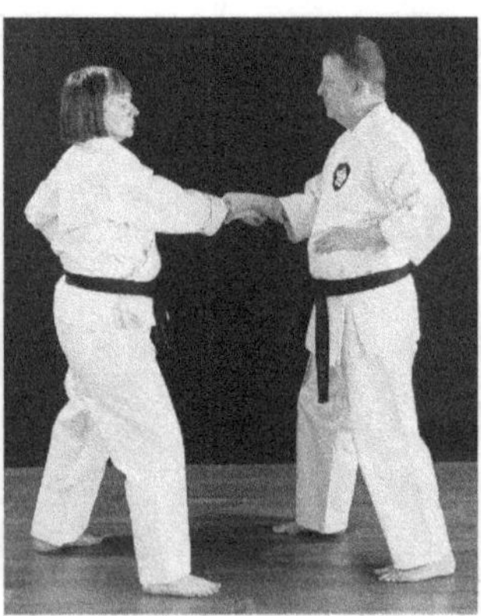

2. (Off - L): Step Forward, Chudan Zuki / (Def - R): Step Back, Chudan Hari to Hiki Uke

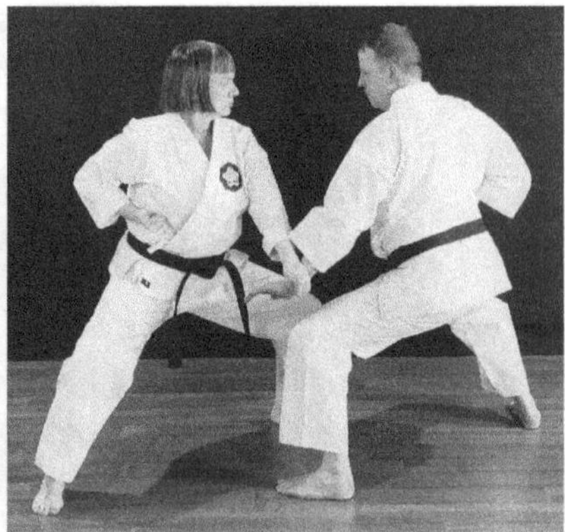

3. (Off - L): Step Forward, Gedan Zuki in Shiko Dachi / (Def - R): Step Back, Gedan Shotei Barai in Shiko Dachi

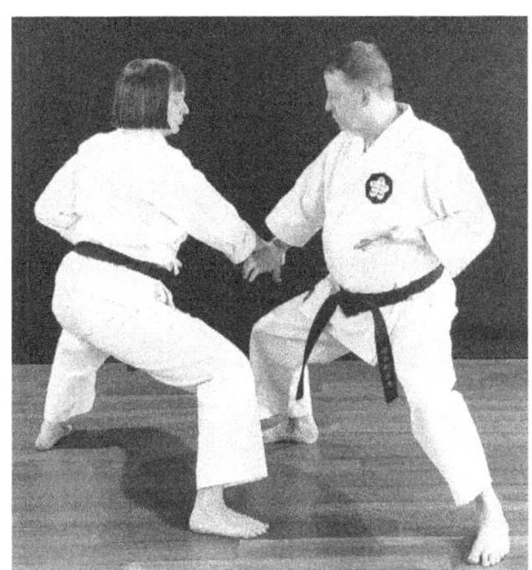

4. (Off - L): Step Forward, Gedan Zuki in Shiko Dachi / (Def - R): Step Back, Gedan Shotei Barai in Shiko Dachi

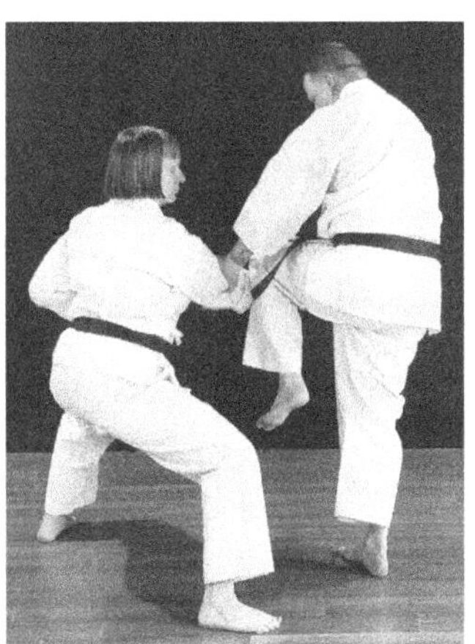

5. (Def - R): Pivot to Right, Grabbing Opponent's Arm, Drive Knee Through Opponent's Arm

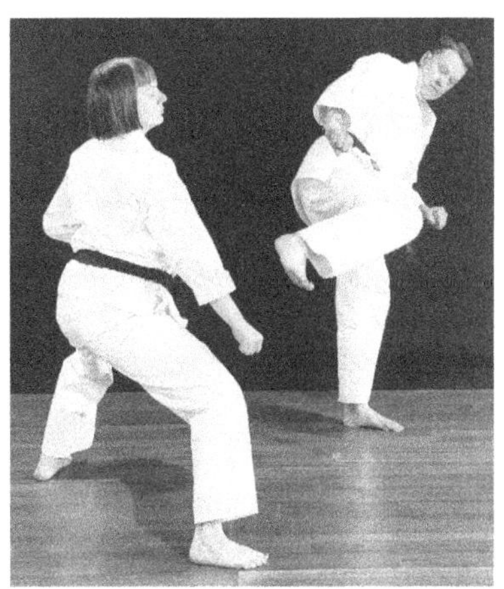

6. (Def - R): Mawatte, Right Jodan Yoko Geri (Kiai)

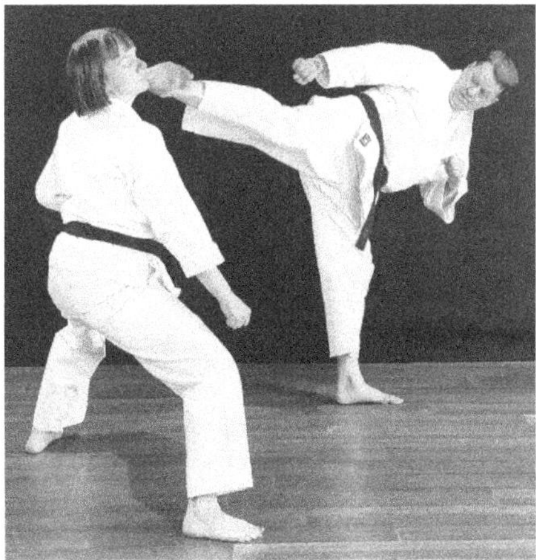

7. (Def - R): Jodan Yoko Geri (Kiai)

(cont.)

Repeat in Other Direction

Kumite Shi - Bag Work

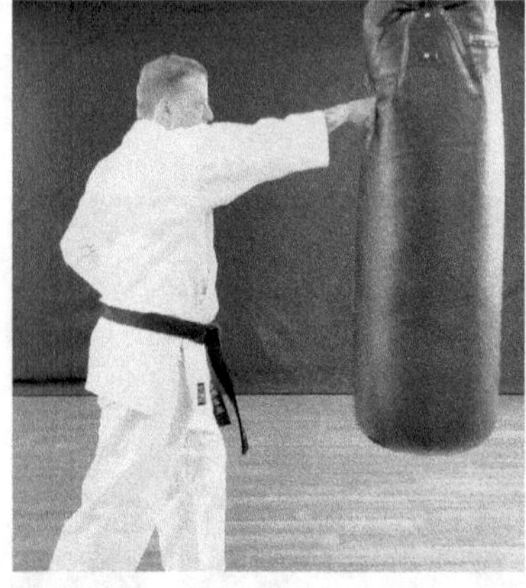
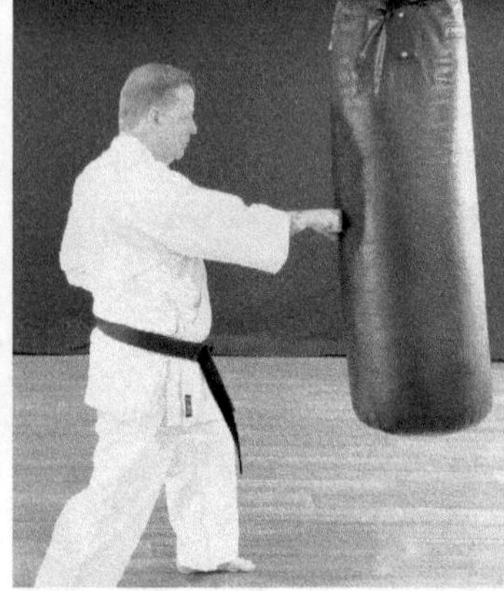
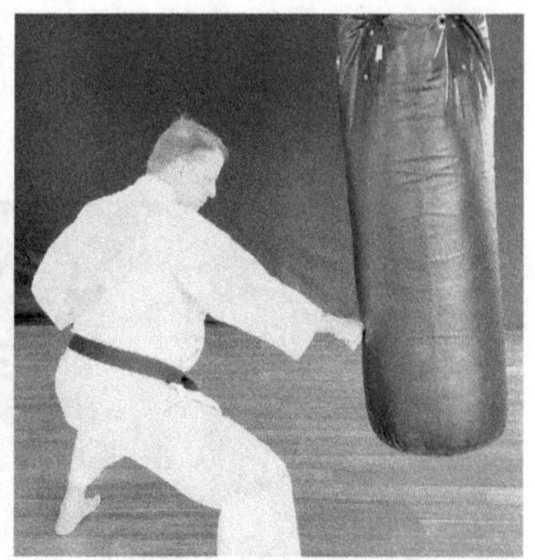

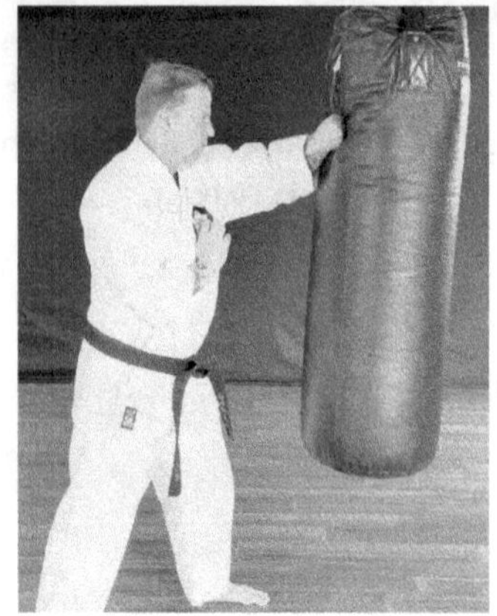

Jodan Zuki (Top) & Jodan Age Ko Uke (Bottom)

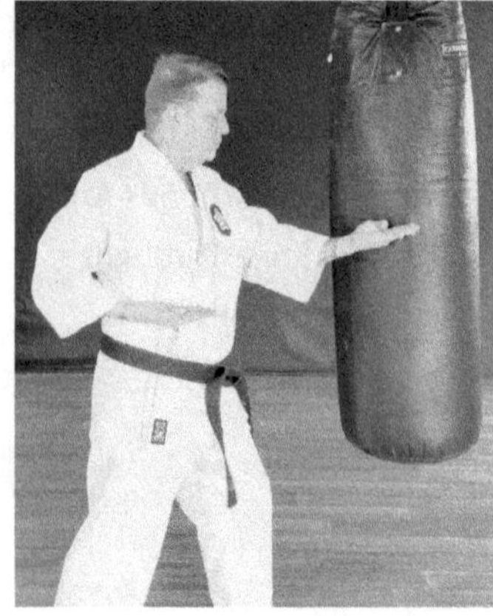

Chudan Zuki (Top) & Hari Uke (Bottom)

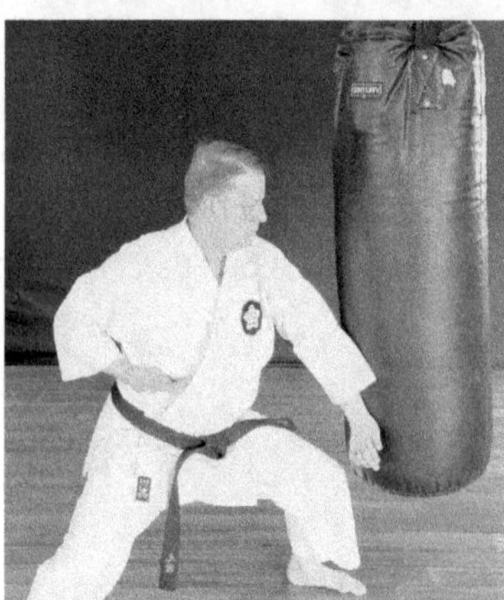

Gedan Zuki (Top) & Gedan Shotei Barai (Bottom)

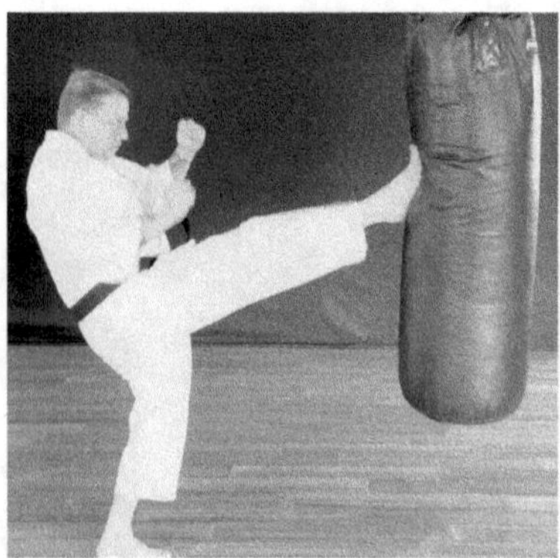
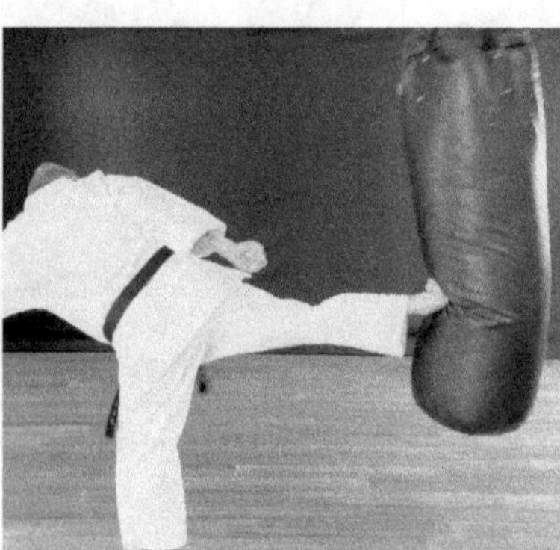

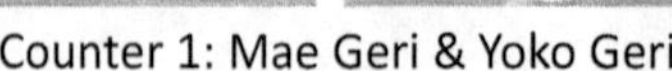

Counter 1: Mae Geri & Yoko Geri

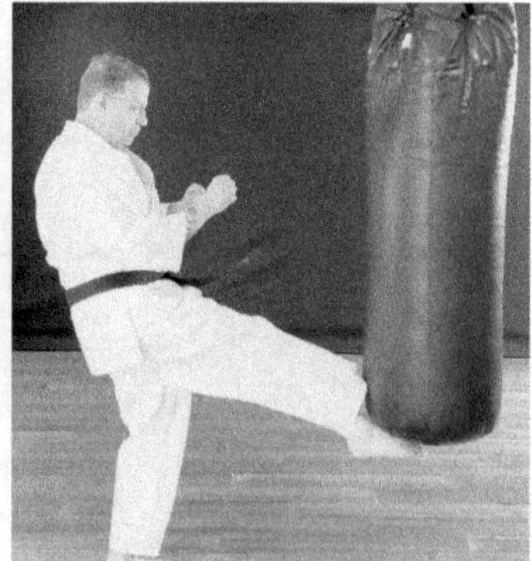

Counter 2: Kin Geri

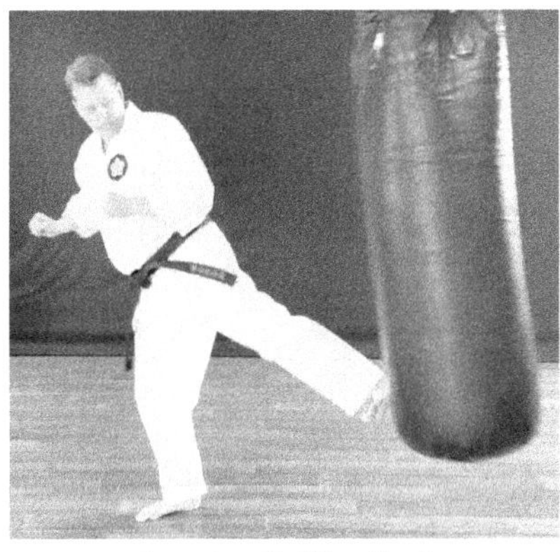
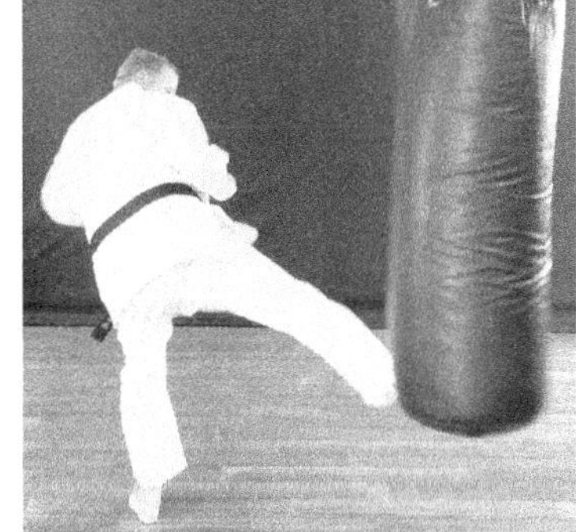
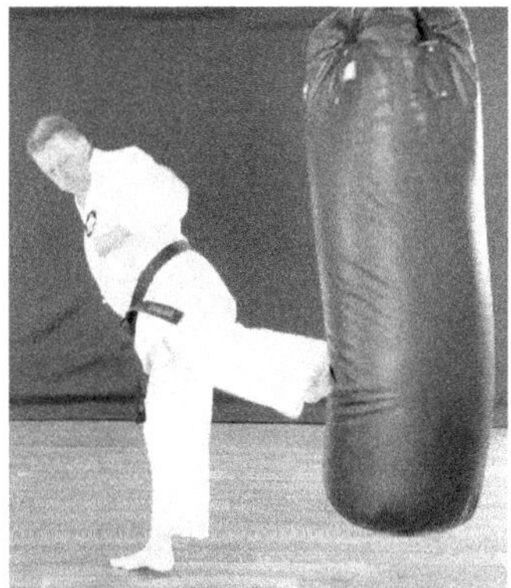

Counter 2: Hiza Geri

Counter 3: Hiza Geri &Yoko Geri

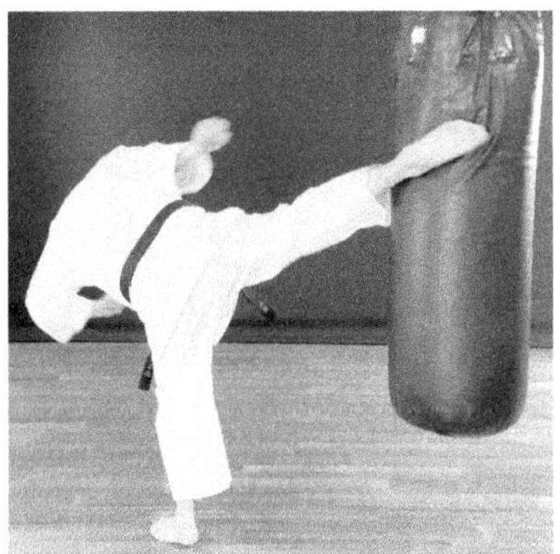
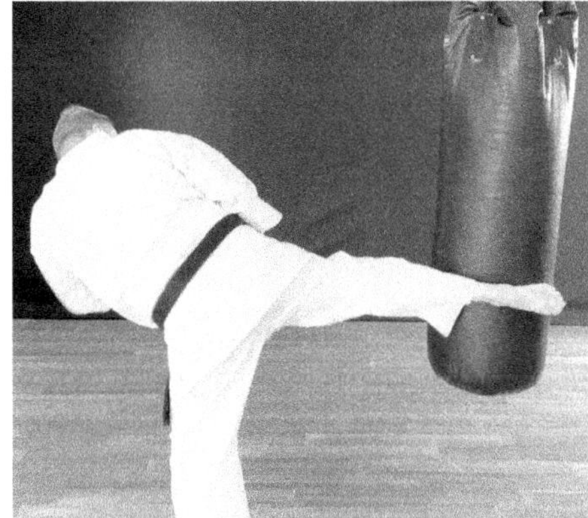

Counter 4: Jodan & Chudan (or Gedan) Mawashi Geri

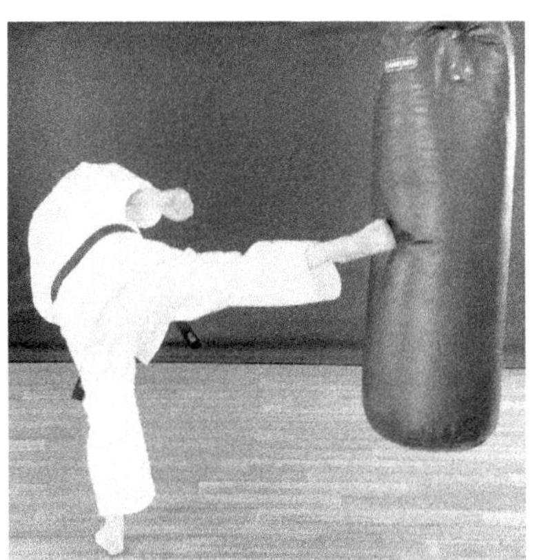
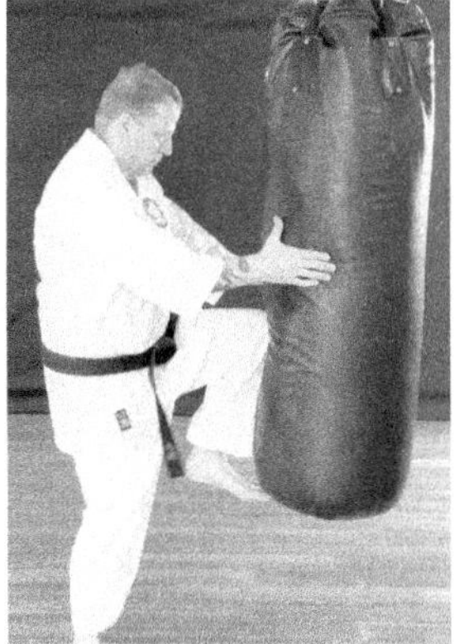
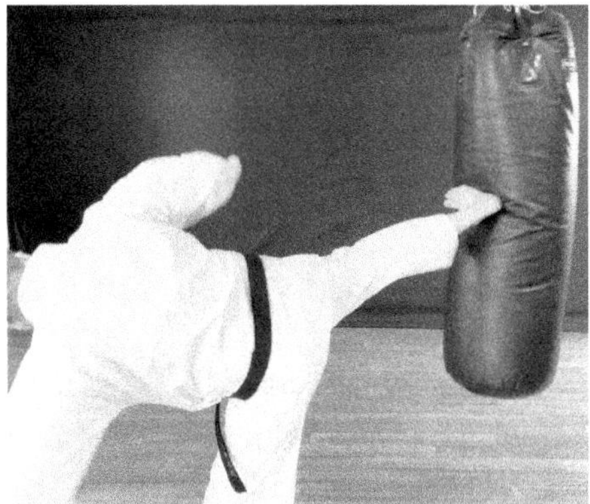

Counter 6: Mawashi Geri with Ball of Foot, Age Hiza Uchi & Yoko Geri

11. Kumite Go (5)

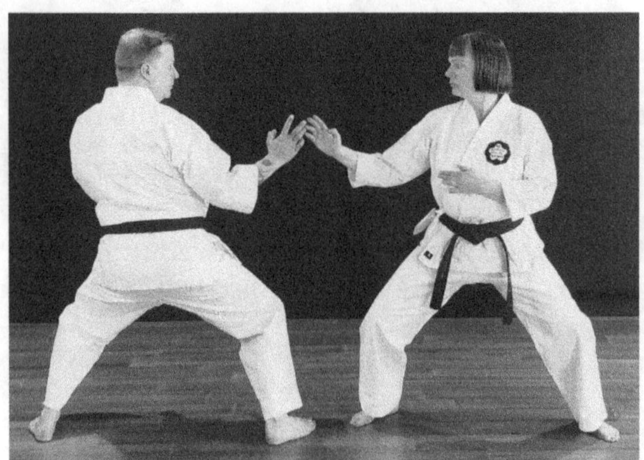

Open Hand Yoko Kumite Dachi

Begin Counter 1

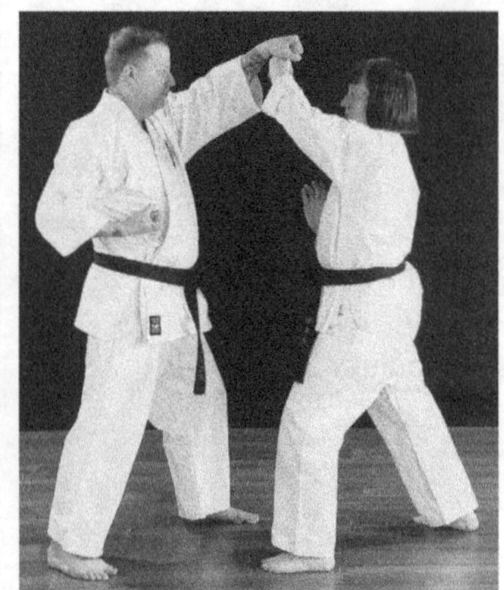

1. (Off - L): Step Forward, Jodan Zuki / (Def - R): Step Back, Jodan Age Ko Uke

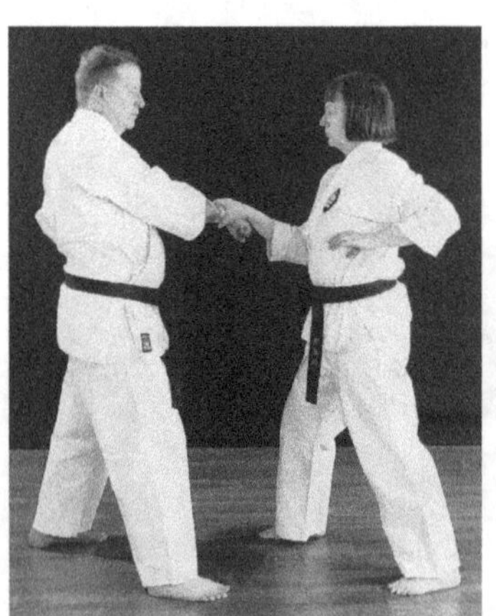

2. (Off - L): Step Forward, Chudan Zuki / (Def - R): Step Back, Chudan Hari to Hiki Uke

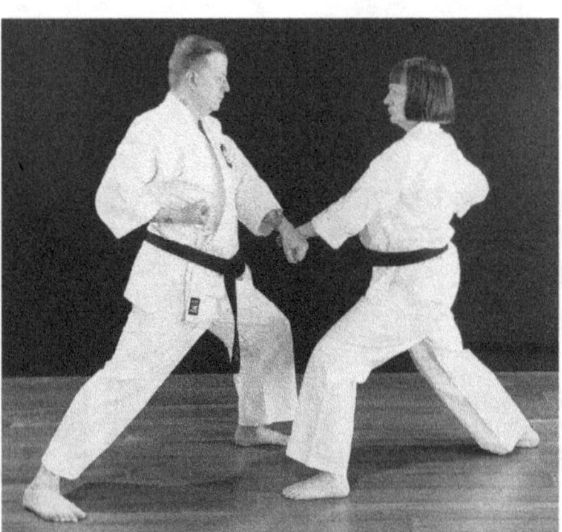

3. (Off - L): Step Forward, Gedan Zuki in Zenkutsu Dachi / (Def - R): Step Back, Gedan Shotei Barai in Zenkutsu Dachi

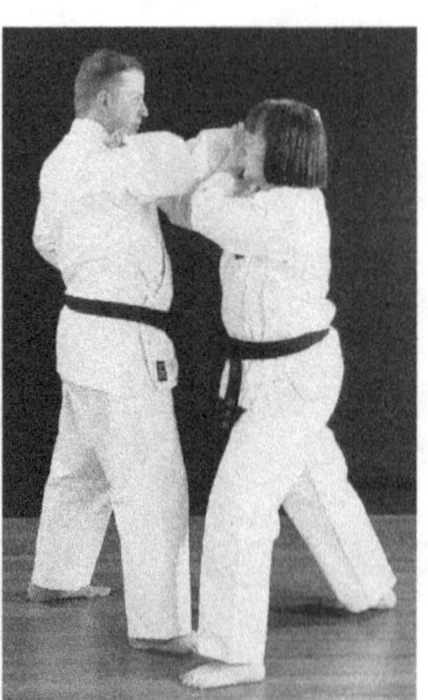

4. (Off - L): Step Forward, Jodan Zuki / (Def - R): Step to Side, Catch Opponent's Arm

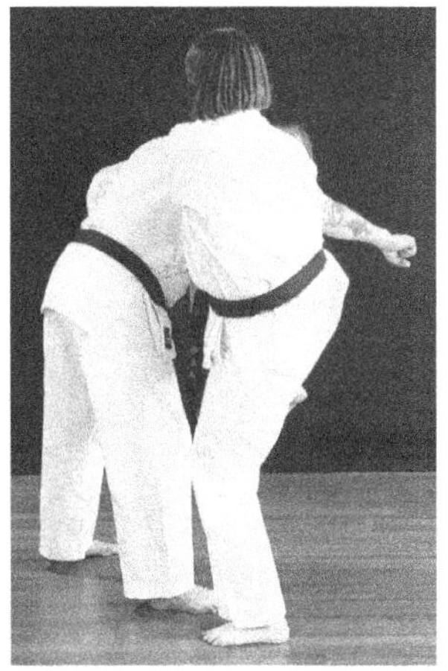
5. (Def - R): Pull Torso Down, Hiza Uchi to Stomach Area

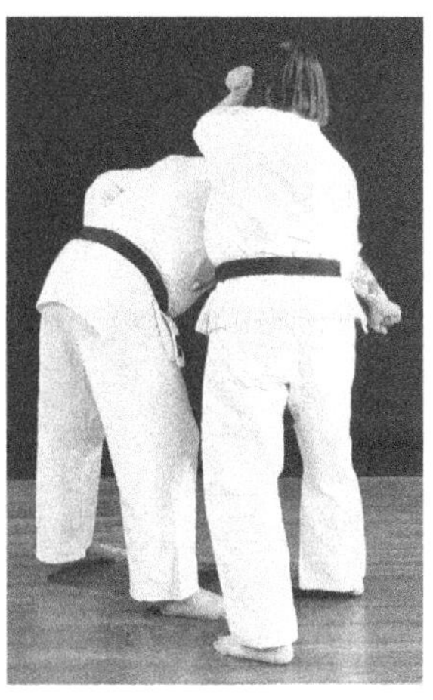
6. (Def - R): Empi Otoshi Uchi to Back (Kiai)

Repeat in Other Direction

Begin Counter 2

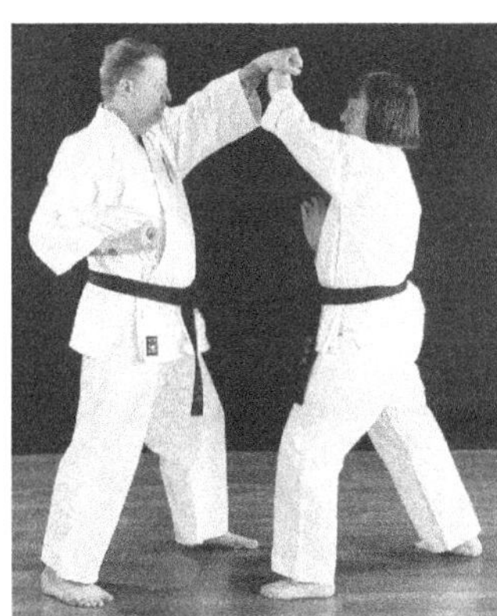
1. (Off - L): Step Forward, Jodan Zuki / (Def - R): Step Back, Jodan Age Ko Uke

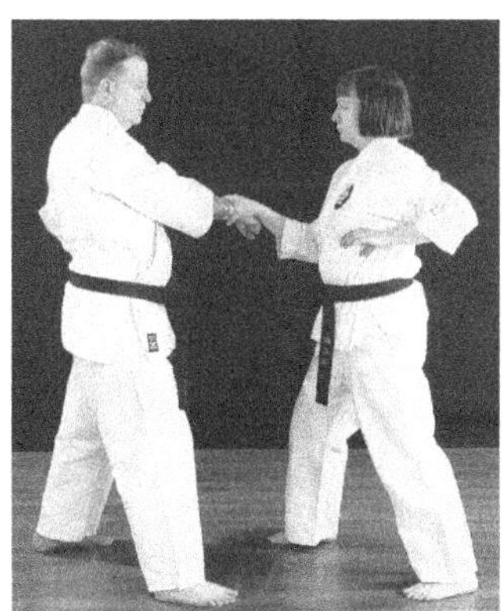
2. (Off - L): Step Forward, Chudan Zuki / (Def - R): Step Back, Chudan Hari to Hiki Uke

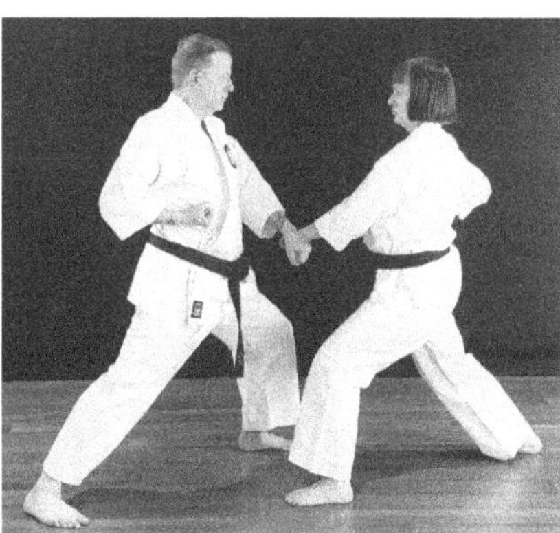
3. (Off - L): Step Forward, Gedan Zuki in Zenkutsu Dachi / (Def - R): Step Back, Gedan Shotei Barai in Zenkutsu Dachi

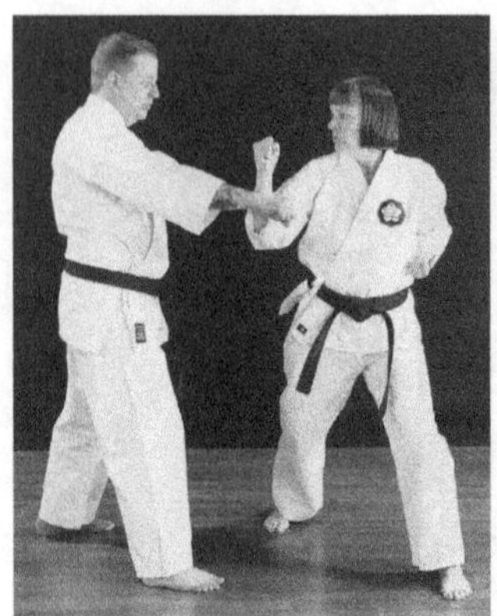
4. (Off - L): Step Forward, Chudan Zuki / (Def - R): Pivot Left, Soto Uchi

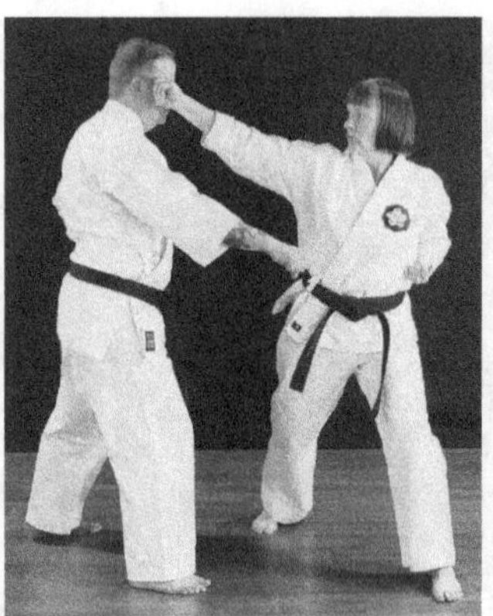
5. (Def - R): Yoko Uraken Uchi

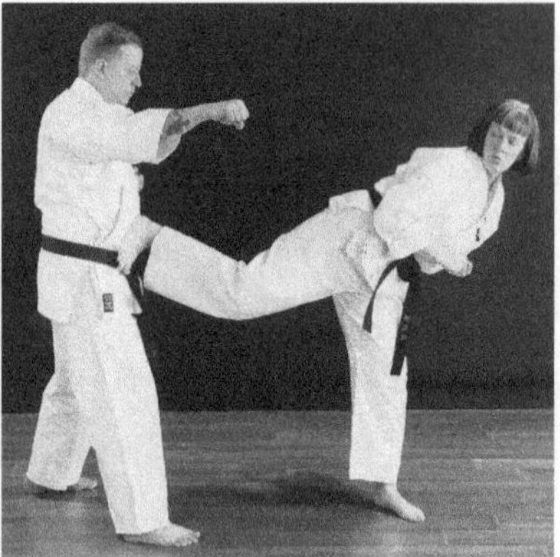
6. (Def - R): Ushiro Kakato Geri (Kiai)

Repeat in Other Direction

Begin Counter 3

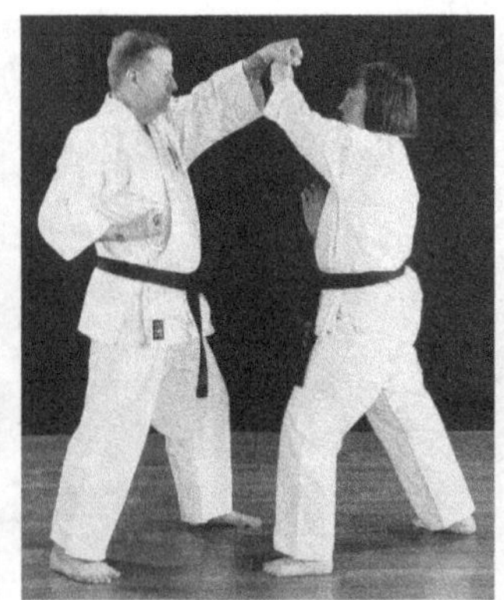
1. (Off - L): Step Forward, Jodan Zuki / (Def - R): Step Back, Jodan Age Ko Uke

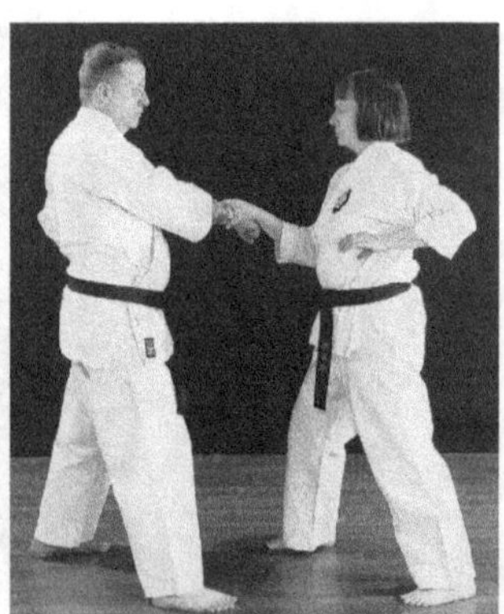
2. (Off - L): Step Forward, Chudan Zuki / (Def - R): Step Back, Chudan Hari to Hiki Uke

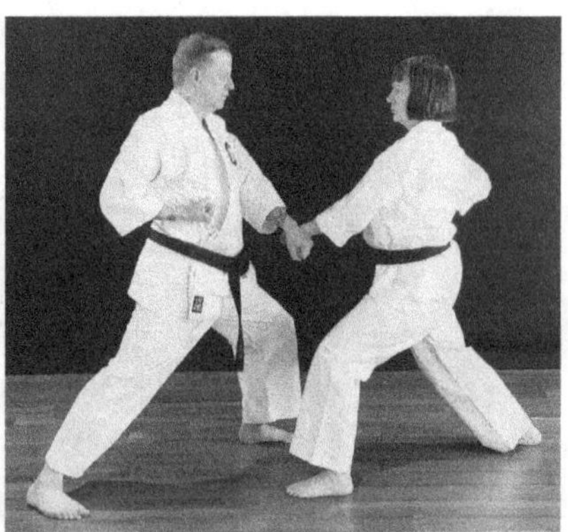
3. (Off - L): Step Forward, Gedan Zuki in Zenkutsu Dachi / (Def - R): Step Back, Gedan Shotei Barai in Zenkutsu Dachi

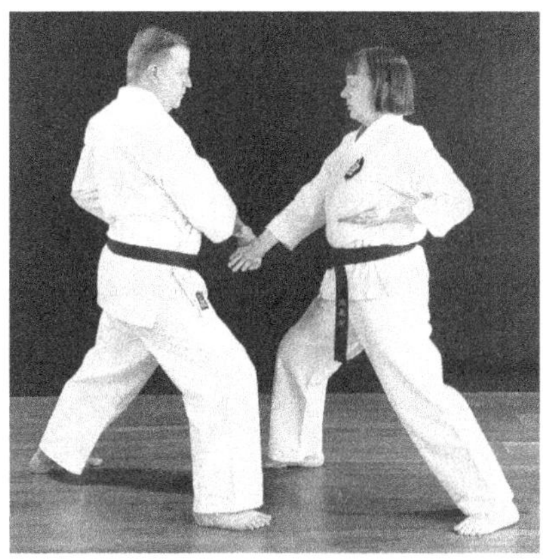

4. (Off - L): Step Forward, Gedan Zuki in Zenkutsu Dachi / (Def - R): Step Back, Gedan Shotei Barai in Zenkutsu Dachi, Grab Wrist

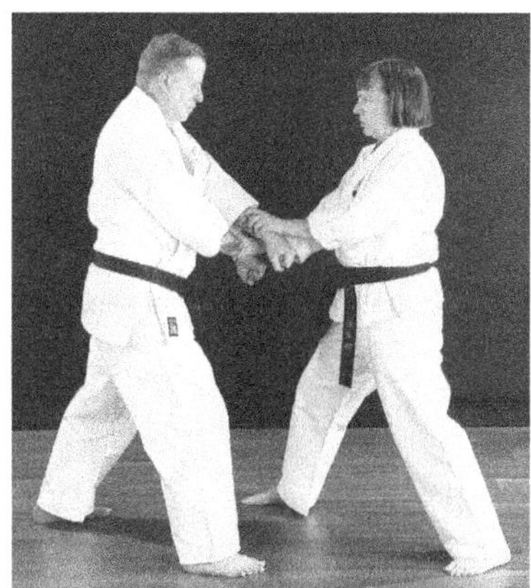

5. (Off - L): Left Gedan Zuki / (Def - R): Gedan Shotei Barai, Grab Wrist

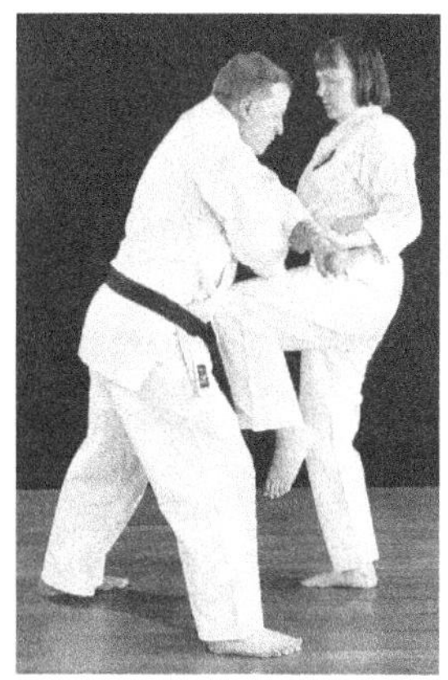

6. (Def - R): Pull Opponents Arms Down, Age Hiza Uchi to Groin or Midsection (Kiai)

Repeat in Other Direction

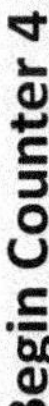

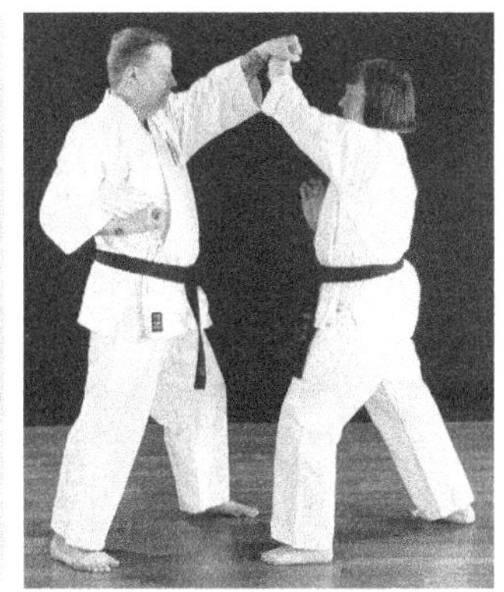

1. (Off - L): Step Forward, Jodan Zuki / (Def - R): Step Back, Jodan Age Ko Uke

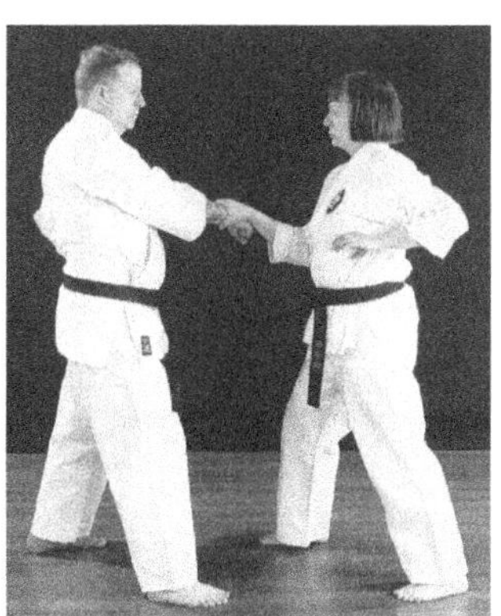

2. (Off - L): Step Forward, Chudan Zuki / (Def - R): Step Back, Chudan Hari to Hiki Uke

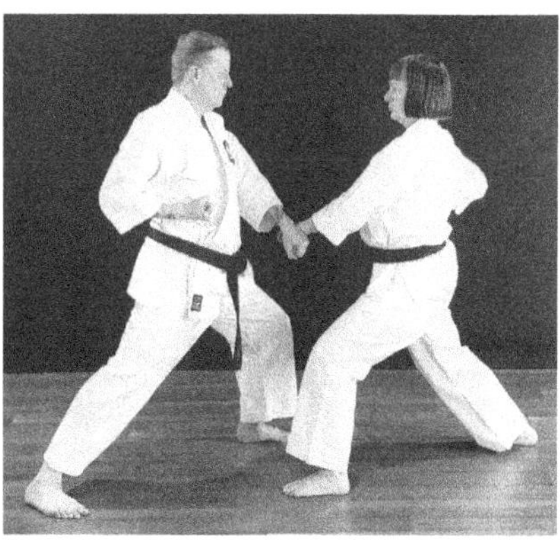

3. (Off - L): Step Forward, Gedan Zuki in Zenkutsu Dachi / (Def - R): Step Back, Gedan Shotei Barai in Zenkutsu Dachi

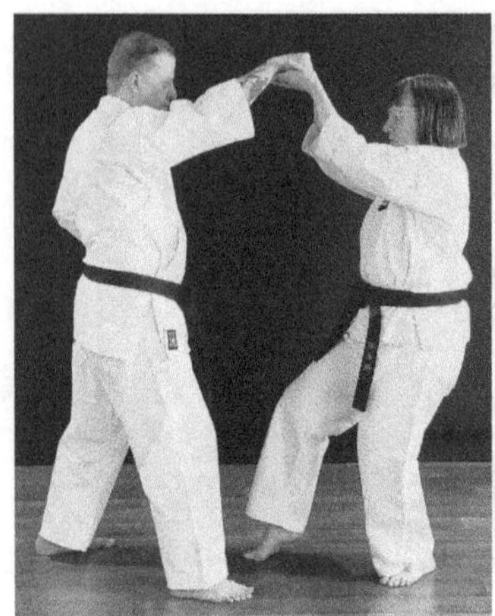

4. (Off - L): Step Forward, Jodan Zuki / (Def - R): Step Back into Neko Ashi Dachi, Morote Sukui Age Uke

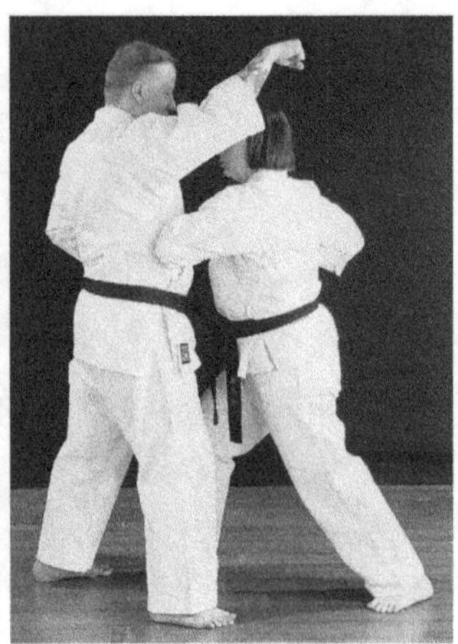

5. (Def - R): Step Forward, Left Kote Uchi to Ribs

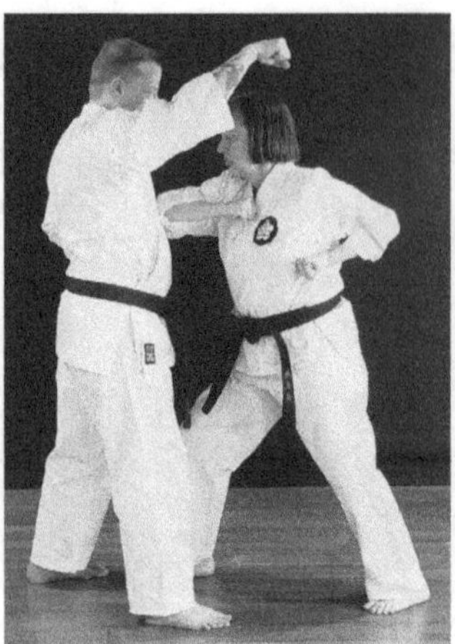

6. (Def - R): Right Chudan Mawashi Empi Uchi (Kiai)

Repeat in Other Direction

Begin Counter 5

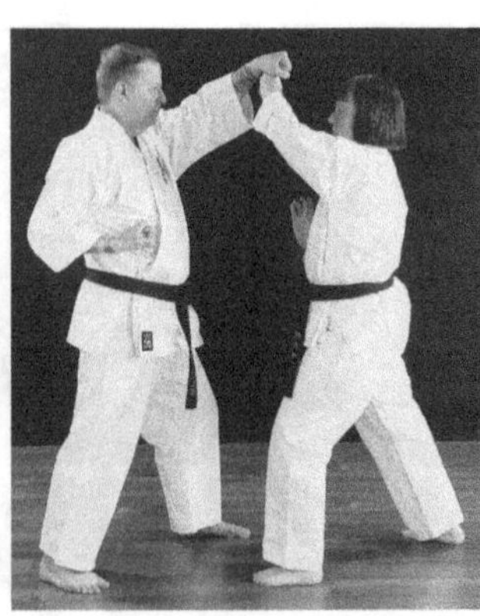

1. (Off - L): Step Forward, Jodan Zuki / (Def - R): Step Back, Jodan Age Ko Uke

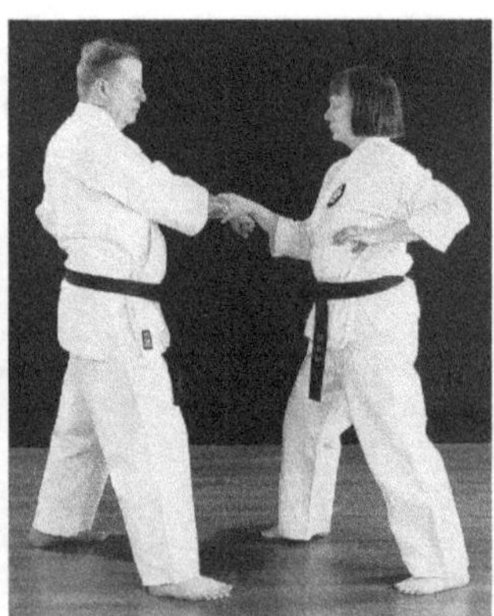

2. (Off - L): Step Forward, Chudan Zuki / (Def - R): Step Back, Chudan Hari to Hiki Uke

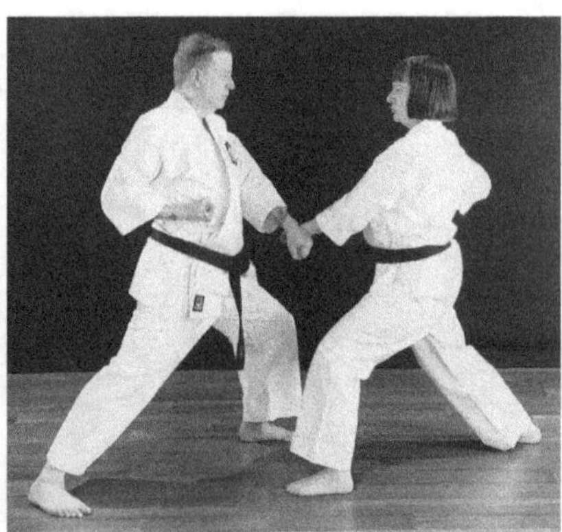

3. (Off - L): Step Forward, Gedan Zuki in Zenkutsu Dachi / (Def - R): Step Back, Gedan Shotei Barai in Zenkutsu Dachi

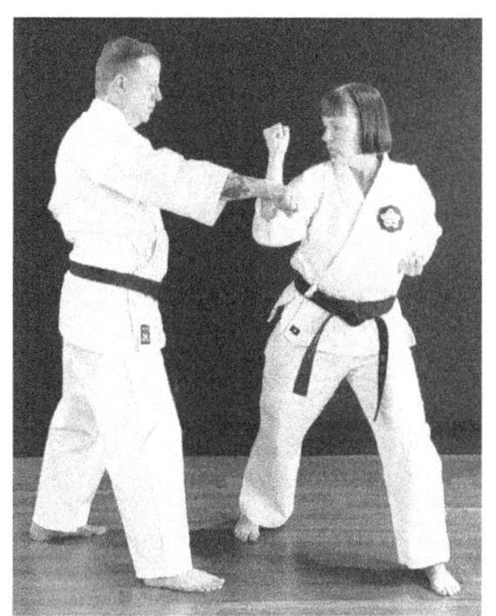

4. (Off - L): Step Forward, Chudan Zuki / (Def - R): Pivot Left, Soto Uchi

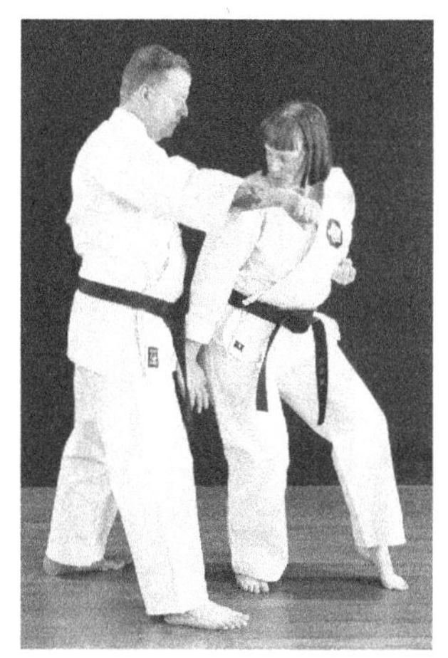

5. (Def - R): Slide into Neko Ashi Dachi, Gedan Shotei Uchi

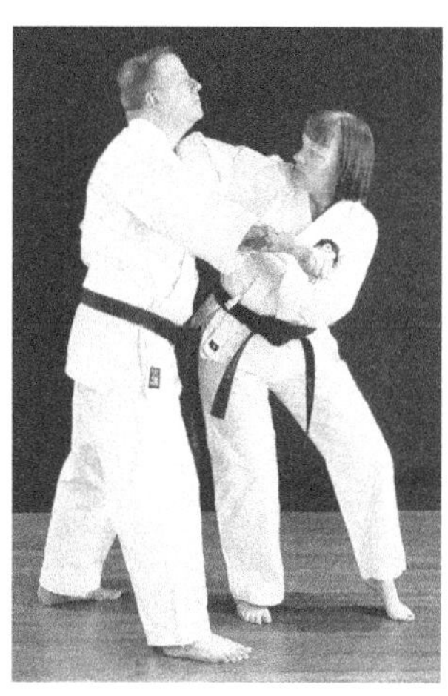

6. (Def - R): Age Empi Uchi to Chin

Repeat in Other Direction

Begin Counter 6

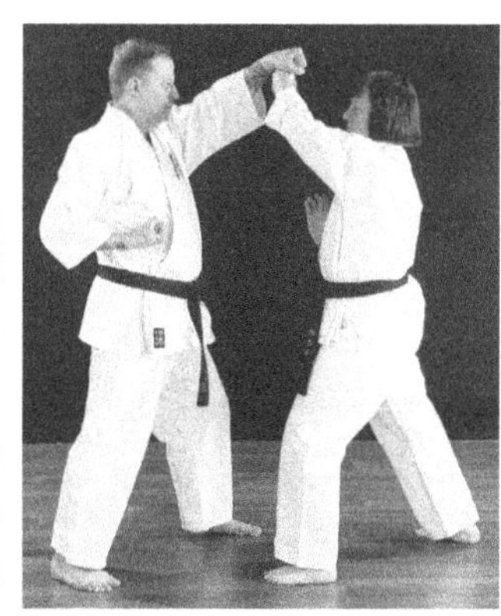

1. (Off - L): Step Forward, Jodan Zuki / (Def - R): Step Back, Jodan Age Ko Uke

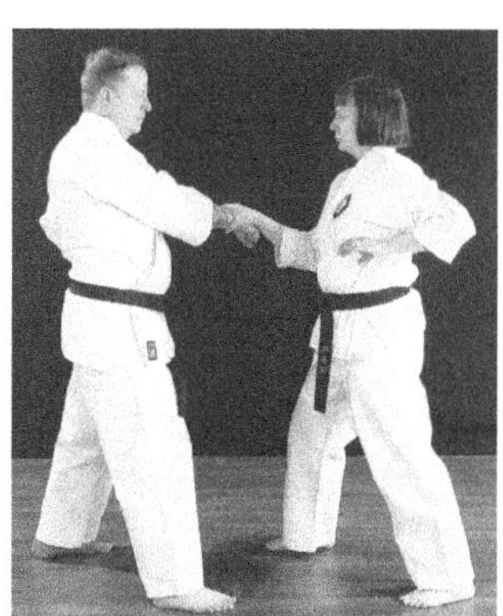

2. (Off - L): Step Forward, Chudan Zuki / (Def - R): Step Back, Chudan Hari to Hiki Uke

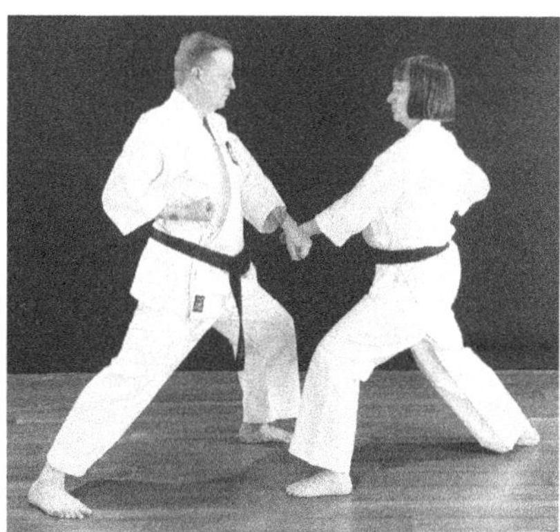

3. (Off - L): Step Forward, Gedan Zuki in Zenkutsu Dachi / (Def - R): Step Back, Gedan Shotei Barai in Zenkutsu Dachi

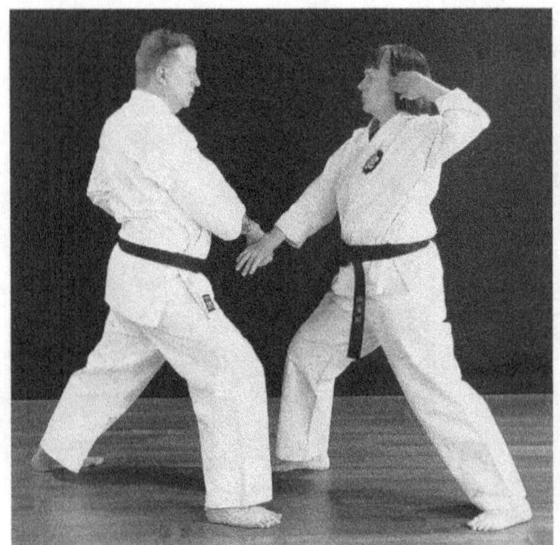

4. (Off - L): Step Forward, Gedan Zuki in Zenkutsu Dachi / (Def - R): Step Back, Gedan Shotei Barai in Zenkutsu Dachi, Chamber Left Hand

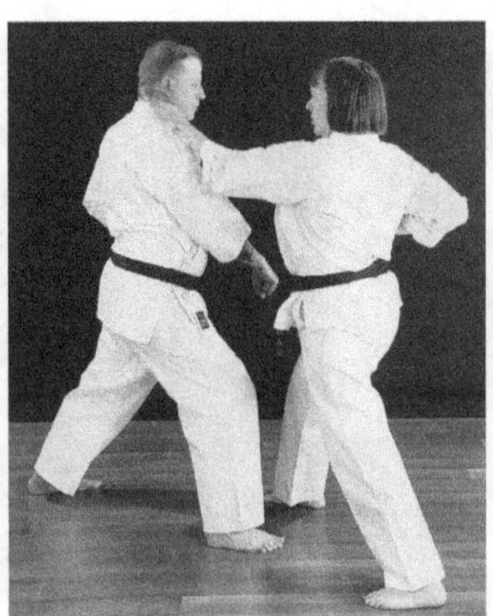

5. (Def - R): Step to Side, Shuto Uchi to Neck

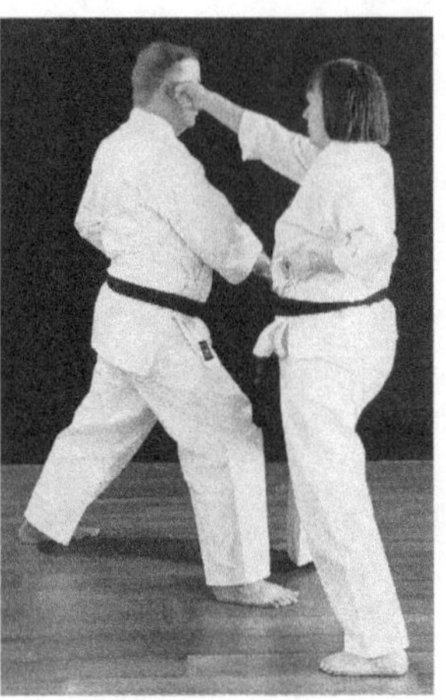

6. (Def - R): Right Tate Uchi to Temple

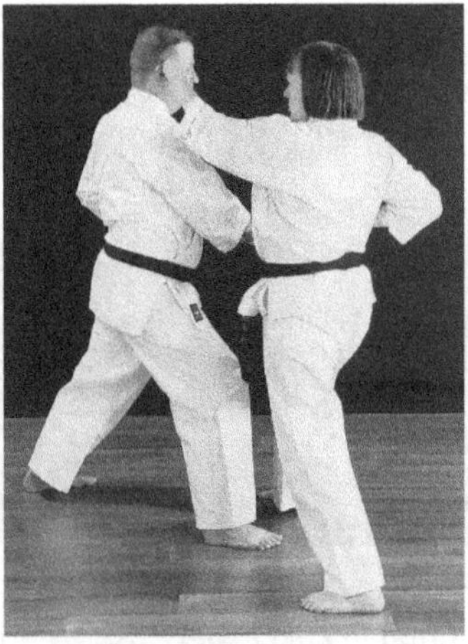

7. (Def - R): Left Tate Uchi (Kiai)

Repeat in Other Direction

Kumite Go - Bag Work

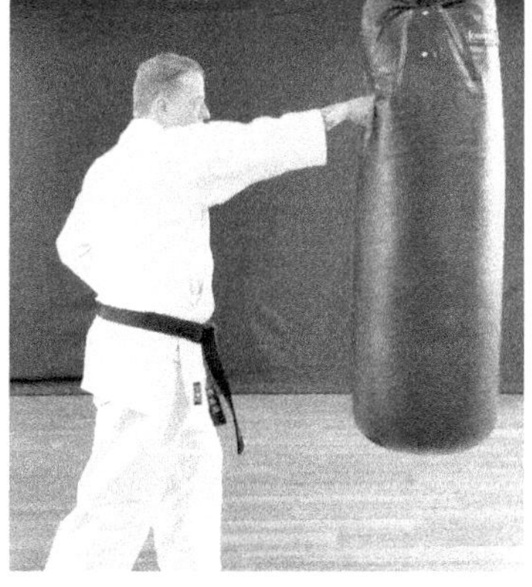
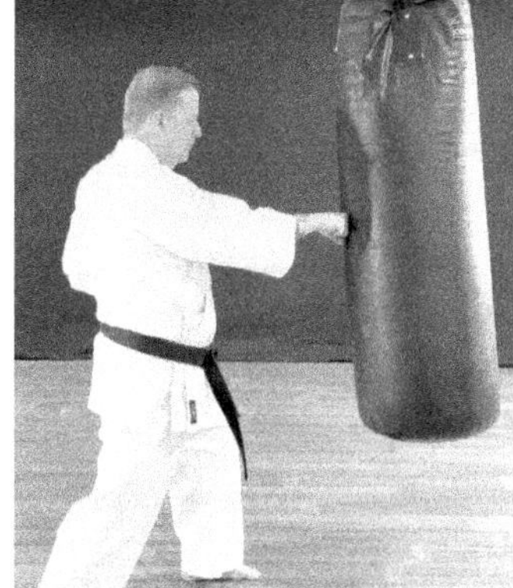
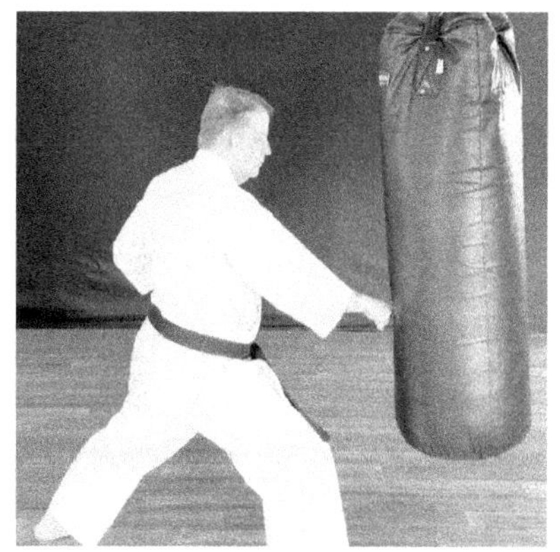
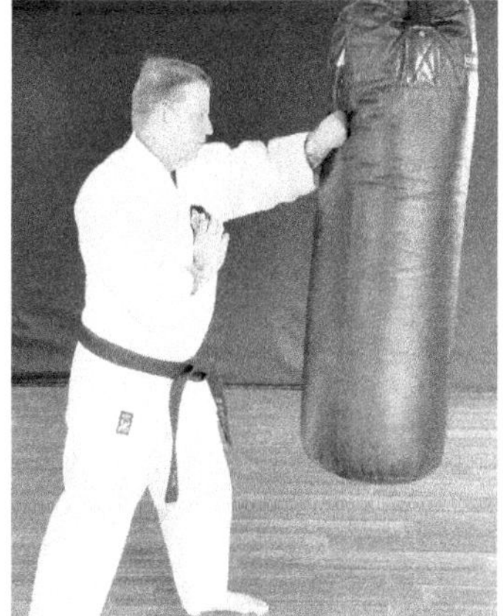

Jodan Zuki (Top) & Jodan Age Ko Uke (Bottom)

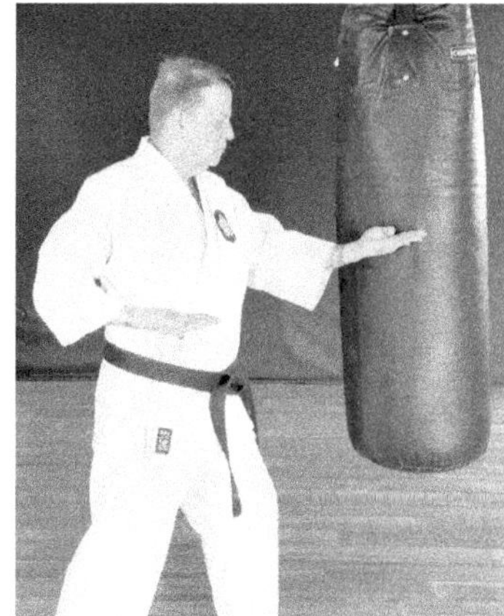

Chudan Zuki (Top) & Chudan Hari Uke (Bottom)

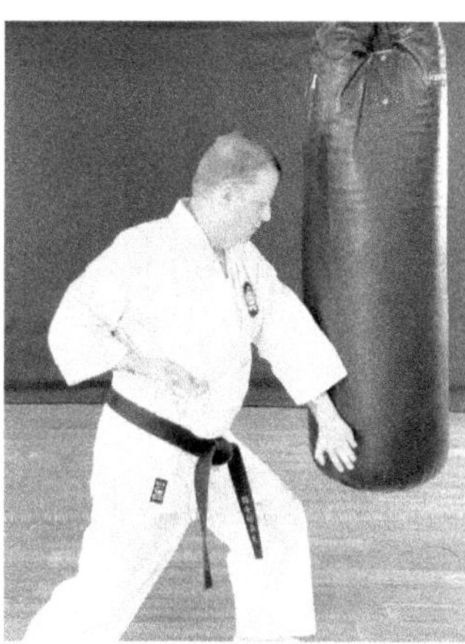

Gedan Zuki (Top) & Gedan Shotei Barai (Bottom)

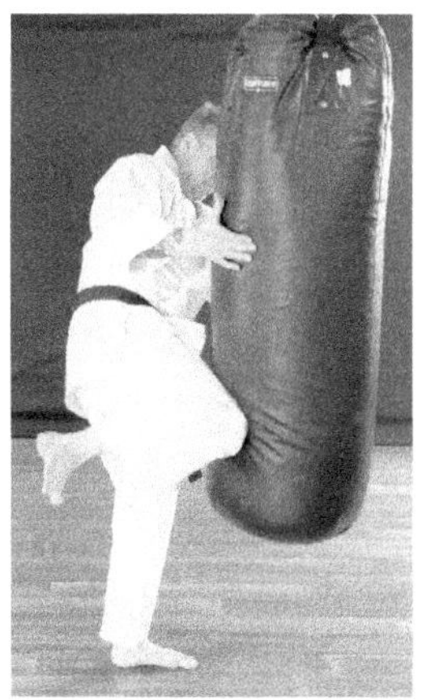
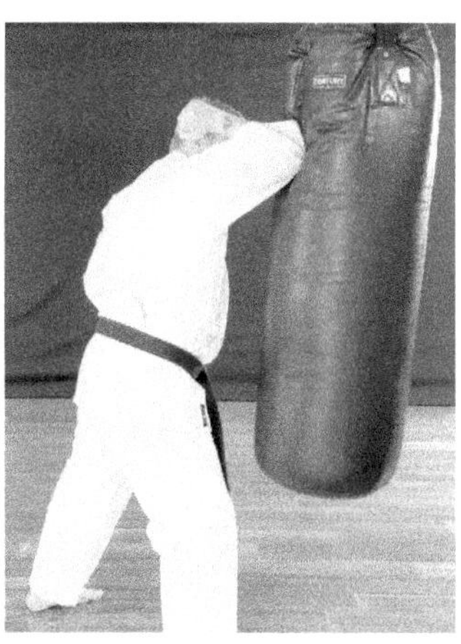

Counter 1: Hiza Uchi & Otoshi Empi Uchi

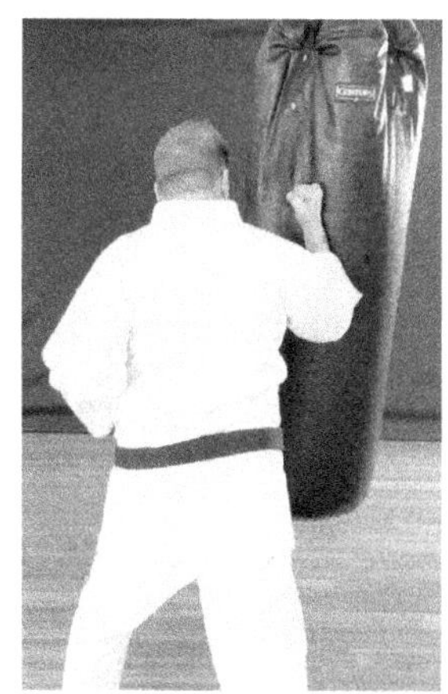

Counter 2: Soko Uke

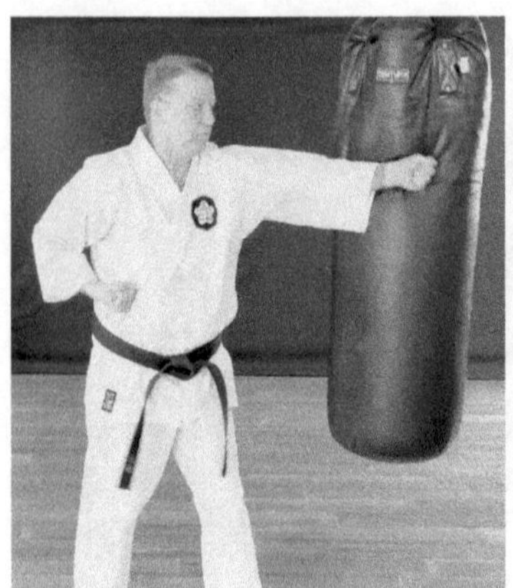
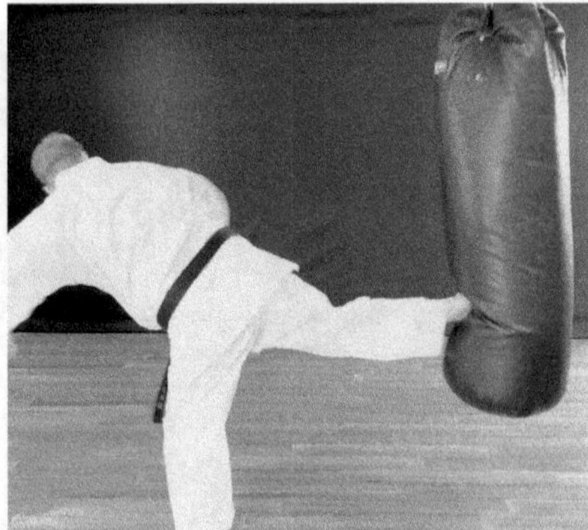

Counter 2: Uraken Uchi & Ushiro Kakato Geri

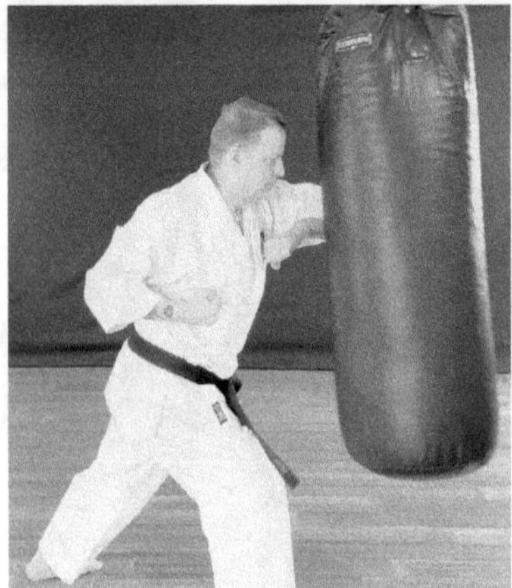
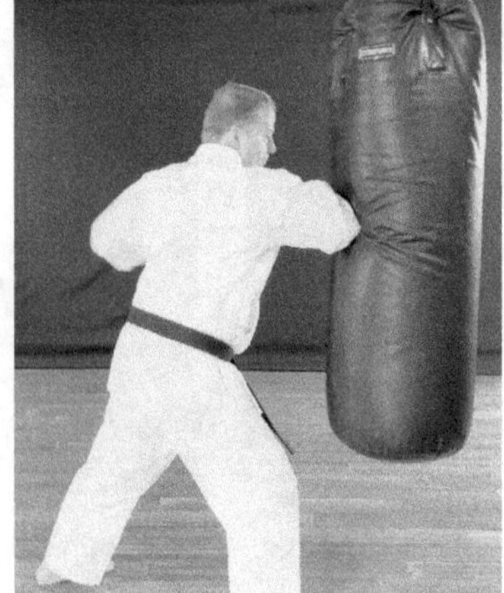

Counter 4: Kote Uchi & Mawashi Empi Uchi

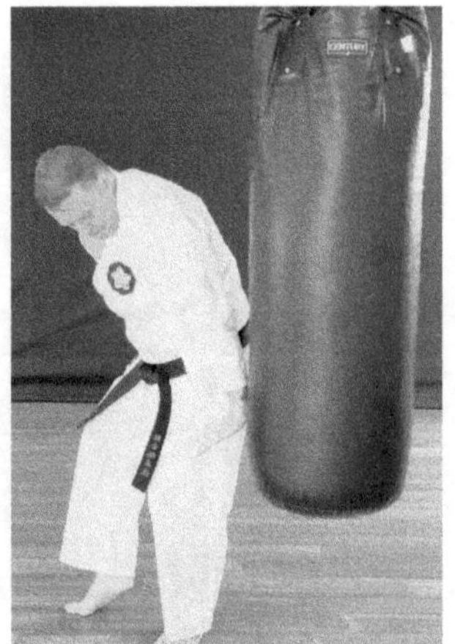
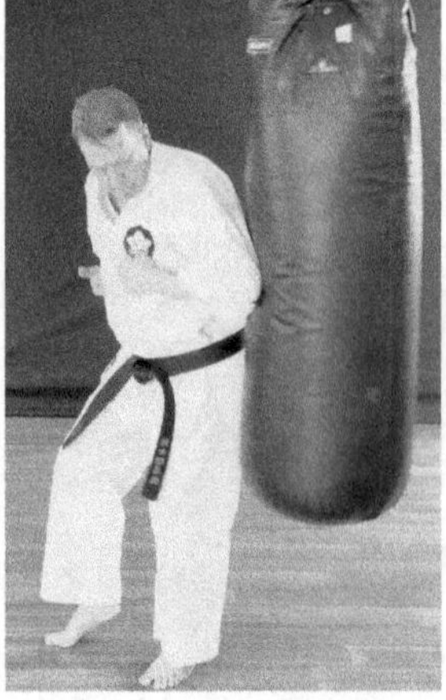

Counter 5: Gedan Shotei Uchi & Ushiro Empi Uchi

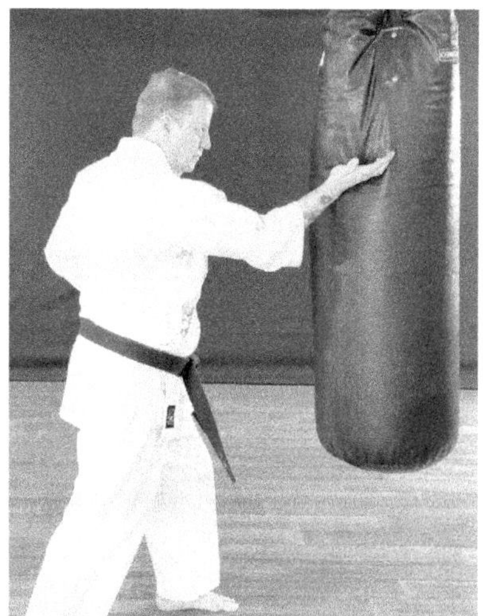

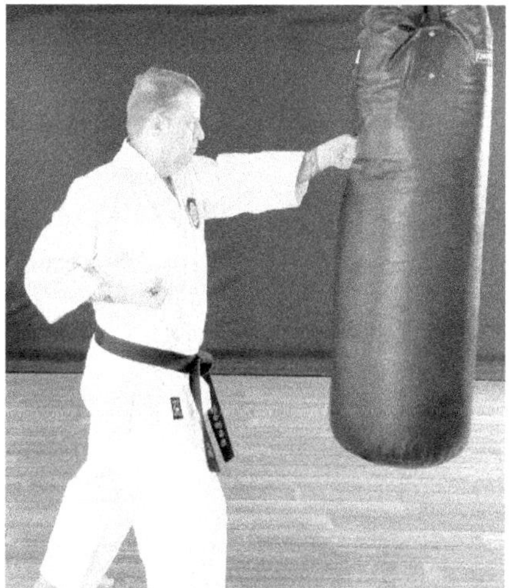

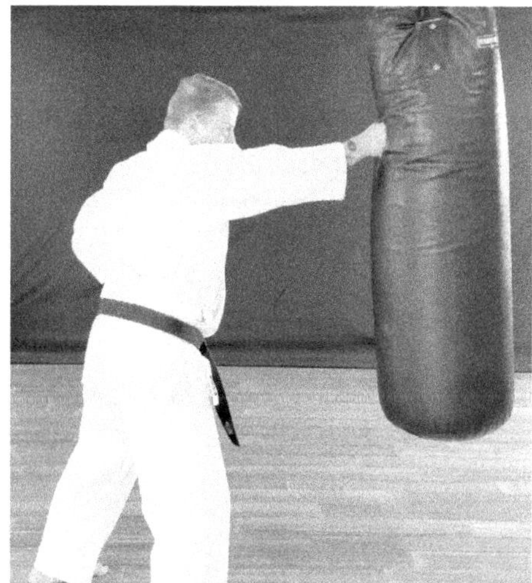

Counter 6: Mae Shuto Uchi & Tate Uchi

12. Kumite Rokyu (6)

Renoji Dachi Kamae
Chamber Hand at Chest,
Palm Up

Begin Counter 1

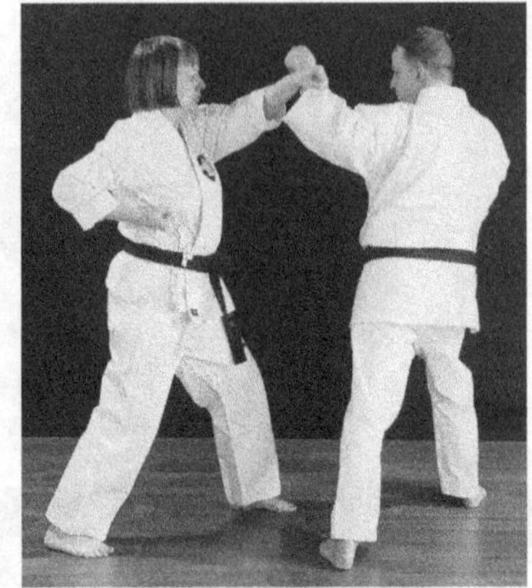

1. (Off - L): Step Forward, Jodan Zuki / (Def - R): Step Back to Side, Jodan Yoko Ko Uke

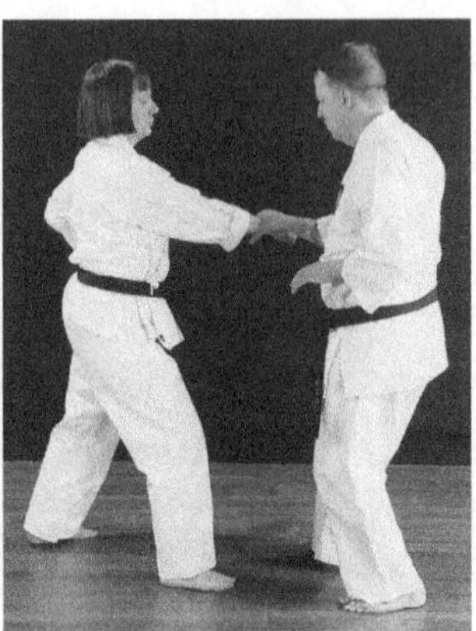

2. (Off - L): Step Forward, Chudan Zuki / (Def - R): Step Back Off Center, Chudan Hari to Hiki Uke

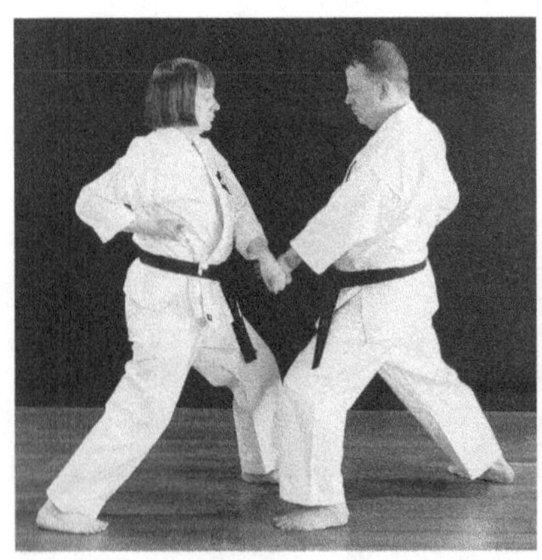

3. (Off - L): Step Forward, Gedan Zuki in Zenkutsu Dachi / (Def - R): Step Back, Gedan Shotei Barai in Zenkutsu Dachi

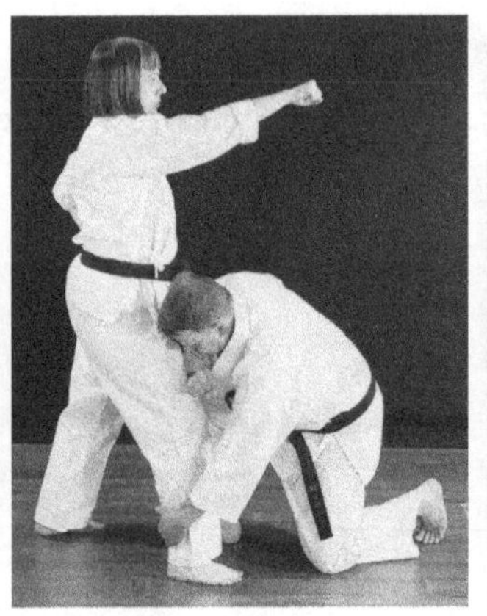

4. (Off - L): Step Forward, Jodan Zuki / (Def - R): Drop to Knee, Kibisu Gaeshi

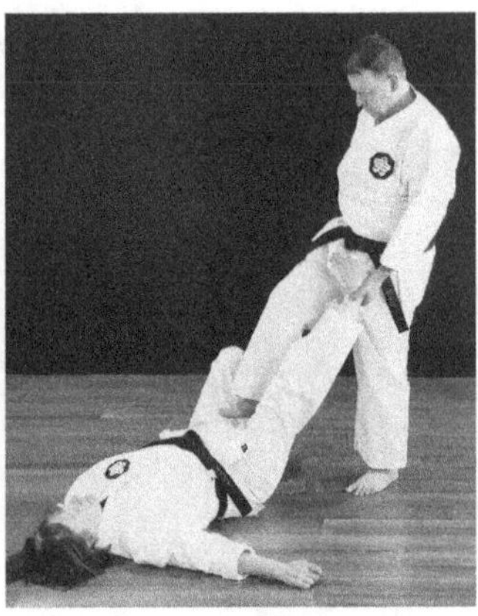

5. (Def - R): Kakato Otoshi Geri (Kiai)

Repeat in Other Direction

Begin Counter 2

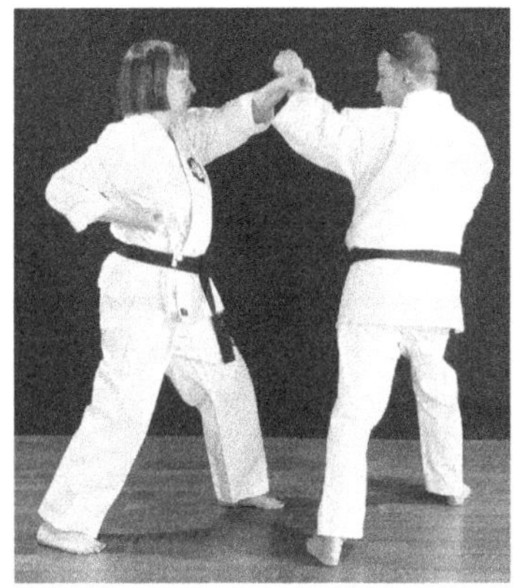

1. (Off - L): Step Forward, Jodan Zuki / (Def - R): Step Back to Side, Jodan Yoko Ko Uke

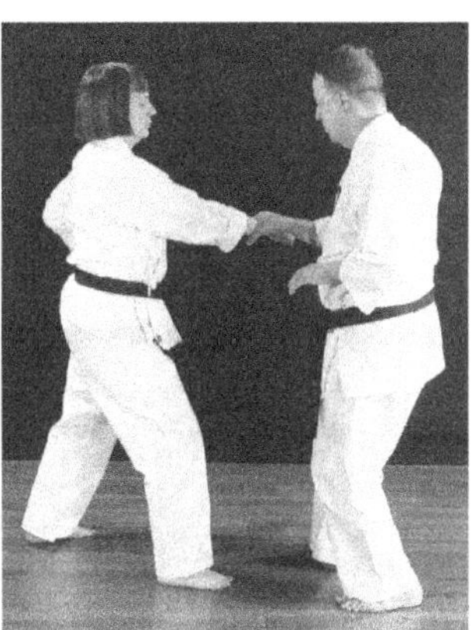

2. (Off - L): Step Forward, Chudan Zuki / (Def - R): Step Back Off Center, Chudan Hari to Hiki Uke

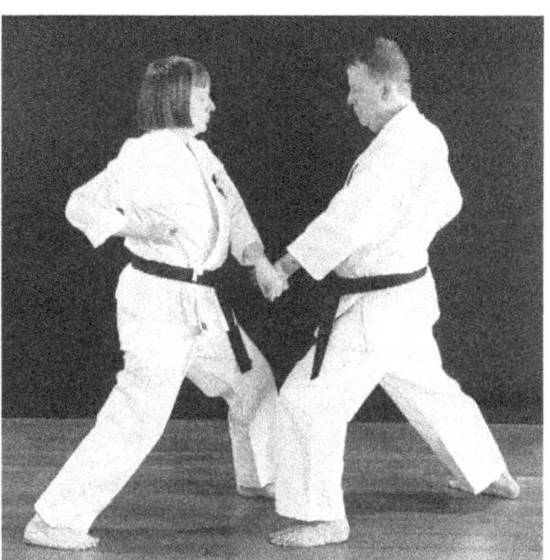

3. (Off - L): Step Forward, Gedan Zuki in Zenkutsu Dachi / (Def - R): Step Back, Gedan Shotei Barai in Zenkutsu Dachi

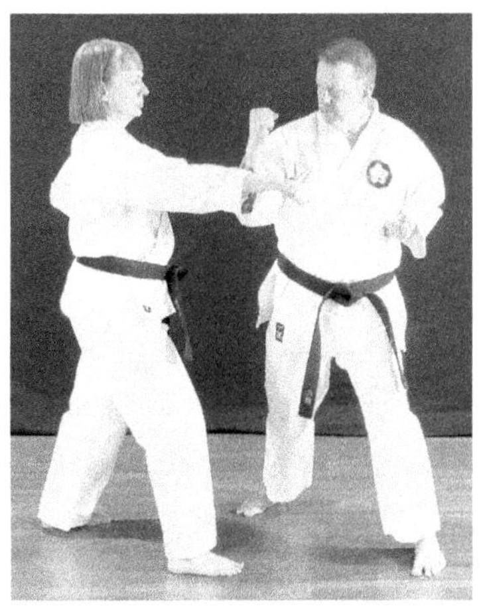

4. (Off - L): Step Forward, Chudan Zuki / (Def - R): Pivot Left, Soto Uchi

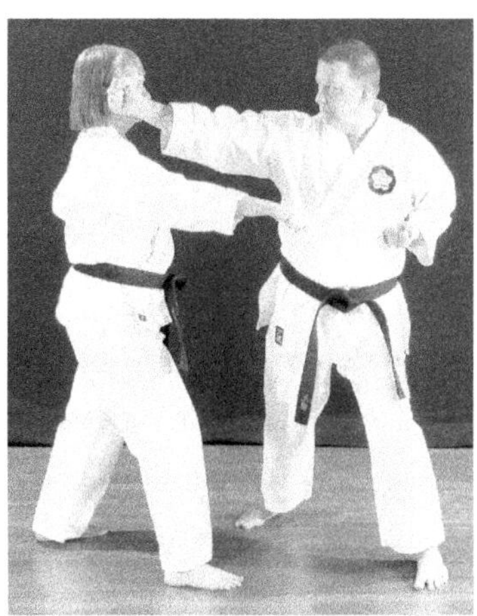

5. (Def - R): Yoko Uraken Uchi

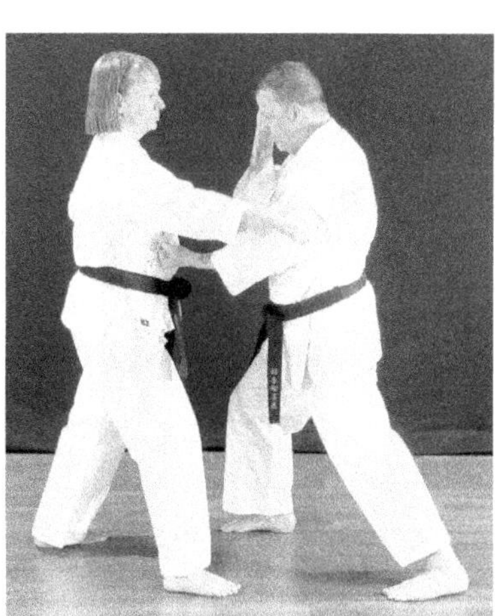

6. (Def - R): Pivot Right, Ura Zuki to Body

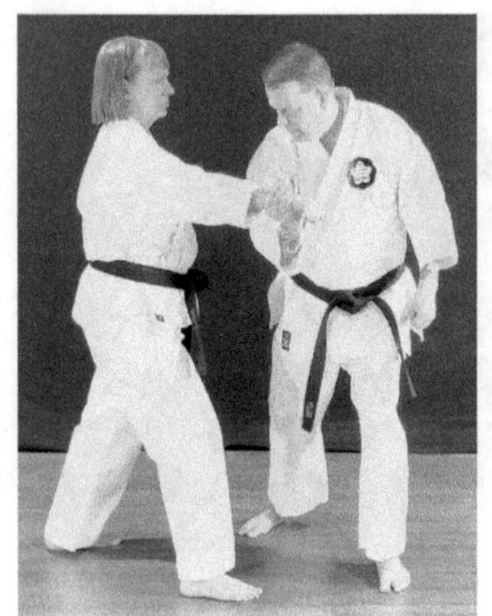

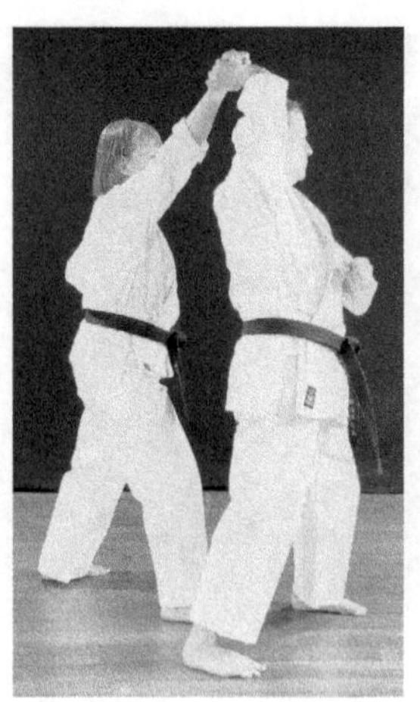

7. (Def - R): Catch Opponent's Wrist, Twist Underneath and Behind

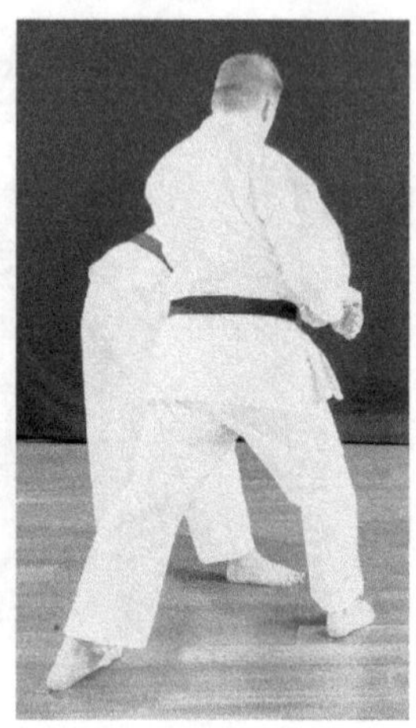

8. (Def - R): Push Down Opponent's Shoulder, Pulling Up on Wrist

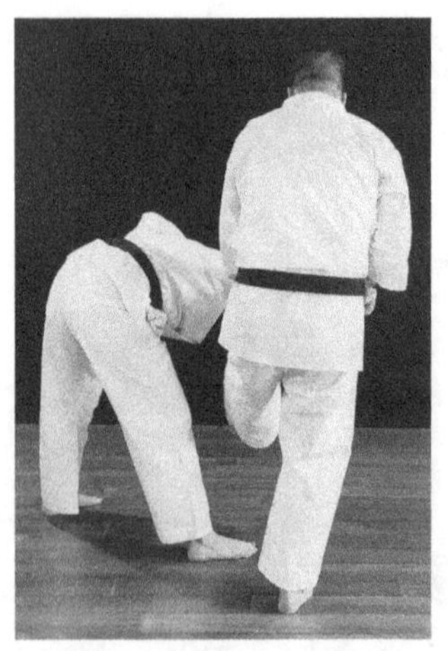

9. (Def - R): Jodan Mae Geri to Face

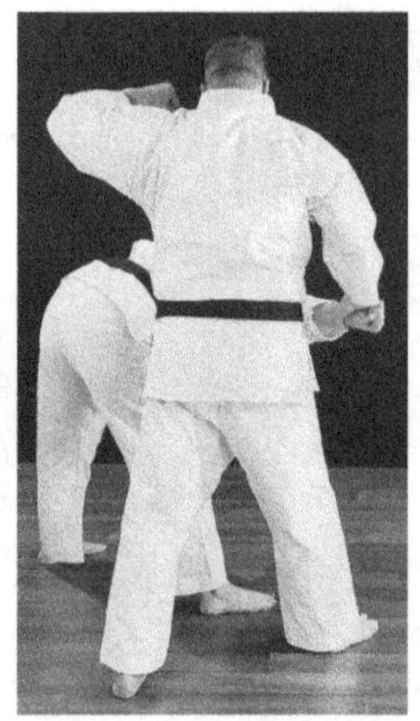

10. (Def - R): Drive Down with Forearm on Opponent's Arm, Pushing Opponent to Floor

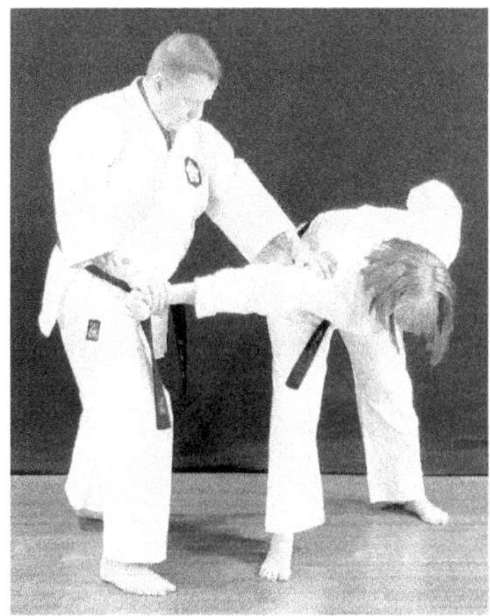
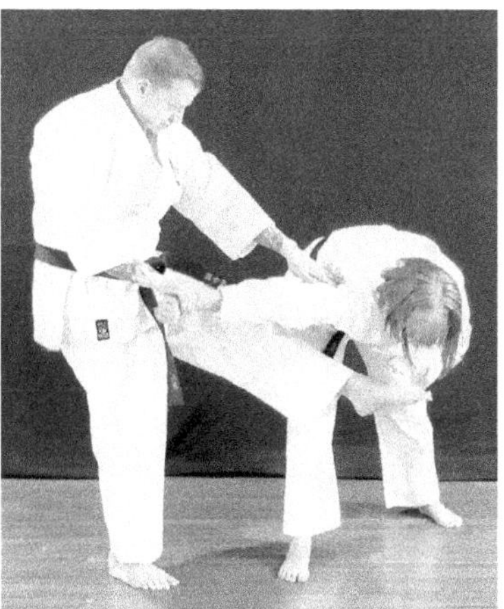
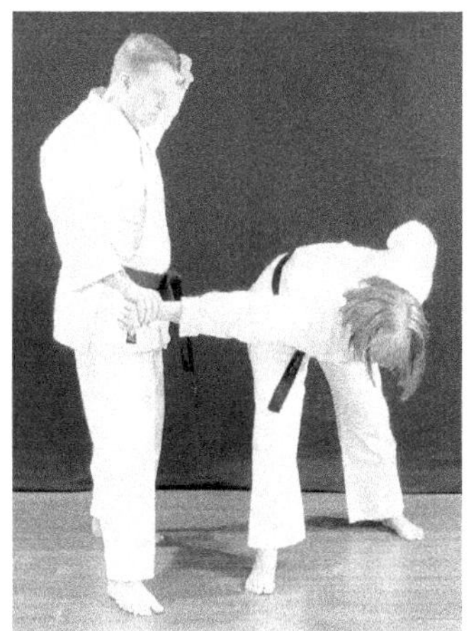

Forward POV of Steps 8 - 10

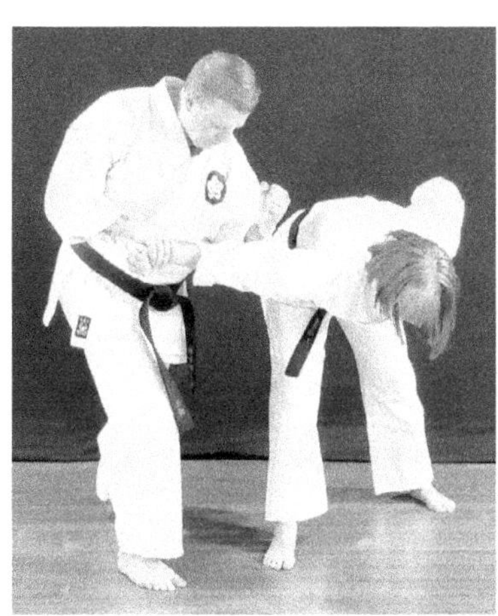

Forward POV of Step 10

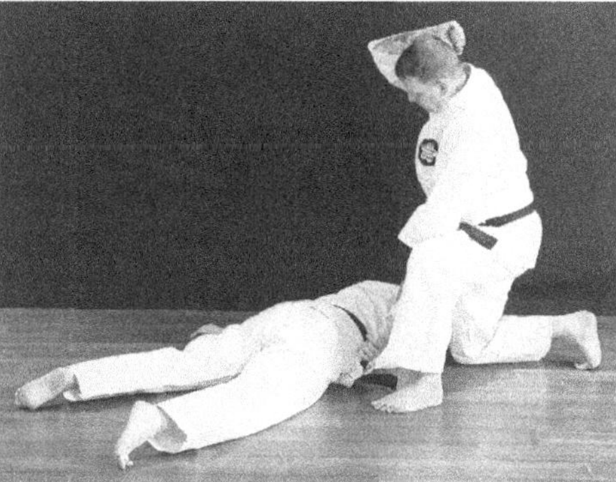
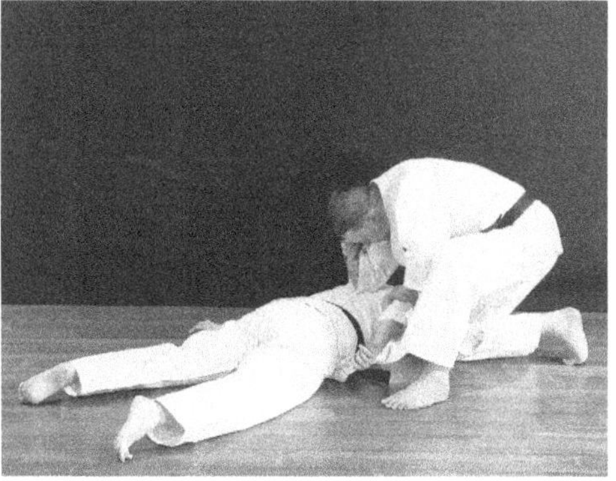

Repeat in Other Direction

11. (Def - R): Empi Otoshi Uchi to Opponent's Middle Upper Back (Kiai)

Begin Counter 3

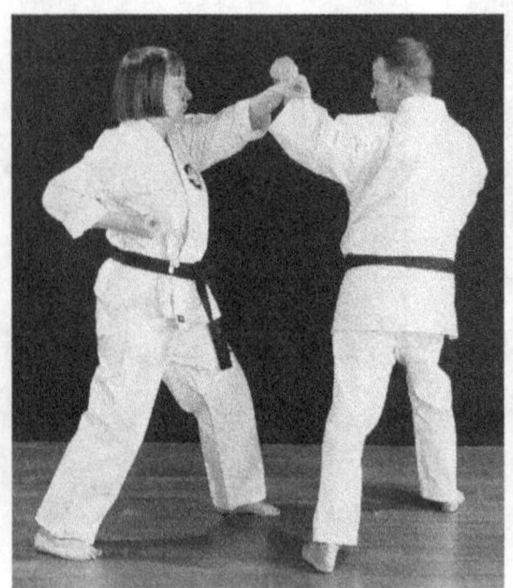
1. (Off - L): Step Forward, Jodan Zuki / (Def - R): Step Back to Side, Jodan Yoko Ko Uke

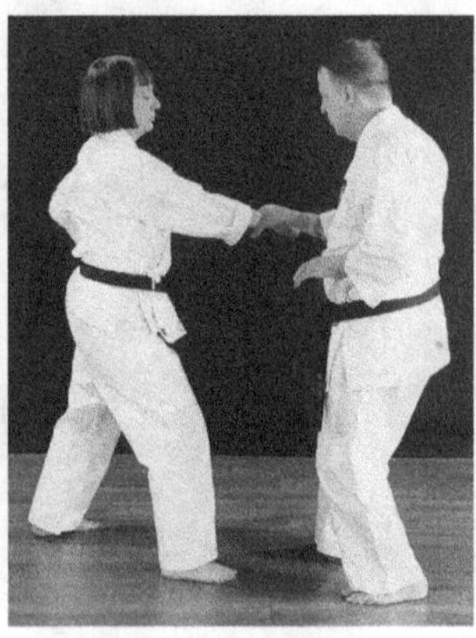
2. (Off - L): Step Forward, Chudan Zuki / (Def - R): Step Back Off Center, Chudan Hari to Hiki Uke

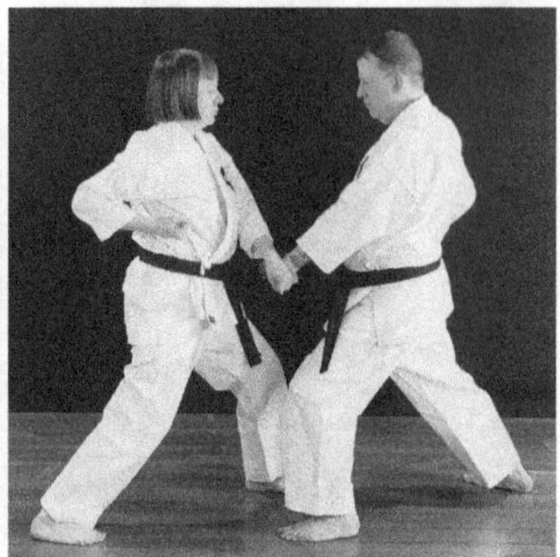
3. (Off - L): Step Forward, Gedan Zuki in Zenkutsu Dachi / (Def - R): Step Back, Gedan Shotei Barai in Zenkutsu Dachi

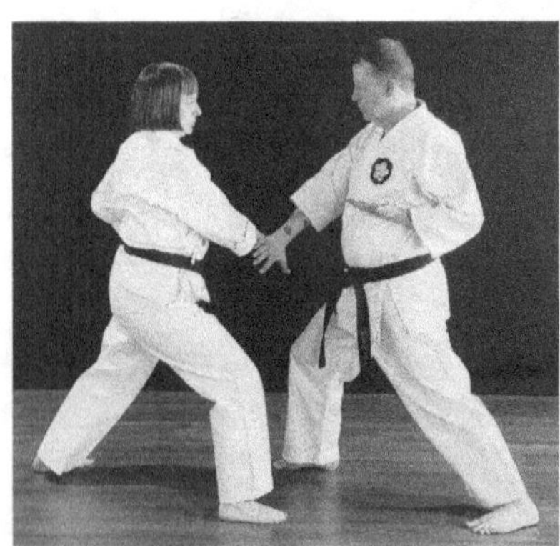
4. (Off - L): Step Forward, Gedan Zuki in Zenkutsu Dachi / (Def - R): Step Back, Gedan Shotei Barai in Zenkutsu Dachi

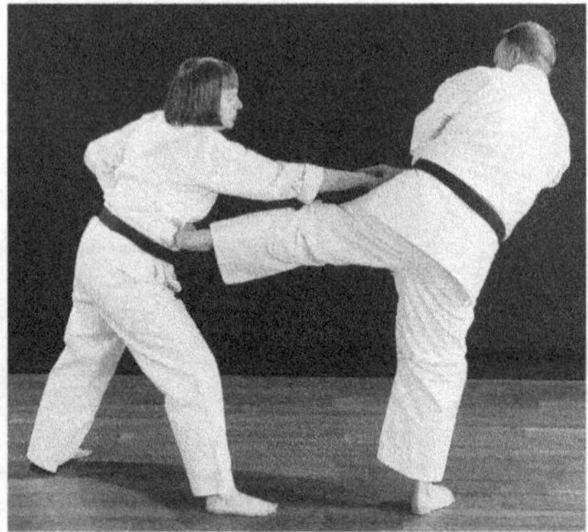
5. (Def - R): Grab Opponent's Wrist, Pivot Right, Reposition on Right Foot, Yoko Geri

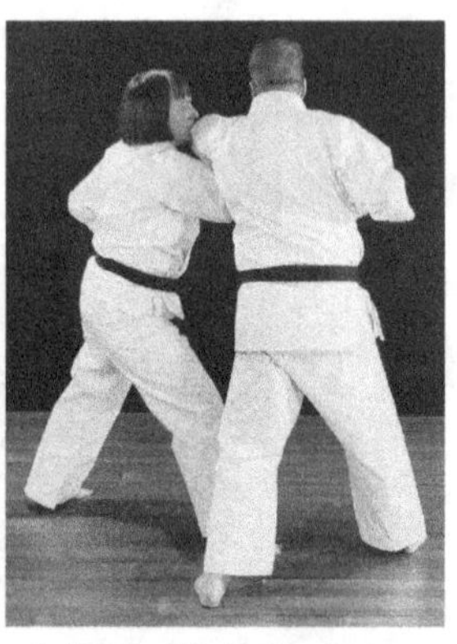
6. (Def - R): Yoko Jodan Empi Uchi

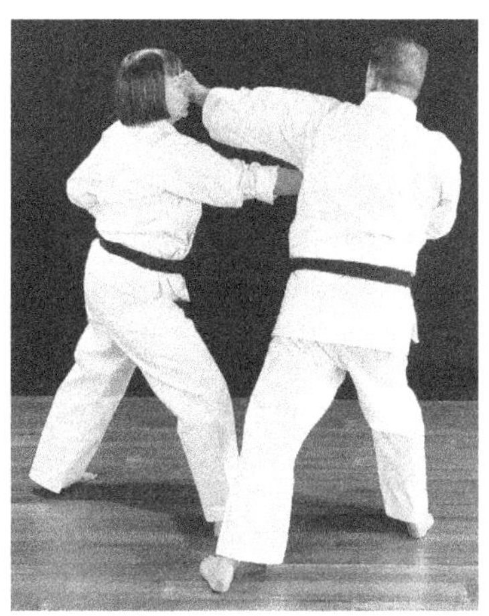

7. (Def - R): Lean Away, Yoko Uraken Uchi

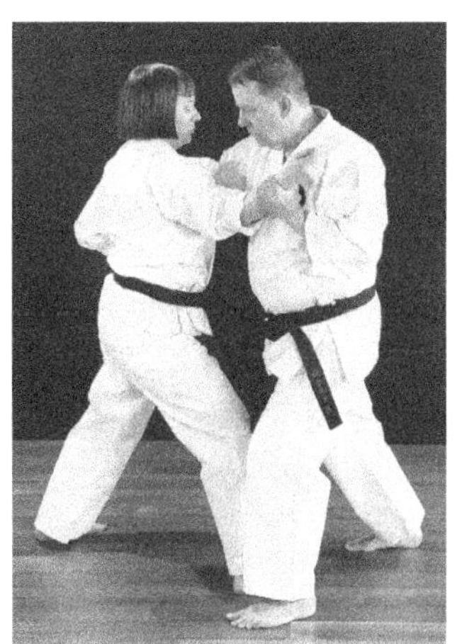

8. (Def - R): Reposition to Side, Put Opponent's Wrist in Left Hand, Osoto-gari

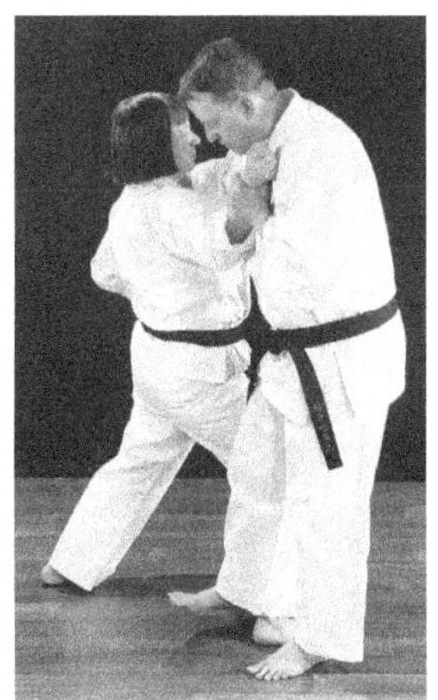

Osoto-gari (cont.)

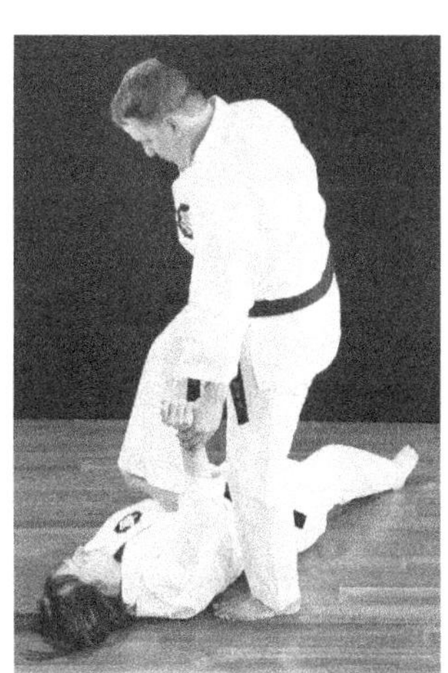

9. (Def - R): Kakato Otoshi Geri to Chest

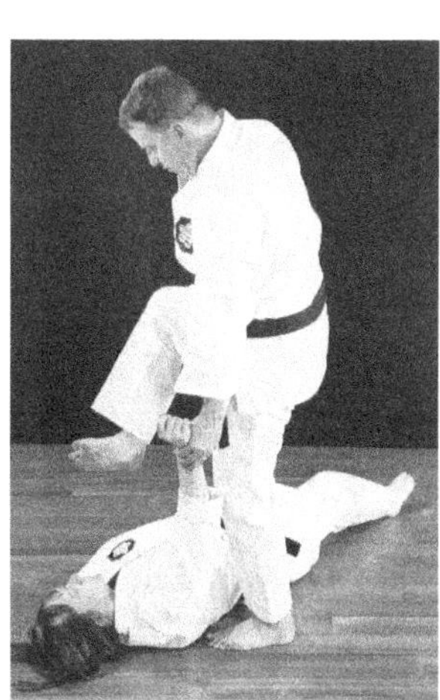

10. (Def - R): Sokuto Otoshi Geri to Throat

Repeat in Other Direction

(Def - R): Sokuto Otoshi Geri (cont.) (Kiai)

Begin Counter 4

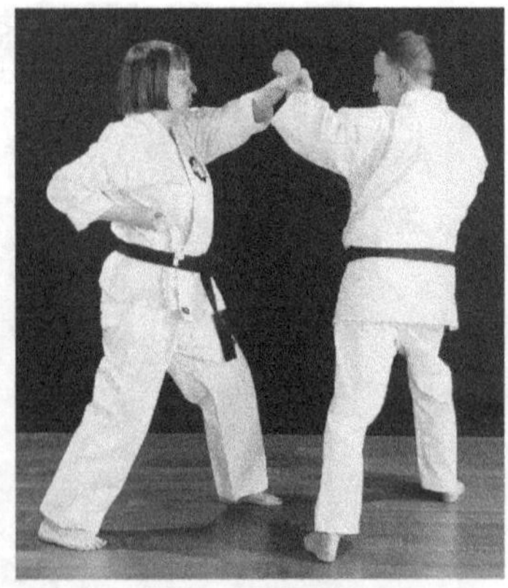

1. (Off - L): Step Forward, Jodan Zuki / (Def - R): Step Back to Side, Jodan Yoko Ko Uke

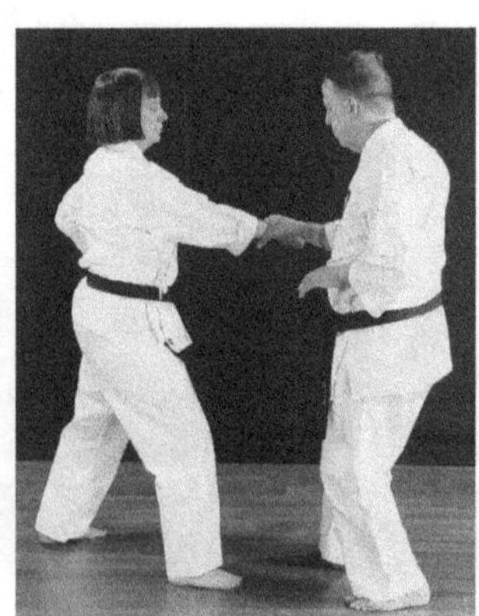

2. (Off - L): Step Forward, Chudan Zuki / (Def - R): Step Back Off Center, Chudan Hari to Hiki Uke

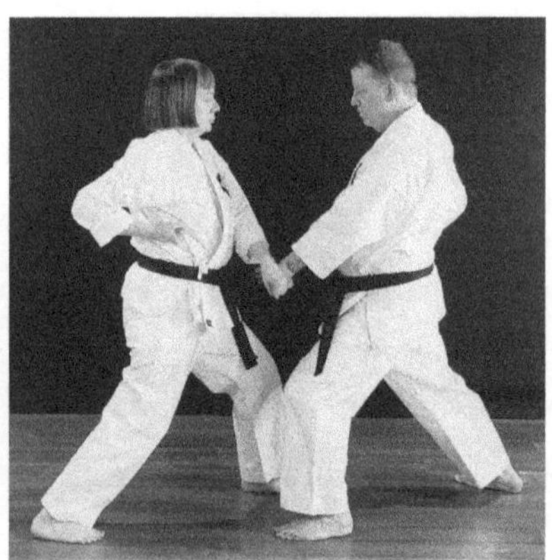

3. (Off - L): Step Forward, Gedan Zuki in Zenkutsu Dachi / (Def - R): Step Back, Gedan Shotei Barai in Zenkutsu Dachi

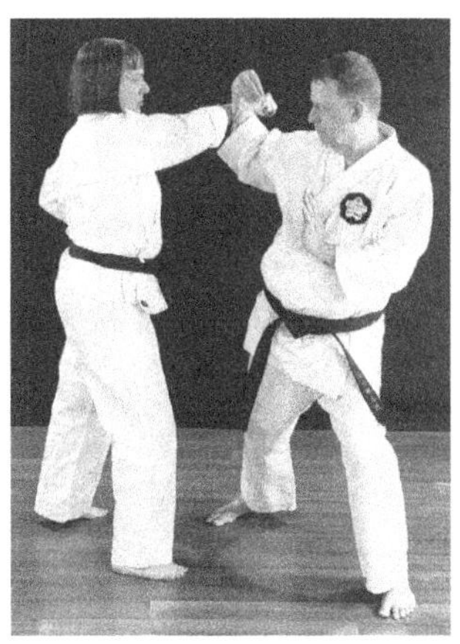

4. (Off - L): Step Forward, Jodan Zuki / (Def - R): Step Back to Side, Jodan Yoko Ko Uke

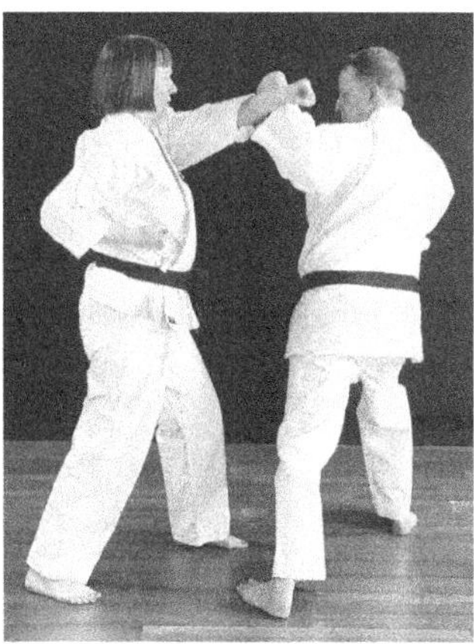

5. (Off - L): Step Forward, Jodan Zuki / (Def - R): Step Back to Side, Jodan Yoko Ko Uke

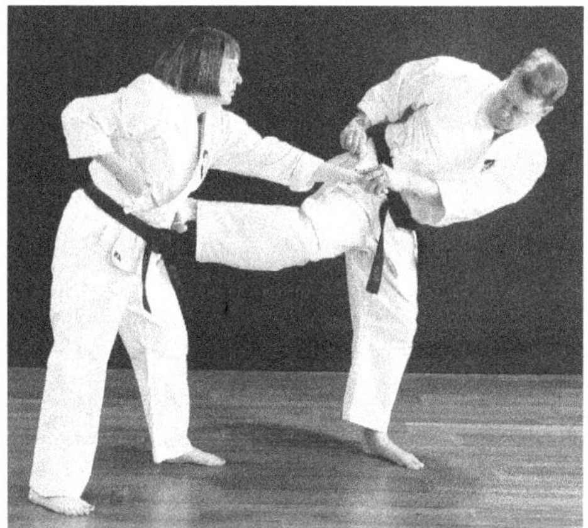

6. (Def - R): Grab Opponent's Wrist, Pivot Right, Reposition Left Foot, Yoko Geri

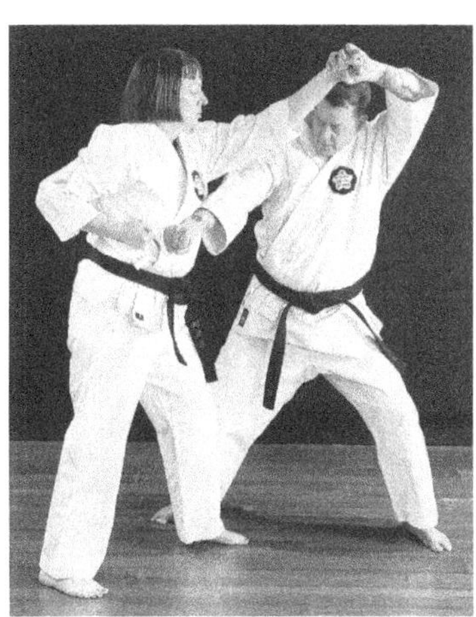

7. (Def - R): Yoko Tettsui Uchi

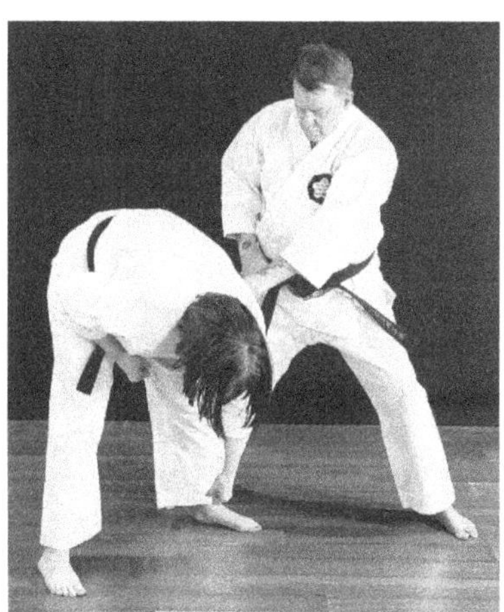

8. (Def - R): Throw Opponent's Left Arm Down

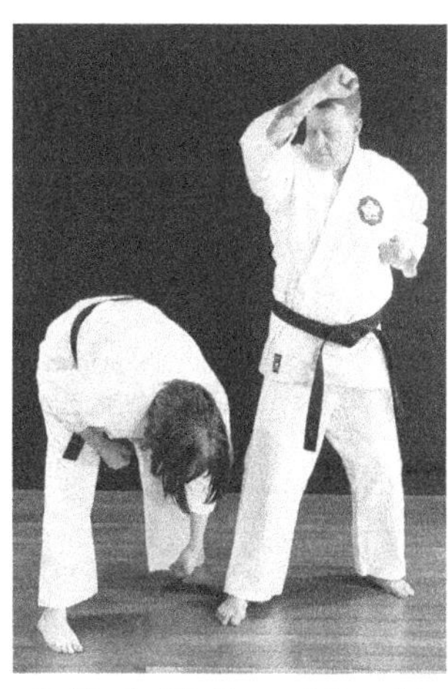

9. (Def - R): Tettsui Otoshi Uchi

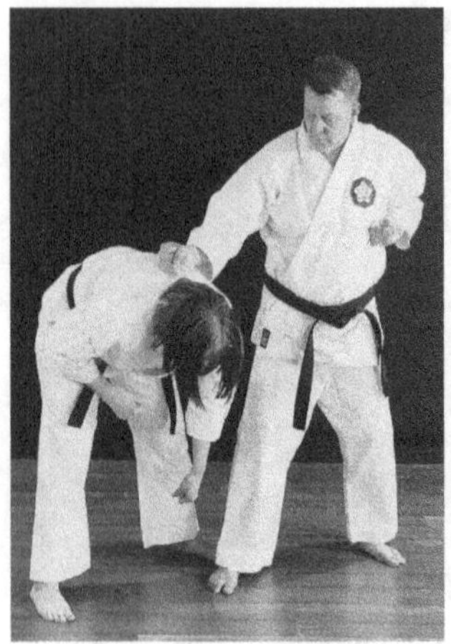

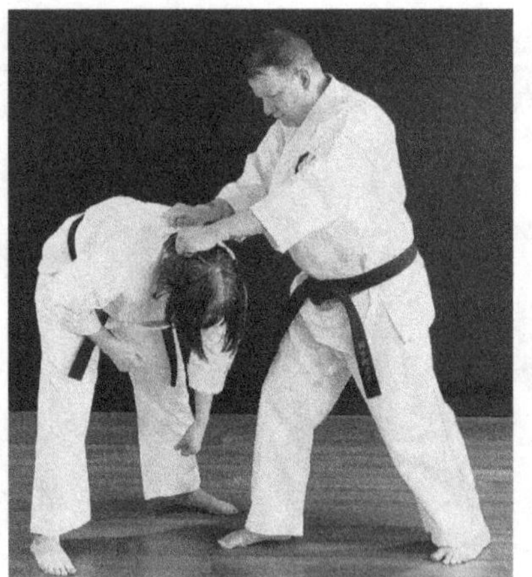

Repeat in Other Direction

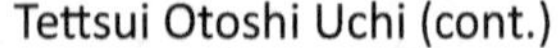

Tettsui Otoshi Uchi (cont.)

10. (Def - R): Hiza Uchi to Head (Kiai), Push Away

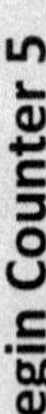

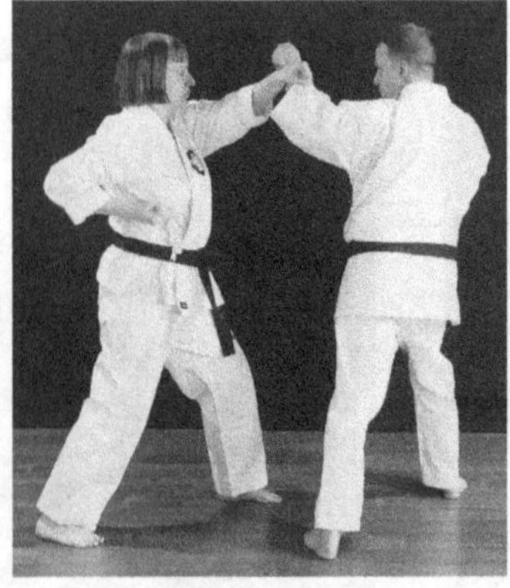

1. (Off - L): Step Forward, Jodan Zuki / (Def - R): Step Back to Side, Jodan Yoko Ko Uke

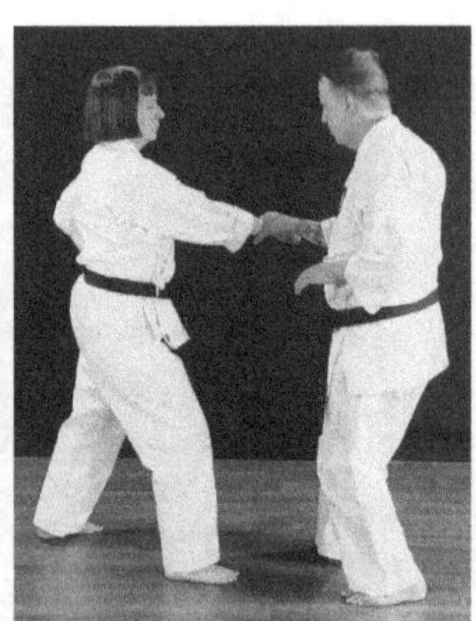

2. (Off - L): Step Forward, Chudan Zuki / (Def - R): Step Back Off Center, Chudan Hari to Hiki Uke

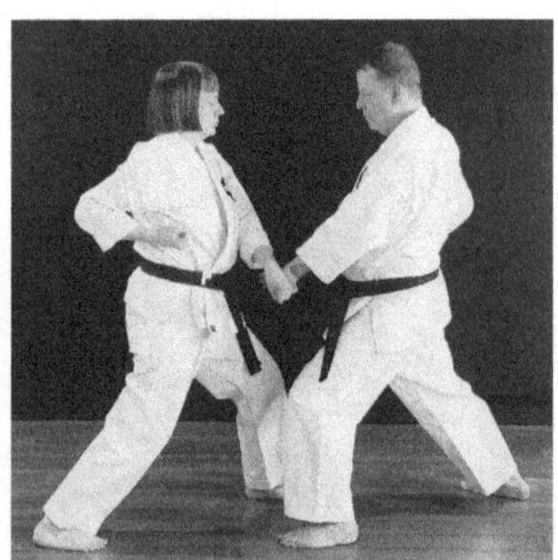

3. (Off - L): Step Forward, Gedan Zuki in Zenkutsu Dachi / (Def - R): Step Back, Gedan Shotei Barai in Zenkutsu Dachi

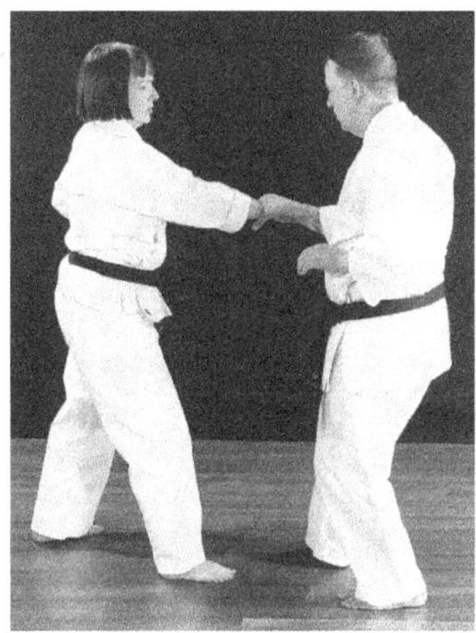

4. (Off - L): Step Forward, Chudan Zuki / (Def - R): Step Back Off Center, Chudan Hari to Hiki Uke

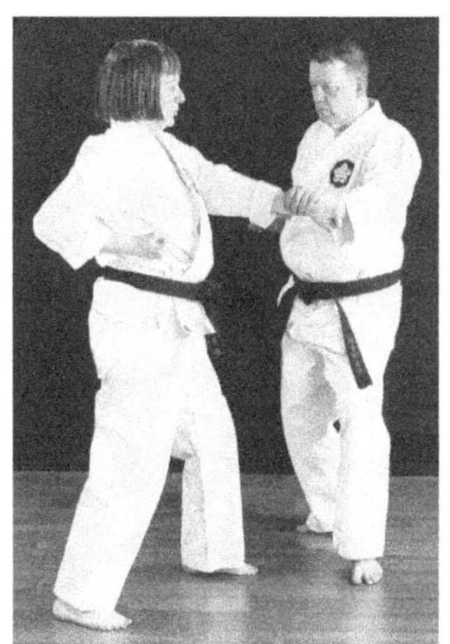

5. (Off - L): Step Forward, Chudan Zuki / (Def - R): Step Back Off Center, Chudan Hari to Hiki Uke, Grab Wrist

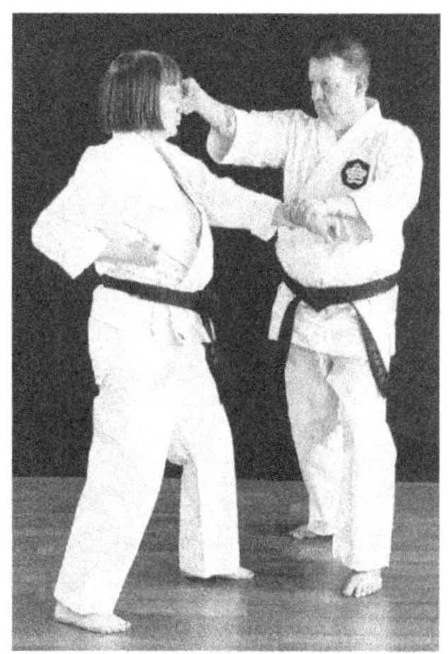

6. (Def - R): Jodan Tate Uchi

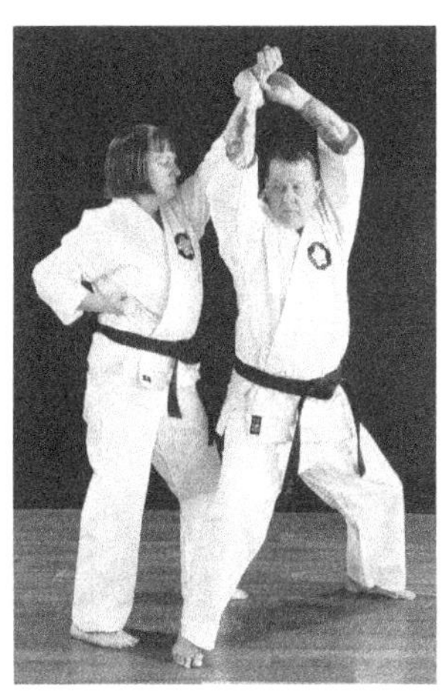

7. (Def - R): Grab Arm with Both Hands, Step in Front of Opponent, Raising Arm

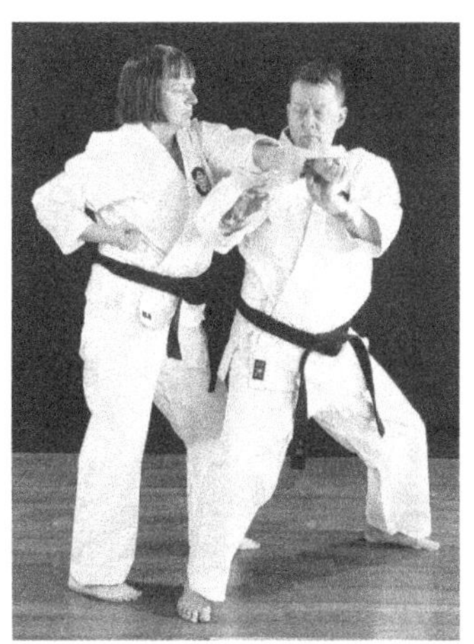

8. (Def - R): Twist Opponent's Arm and Bring Down on Shoulder

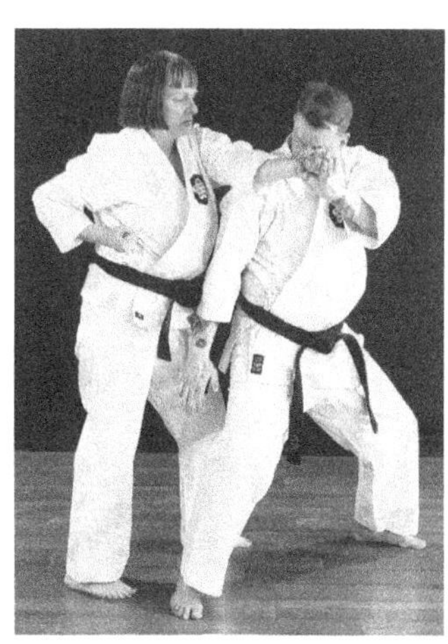

9. (Def - R): Ushiro Shuto Uchi to Groin

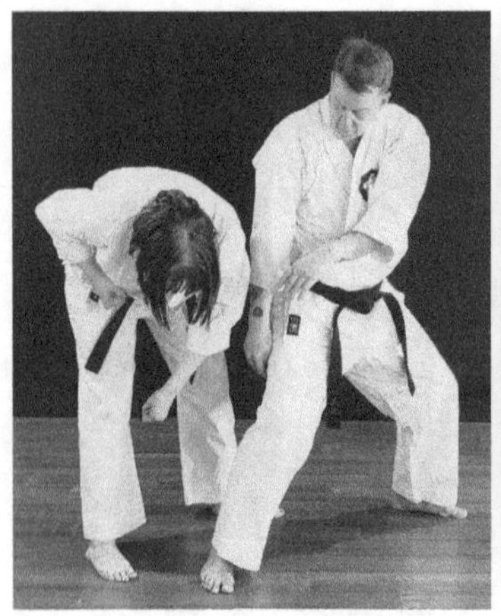

10. (Def - R): Throw Opponent's Left Arm Down

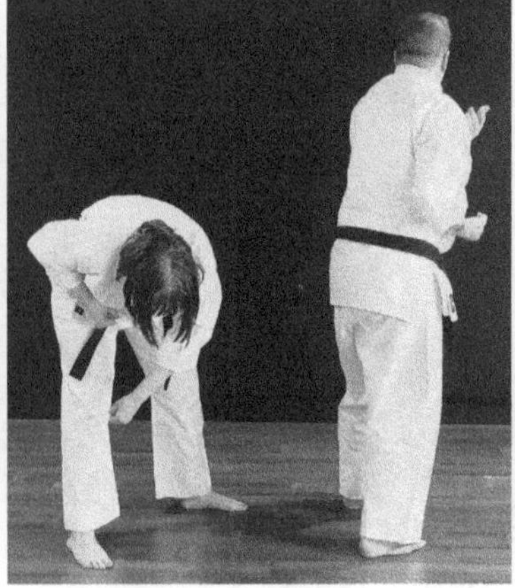

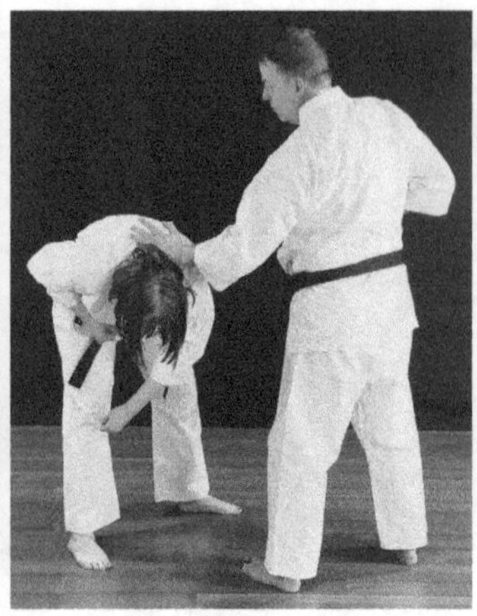

11. (Def - R): Mawatte, Shuto Otoshi Uchi to Base of Skull (Kiai)

Repeat in Other Direction

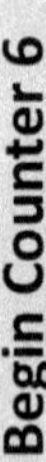

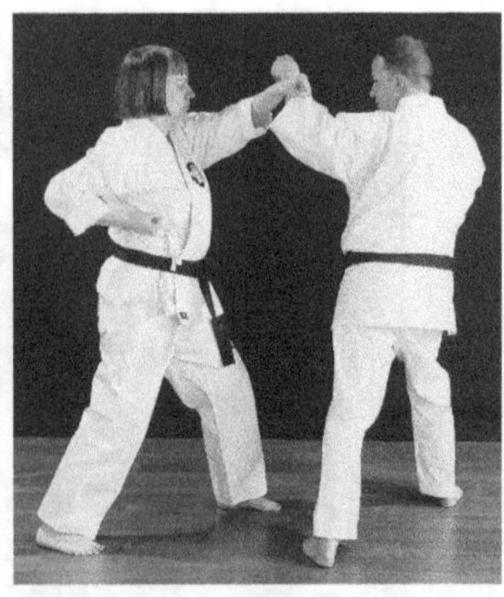

1. (Off - L): Step Forward, Jodan Zuki / (Def - R): Step Back to Side, Jodan Yoko Ko Uke

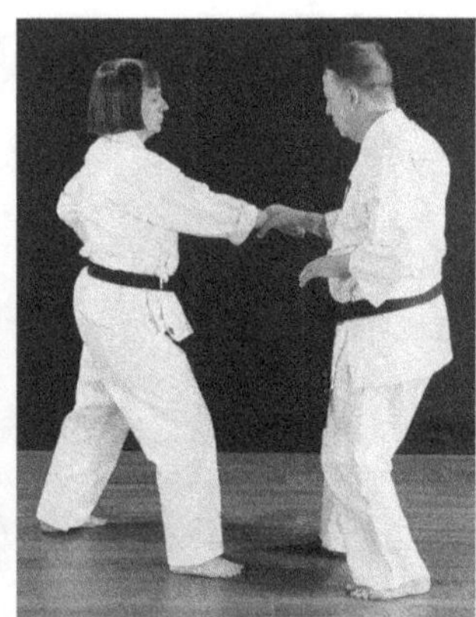

2. (Off - L): Step Forward, Chudan Zuki / (Def - R): Step Back Off Center, Chudan Hari to Hiki Uke

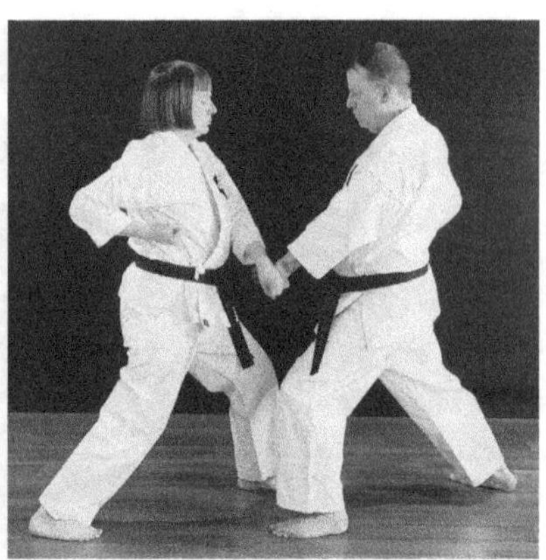

3. (Off - L): Step Forward, Gedan Zuki in Zenkutsu Dachi / (Def - R): Step Back, Gedan Shotei Barai in Zenkutsu Dachi

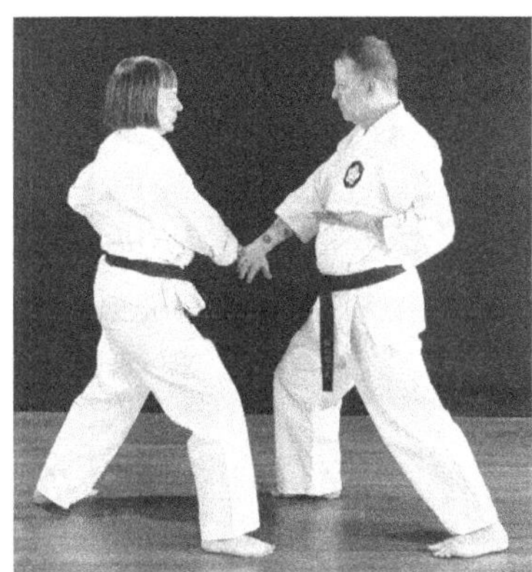
4. (Off - L): Step Forward, Gedan Zuki in Zenkutsu Dachi / (Def - R): Step Back, Gedan Shotei Barai in Zenkutsu Dachi

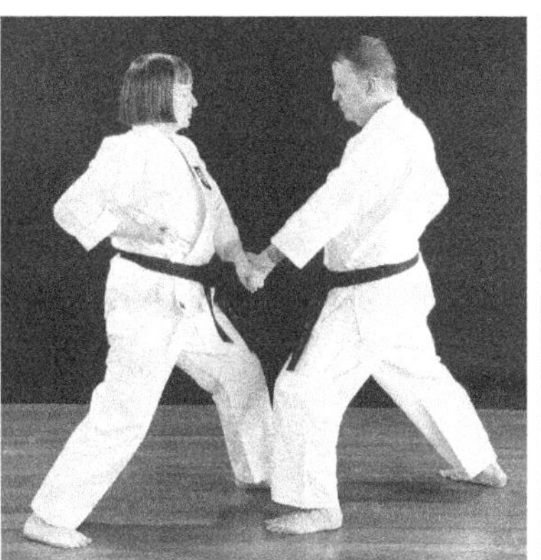
5. (Off - L): Step Forward, Gedan Zuki in Zenkutsu Dachi / (Def - R): Step Back, Gedan Shotei Barai in Zenkutsu Dachi

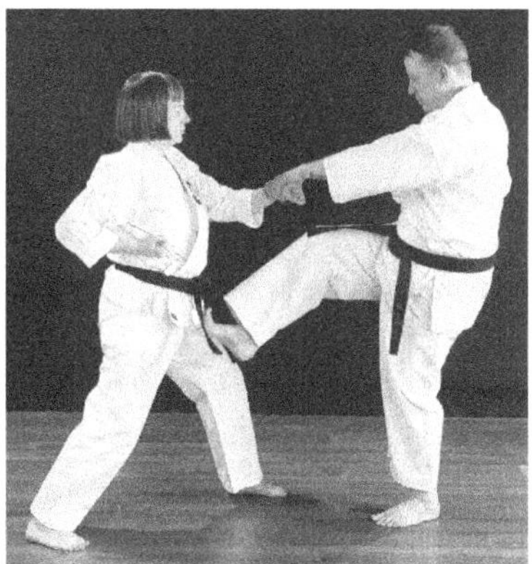
6. (Def - R): Grab Wrist, Gedan Mae Geri

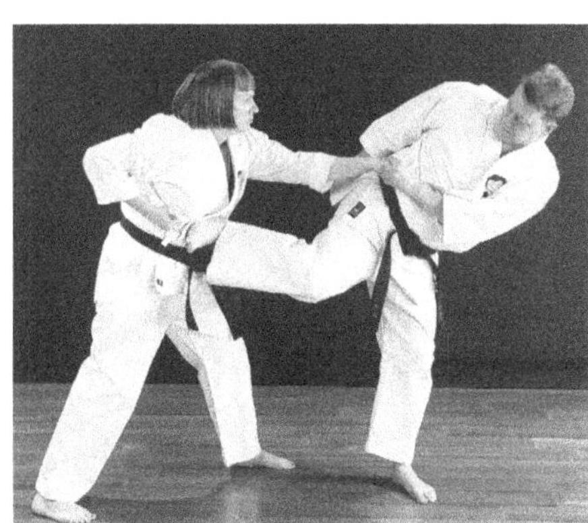
7. (Def - R): Pivot Left, Yoko Geri

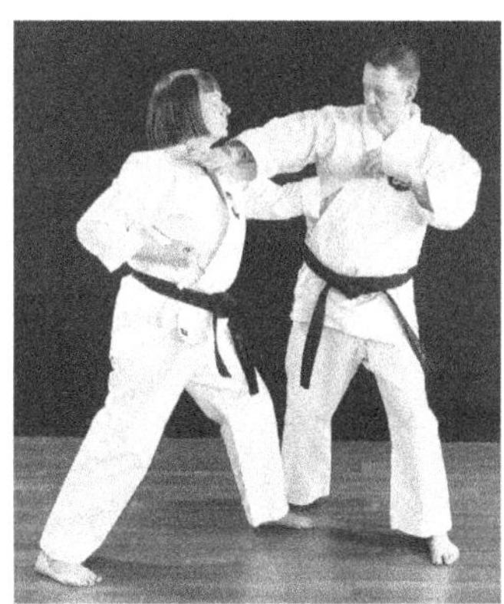
8. (Def - R): Shuto Uchi to Throat

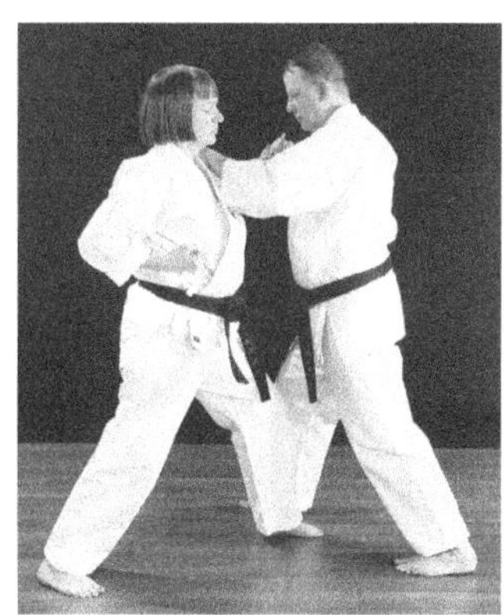
9. (Def - R): Osoto-gari

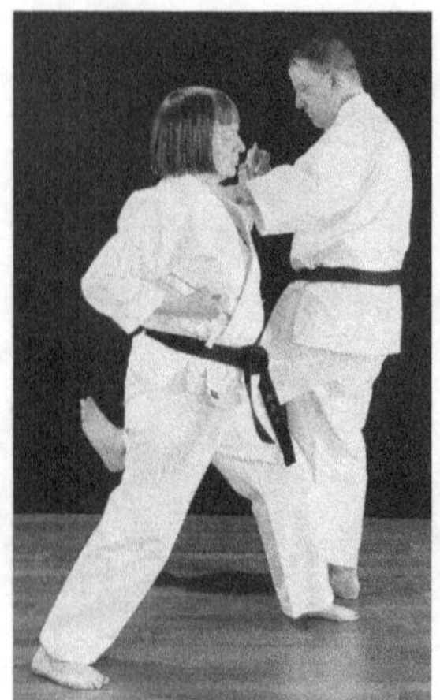

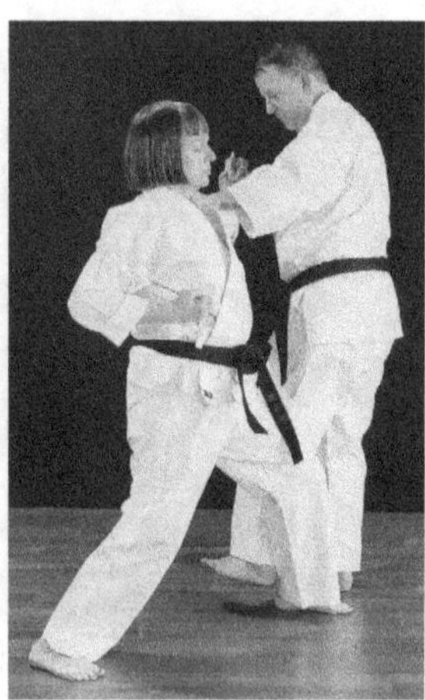

Osoto-gari (cont.)

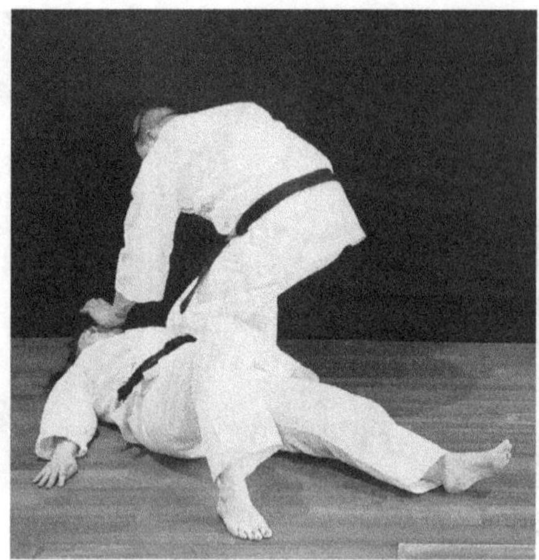

10. (Def - R): Follow Opponent Down with Left Knee on Ribs, Shotei Otoshi Uchi to Face (Kiai)

Repeat in Other Direction

Kumite Rokyu - Bag Work

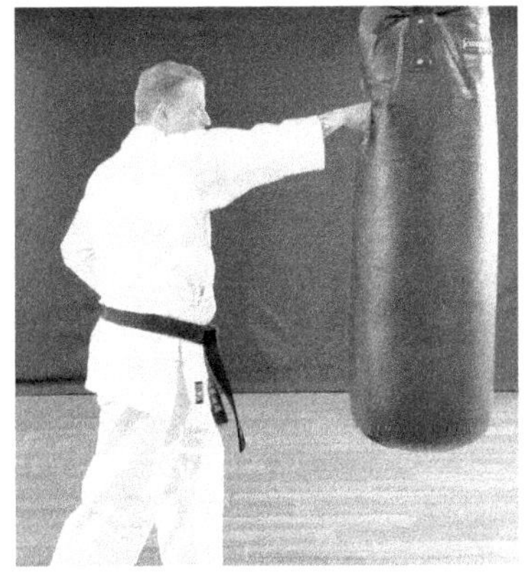
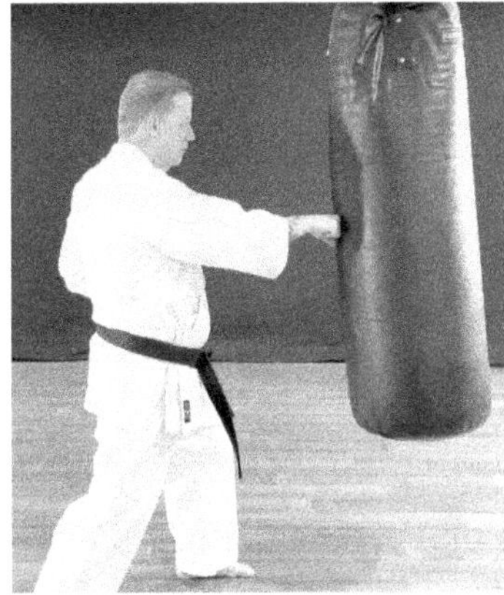
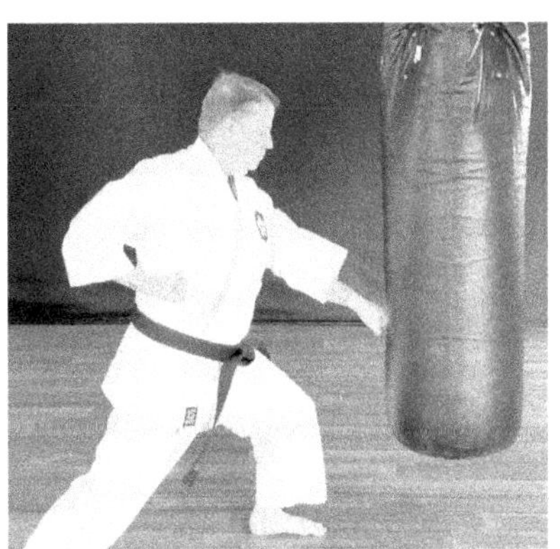

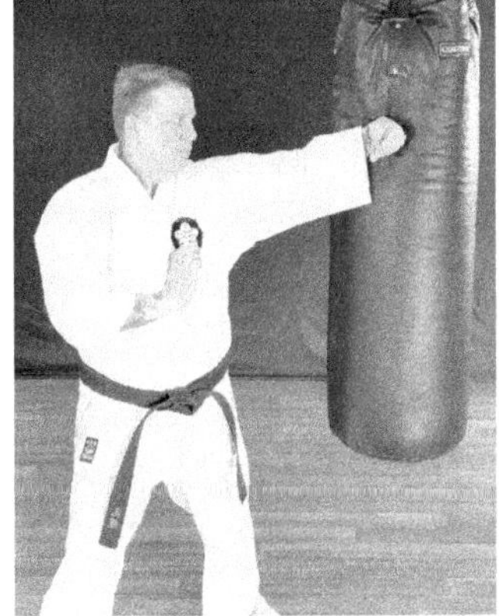

Jodan Zuki (Top) & Jodan Yoko Ko Uke (Bottom)

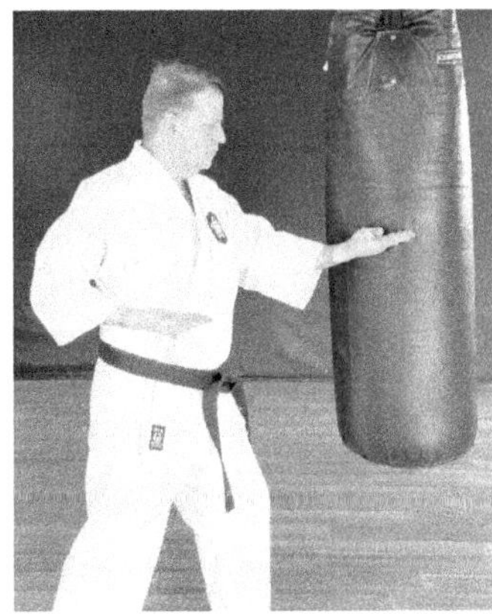

Chudan Zuki (Top) & Chudan Hari Uke (Bottom)

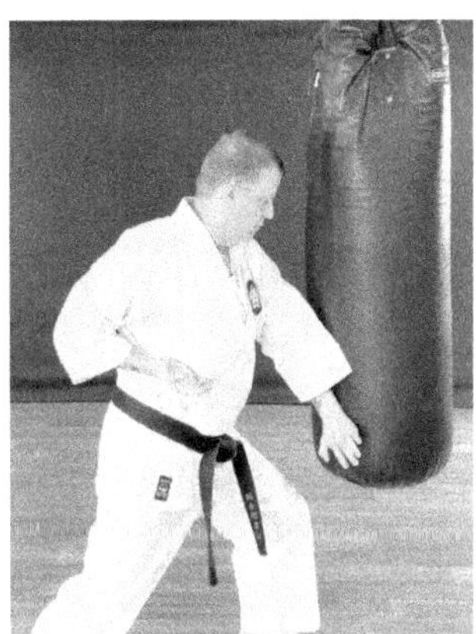

Gedan Zuki (Top) & Shotei Barai (Bottom)

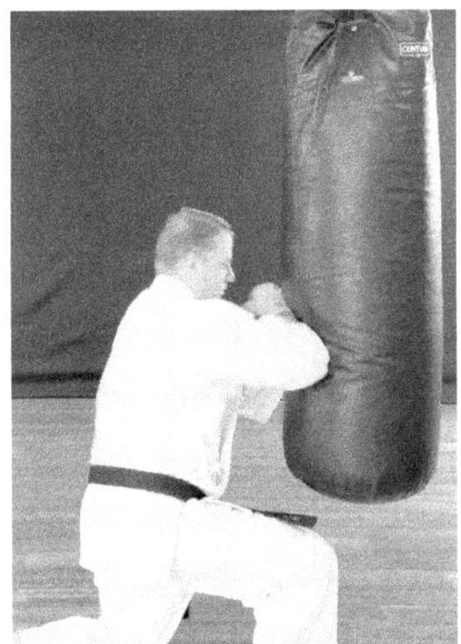
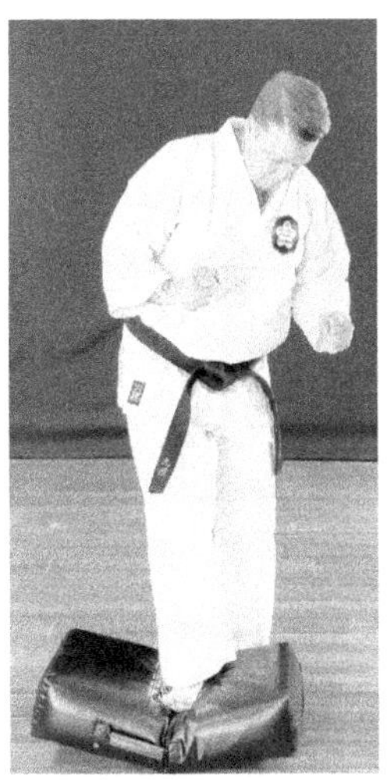

Counter 1: Kote Uchi & Kakato Otoshi Geri

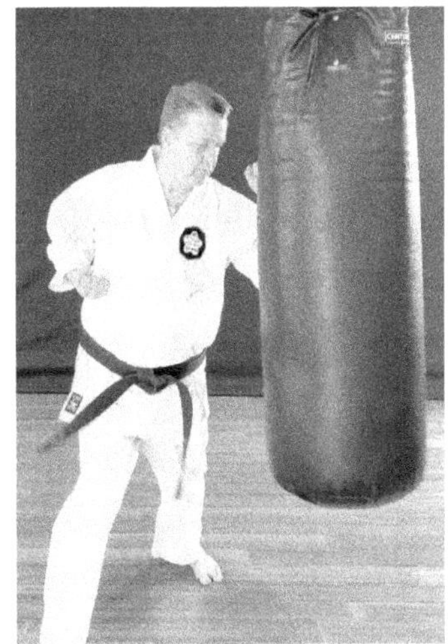

Counter 2: Soto Uke

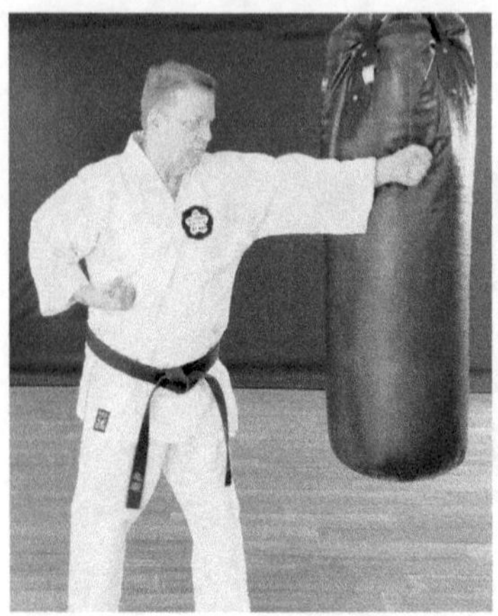
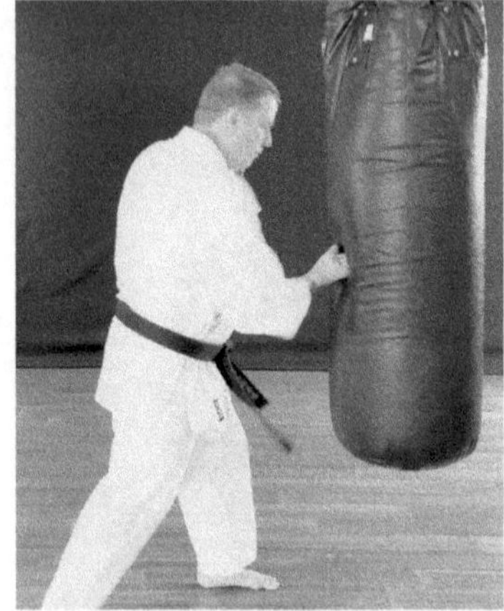
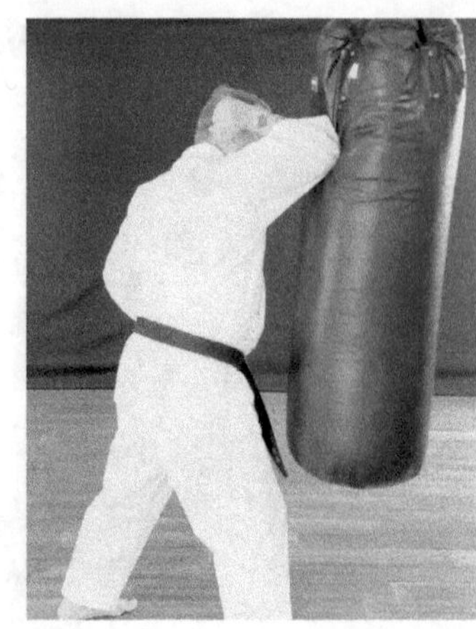

Counter 2: Yoko Uraken Uchi, Ura Zuki, & Empi Otoshi Uchi

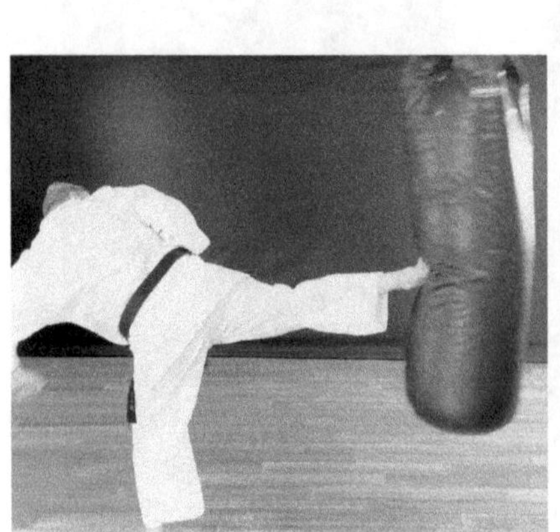
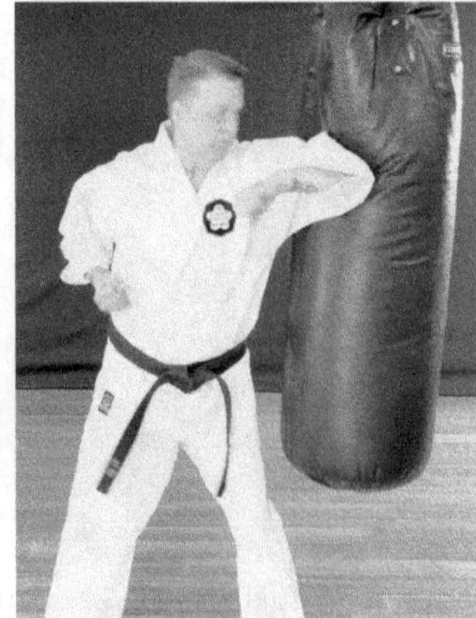
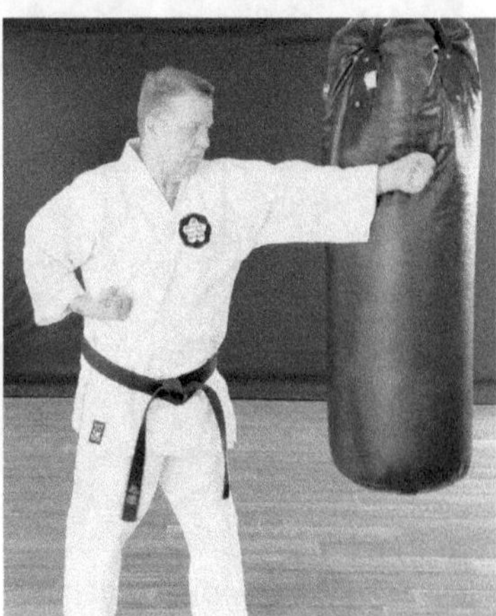

Counter 3: Yoko Geri, Ushiro Empi Uchi, & Yoko Uraken Uchi

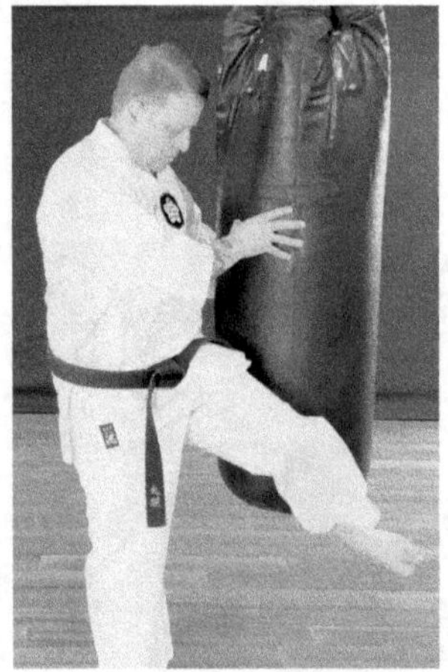
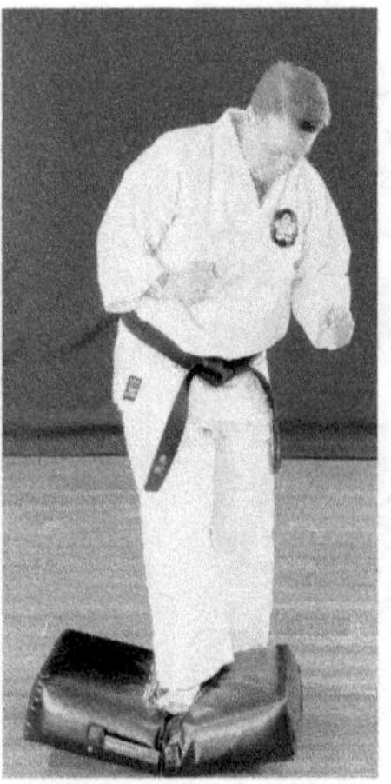

Counter 3: Osoto-gari & Kakato Otoshi Geri

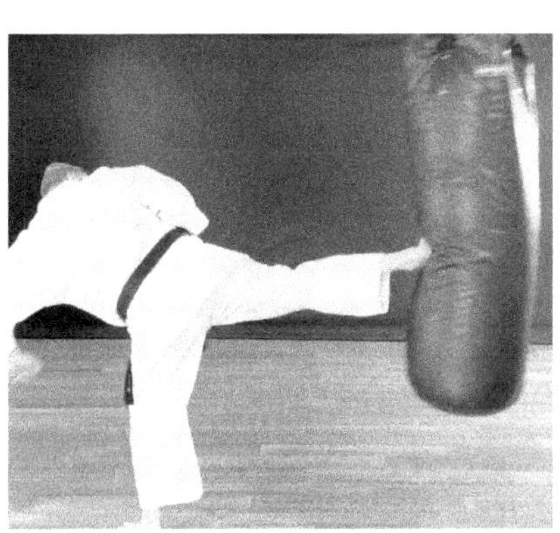
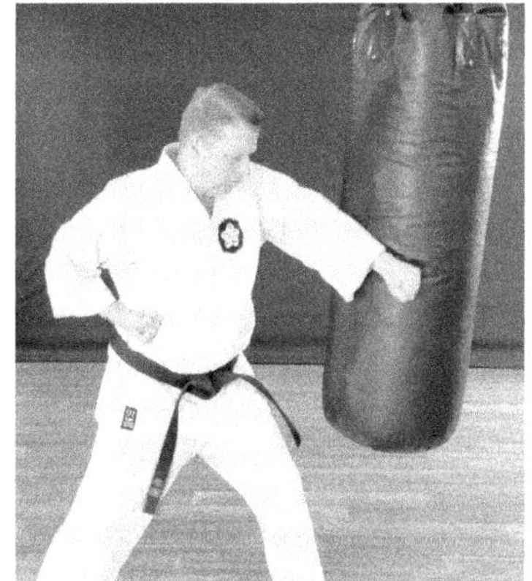
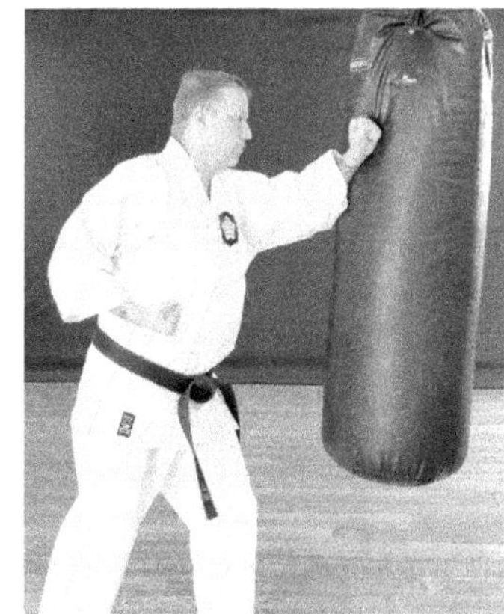

Counter 4: Yoko Geri, Yoko Tettsui Uchi & Tettsui Otoshi Uchi

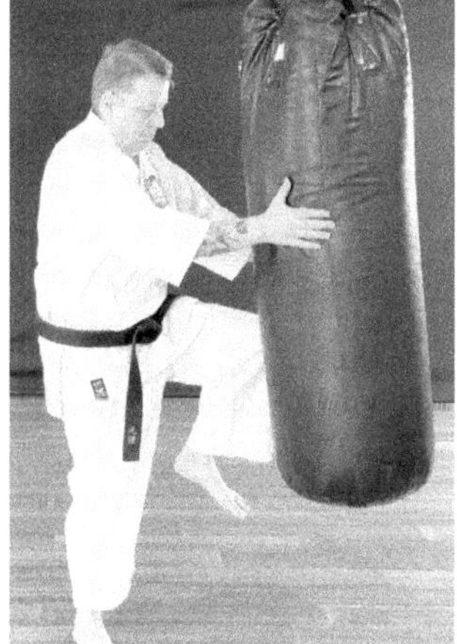

Counter 4: Hiza Uchi

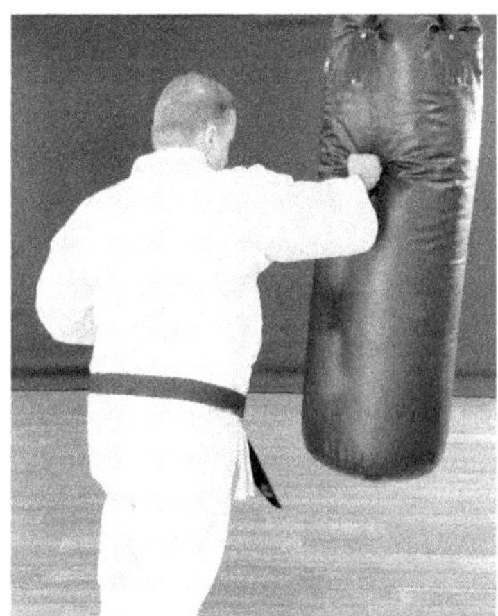

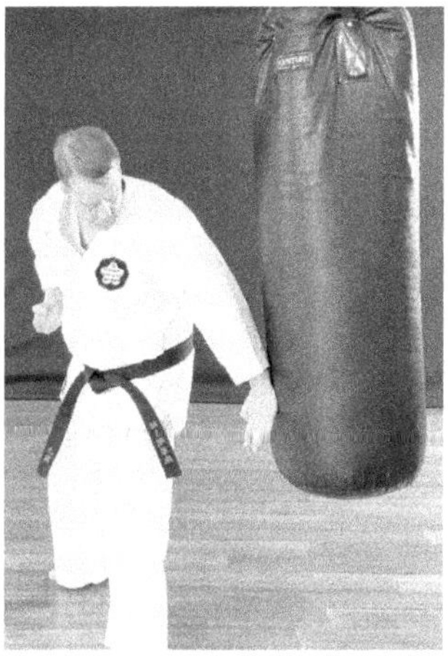

Counter 5: Tate Uchi & Ushiro Shuto Uchi

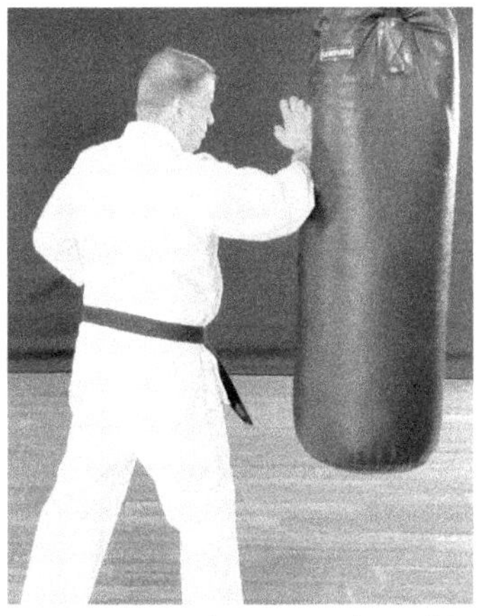

Counter 5: Shuto Otoshi Uchi

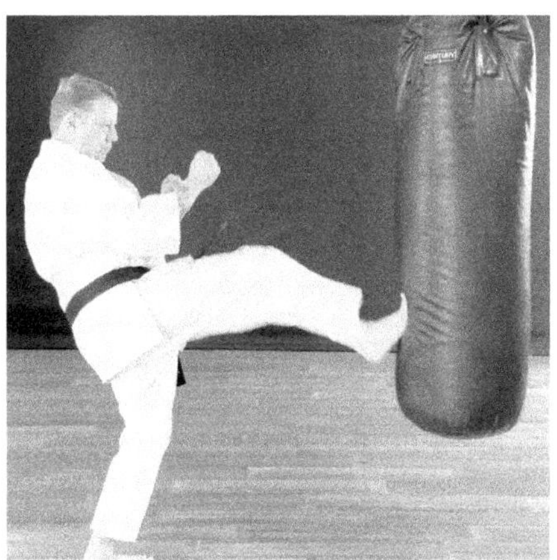

Counter 6: Gedan Mae Geri

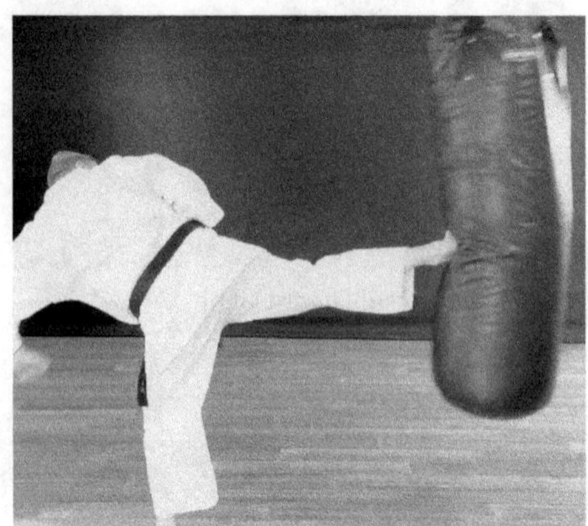
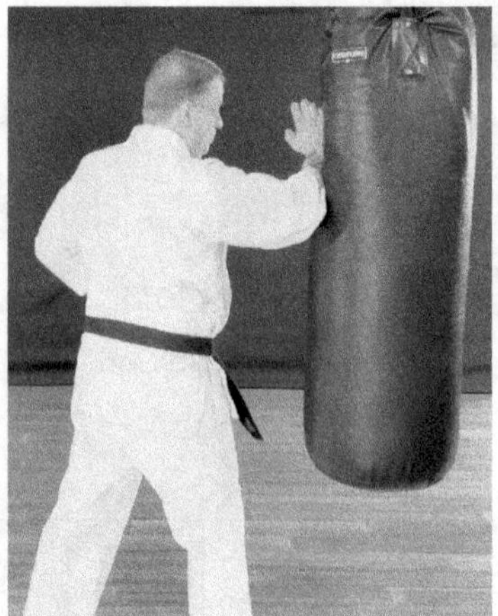
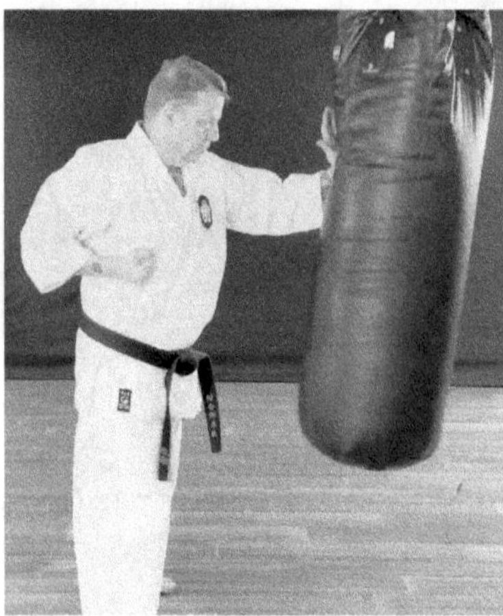

Counter 6: Yoko Geri, Mae Shuto Uchi, & Shotei Uchi

13. Kumite Shichi (7)

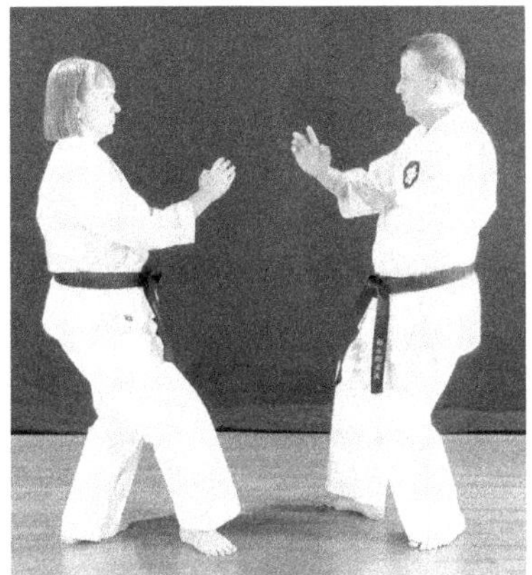

Renoji Dachi Kamae
Chamber Hand at Chest,
Palm Up

Begin Counter 1

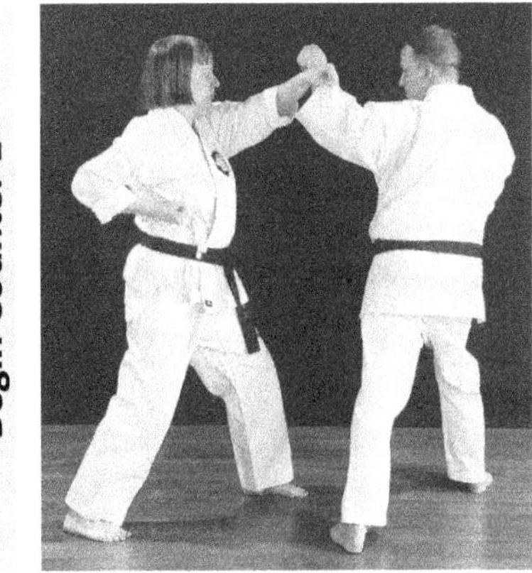

1. (Off - L): Step Forward, Jodan Zuki / (Def - R): Step Back to Side, Jodan Yoko Ko Uke

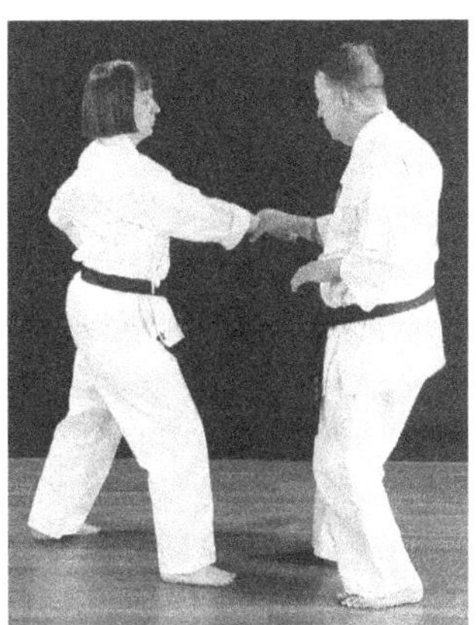

2. (Off - L): Step Forward, Chudan Zuki / (Def - R): Step Back Off Center, Chudan Hari to Hiki Uke

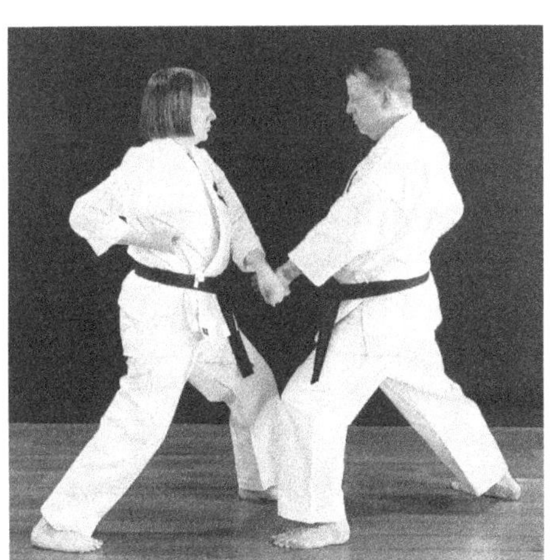

3. (Off - L): Step Forward, Gedan Zuki in Zenkutsu Dachi / (Def - R): Step Back, Gedan Shotei Barai in Zenkutsu Dachi

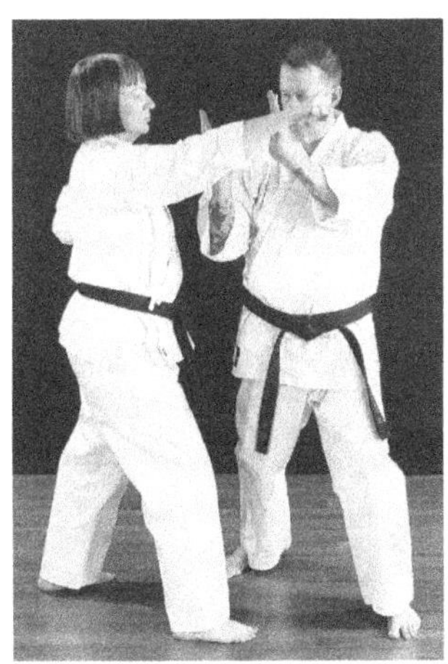

4. (Off - L): Step Forward, Jodan Zuki / (Def - R): Morote Yoko Shuto Uke

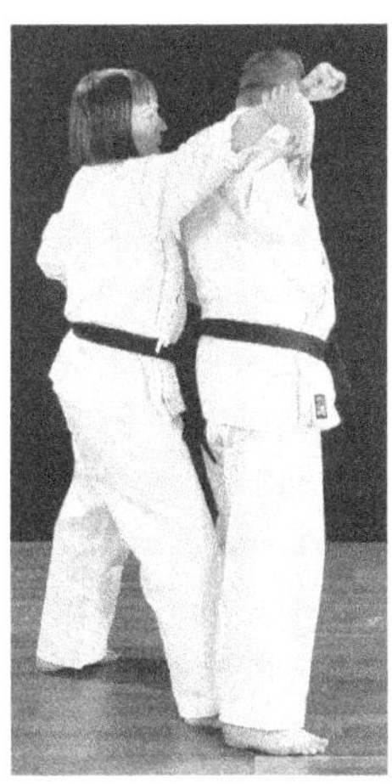

5. (Def - R): Grab Opponents Arm, Step in Front of Opponent, Ushiro Empi Uchi

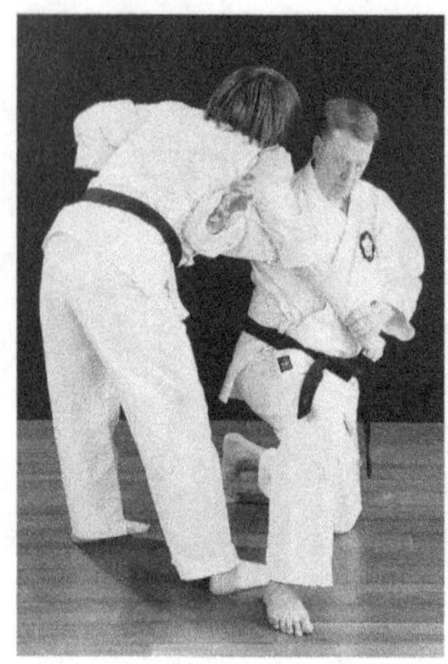

6. (Def - R): Drop Down to Knee While Pulling Opponent Down

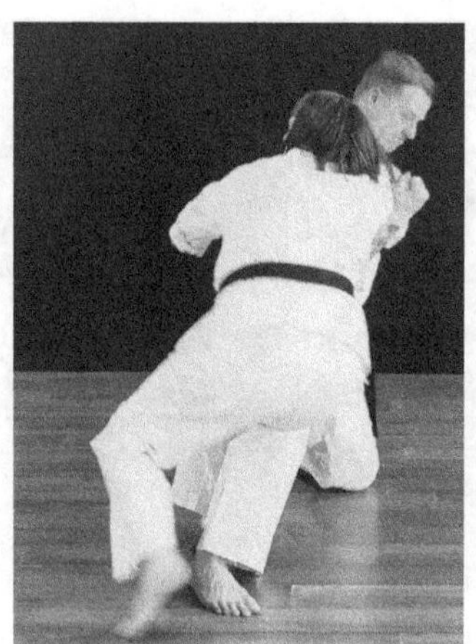

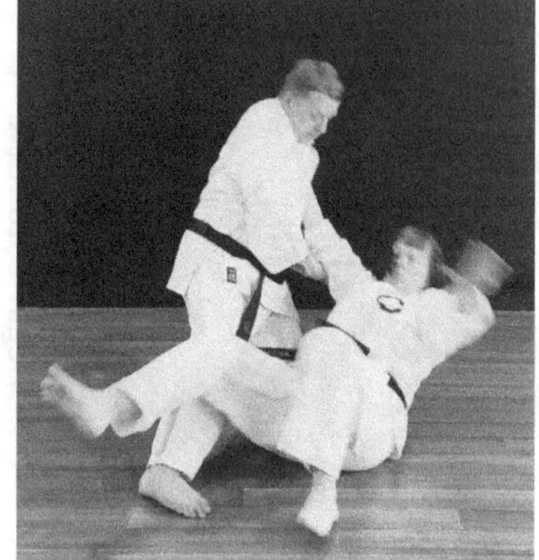

7. (Def - R): Tai Otoshi

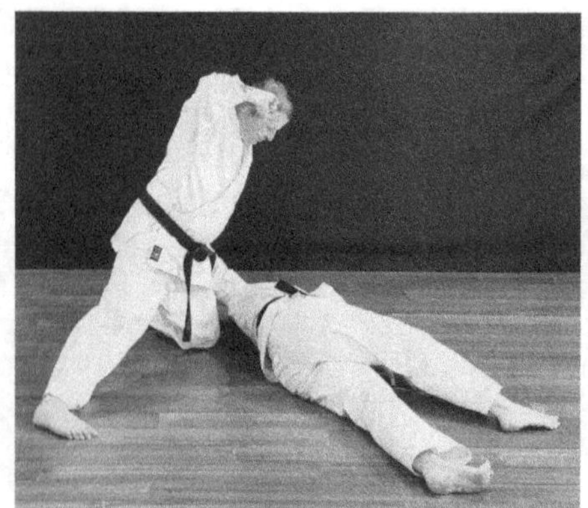

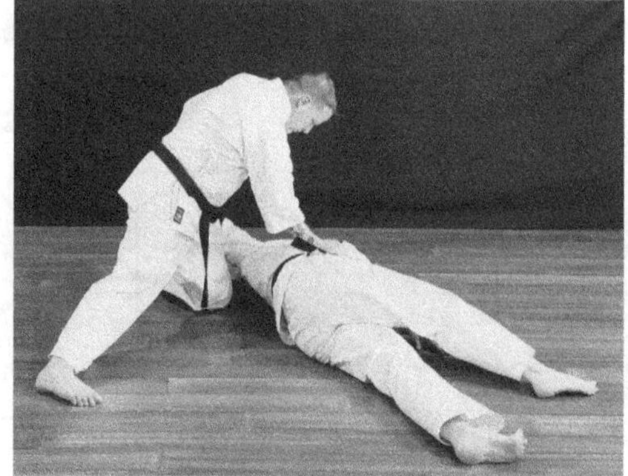

8. (Def - R): Tettsui Otoshi Uchi to Chest

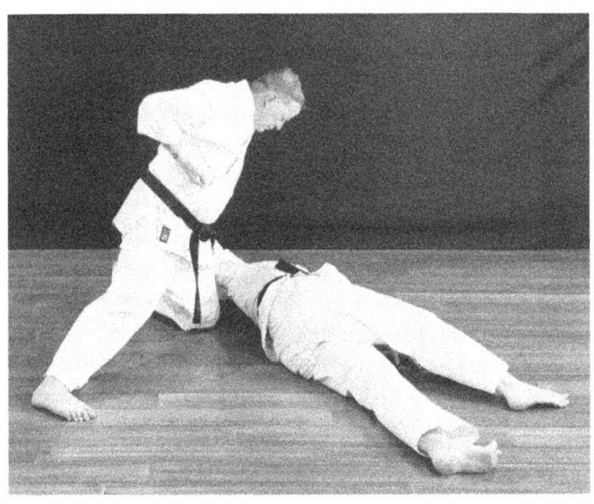

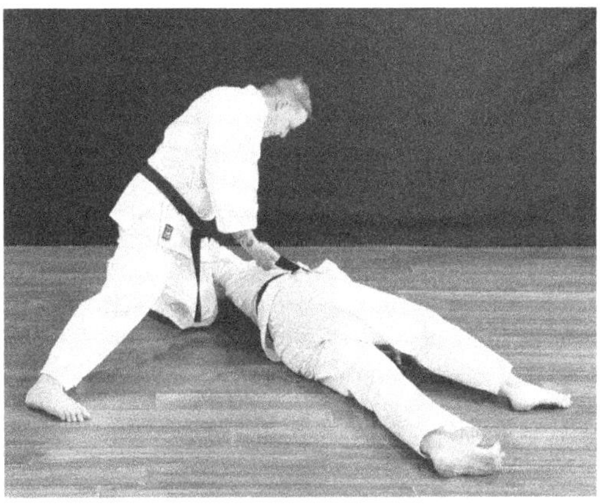

Repeat in Other Direction

9. (Def - R): Ura Zuki to Ribs (Kiai)

Begin Counter 2

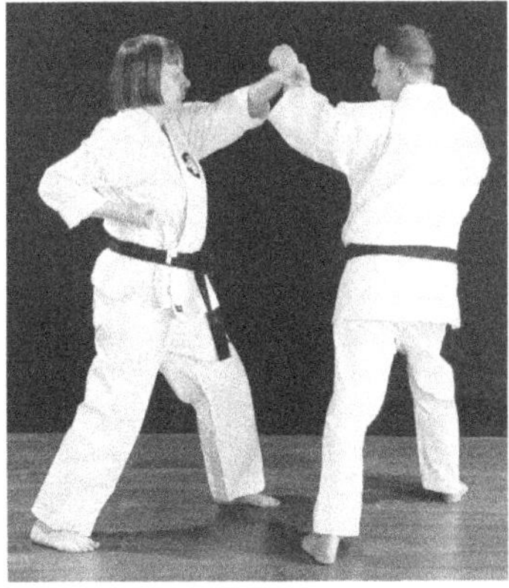

1. (Off - L): Step Forward, Jodan Zuki / (Def - R): Step Back to Side, Jodan Yoko Ko Uke

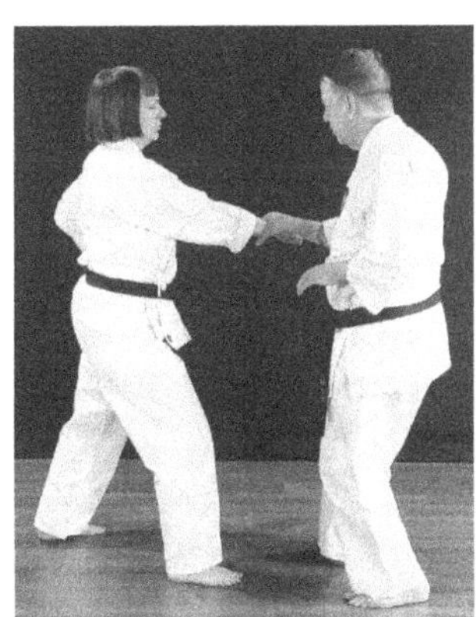

2. (Off - L): Step Forward, Chudan Zuki / (Def - R): Step Back Off Center, Chudan Hari to Hiki Uke

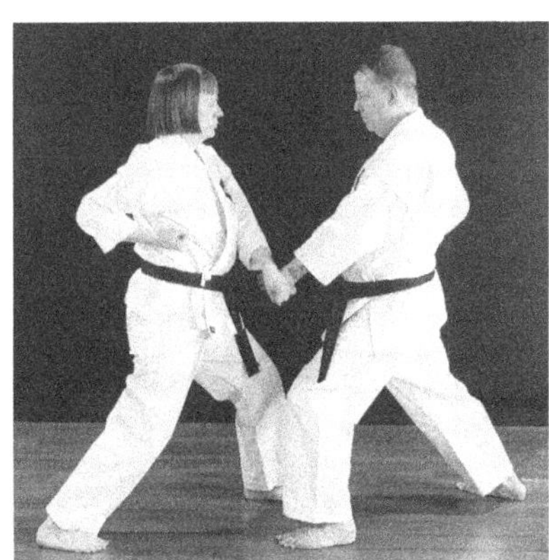

3. (Off - L): Step Forward, Gedan Zuki in Zenkutsu Dachi / (Def - R): Step Back, Gedan Shotei Barai in Zenkutsu Dachi

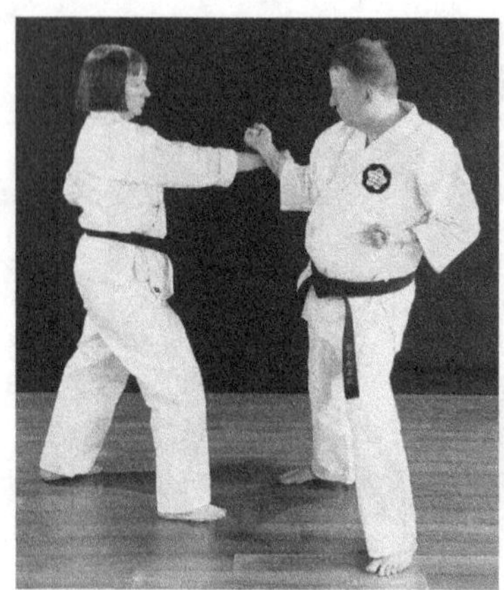

4. (Off - L): Step Forward, Chudan Zuki / (Def - R): Step Back to Side, Chudan Uchi Uke

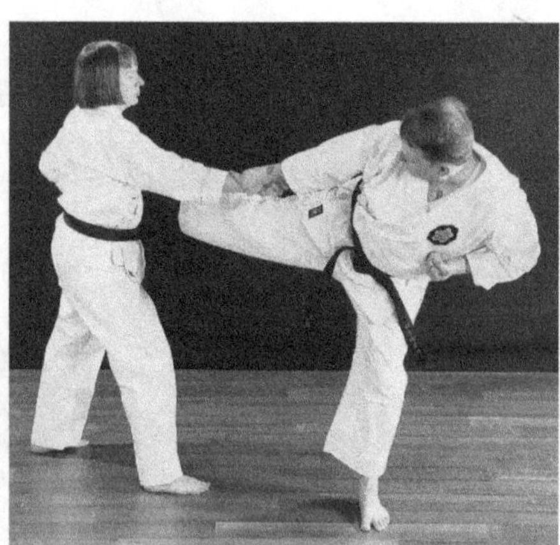

5. (Def - R): Grab Opponent's Wrist, Mawashi Geri with Ball of Foot to Chest

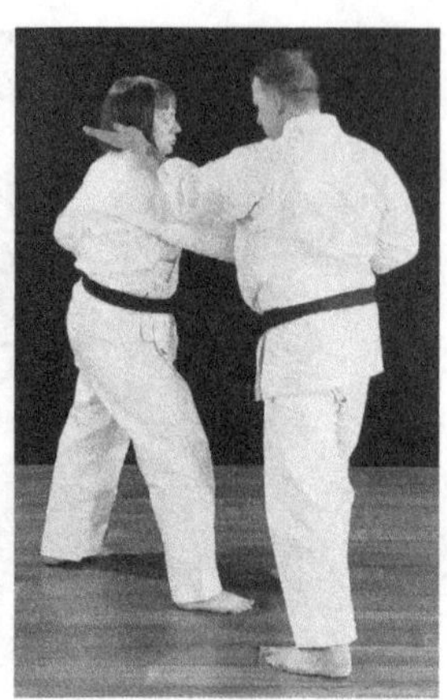

6. (Def - R): Shuto Uchi to Neck

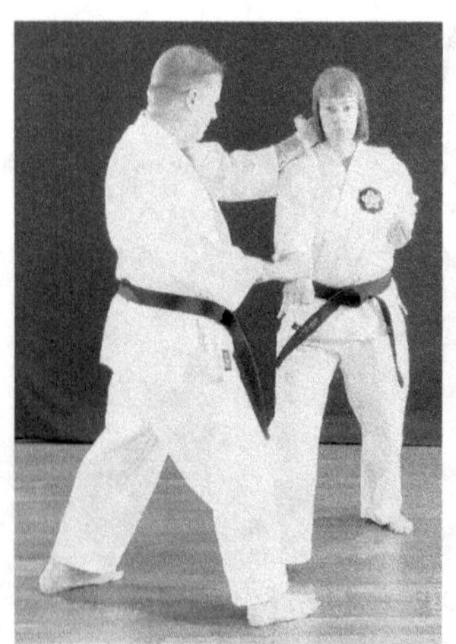

Front POV of Step 6

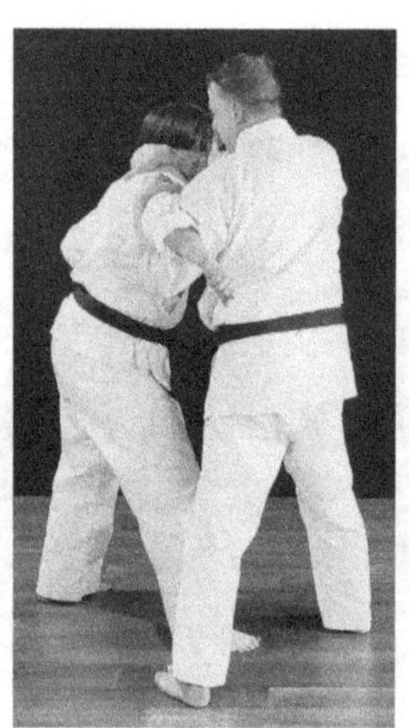

7. (Def - R): Slide Arm Down into Arm Bar, Pushing Opponent Down

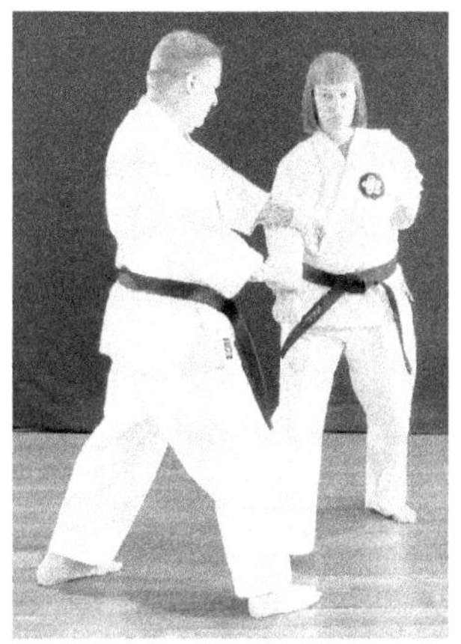
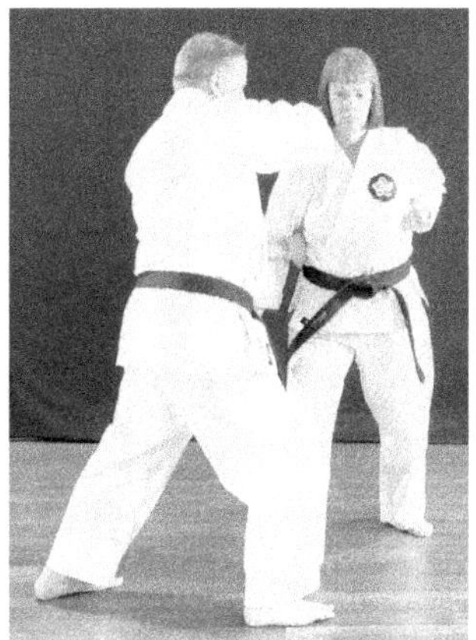
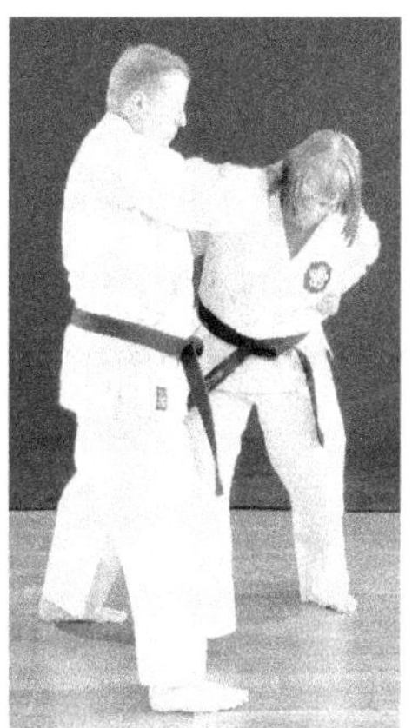
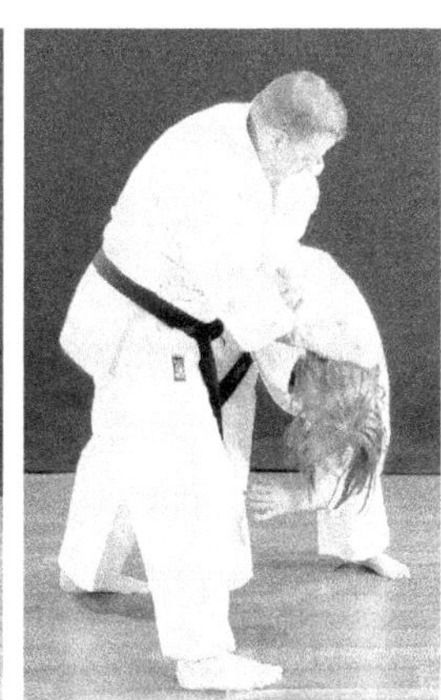

Front POV of Step 7

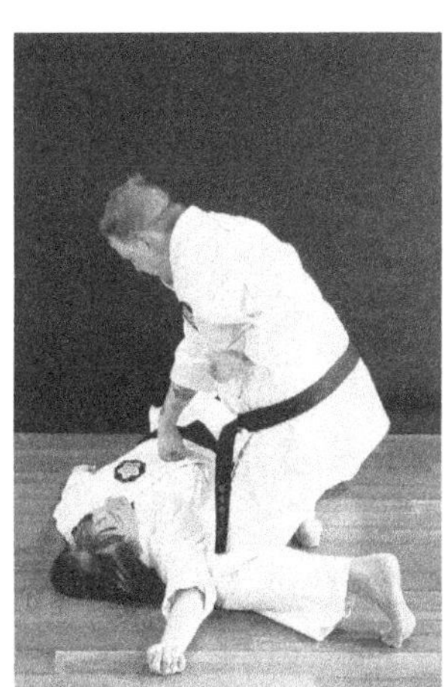
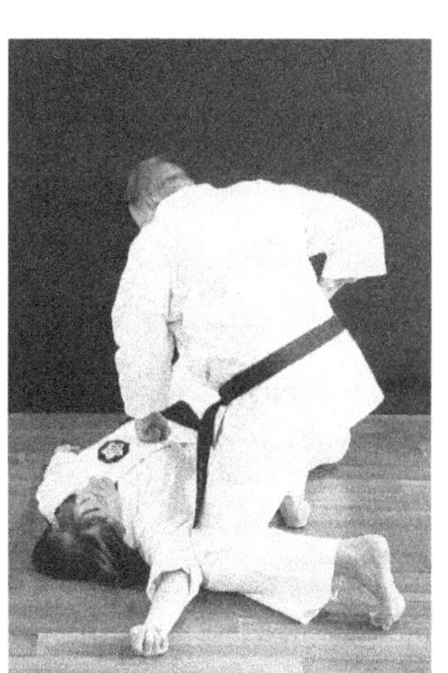
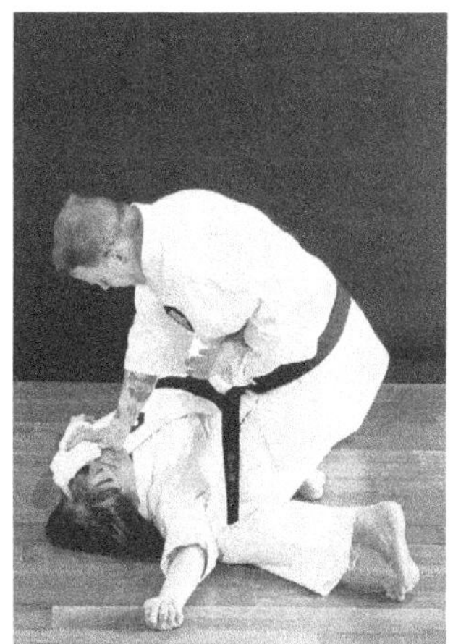

Repeat in Other Direction

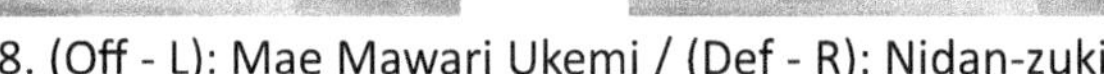

8. (Off - L): Mae Mawari Ukemi / (Def - R): Nidan-zuki

9. (Def - R): Otoshi Shotei Uchi to Face (Kiai)

Begin Counter 3

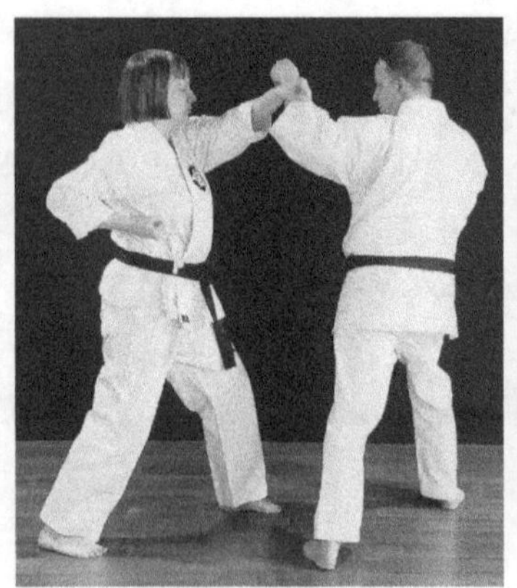

1. (Off - L): Step Forward, Jodan Zuki / (Def - R): Step Back to Side, Jodan Yoko Ko Uke

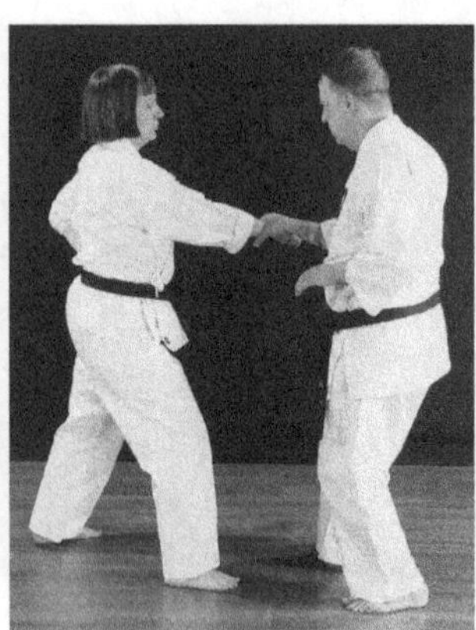

2. (Off - L): Step Forward, Chudan Zuki / (Def - R): Step Back Off Center, Chudan Hari to Hiki Uke

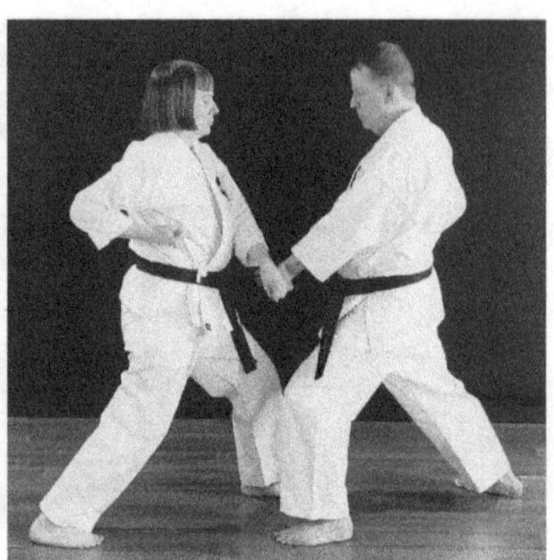

3. (Off - L): Step Forward, Gedan Zuki in Zenkutsu Dachi / (Def - R): Step Back, Gedan Shotei Barai in Zenkutsu Dachi

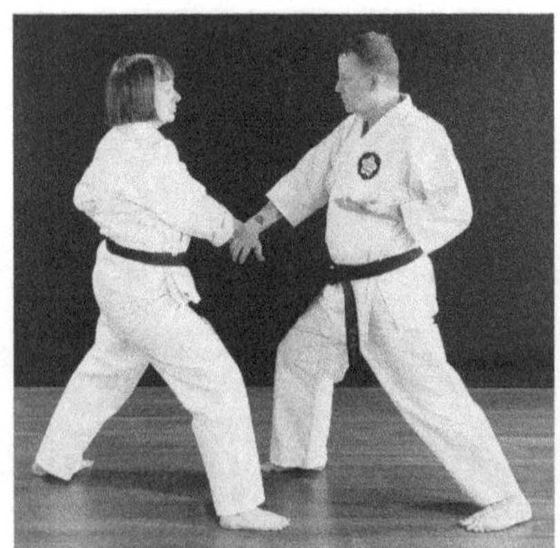

4. (Off - L): Step Forward, Gedan Zuki in Zenkutsu Dachi / (Def - R): Step Back, Gedan Shotei Barai in Zenkutsu Dachi

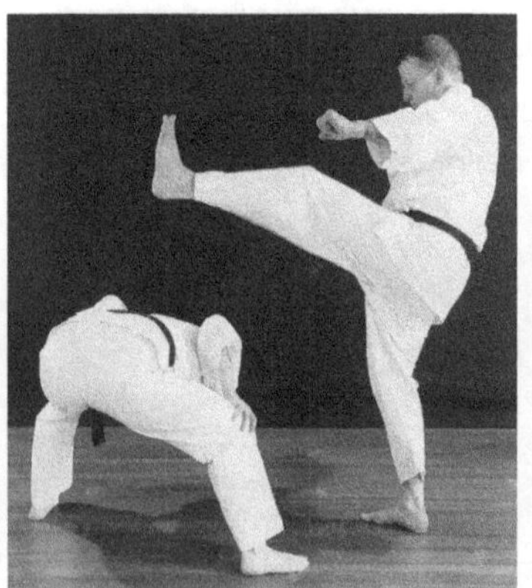

5. (Off - L): Duck Down / (Def - R): Left Mikazuki Geri

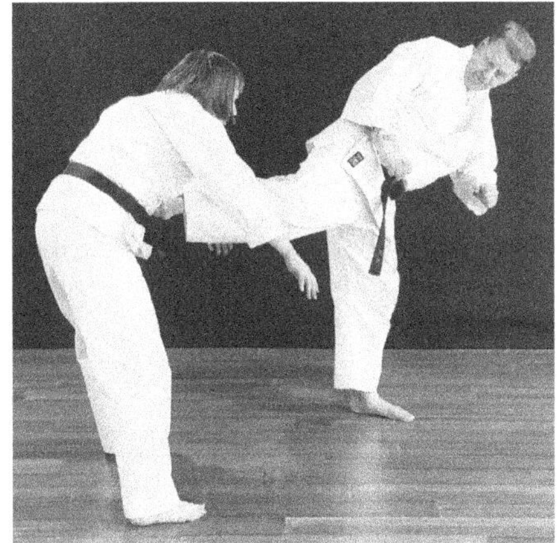

6. (Def - R): Yoko Geri

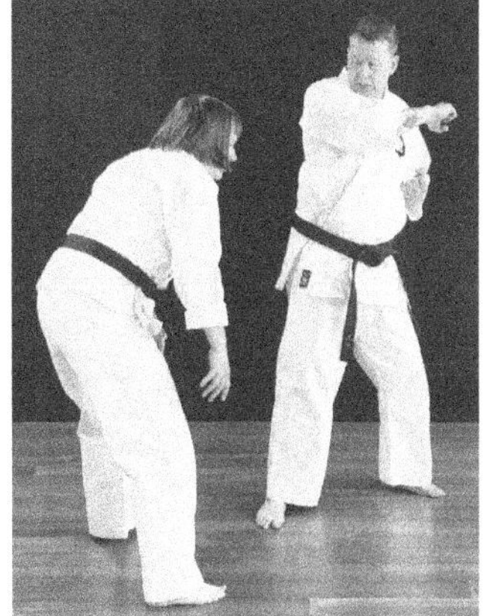

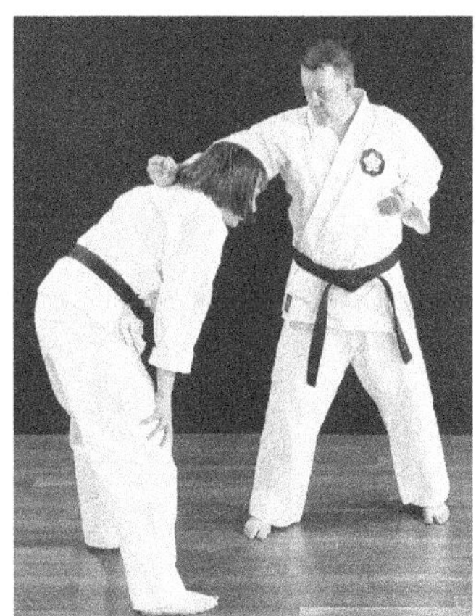

7. (Def - R): Tettsui Otoshi Uchi to Opponent's Upper Back

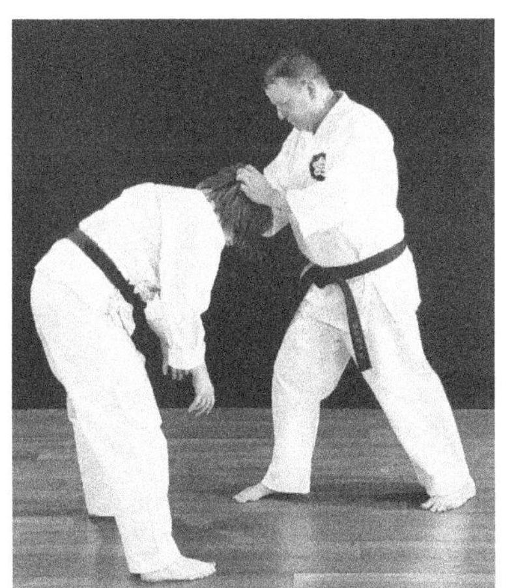

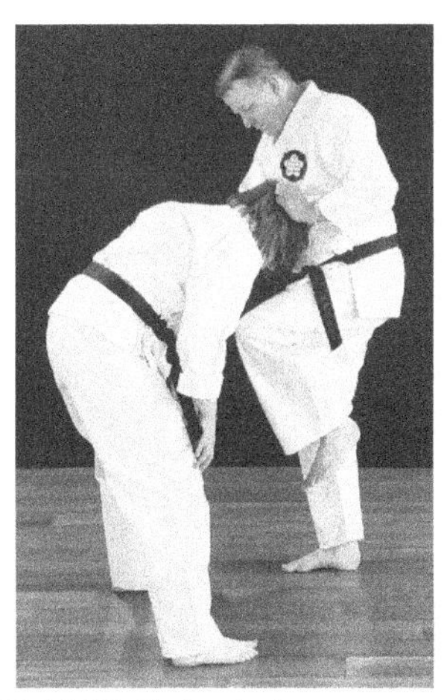

Repeat in Other Direction

8. (Def - R): Grab Head, Age Hiza Uchi (Kiai), Push Away

Begin Counter 4

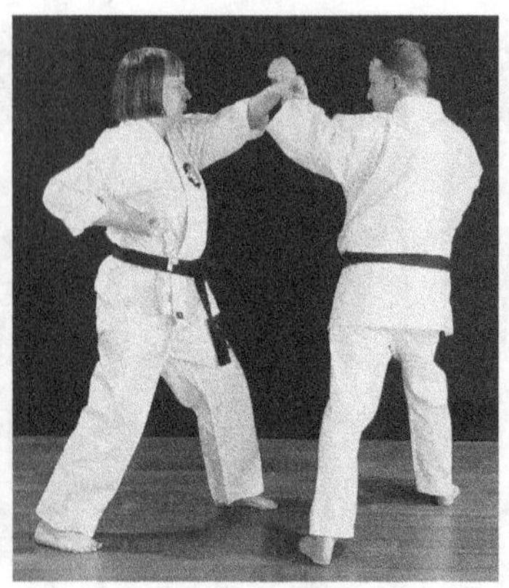

1. (Off - L): Step Forward, Jodan Zuki / (Def - R): Step Back to Side, Jodan Yoko Ko Uke

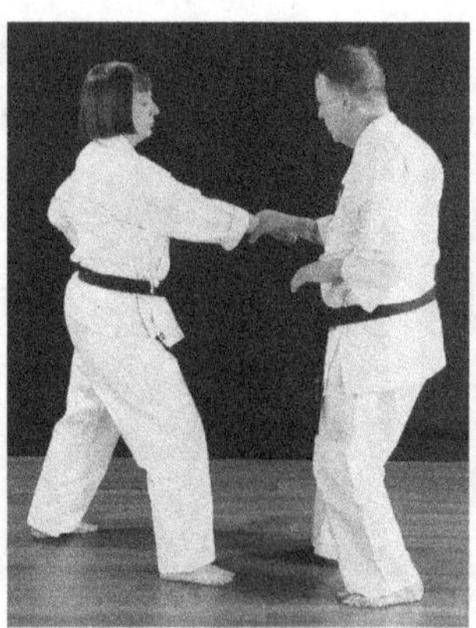

2. (Off - L): Step Forward, Chudan Zuki / (Def - R): Step Back Off Center, Chudan Hari to Hiki Uke

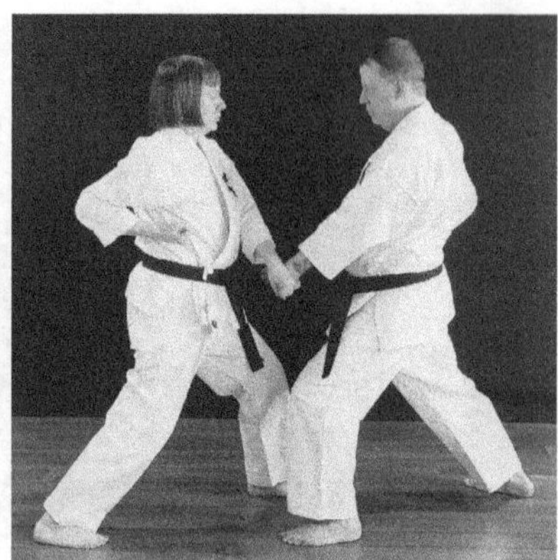

3. (Off - L): Step Forward, Gedan Zuki in Zenkutsu Dachi / (Def - R): Step Back, Gedan Shotei Barai in Zenkutsu Dachi

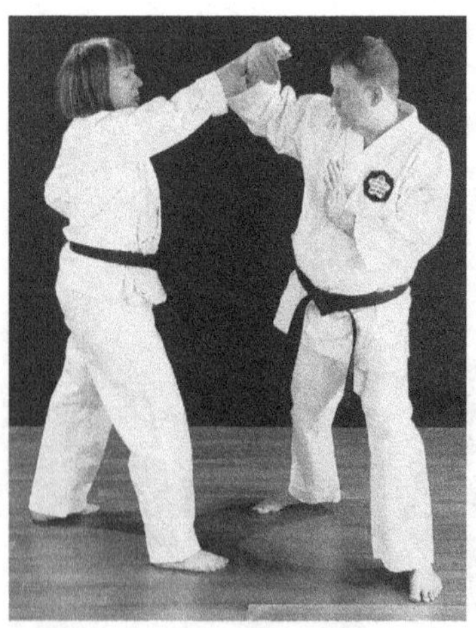

4. (Off - L): Step Forward, Jodan Zuki / (Def - R): Step Back to Side, Jodan Yoko Ko Uke

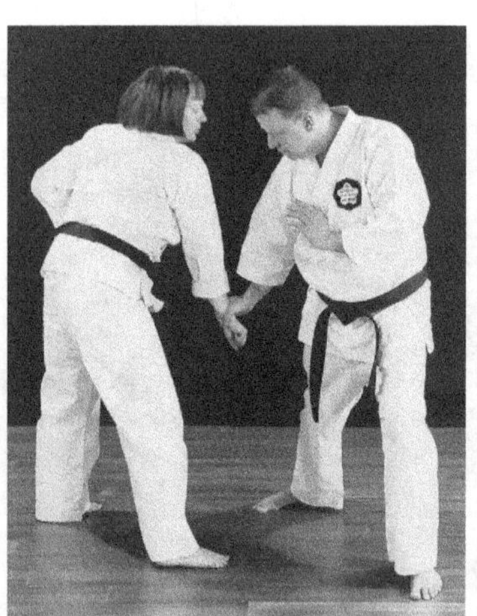

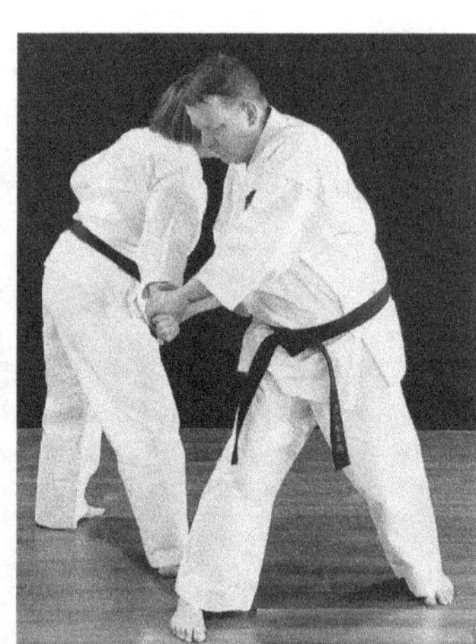

5. (Def - R): Grab Opponent's Wrist, Twist Underneath

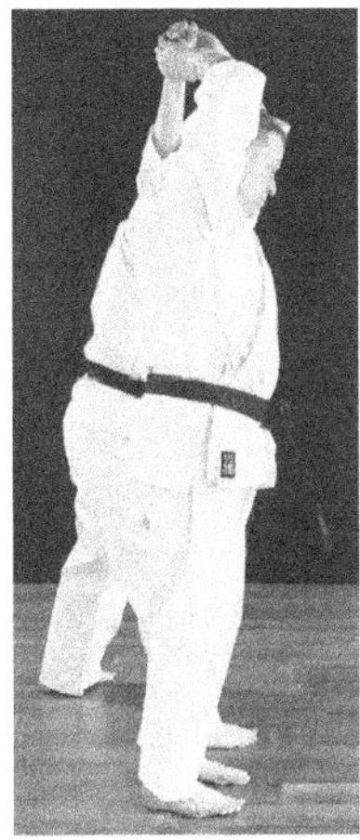

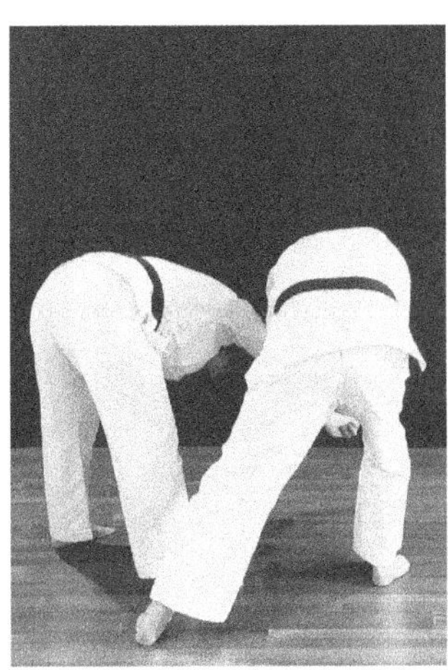

6. (Def - R): Twist Opponent's Wrist, Step Forward, Pulling Opponent Down, Then Pull Up Quickly with Both Hands on Wrist (Te-nage), Opponent Flips Onto Back

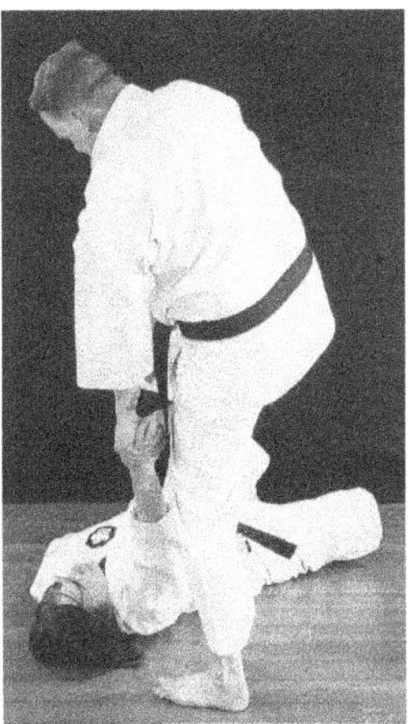

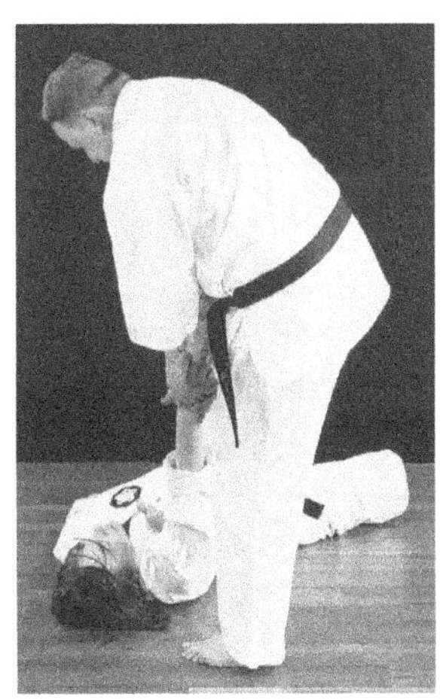

Repeat in Other Direction

7. (Def - R): Kakato Otoshi Geri into Opponent's Arm Pit (Kiai)

Begin Counter 5

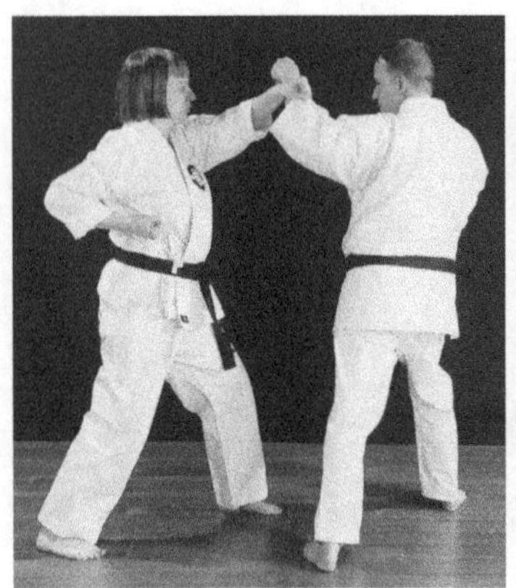

1. (Off - L): Step Forward, Jodan Zuki / (Def - R): Step Back to Side, Jodan Yoko Ko Uke

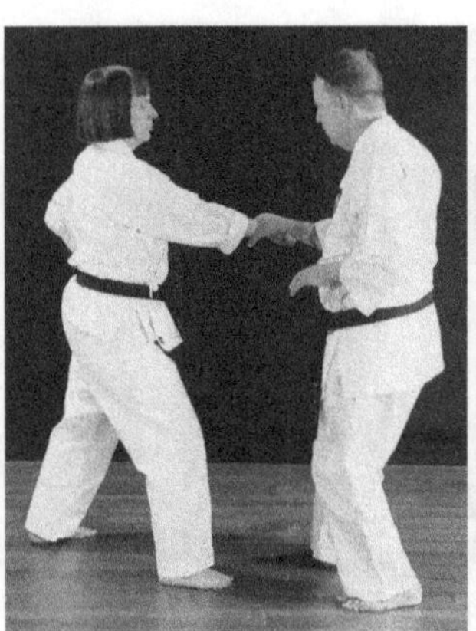

2. (Off - L): Step Forward, Chudan Zuki / (Def - R): Step Back Off Center, Chudan Hari to Hiki Uke

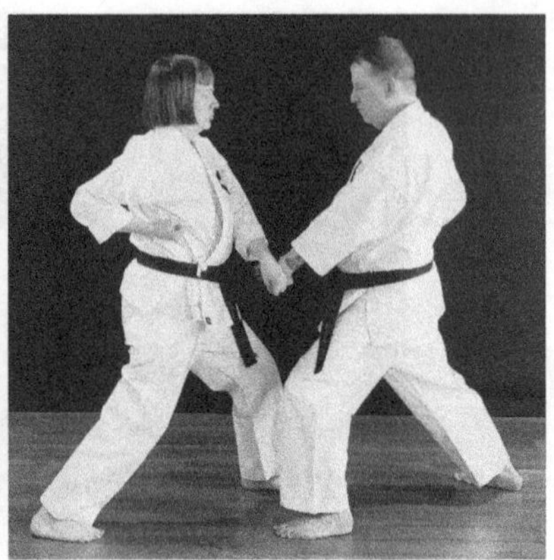

3. (Off - L): Step Forward, Gedan Zuki in Zenkutsu Dachi / (Def - R): Step Back, Gedan Shotei Barai in Zenkutsu Dachi

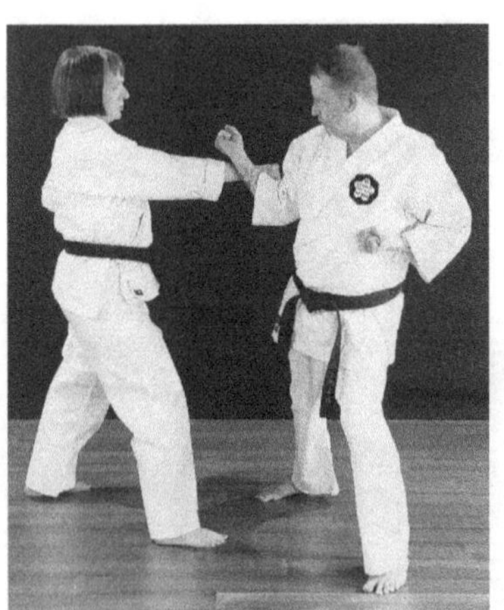

4. (Off - L): Step Forward, Chudan Zuki / (Def - R): Step Back to Side, Chudan Uchi Uke

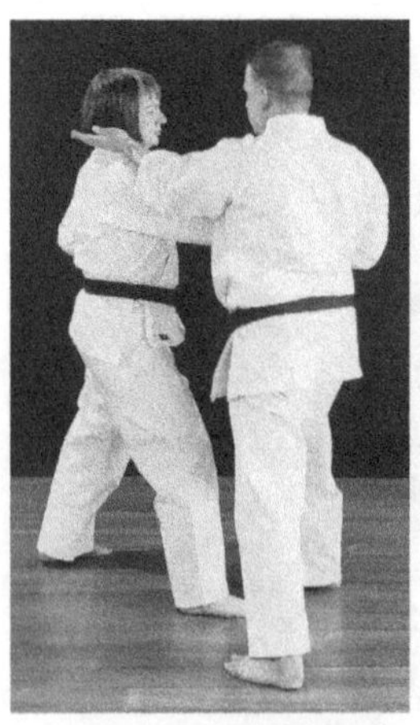

5. (Def - R): Shuto Uchi to Neck

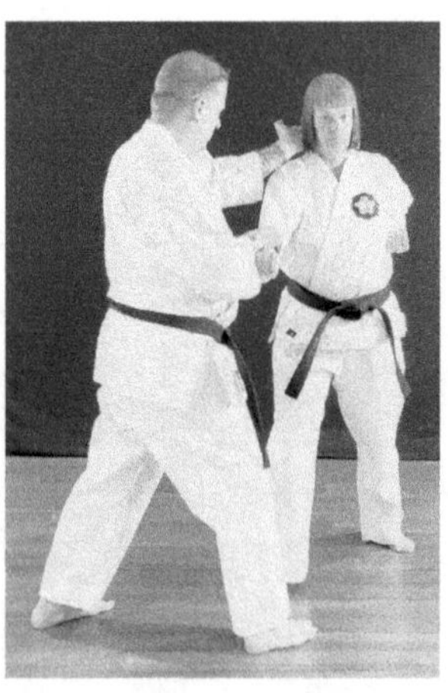

Front POV of Step 5

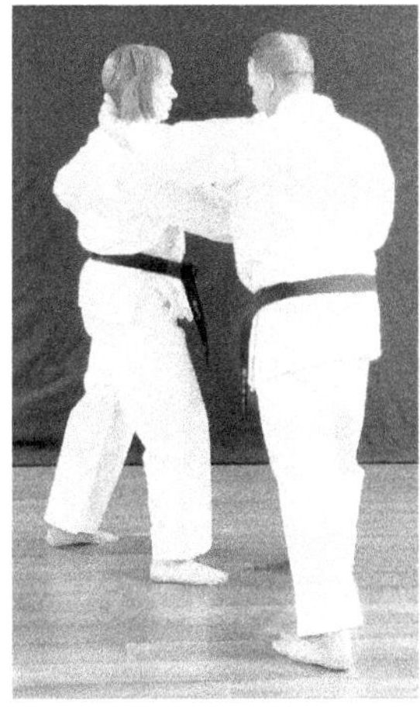
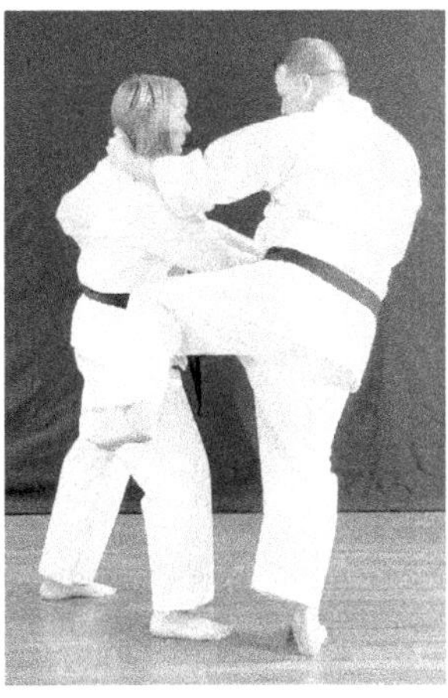

6. (Def - R): Grab Opponent's Neck, Left Hiza Uchi to Ribs

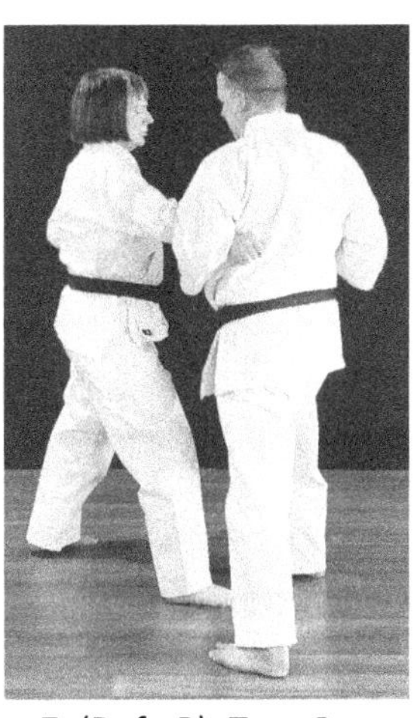
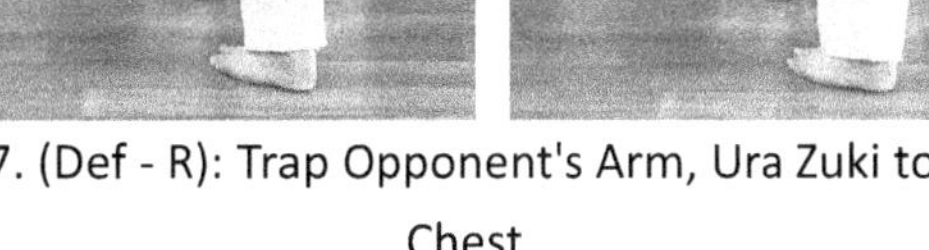

7. (Def - R): Trap Opponent's Arm, Ura Zuki to Chest

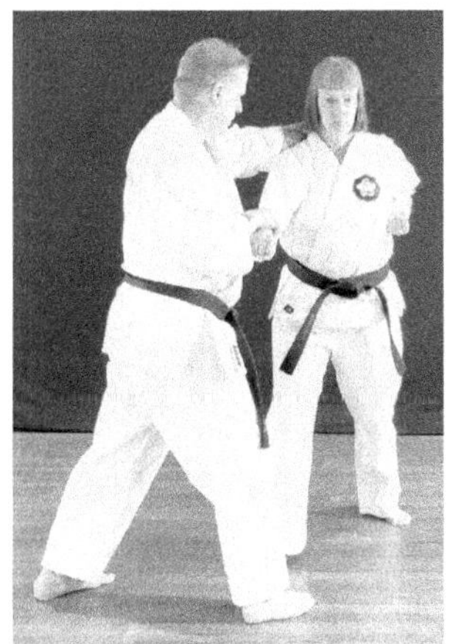
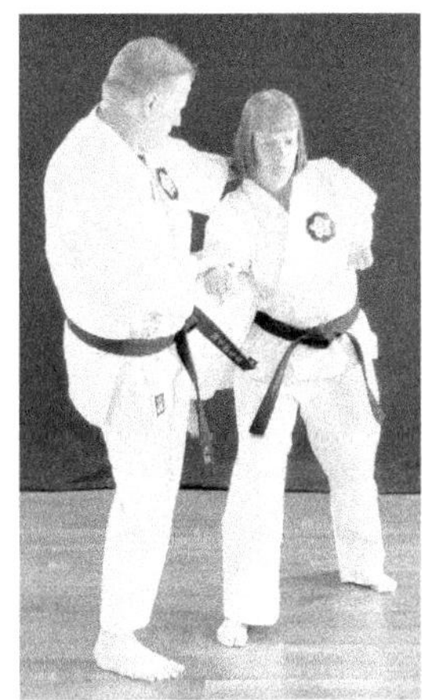

Forward POV of Step 6

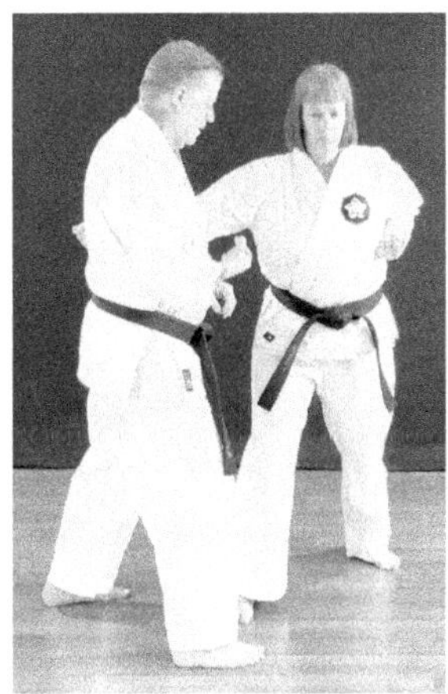
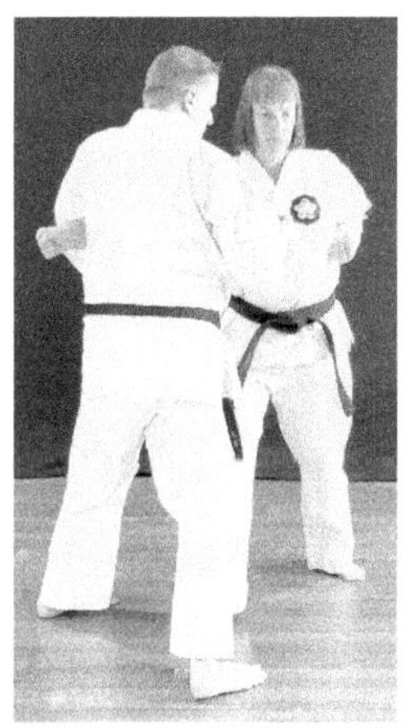

Forward POV of Step 7

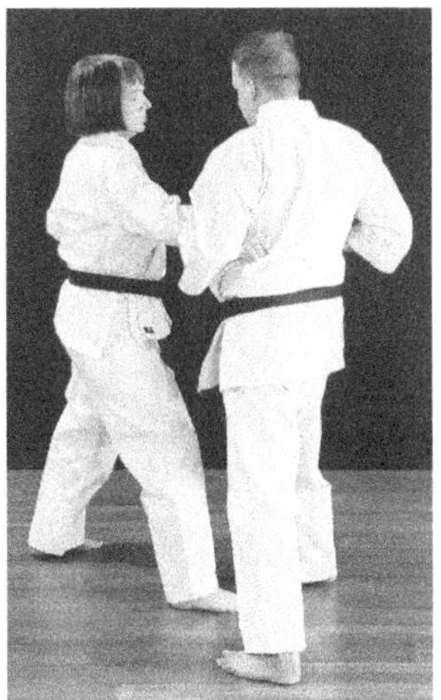
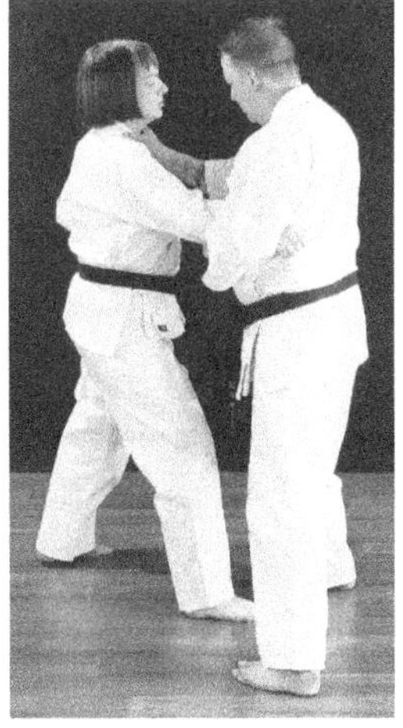

8. (Def - R): Shotei Uchi to Throat

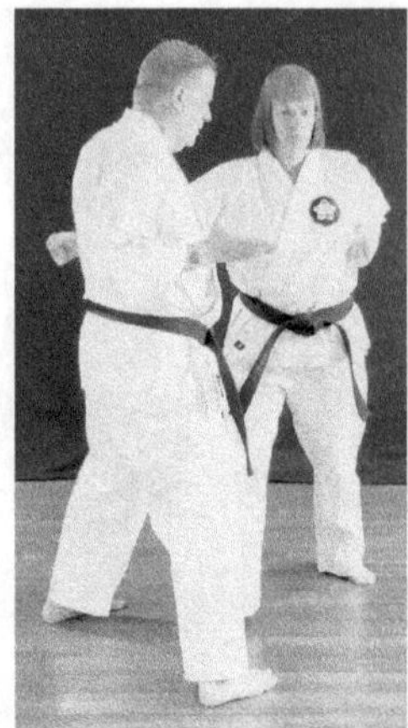

Forward POV of Step 8

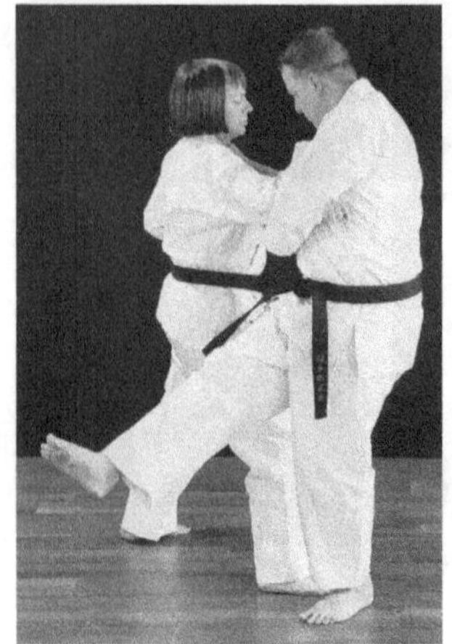

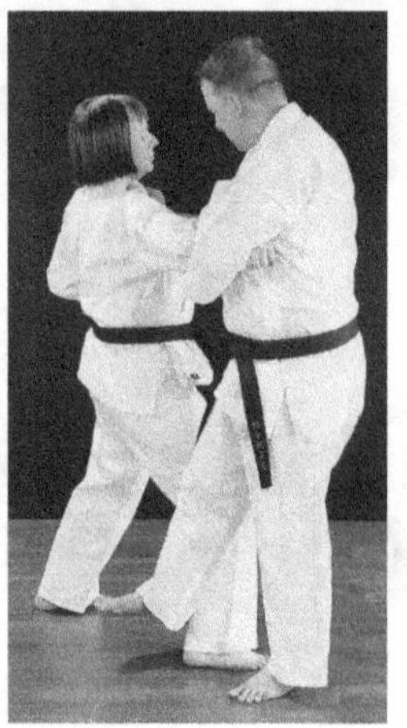

9. (Def - R): Osoto-gari

10. (Def - R): Arm Bar (Kiai)

Repeat in Other Direction

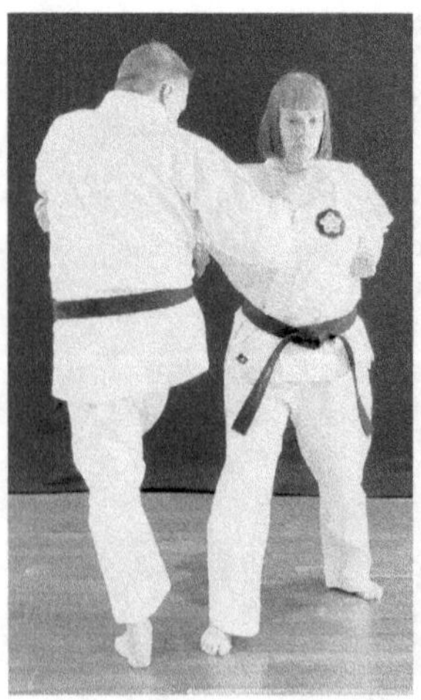

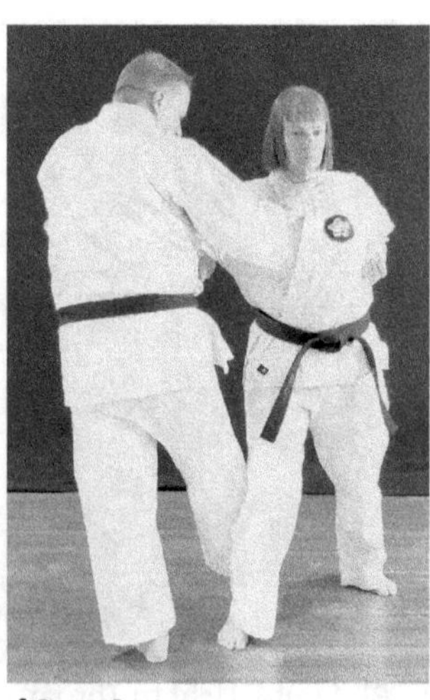

Forward POV of Step 9

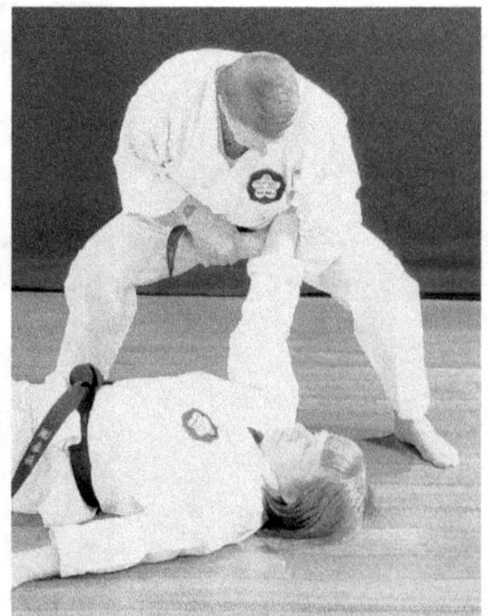

Forward POV of Step 10

Begin Counter 6

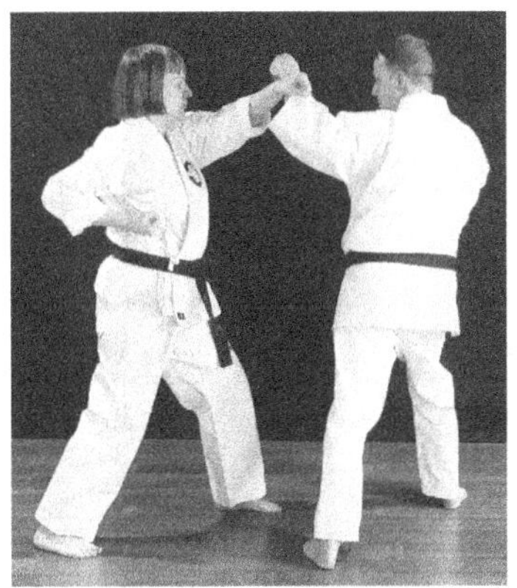
1. (Off - L): Step Forward, Jodan Zuki / (Def - R): Step Back to Side, Jodan Yoko Ko Uke

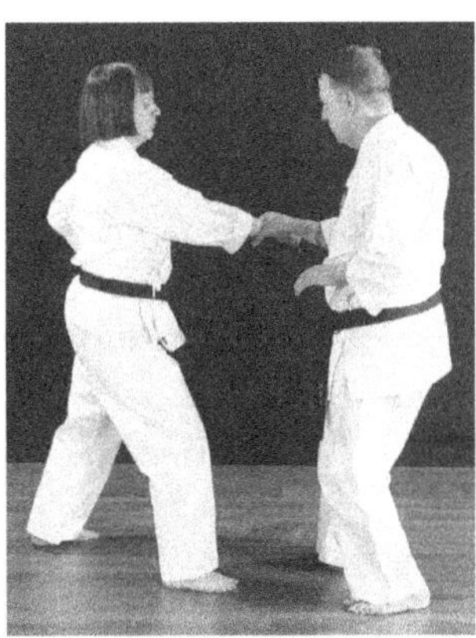
2. (Off - L): Step Forward, Chudan Zuki / (Def - R): Step Back Off Center, Chudan Hari to Hiki Uke

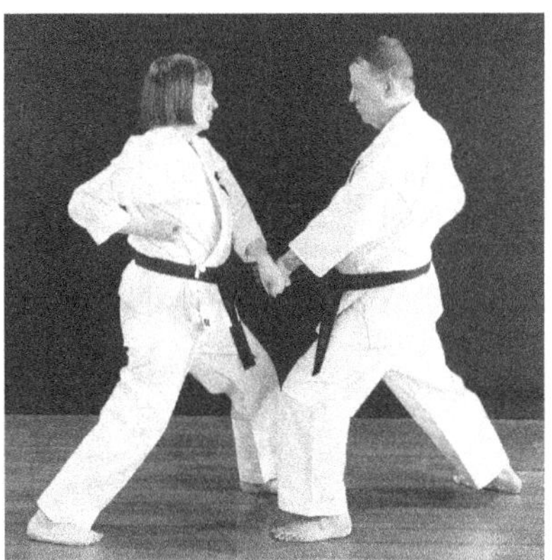
3. (Off - L): Step Forward, Gedan Zuki in Zenkutsu Dachi / (Def - R): Step Back, Gedan Shotei Barai in Zenkutsu Dachi

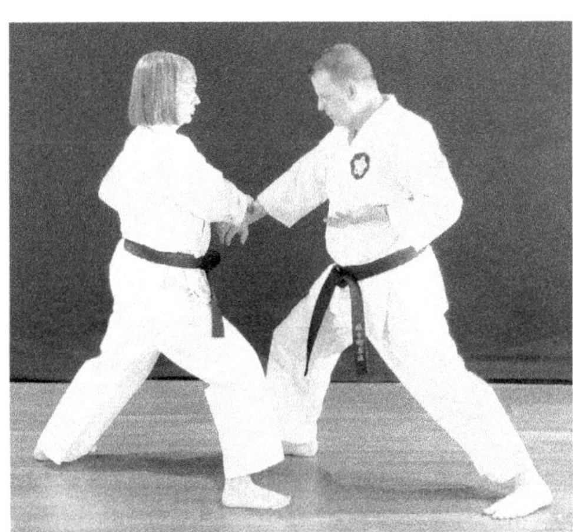
4. (Off - L): Step Forward, Gedan Zuki in Zenkutsu Dachi / (Def - R): Step Back, Gedan Shotei Barai in Zenkutsu Dachi

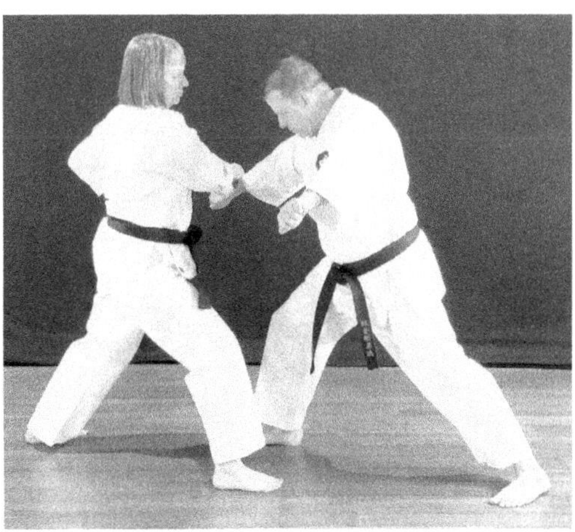
5. (Def - R): Morote Oyayubi Ate

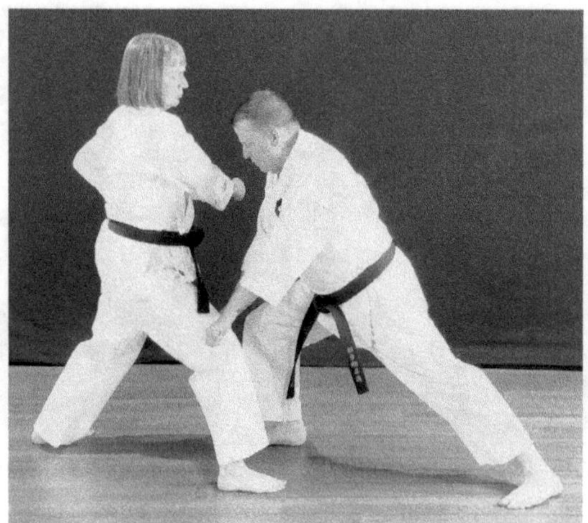

Morote Oyayubi Ate (cont.)

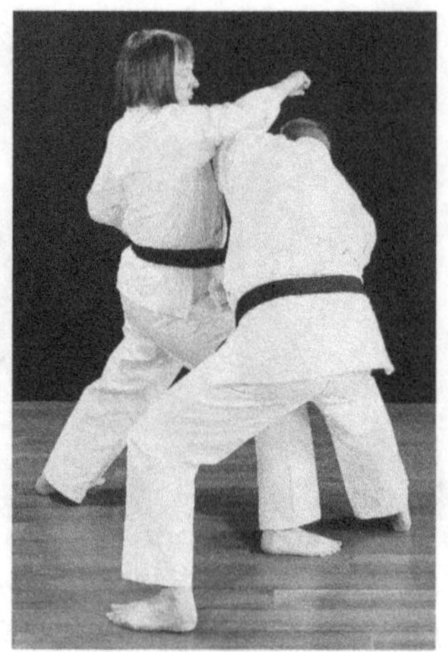

6. (Def - R): Step Around in Shiko Dachi, Grab Behind Knee With Right Hand & Left Arm Across Torso

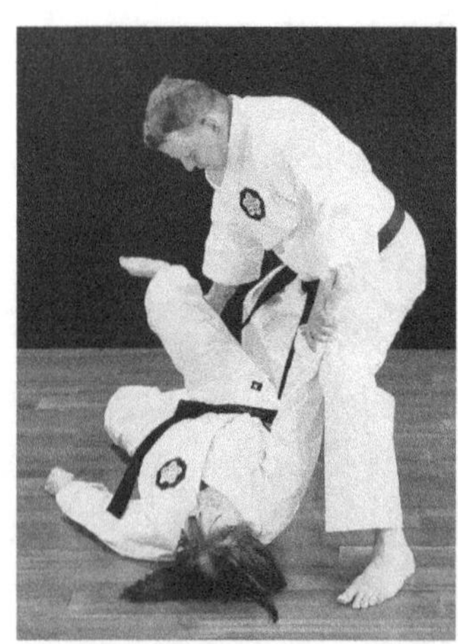

7. (Def - R): Use Knee Pick to Pull Opponent Onto Back (Sukui-nage)

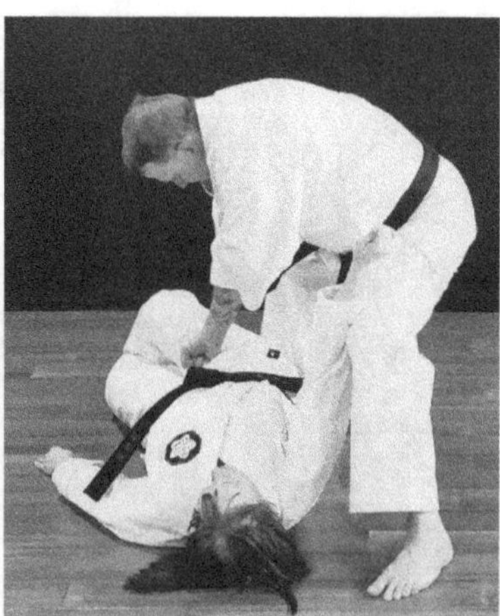

8. (Def - R): Tettsui Otoshi Uchi to Groin

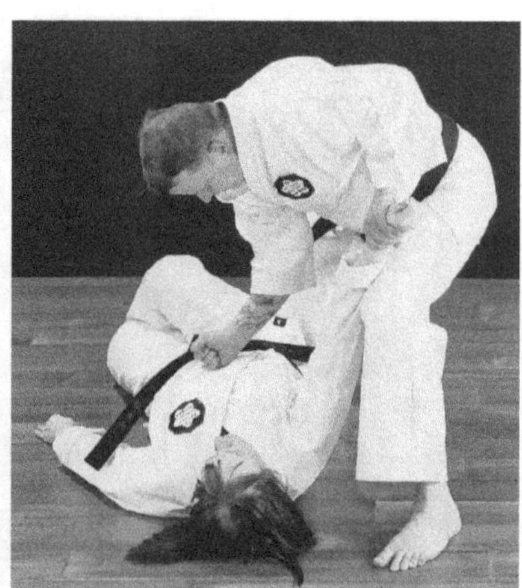

9. (Def - R): Tettsui Otoshi Uchi to Solar Plexus

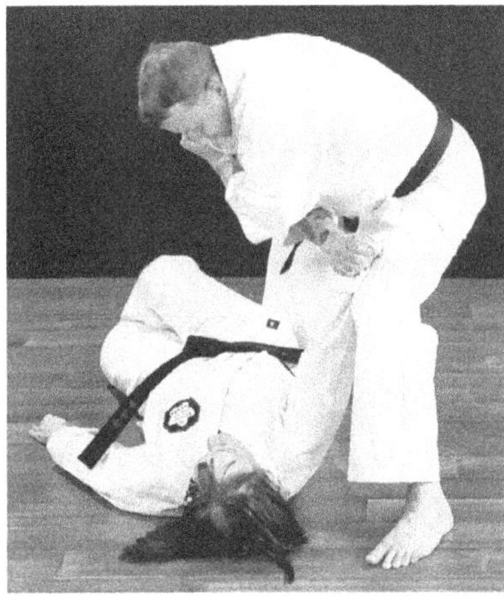
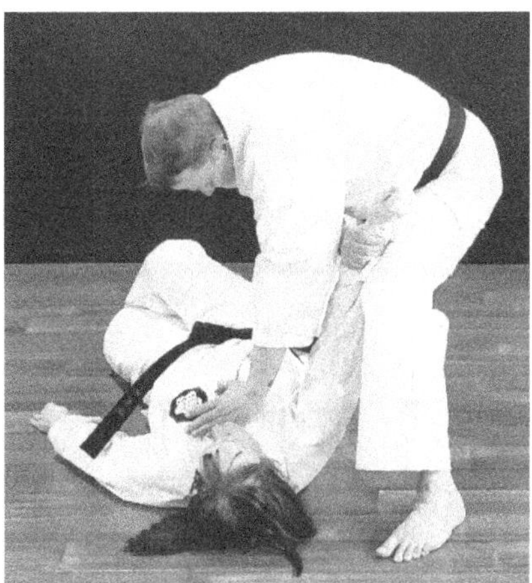

10. (Def - R): Change Grip of Opponent's Left Wrist to Right Hand, Shuto Otoshi Uchi to Throat

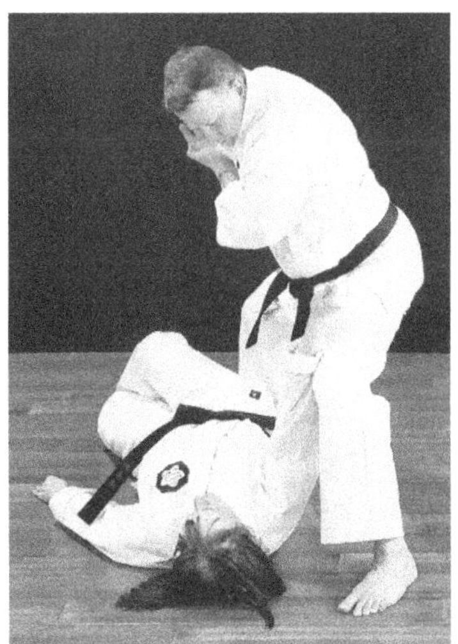
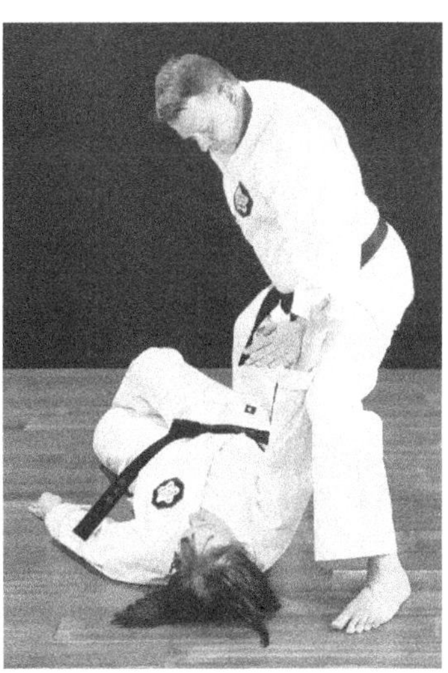

Repeat in Other Direction

11. (Def - R): Shuto Uchi to Opponent's Forearm Using Knee as a Fulcrum (Kiai)

Kumite Shichi - Bag Work

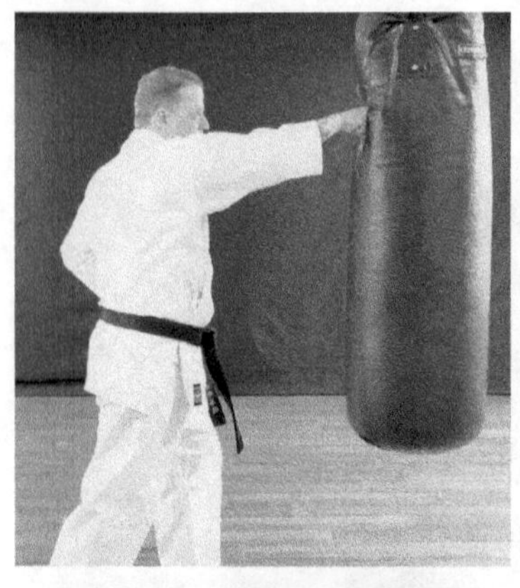
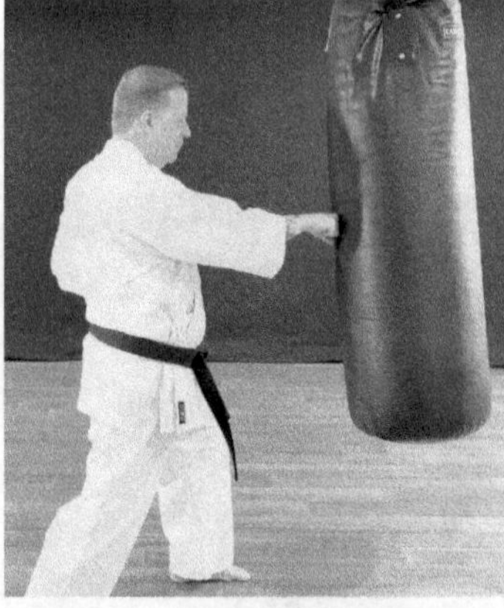
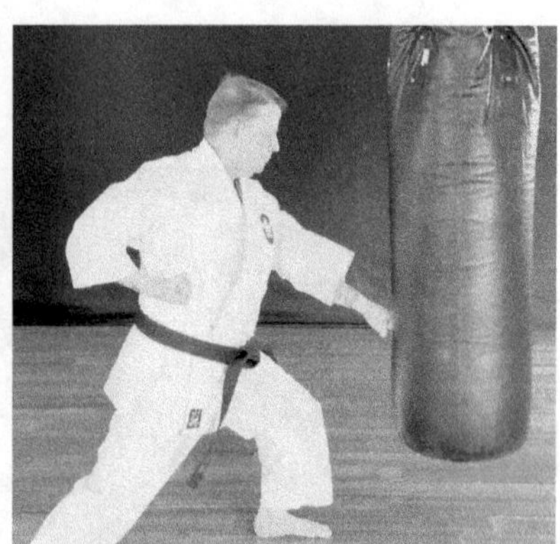
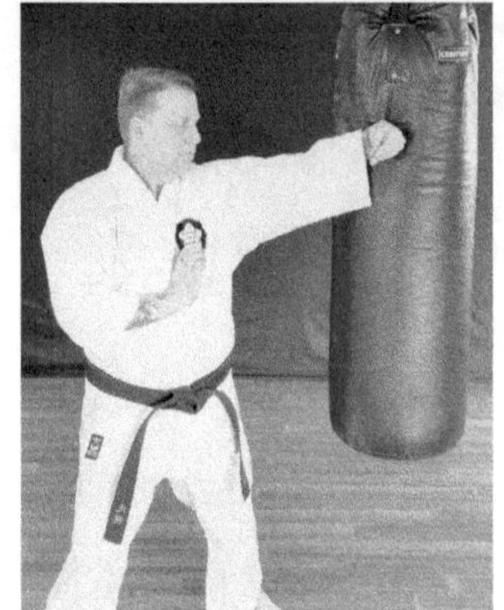

Jodan Zuki (Top) & Jodan Ko Uke (Bottom)

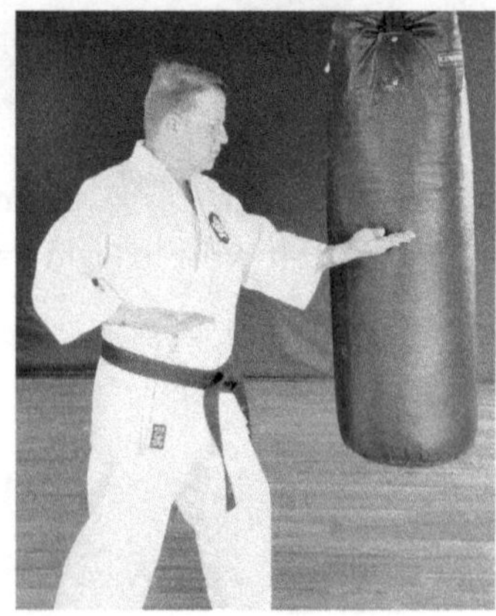

Chudan Zuki (Top) & Chudan Hari Uke (Bottom)

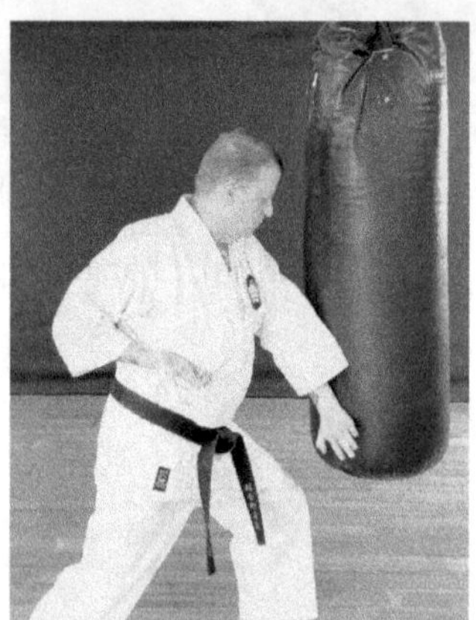

Gedan Zuki (Top) & Shotei Barai (Bottom)

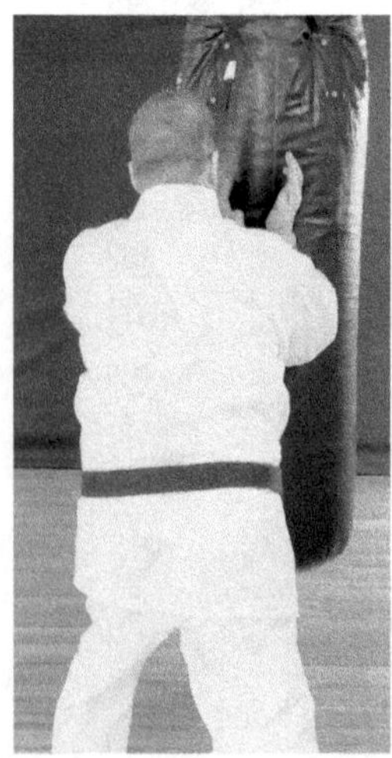
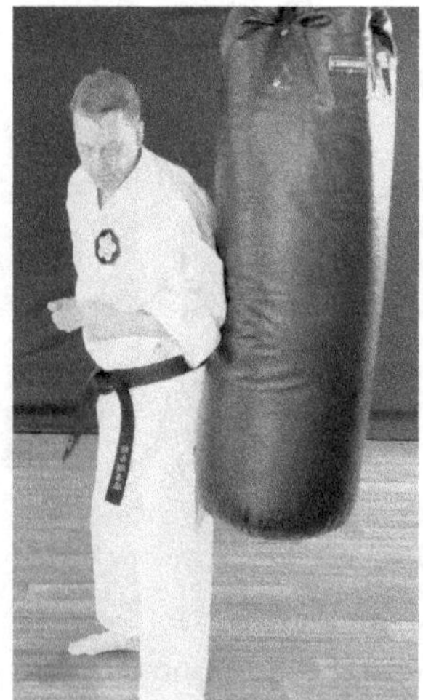
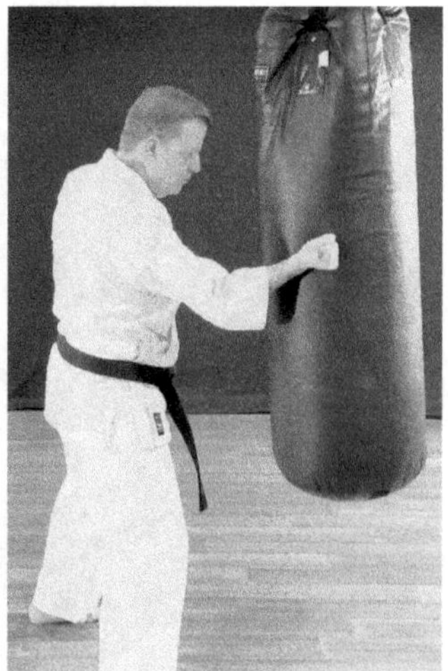

Counter 1: Morote Yoko Shuto Uke, Ushiro Empi Uchi, & Tettsui Uchi

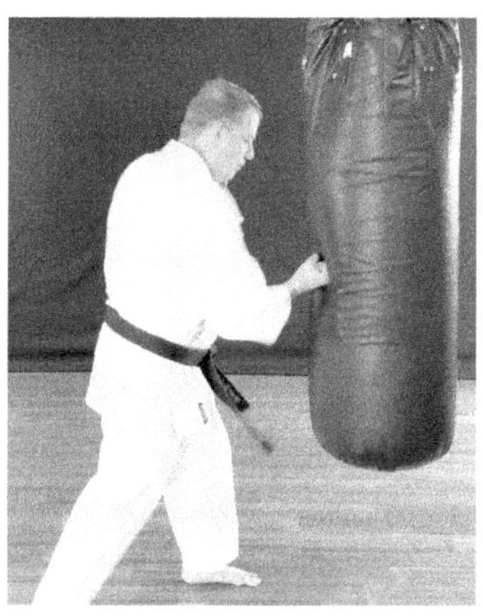
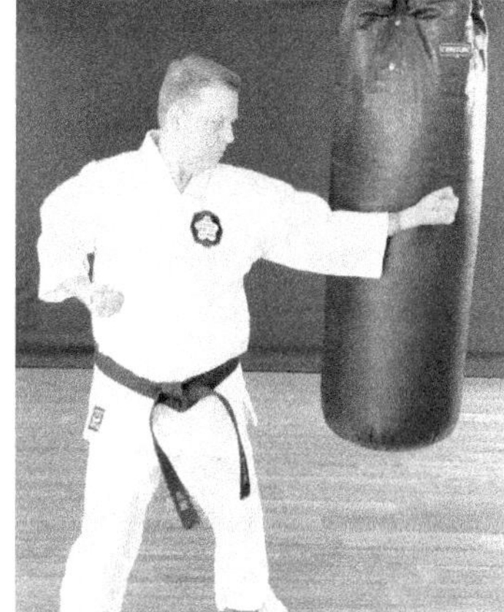
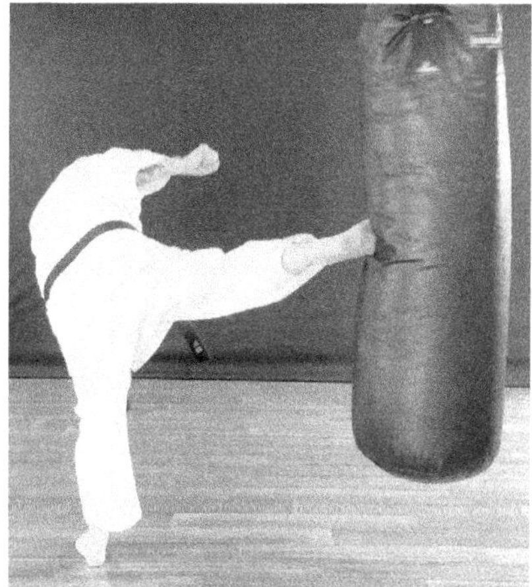

Counter 1: Ura Zuki

Counter 2: Uchi Uke & Mawashi Geri

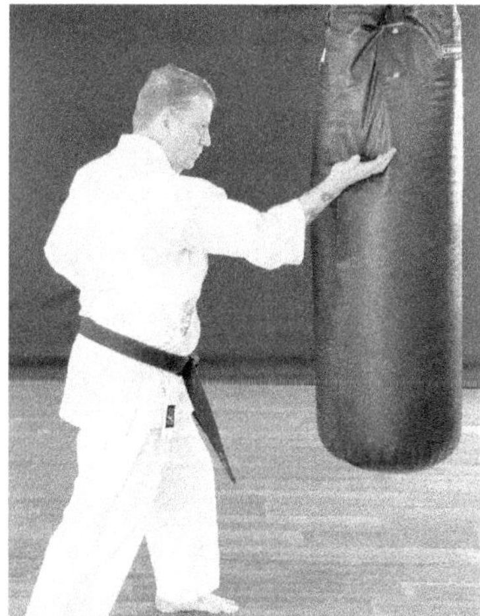

Counter 2: Shuto Uchi

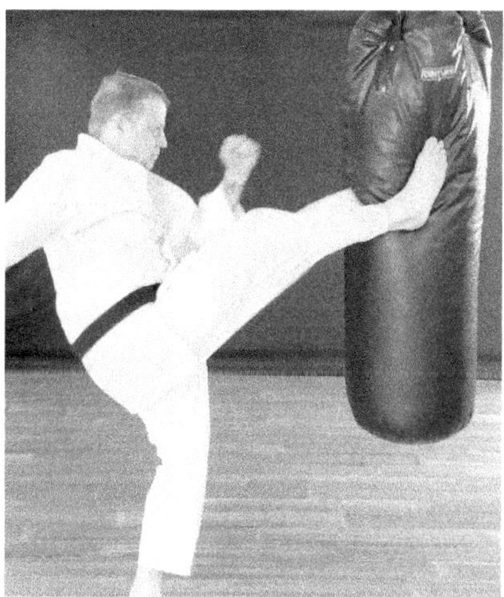

Counter 3: Mikazuki Geri

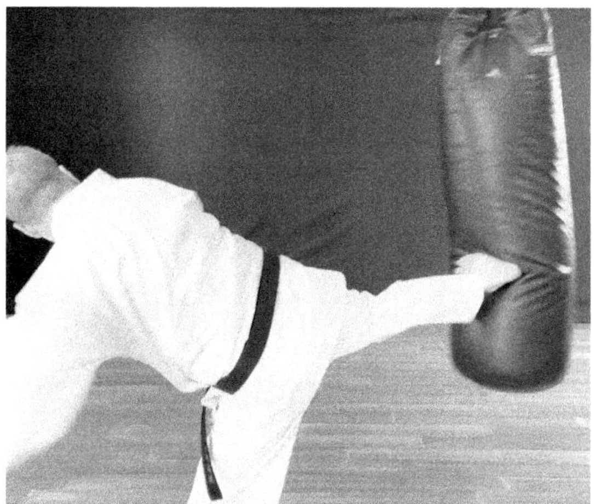
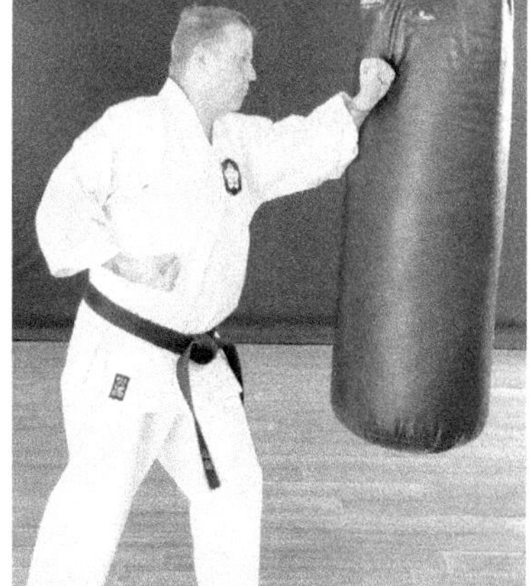

Counter 3: Yoko Geri & Tettsui Otoshi Uchi

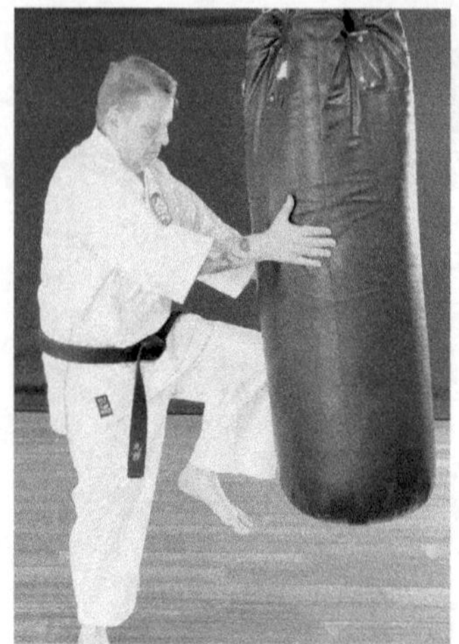

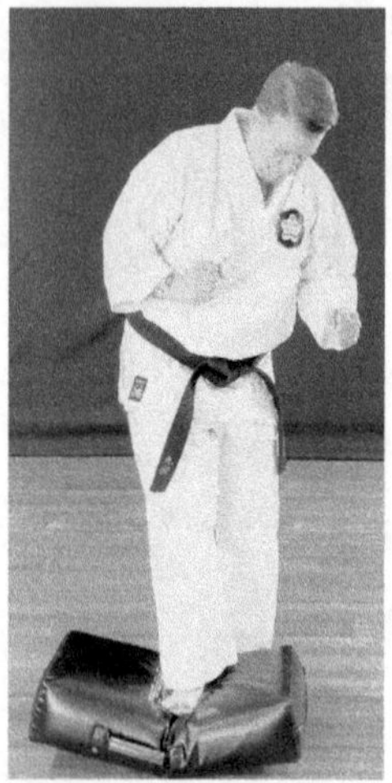

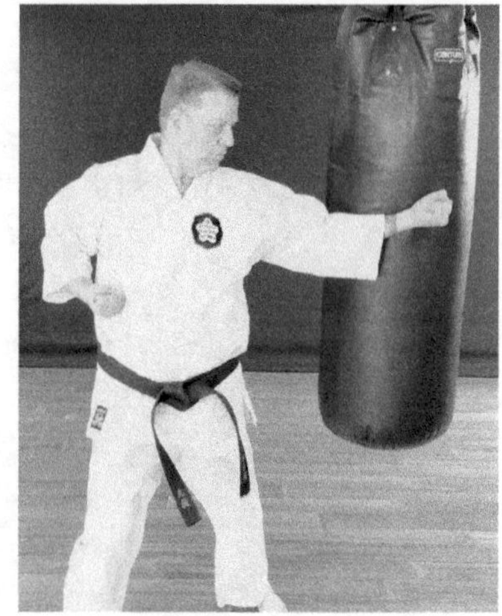

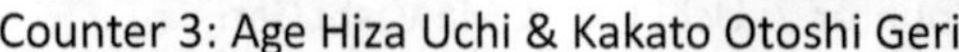

Counter 3: Age Hiza Uchi & Kakato Otoshi Geri

Counter 5: Uchi Uke

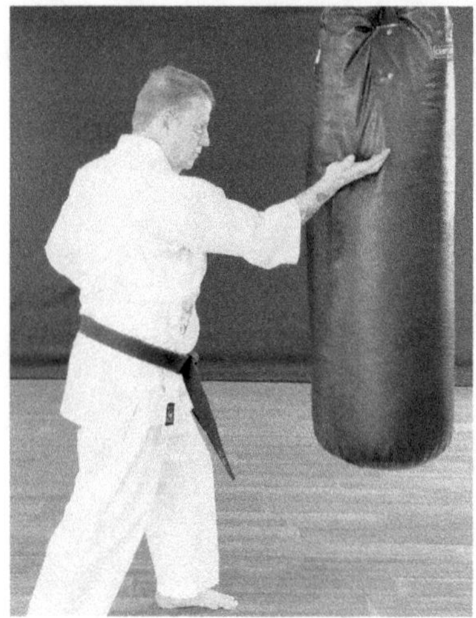

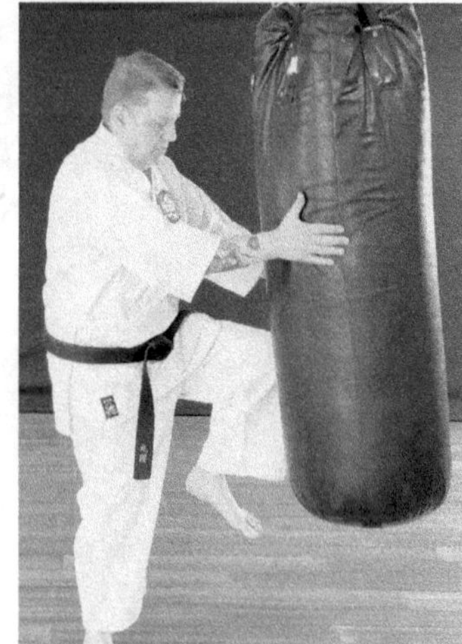

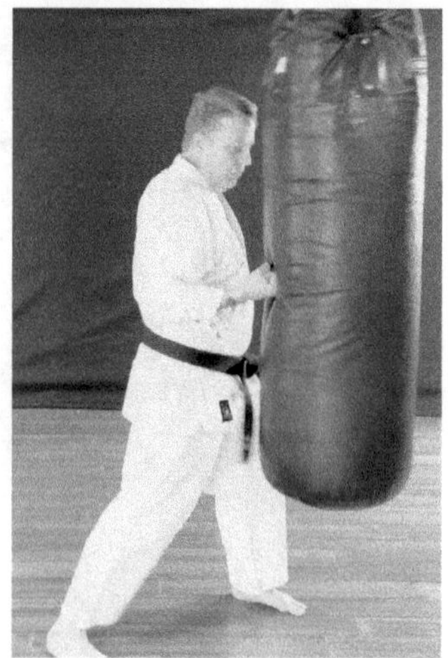

Counter 5: Shuto Uchi, Hiza Uchi, & Ura Zuki

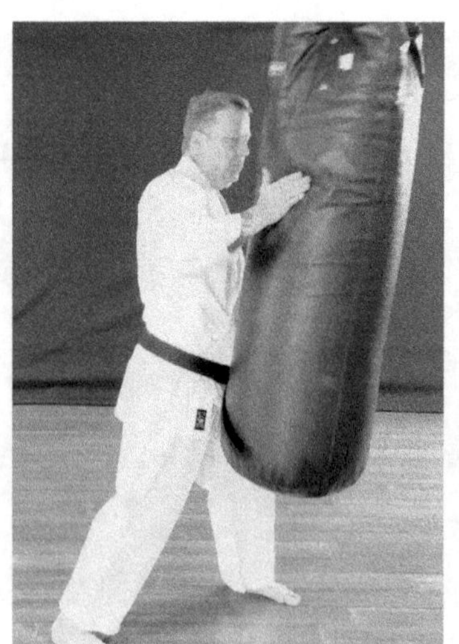

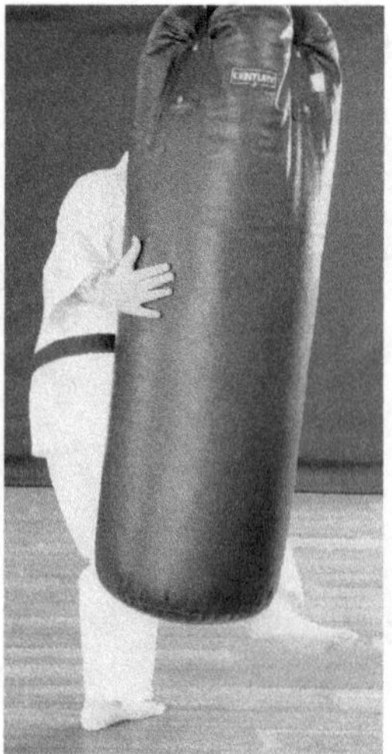

Counter 5: Shotei Uchi & Osoto-gari

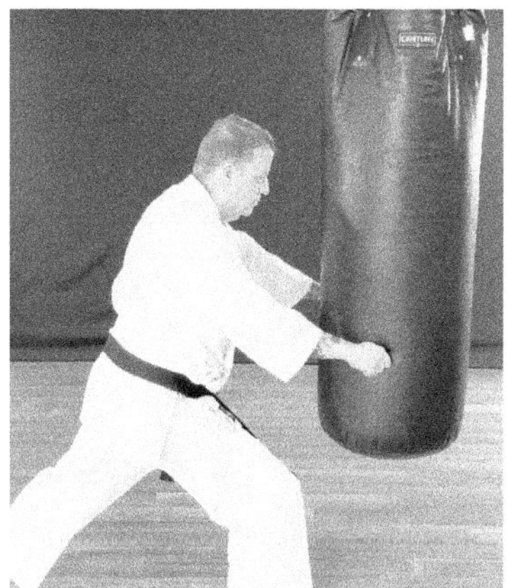

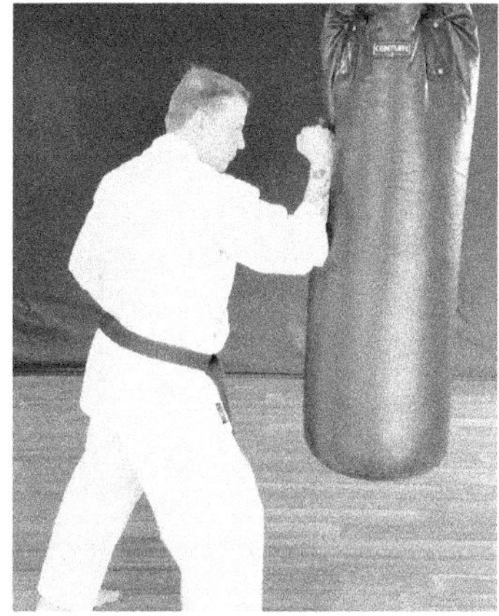

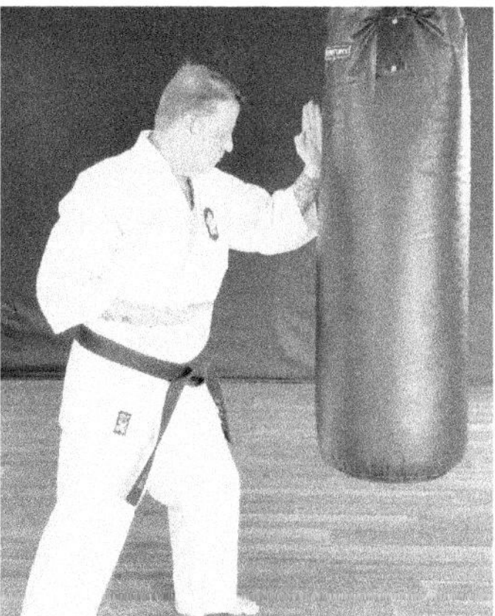

Counter 6: Morote Oyayubi Ippon Ken Uchi, Tettsui Otoshi Uchi, & Shuto Otoshi Uchi

14. Kumite Hachi (8)

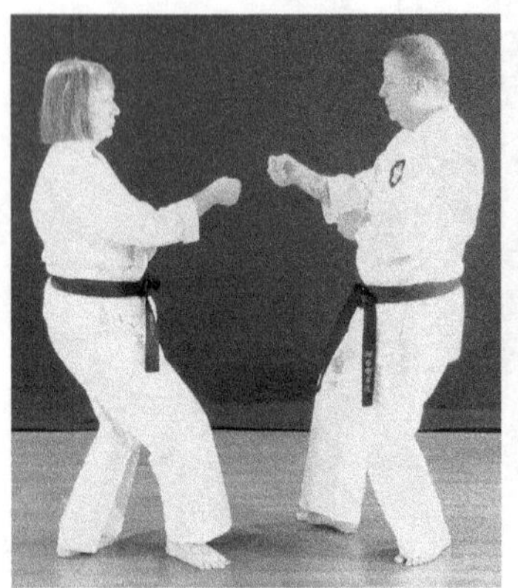

Renoji Dachi Kamae, Hands in Fists Held Vertically, Chamber Hand at Chest

Begin Counter 1

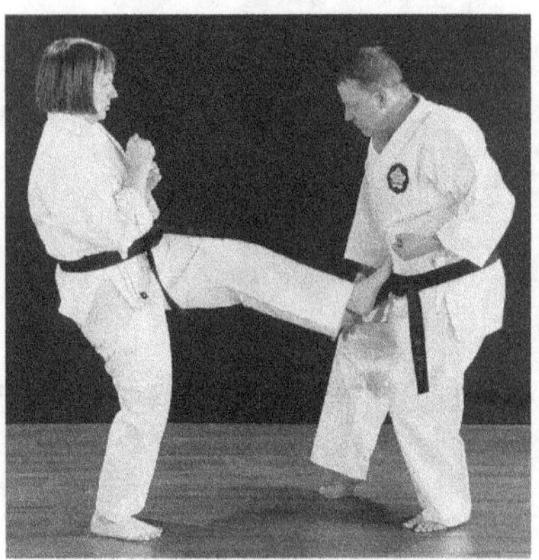

1. (Off - L): Gedan Mae Geri / (Def - R): Step Back into Neko Ashi Dachi, Sukui Uke

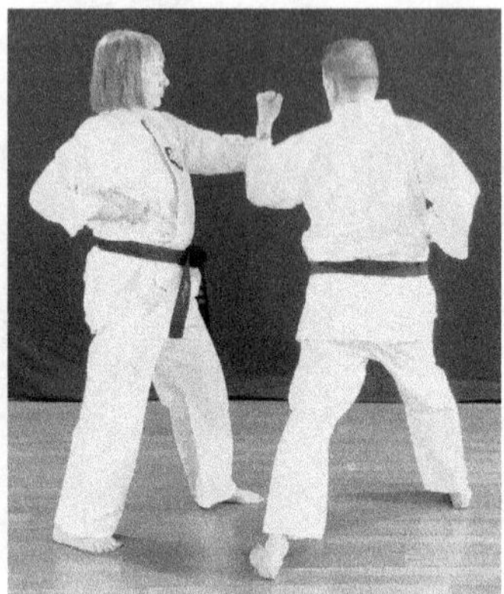

2. (Off - L): Step Forward, Chudan Zuki / (Def - R): Step Back to Side, Pivot Right, Soto Uke

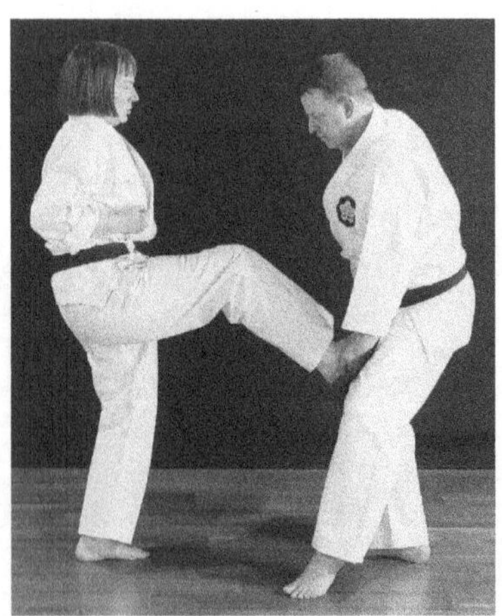

3. (Off - L): Gedan Mae Geri / (Def - R): Step Back into Neko Ashi Dachi, Sukui Uke

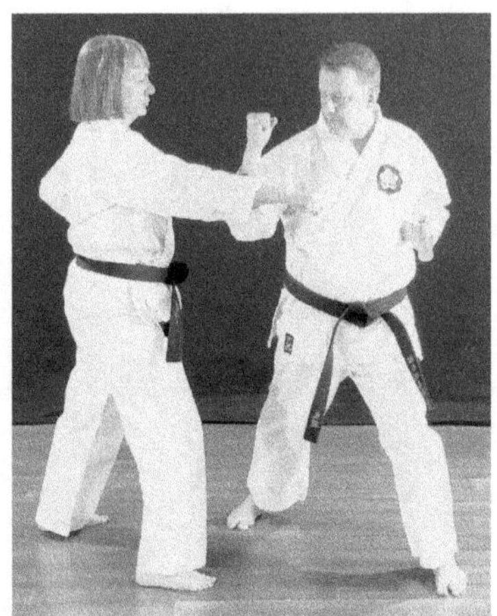

4. (Off - L): Step Forward, Chudan Zuki / (Def - R): Step Back to Side, Pivot Left, Soto Uke

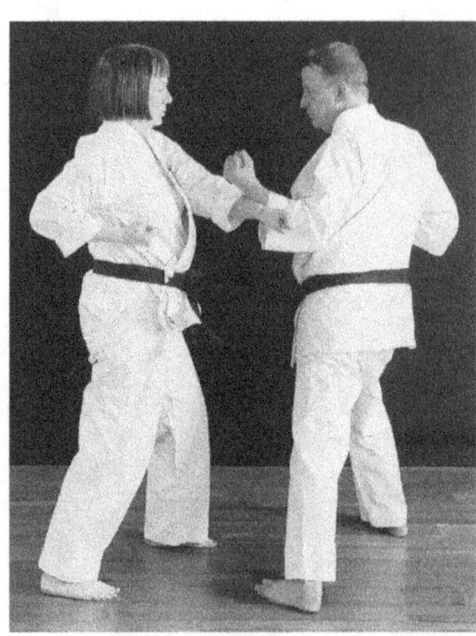

5. (Off - L): Step Forward, Chudan Zuki / (Def - R): Step Back to Side, Chudan Uchi Uke

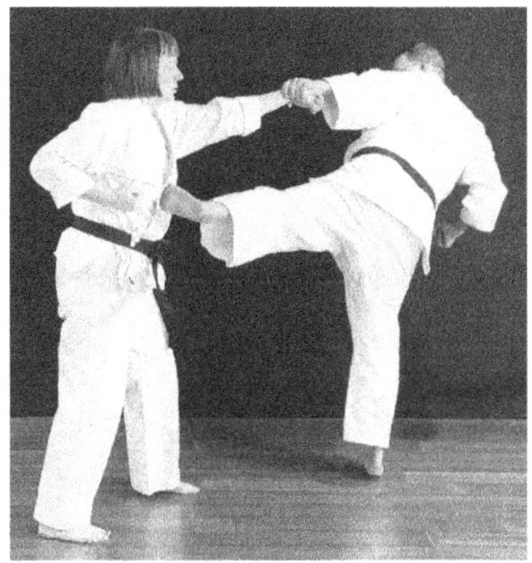

6. (Def - R): Grab Opponent's Wrist, Mawashi Geri to Chest with Ball of Foot

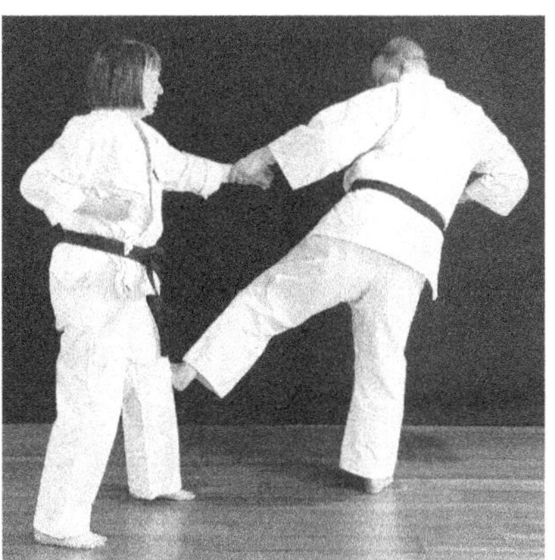

7. (Def - R): Hiza Geri

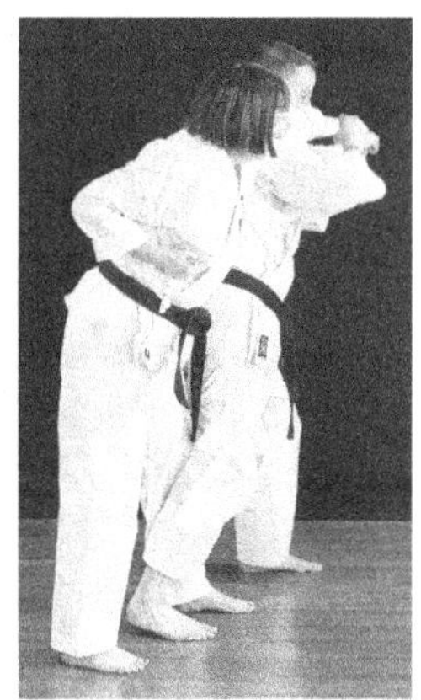

8. (Def - R): Step in Front of Opponent's Left Leg, Pull Arm Over Shoulder for Throw (Seoi-nage) (Kiai)

Repeat in Other Direction

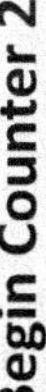

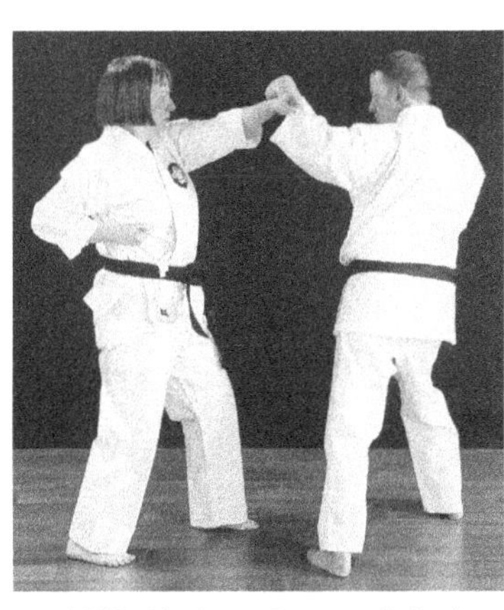

1. (Off - L): Step Forward, Jodan Zuki / (Def - R): Step Back to Side, Jodan Yoko Ko Uke

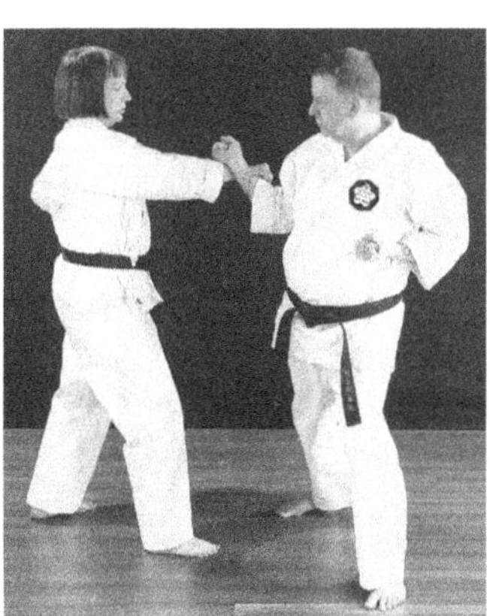

2. (Off - L): Step Forward, Chudan Zuki / (Def - R): Step Back to Side, Chudan Uchi Uke

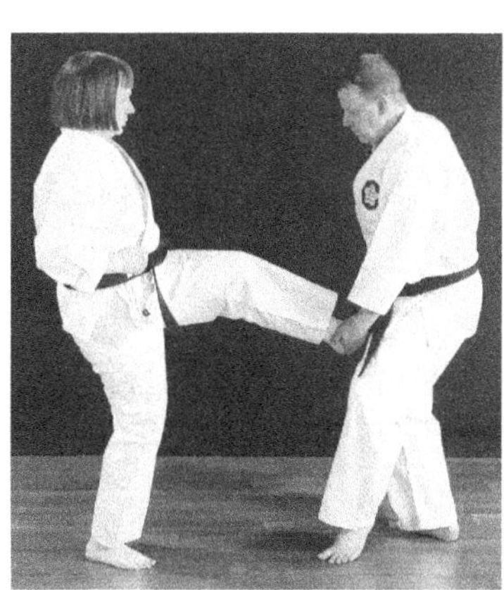

3. (Off - L): Gedan Mae Geri / (Def - R): Step Back into Neko Ashi Dachi, Sukui Uke

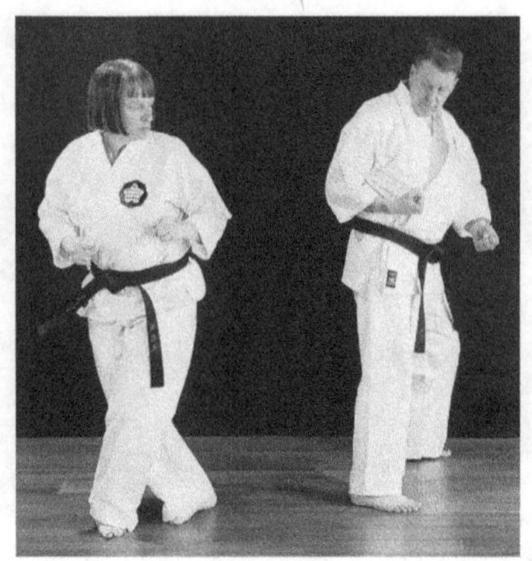
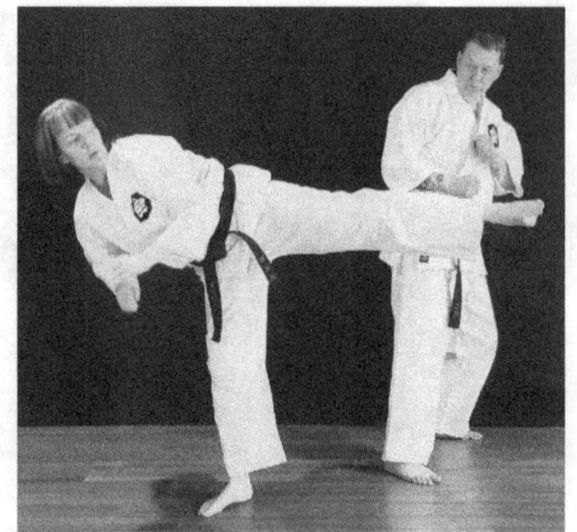

4. (Off - L): Step Behind Yoko Geri / (Def - R): Mawatte, Behind Opponent

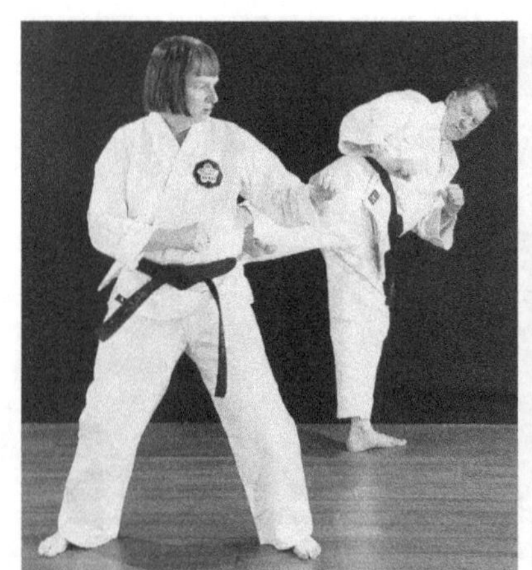

5. (Def - R): Yoko Geri

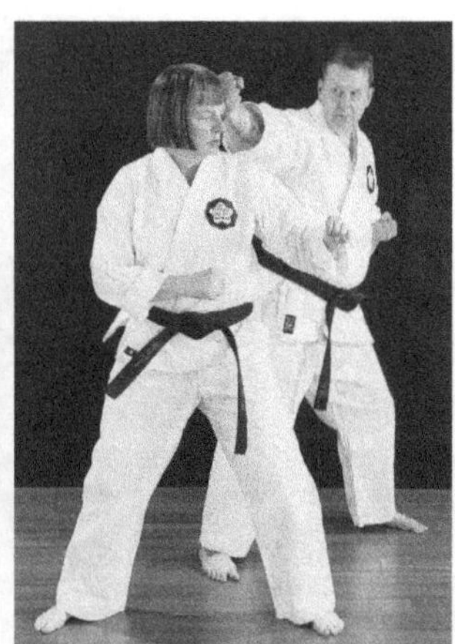

6. (Def - R): Uraken Uchi

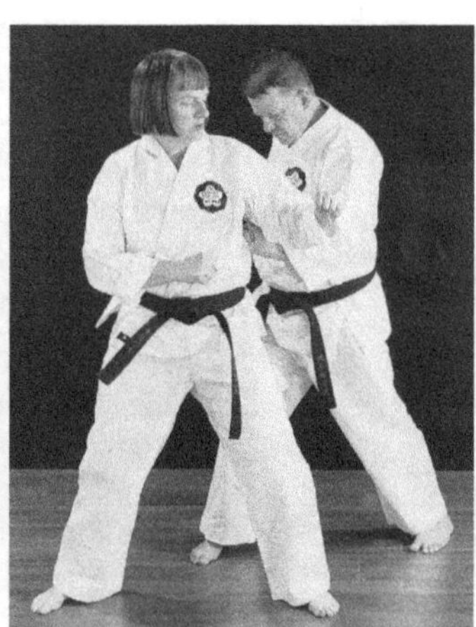

7. (Def - R): Ura Zuki (Kiai)

Repeat in Other Direction

Begin Counter 3

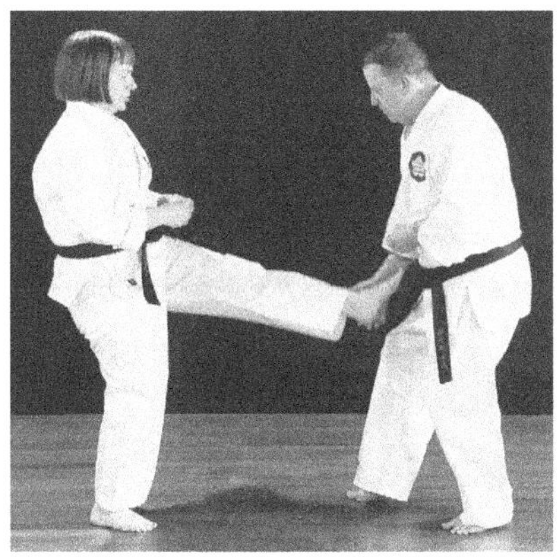

1. (Off - L): Gedan Mae Geri / (Def - R): Step Back into Neko Ashi Dachi, Sukui Uke

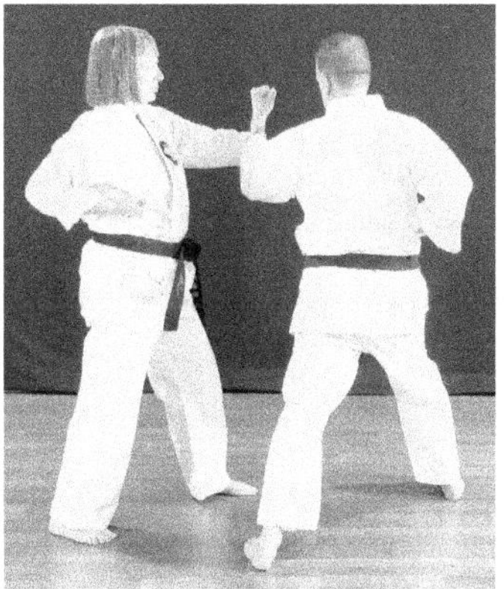

2. (Off - L): Step Forward, Chudan Zuki / (Def - R): Step Back to Side, Pivot Right, Soto Uke

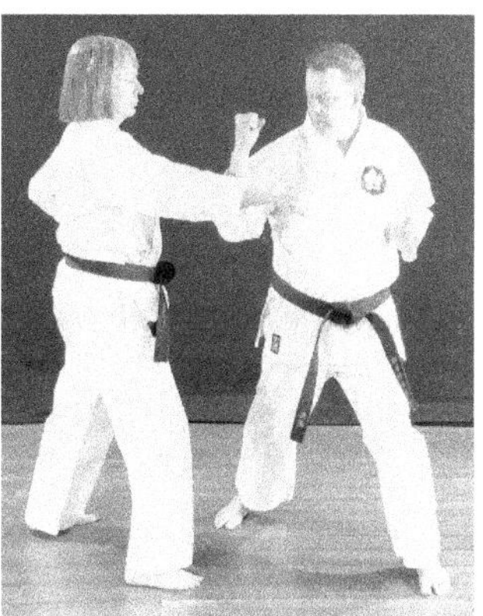

3. (Off - L): Step Forward, Chudan Zuki / (Def - R): Step Back to Side, Pivot Left, Soto Uke

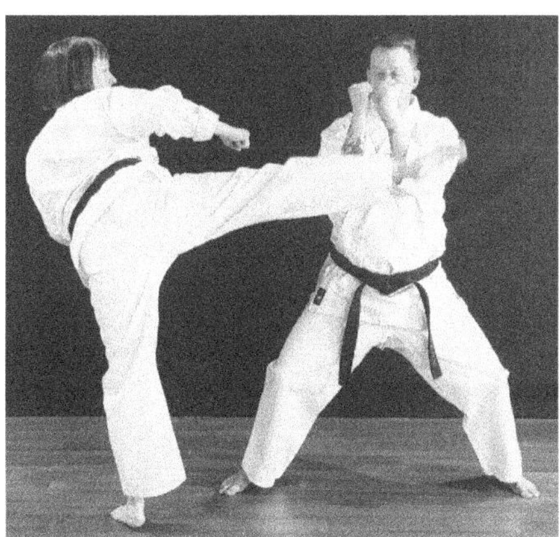

4. (Off - L): Jodan Tobi Mawashi Geri / (Def - R): Stutter Step Back, Morote Yoko Kote Uchi

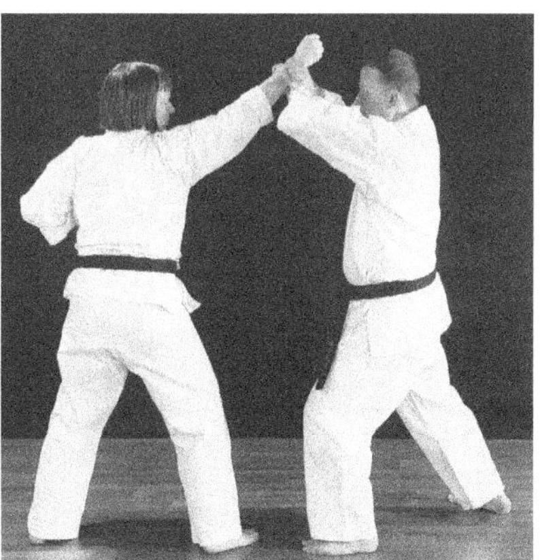

5. (Off - L): Step Behind Tettsui Otoshi Uchi / (Def - R): Step Back, Juji Age Uke

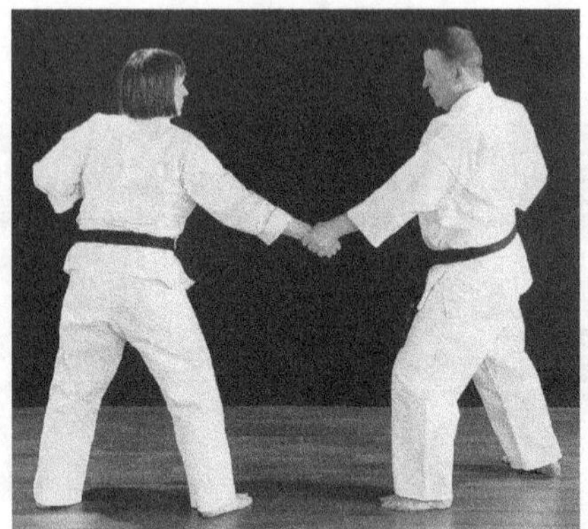

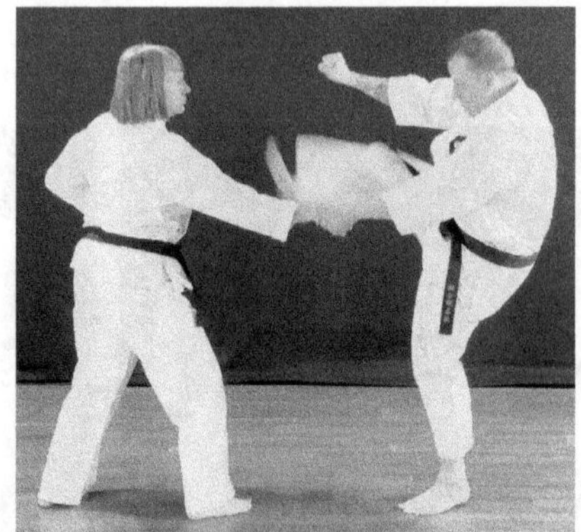

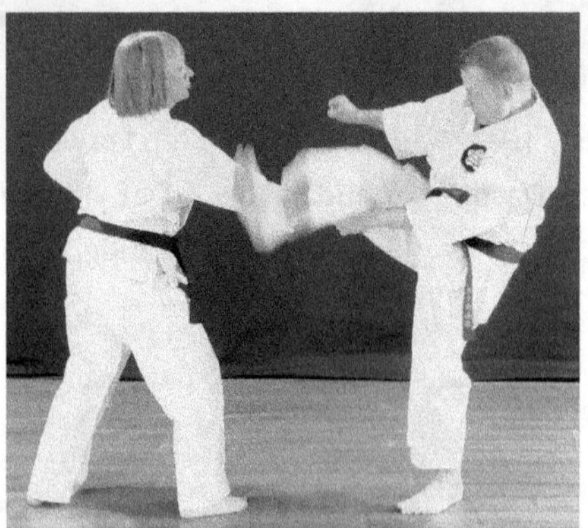

6. (Def - R): Grab Wrist, Right Mikazuki Geri Over Arm

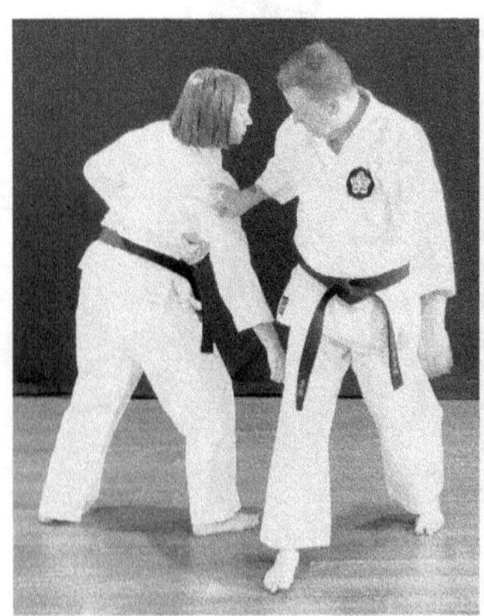

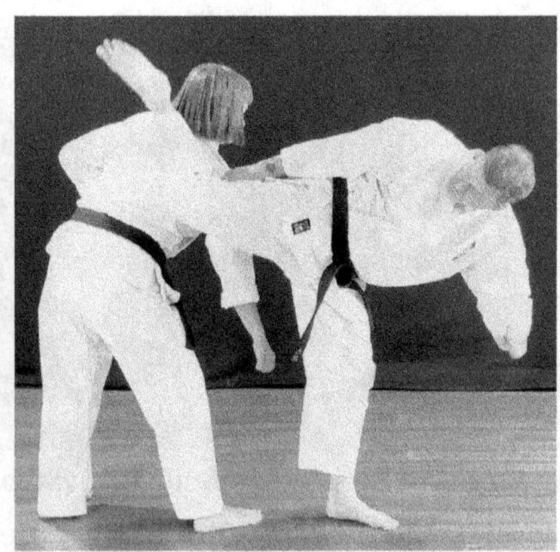

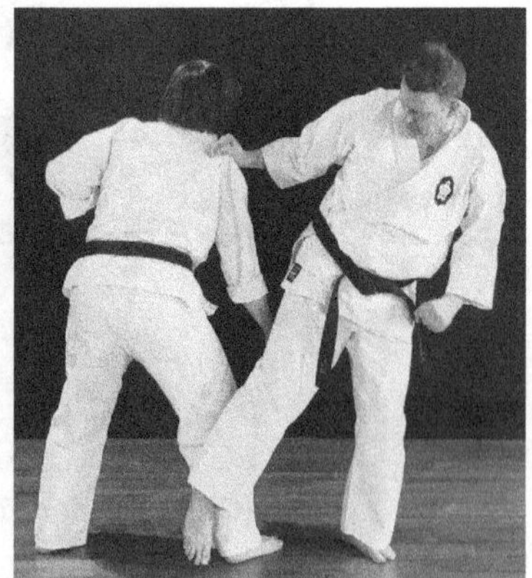

7. (Def - R): Grab Shoulder Area, Jodan Ushiro Mawashi Geri, then Ashi Kake Nage

Repeat in Other Direction

8. (Def - R): Sokuto Otoshi Geri to Throat (Kiai)

Begin Counter 4

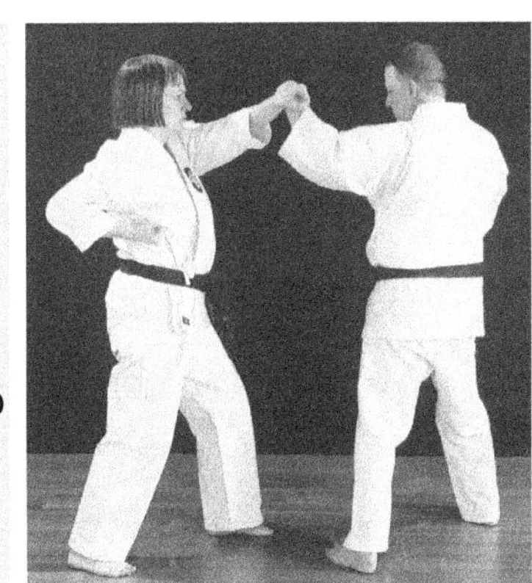

1. (Off - L): Step Forward, Jodan Zuki / (Def - R): Step Back to Side, Jodan Yoko Ko Uke

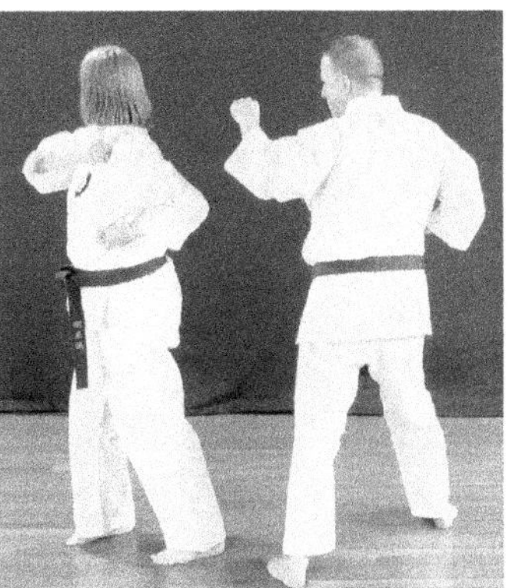

2. (Off - L): Jodan Ushiro Mawashi Uraken Uchi / (Def - R): Stutter Step Back, Soto Uke

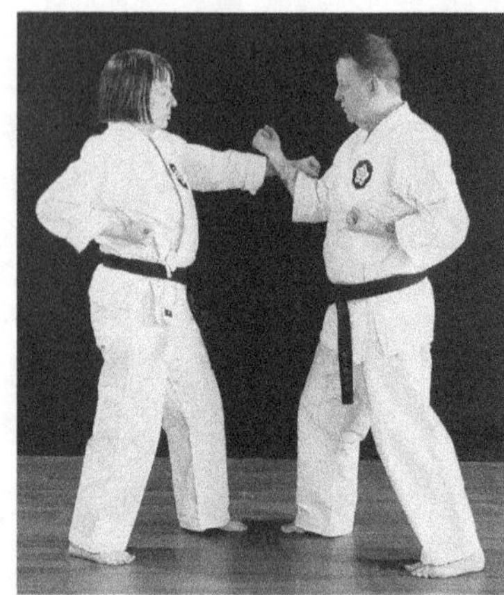

3. (Off - L): Step Forward, Chudan Zuki / (Def - R): Stutter Step Back, Chudan Uke

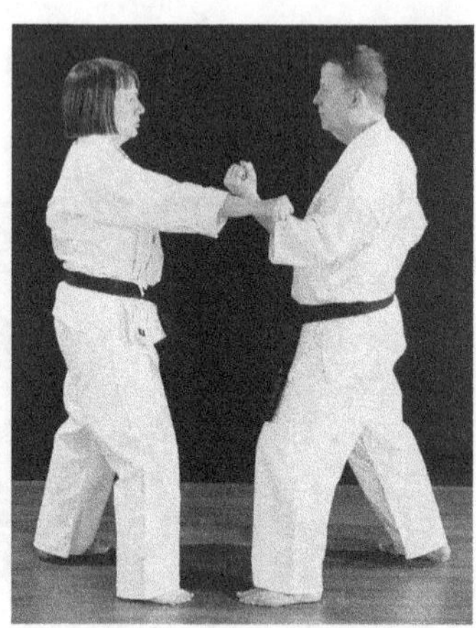

4. (Off - L): Step Forward, Chudan Zuki / (Def - R): Step Back, Chudan Uke

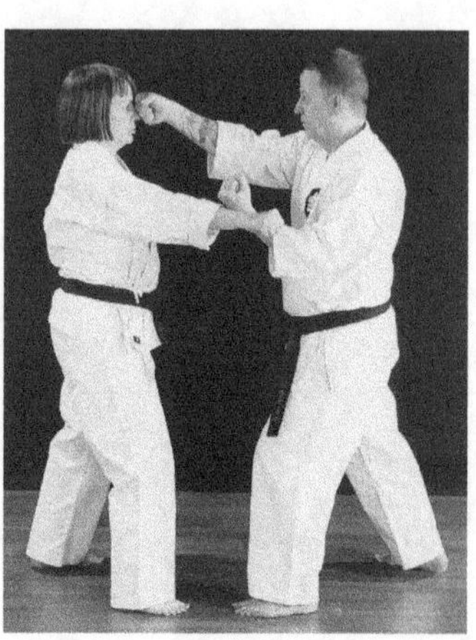

5. (Def - R): Jodan Tate Uchi

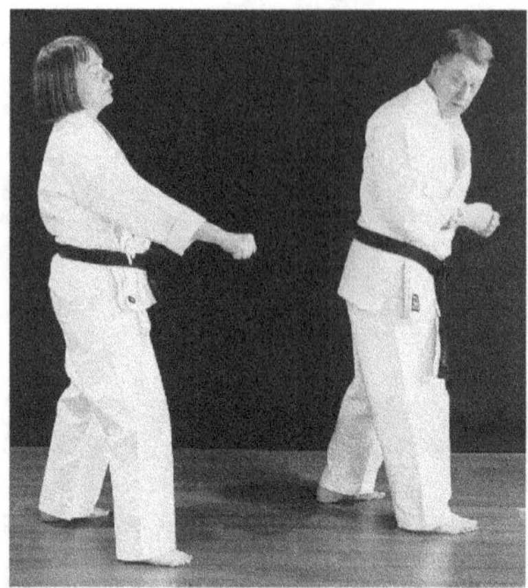

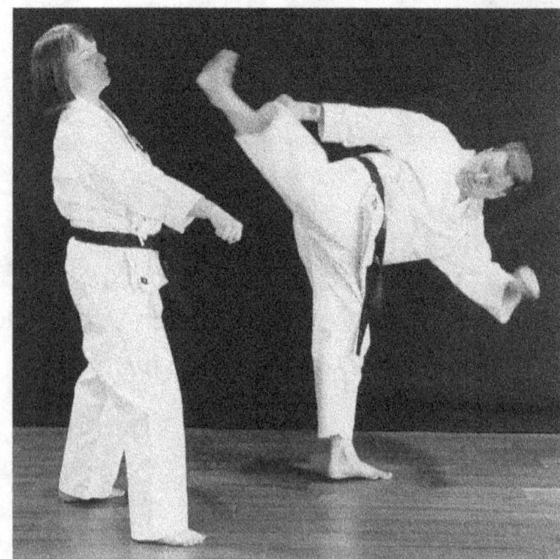

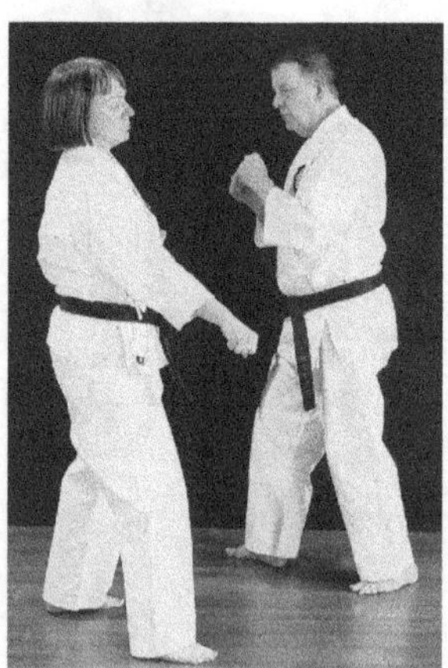

6. (Def - R): Mawatte, Right Jodan Kake Geri

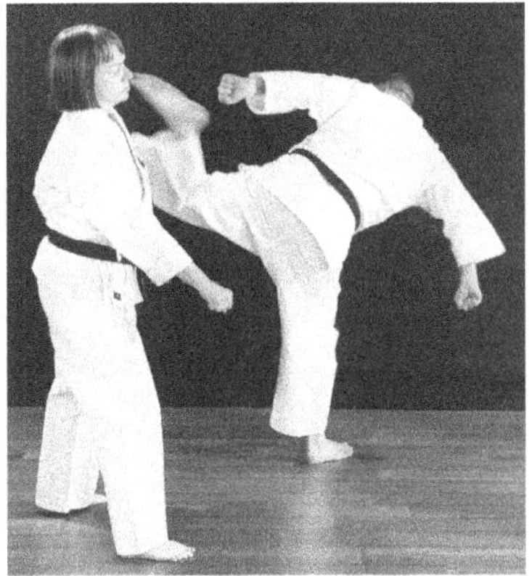

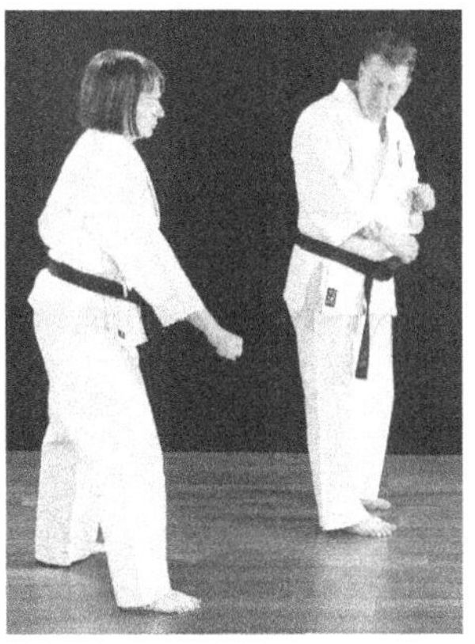

7. (Def - R): Left Jodan Kake Geri

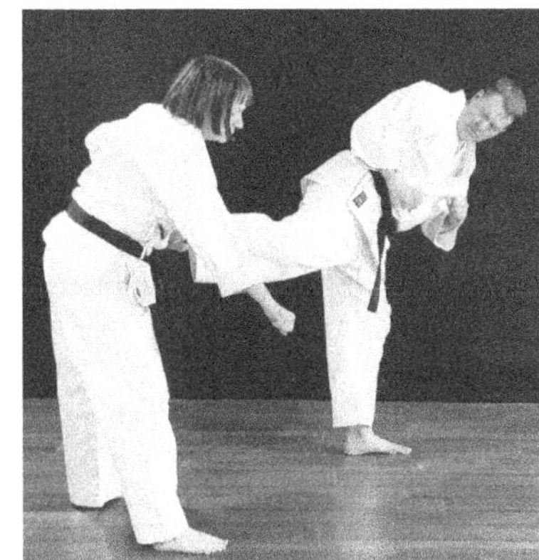

8. (Def - R): Yoko Geri (Kiai)

Repeat in Other Direction

Begin Counter 5

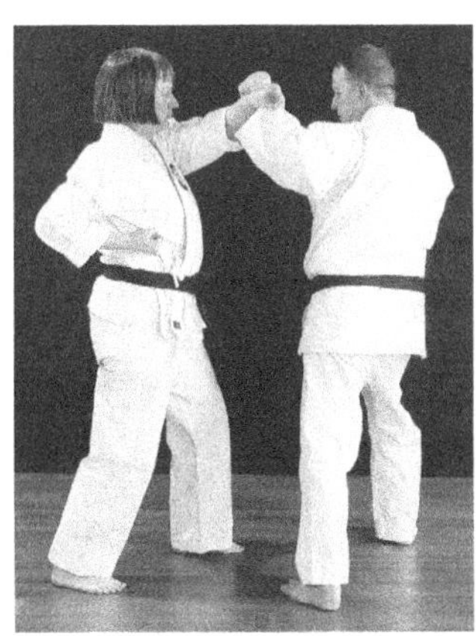

1. (Off - L): Step Forward, Jodan Zuki / (Def - R): Step Back to Side, Jodan Yoko Ko Uke

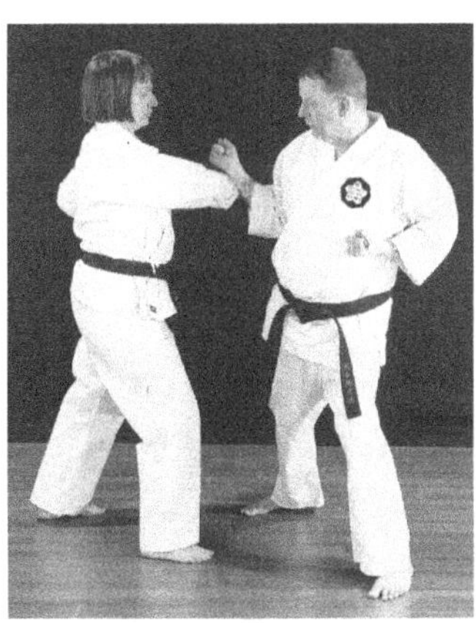

2. (Off - L): Step Forward, Chudan Zuki / (Def - R): Step Back to Side, Chudan Uchi Uke

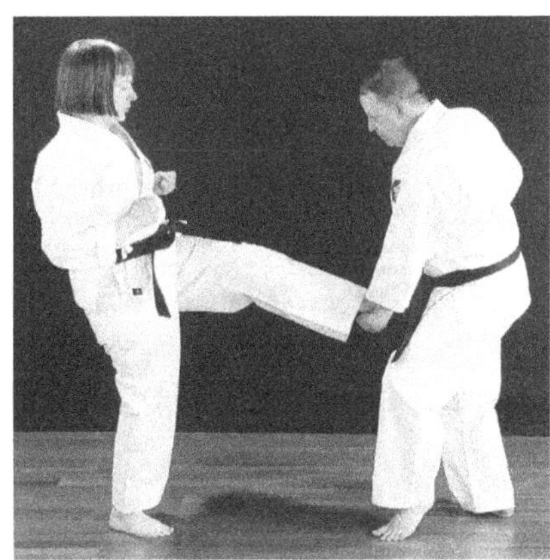

3. (Off - L): Left Gedan Mae Geri / (Def - R): Step Back into Neko Ashi Dachi, Sukui Uke

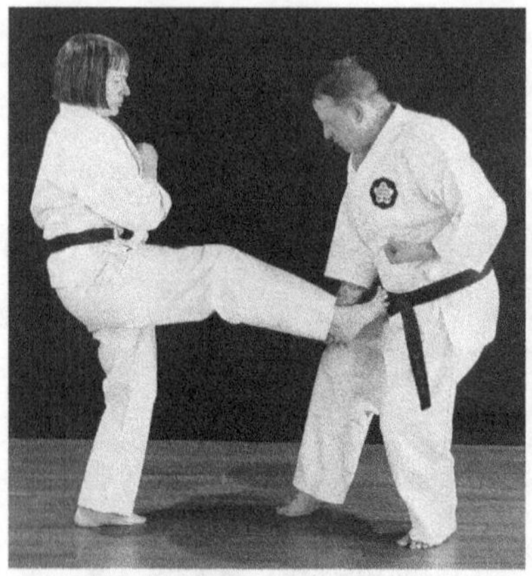

4. (Off - L): Right Gedan Mae Geri / (Def - R): Step Back into Neko Ashi Dachi, Sukui Uke

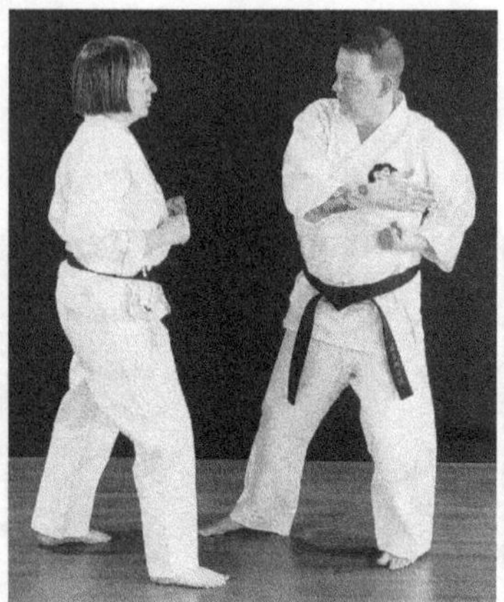

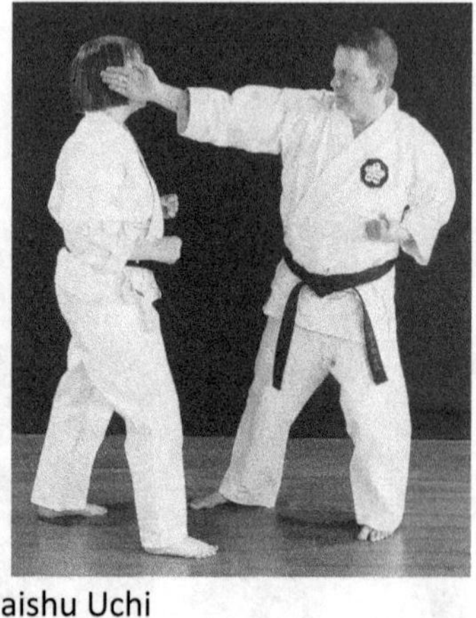

5. (Def - R): Haishu Uchi

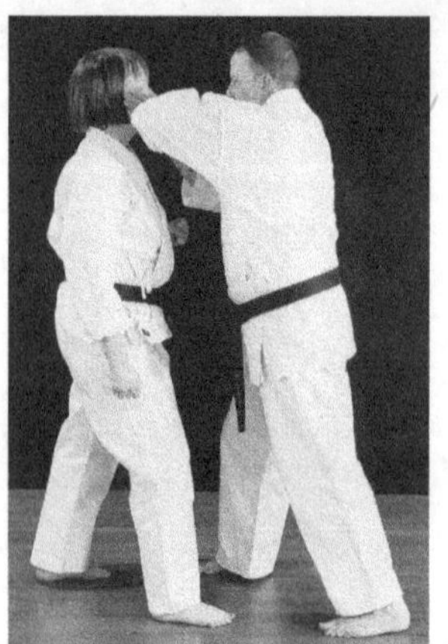

6. (Def - R): Jodan Mawashi Empi Uchi

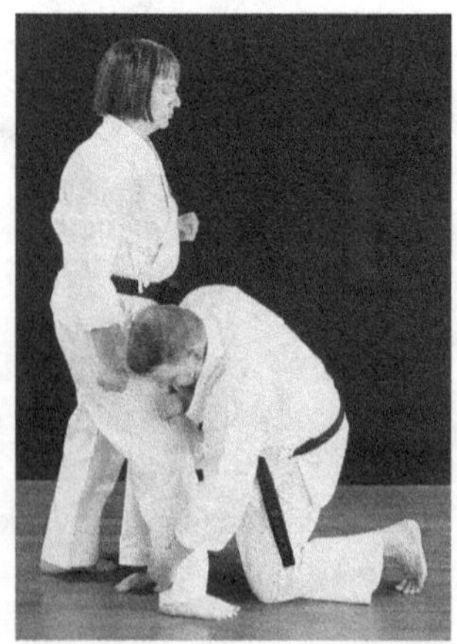

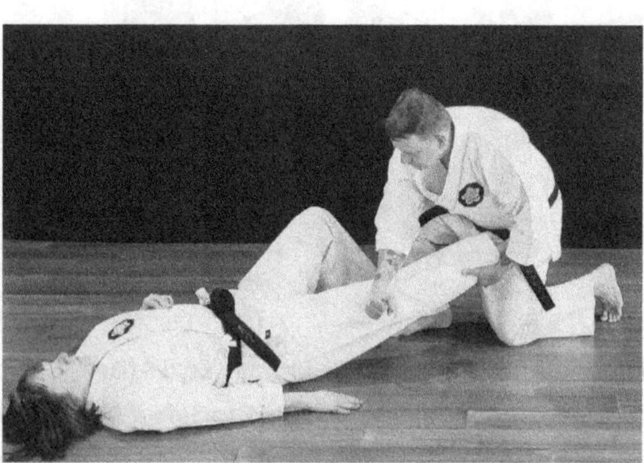

7. (Def - R): Drop Down to Knee, Kibisu Gaeshi

Repeat in Other Direction

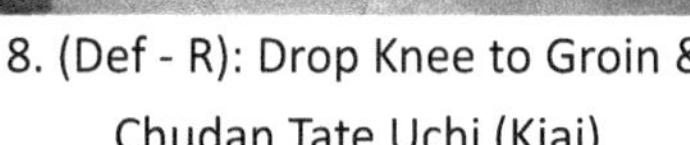

8. (Def - R): Drop Knee to Groin & Chudan Tate Uchi (Kiai)

Begin Counter 6

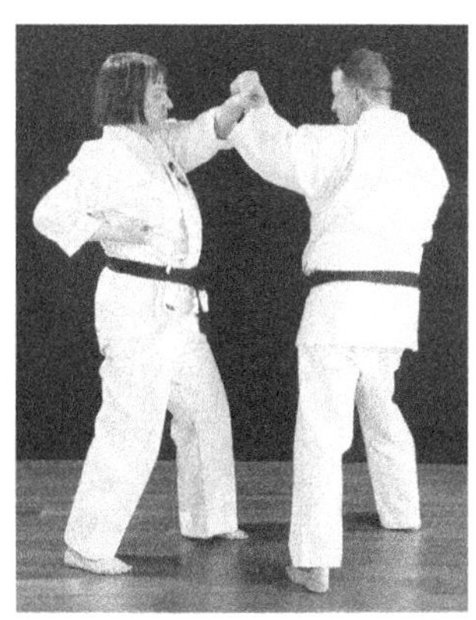

1. (Off - L): Step Forward, Jodan Zuki / (Def - R): Step Back to Side, Jodan Yoko Ko Uke

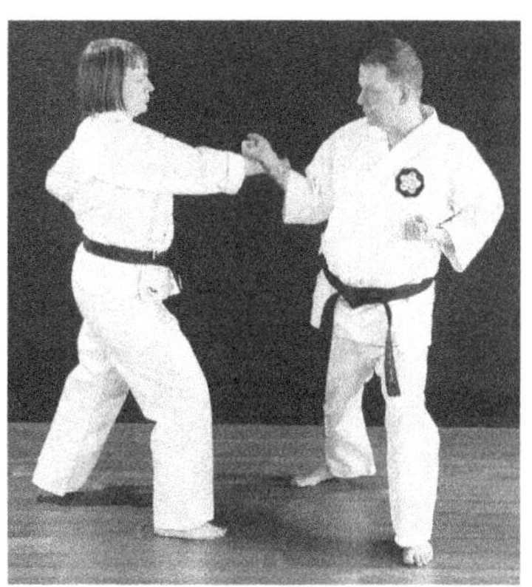

2. (Off - L): Step Forward, Chudan Zuki / (Def - R): Step Back to Side, Chudan Uchi Uke

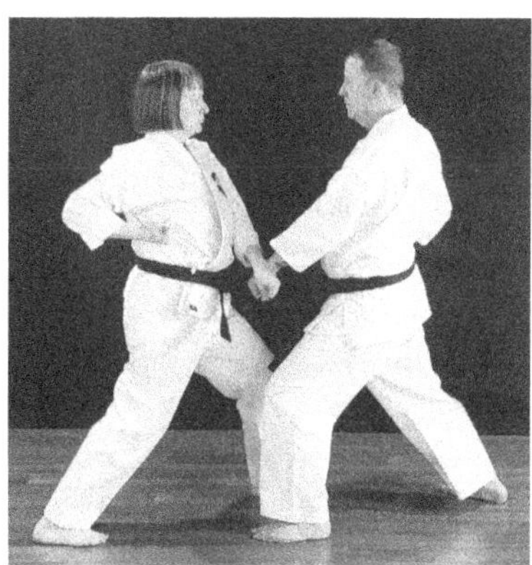

3. (Off - L): Step Forward, Gedan Zuki in Zenkutsu Dachi / (Def - R): Step Back, Gedan Shotei Barai in Zenkutsu Dachi

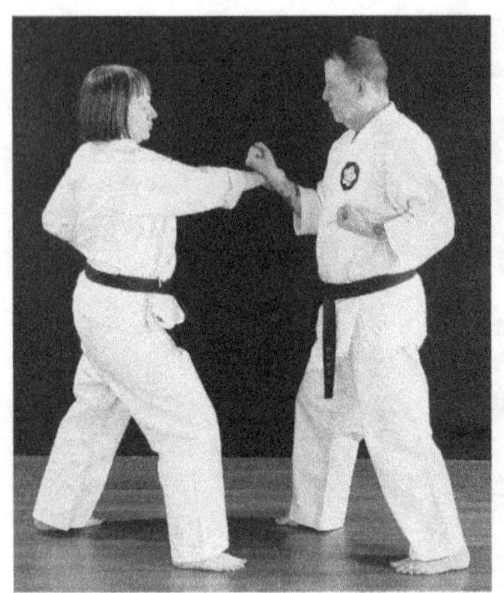

4. (Off - L): Step Forward, Chudan Zuki / (Def - R): Step Back, Chudan Uke

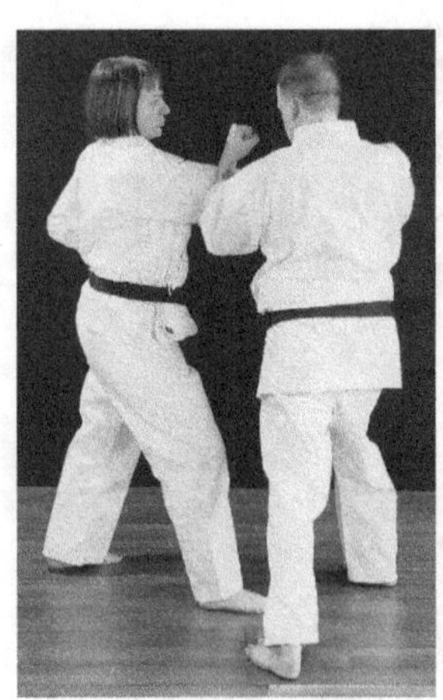

5. (Def - R): Grab Arm, Step Around to Side, Kote Uchi on Opponent's Arm, Just Above the Elbow

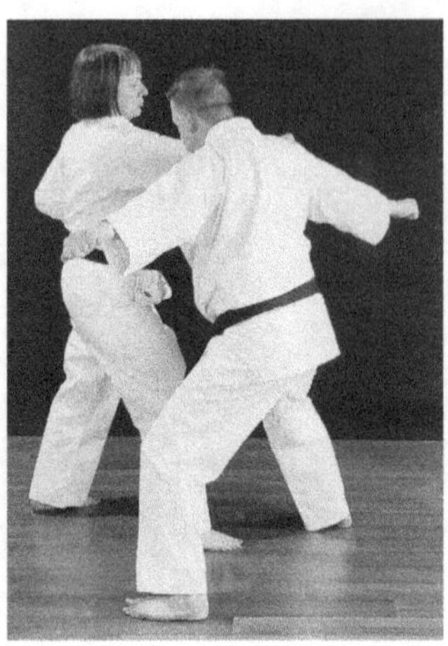

6. (Def - R): Morote Oyayubi Ate

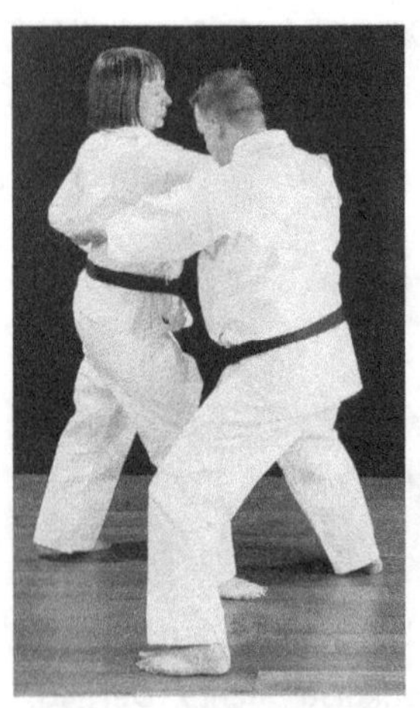

Morote Oyayubi Ate (cont.)

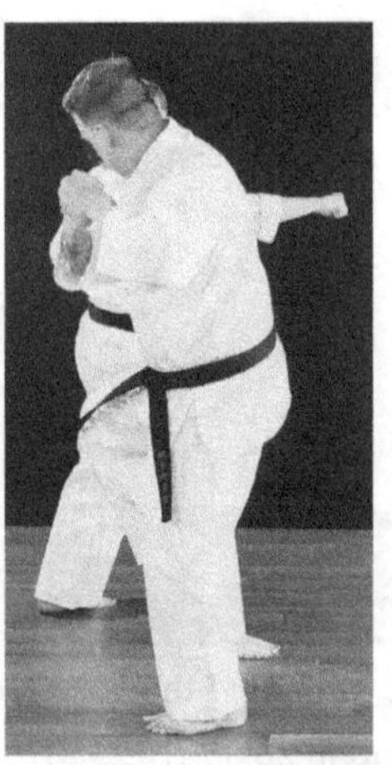

7. (Def - R): Step Inside, Yoko Empi Uchi to Opponent's Ribs

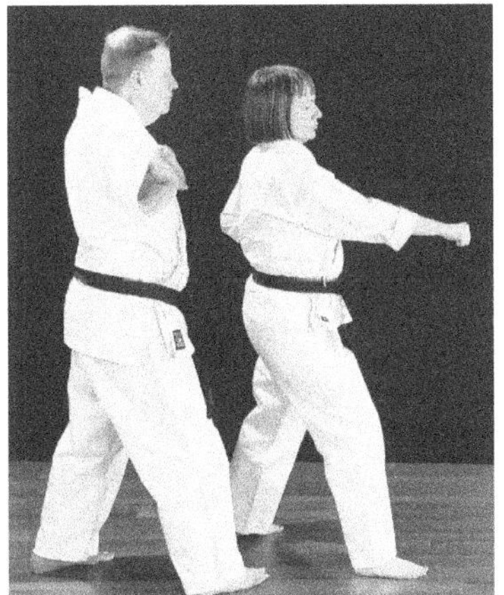

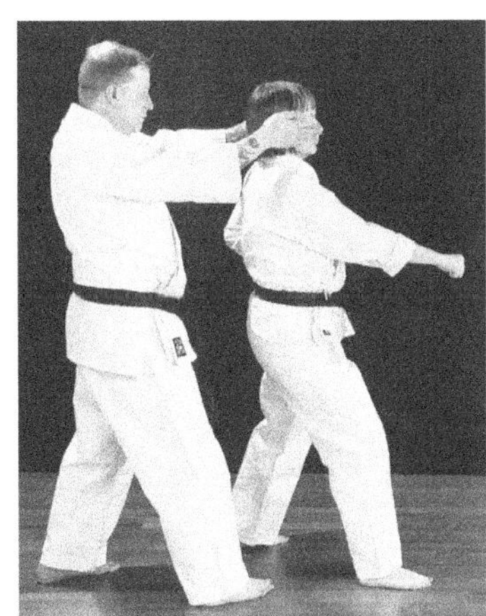

8. (Def - R): Mawatte, Morote Mimi Uchi

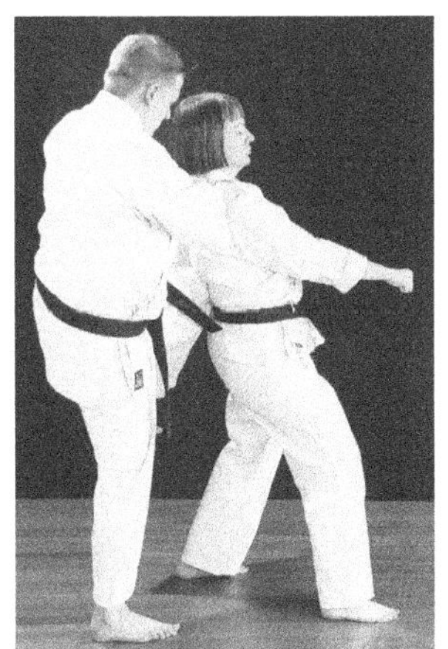

9. (Def - R): Pull Opponent's Shoulders Down, Hiza Uchi to Opponent's Back

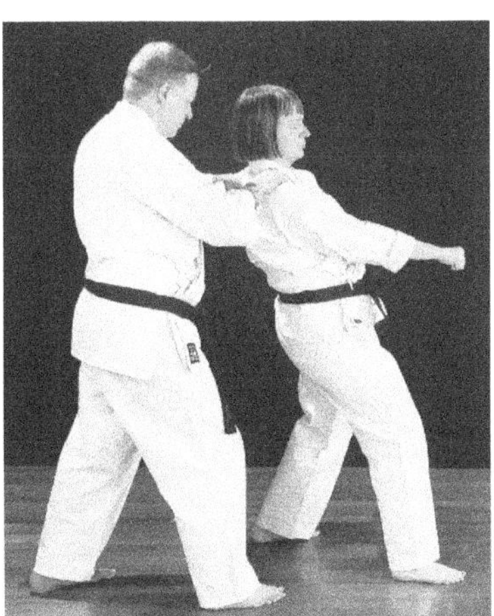

10. (Def - R): Pull Opponent Down to Ground

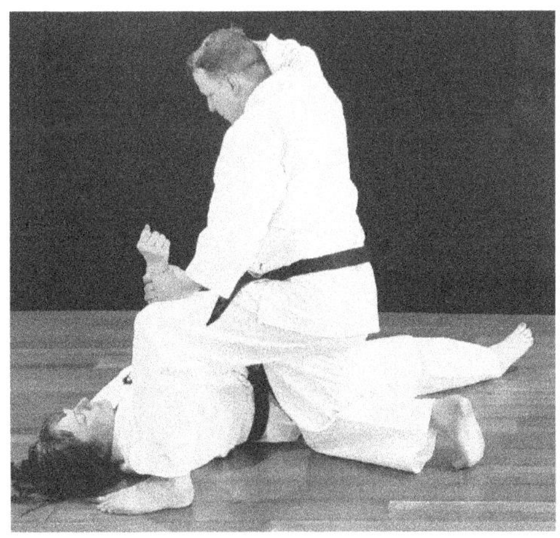

11. (Def - R): Nodo Kaki (Kiai)

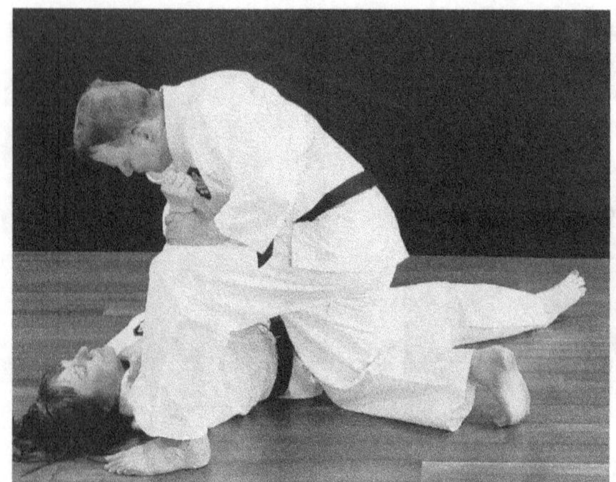

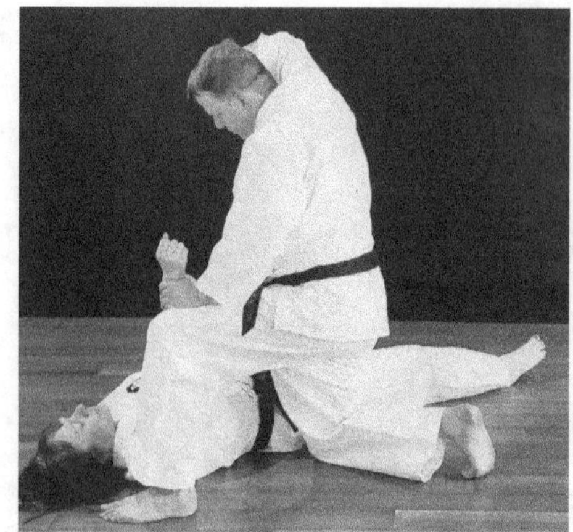

Repeat in Other Direction

Nodo Kaki (cont.)

Kumite Hachi - Bag Work

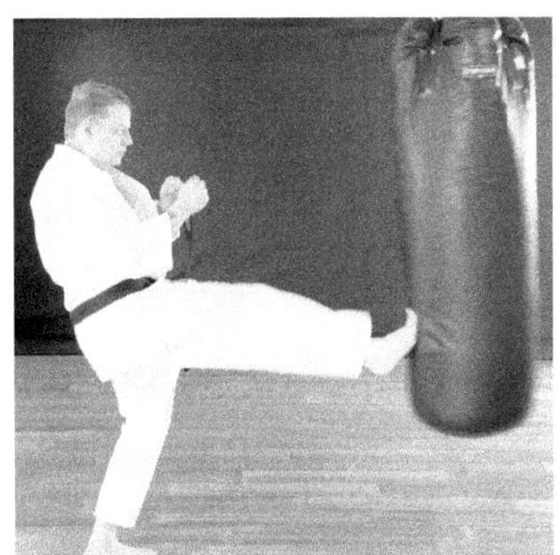

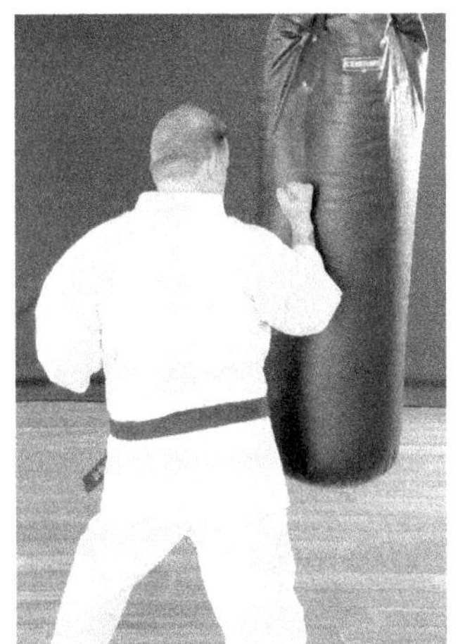

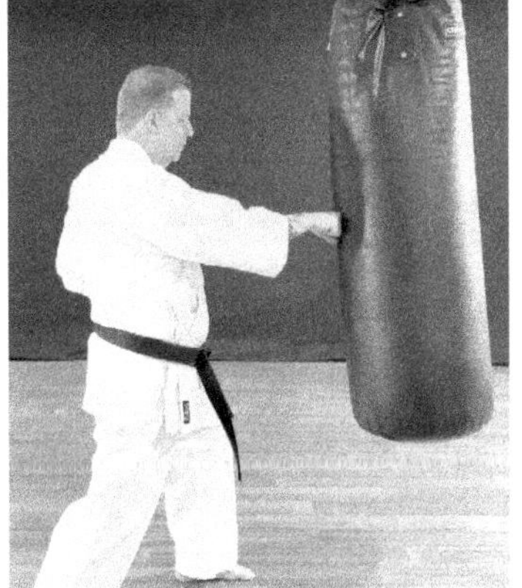

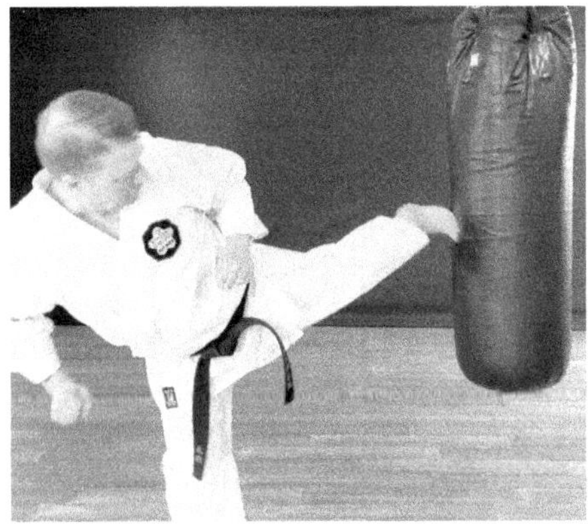

Counter 1: Gedan Mae Geri (Top) & Chudan Zuki (Bottom)

Counter 1: Soto Uke (Top) & Mawashi Geri (Ball of Foot) (Bottom)

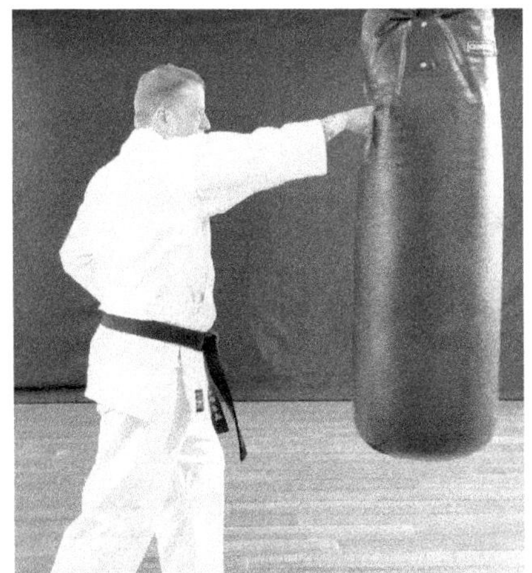

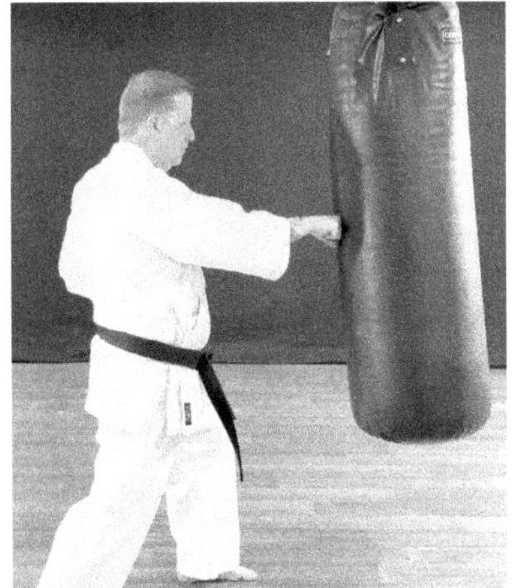

Counter 2: Jodan Zuki & Chudan Zuki

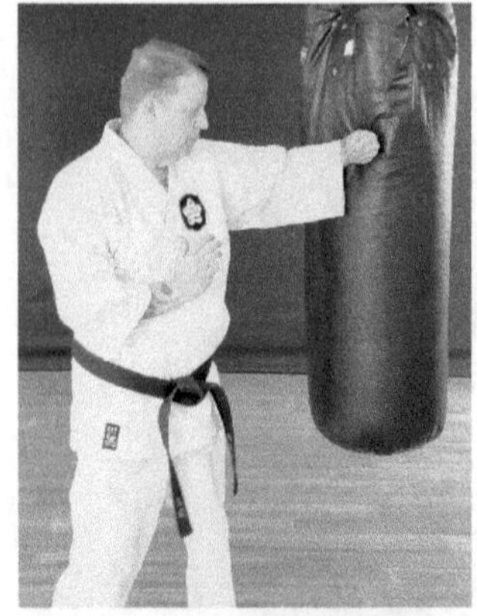

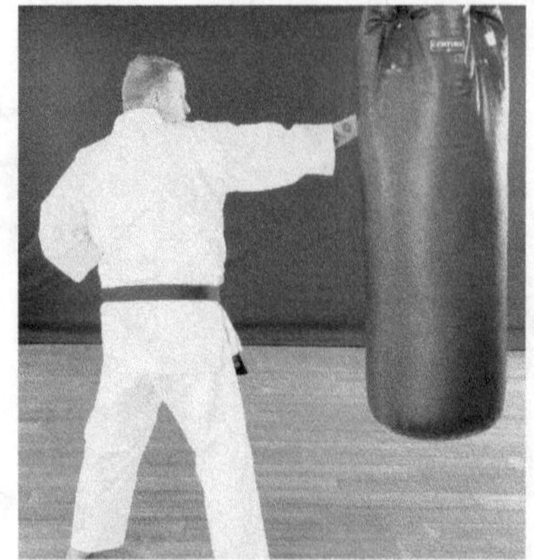

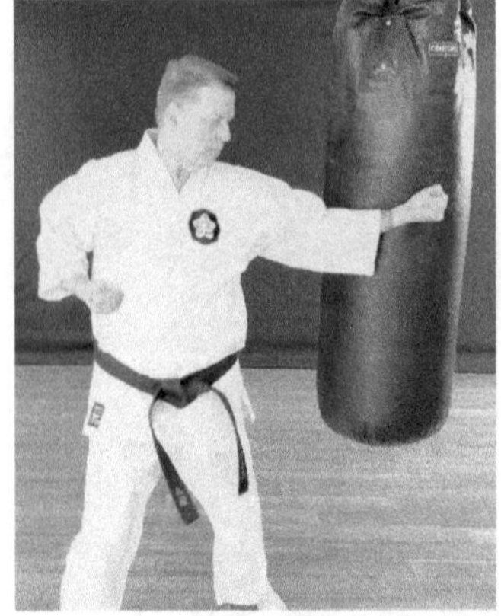

Counter 2: Ko Uke (Top) & Uchi Uke (Bottom)

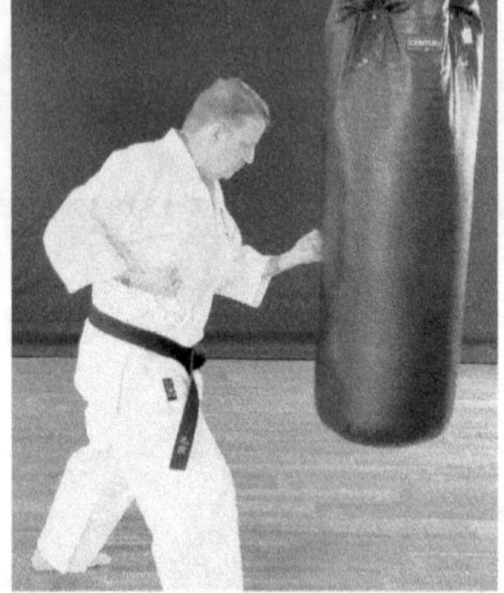

Counter 2: Uraken Uchi (Top) & Ura Zuki (Bottom)

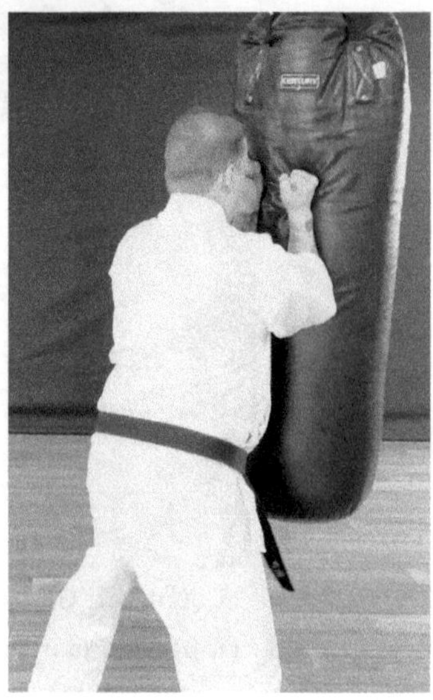

Counter 3: Morote Yoko Kote Uchi

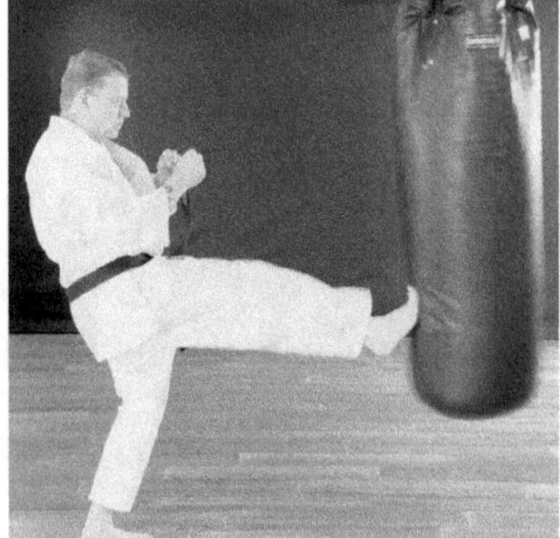

Counter 2: Gedan Mae Geri (Top) & Yoko Geri (Right)

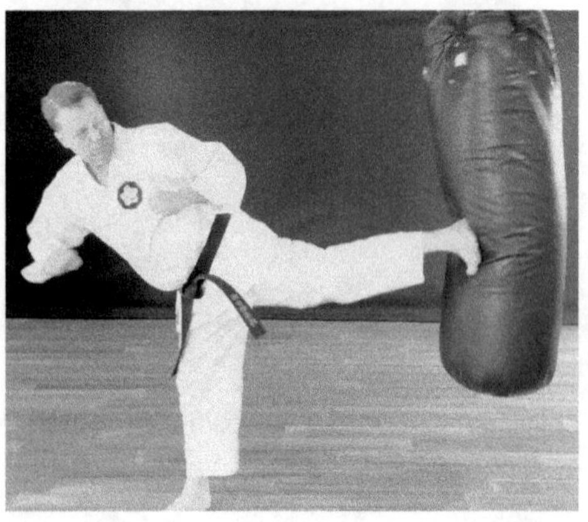

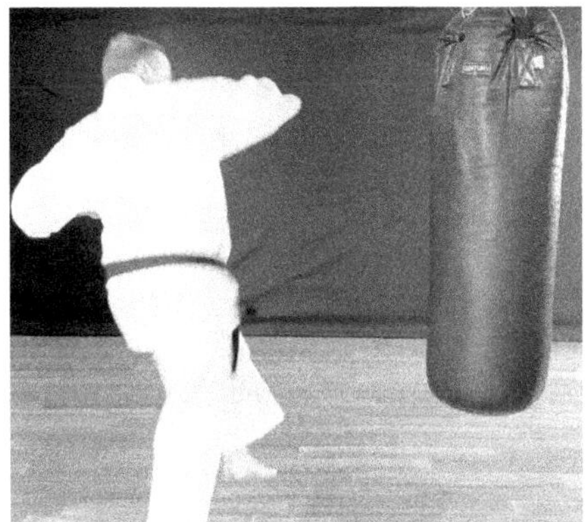

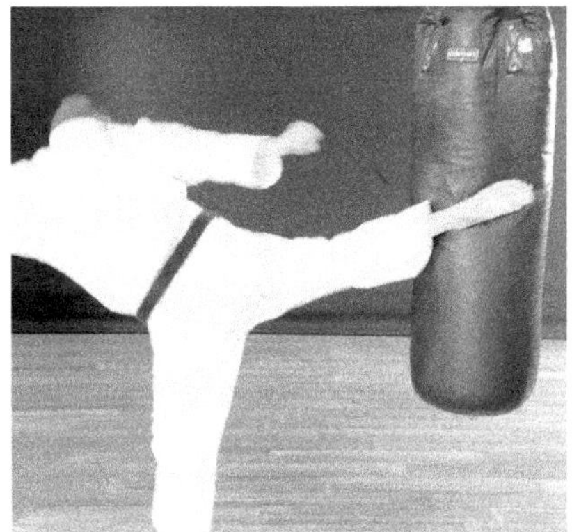

Counter 3: Tobi Mawashi Geri

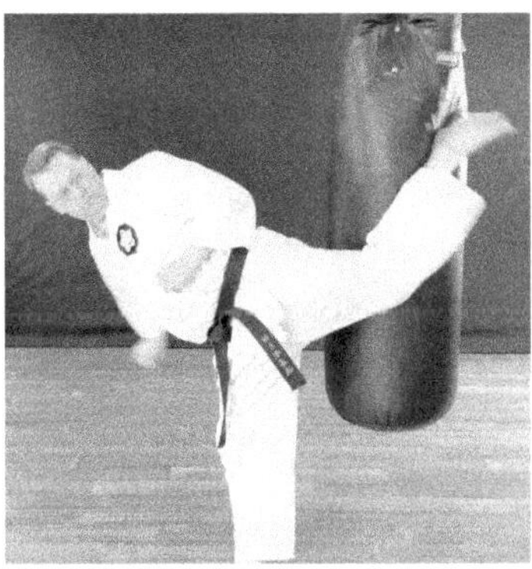

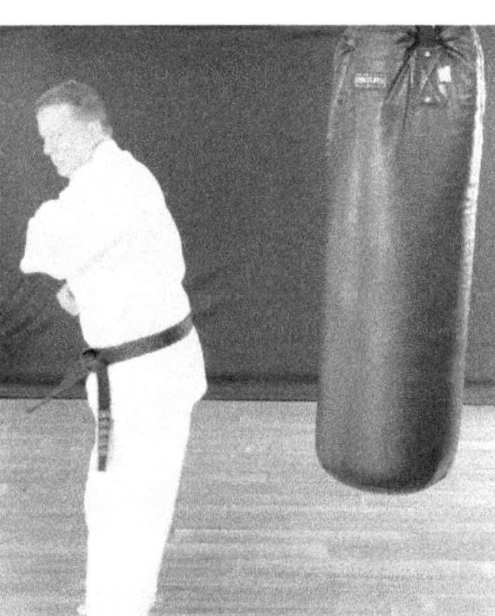

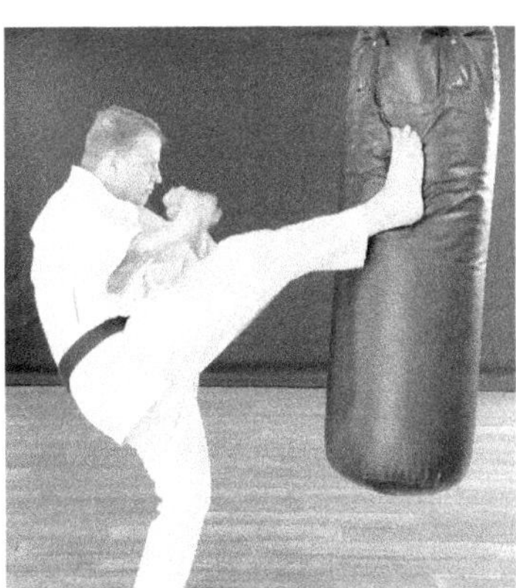

Counter 3: Mikazuki Geri

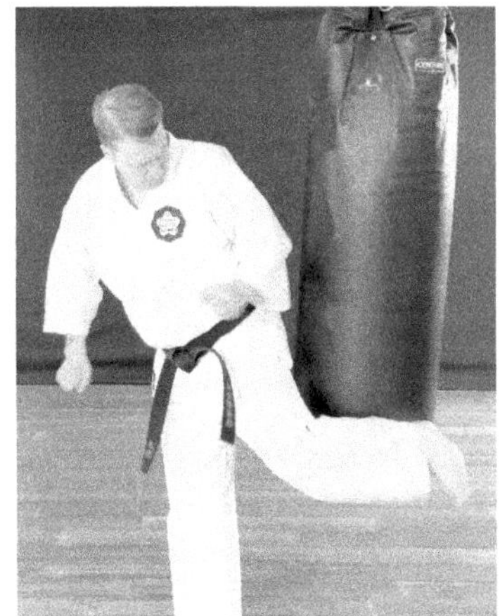

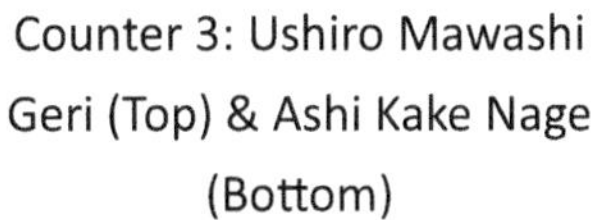

Counter 3: Ushiro Mawashi Geri (Top) & Ashi Kake Nage (Bottom)

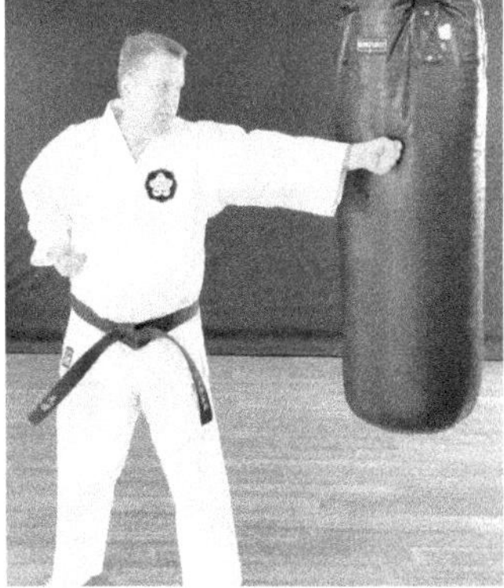

Counter 4: Ushiro Mawashi Uraken Uchi

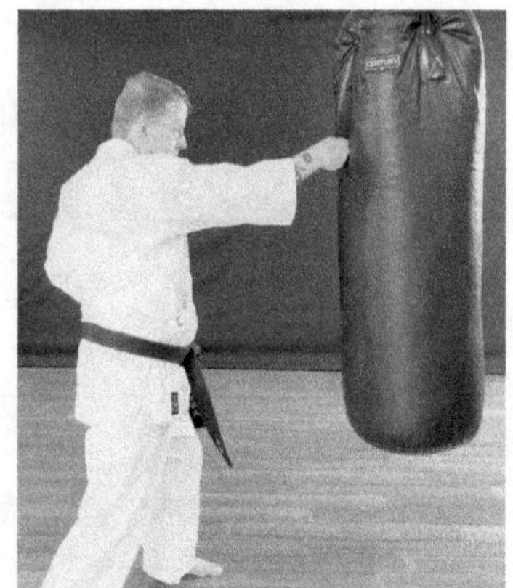
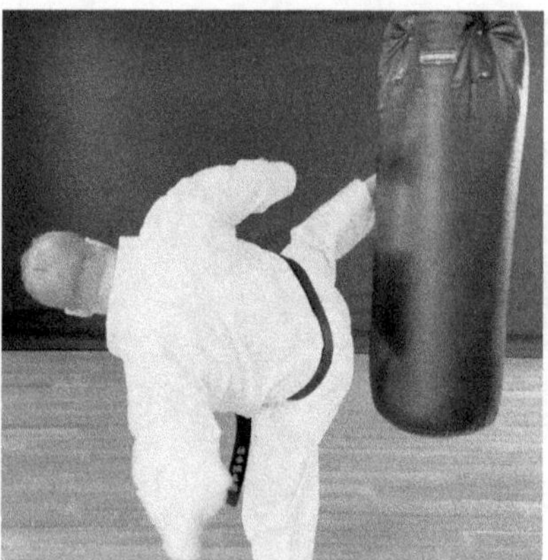

Counter 4: Tate Uchi & Jodan Kake Geri

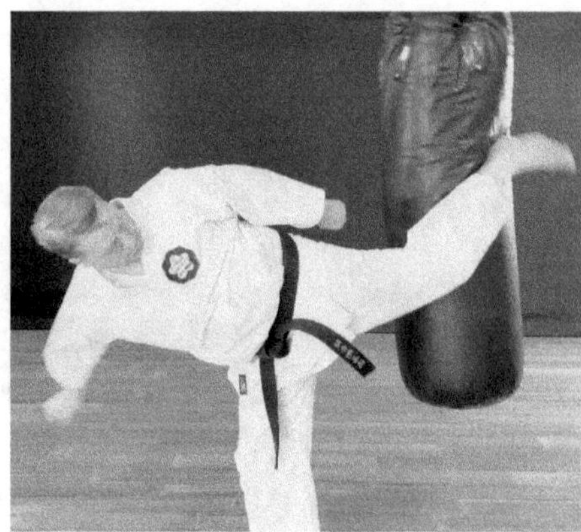
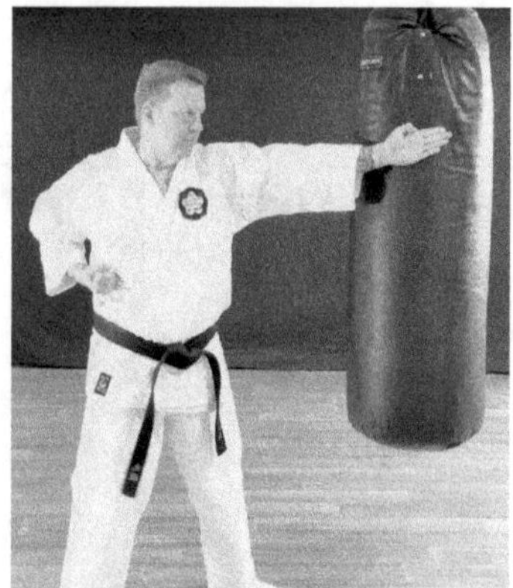
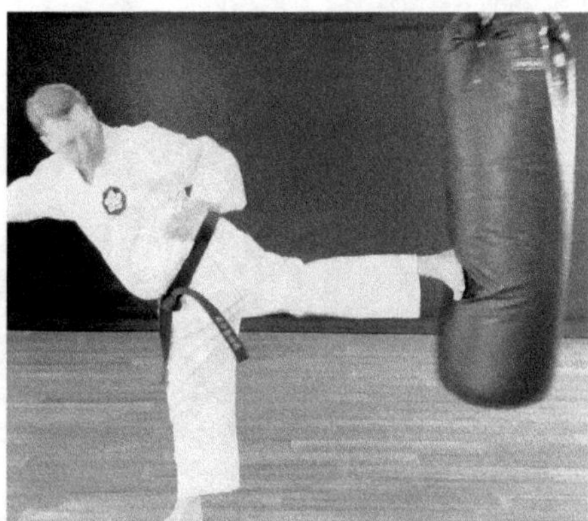

Counter 4: Kake Geri (Top) & Yoko Geri (Bottom)

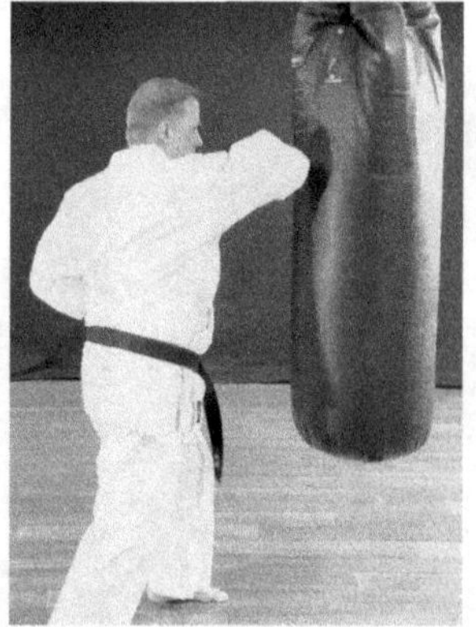

Counter 5: Haishu Uchi (Top) & Mawashi Empi Uchi (Bottom)

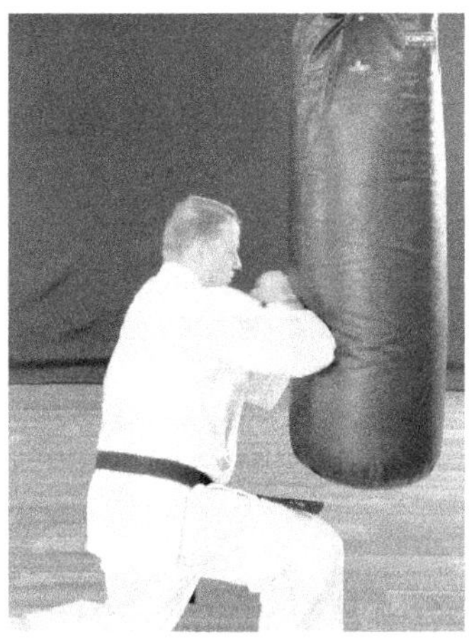

Counter 5: Single Leg Takedown (Kote Uchi)

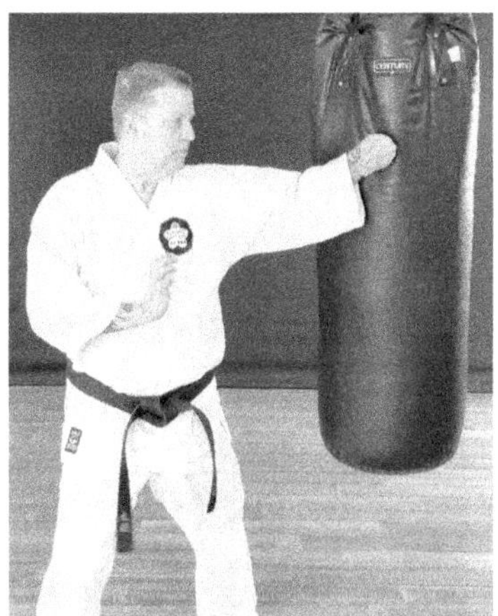

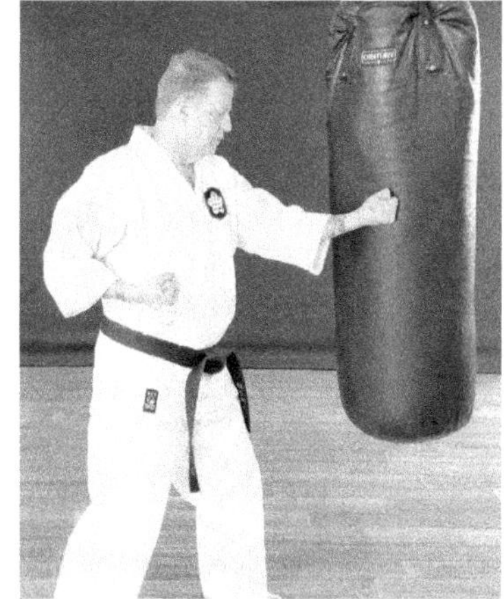

Counter 6: Jodan Yoko Ko Uke & Uchi Uke

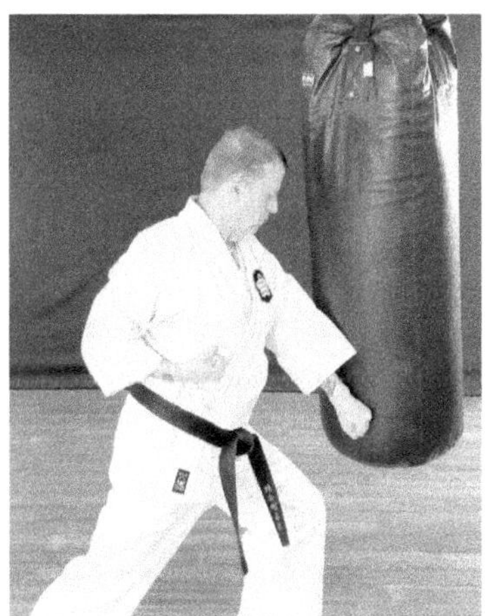

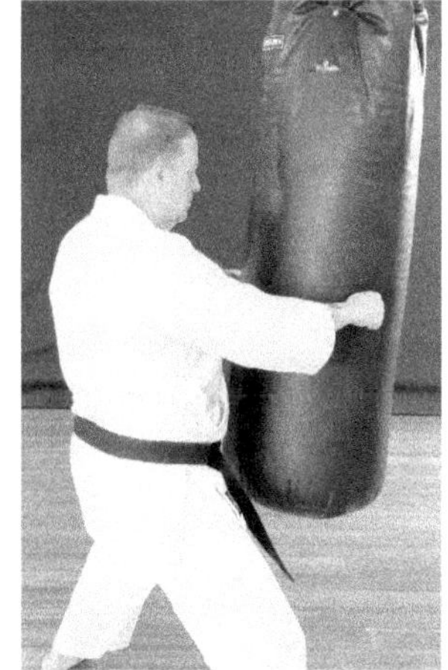

Counter 6: Gedan Barai & Morote Oyayubi Ate

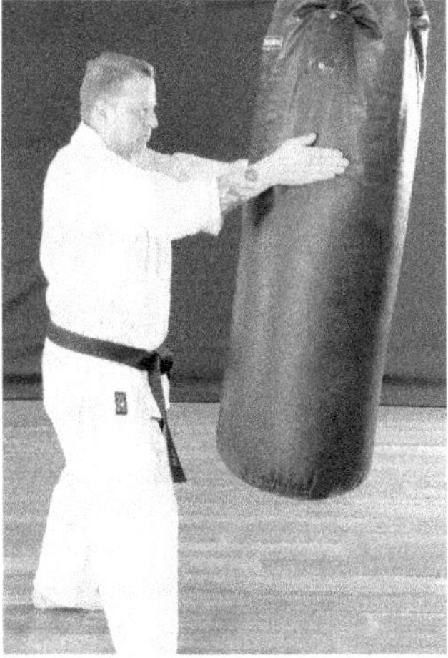

Counter 6: Morote Mimi Uchi

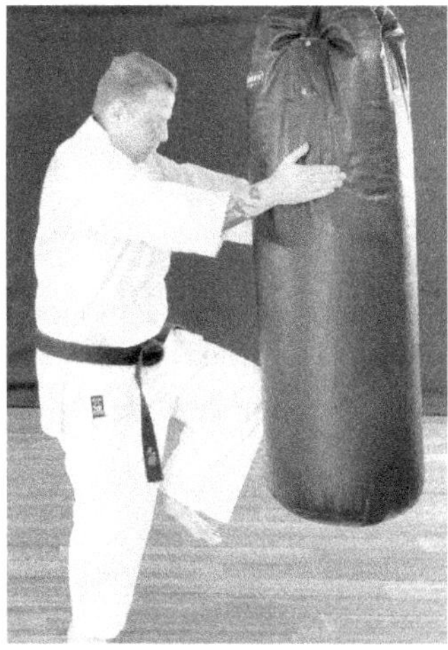

Counter 6: Hiza Uchi

15. Kumite Ku (9)

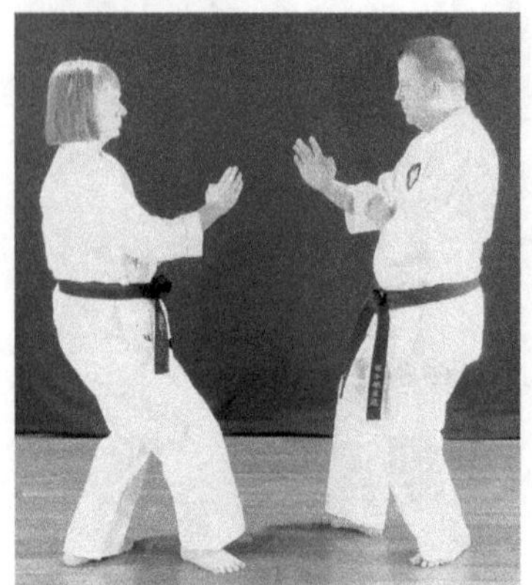

Renoji Dachi Kamae
Lead Hand Held Open at an Angle, Chamber Hand in Fist, Held at Chest, Palm Up

Begin Counter 1

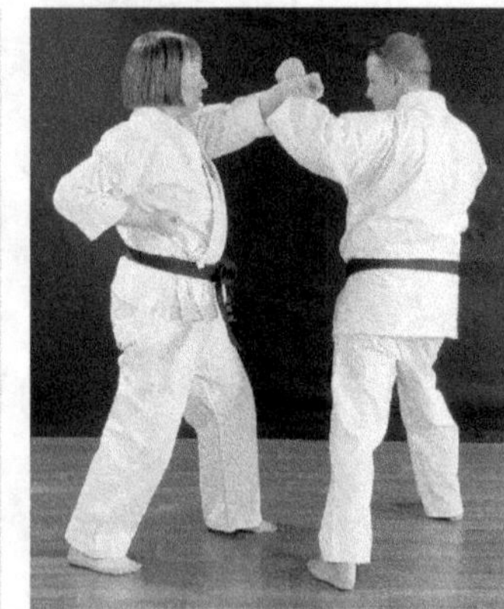

1. (Off - L): Step Forward, Jodan Zuki / (Def - R): Step Back to Side, Jodan Yoko Ko Uke

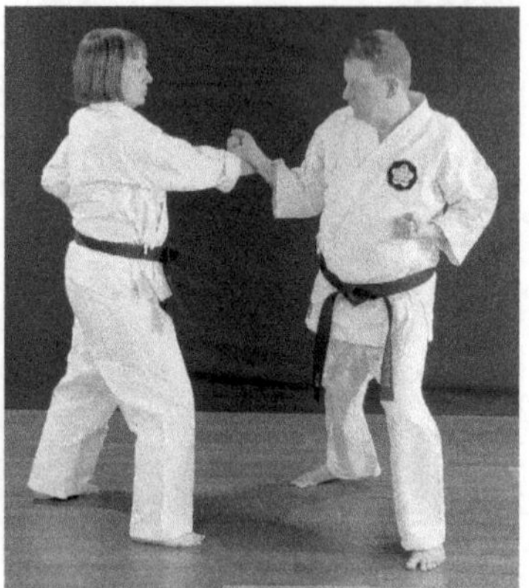

2. (Off - L): Step Forward, Chudan Zuki / (Def - R): Step Back to Side, Chudan Uchi Uke

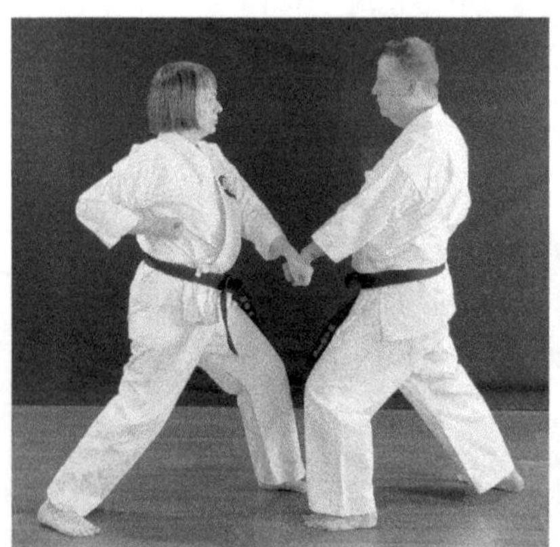

3. (Off - L): Step Forward, Zenkutsu Dachi Gedan Zuki / (Def - R): Step Back, Zenkutsu Dachi Gedan Shotei Barai

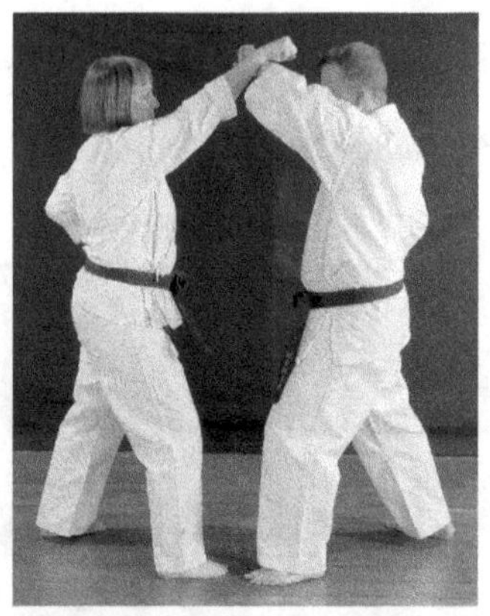

4. (Off - L): Step Forward, Jodan Zuki / (Def - R): Stutter Step Back, Jodan Age Uke

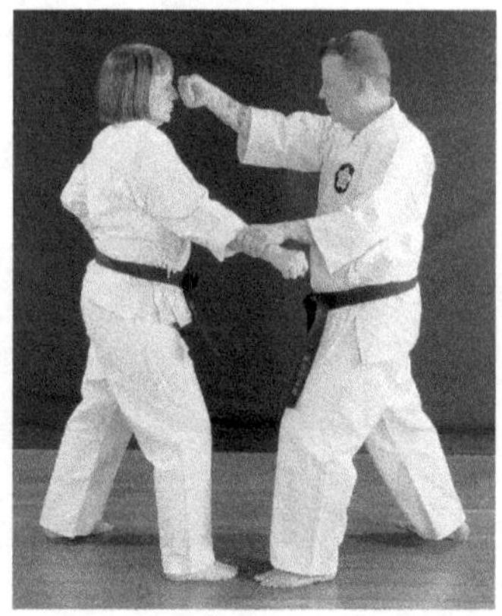

5. (Def - R): Grab Opponent's Wrist, Jodan Tate Zuki

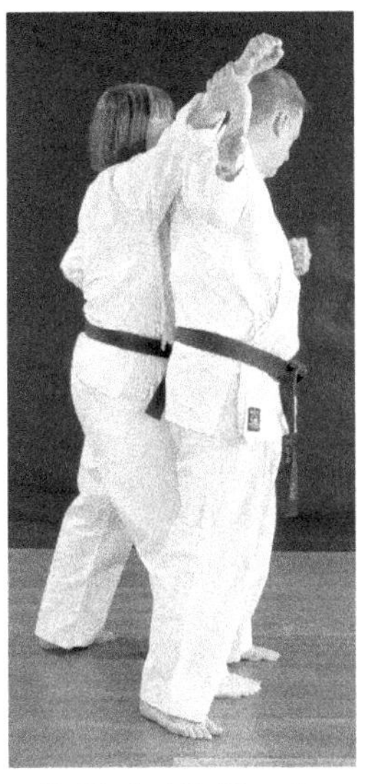

6. (Def - R): Step in Front of Opponent, Ushiro Empi Uchi

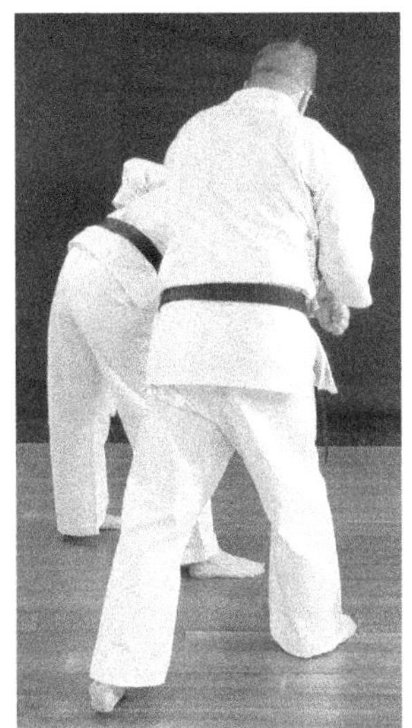

7. (Def - R): Step Behind Opponent, Mae Geri with Instep of Foot to Face

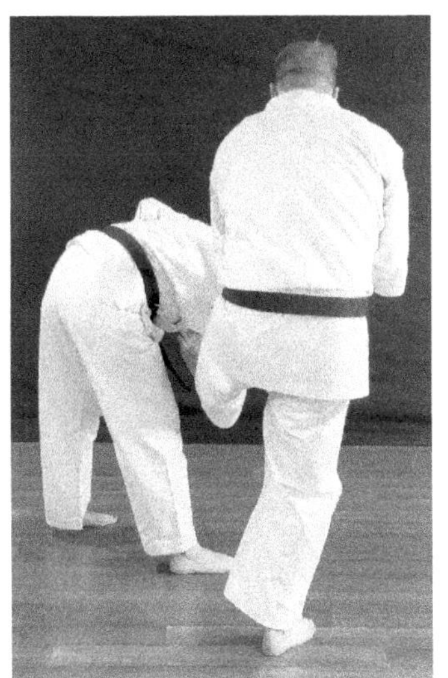

8. (Def - R): Without Putting Foot Down, Mae Geri with Ball of Foot to Chest

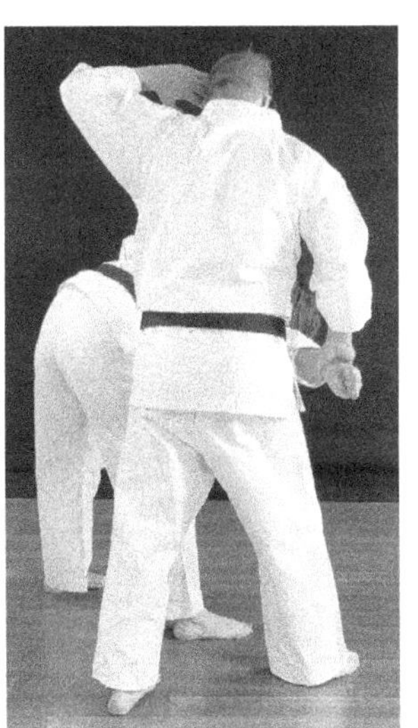

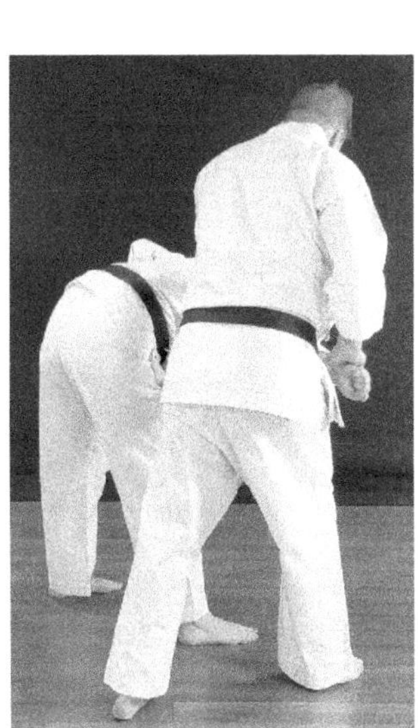

9. (Def - R): Shuto Otoshi Uchi to Base of Skull (Kiai)

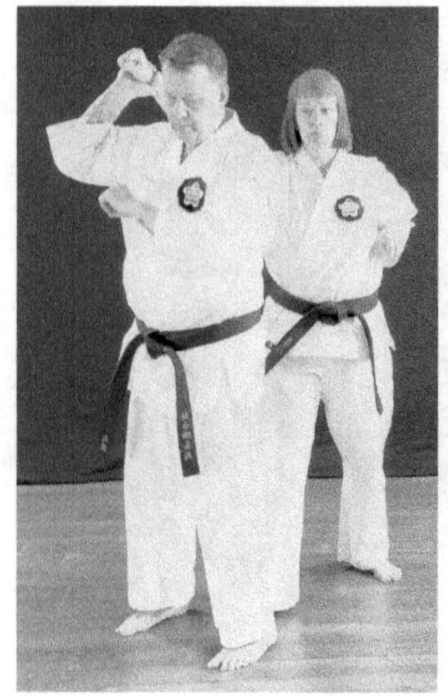

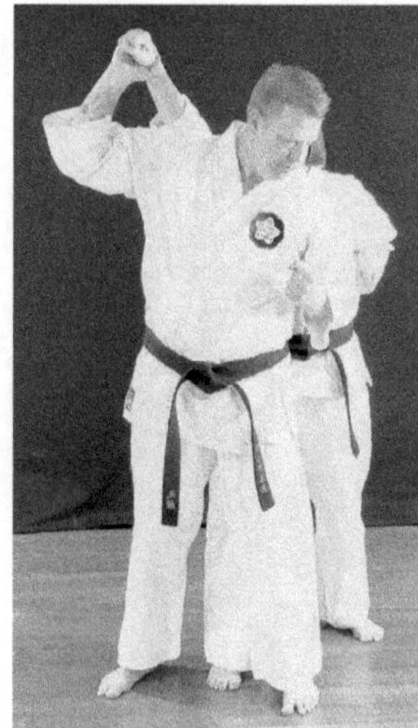

Front POV of Step 6

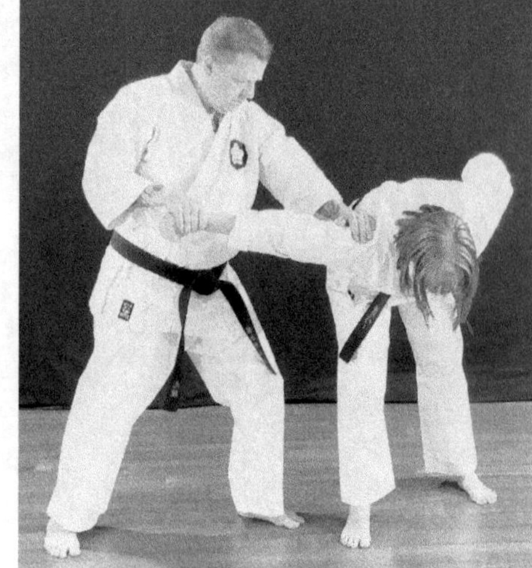

Front POV of Step 7

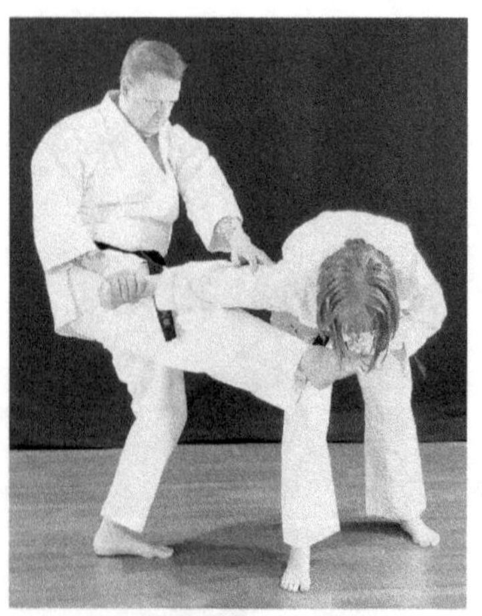

Front POV of Step 7

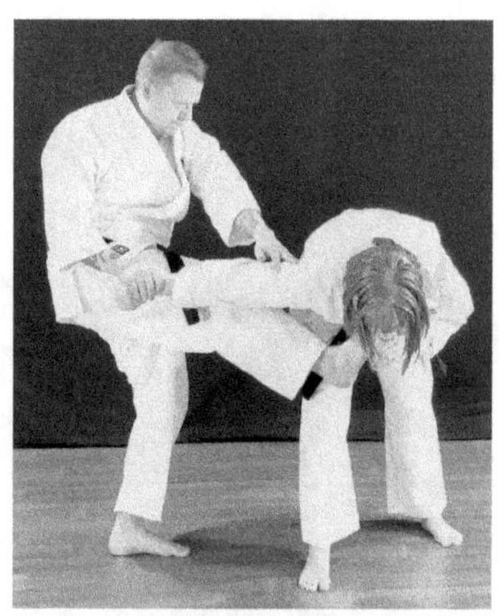

Front POV of Step 8

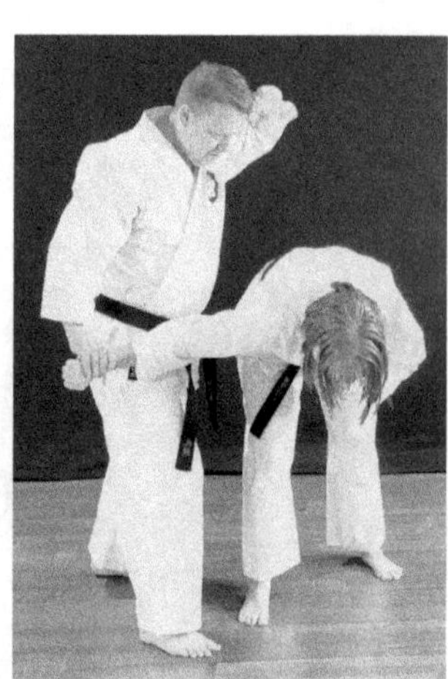

Front POV of Step 9

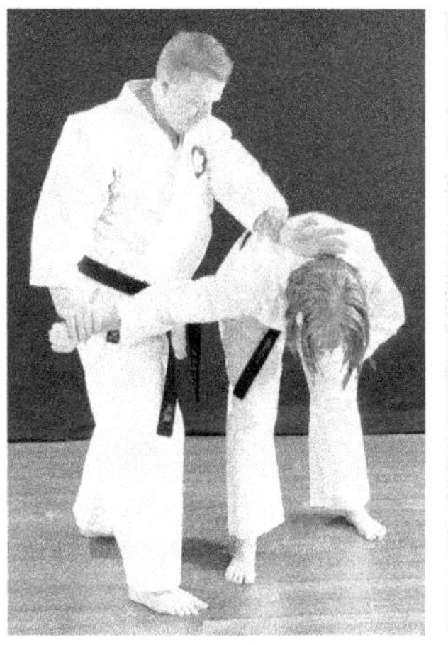
Front POV of Step 9

Repeat in Other Direction

Begin Counter 2

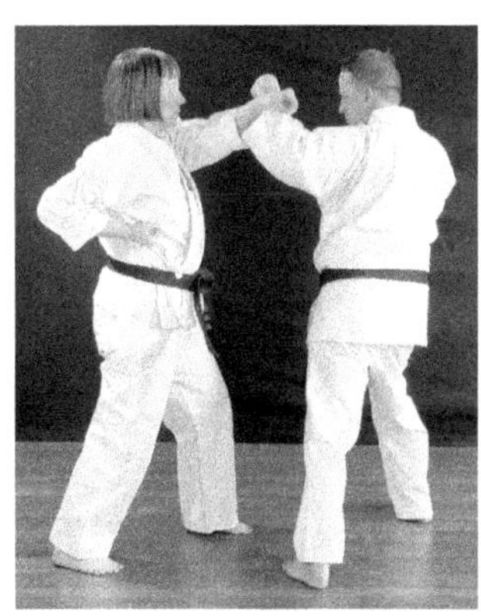
1. (Off - L): Step Forward, Jodan Zuki / (Def - R): Step Back to Side, Jodan Yoko Ko Uke

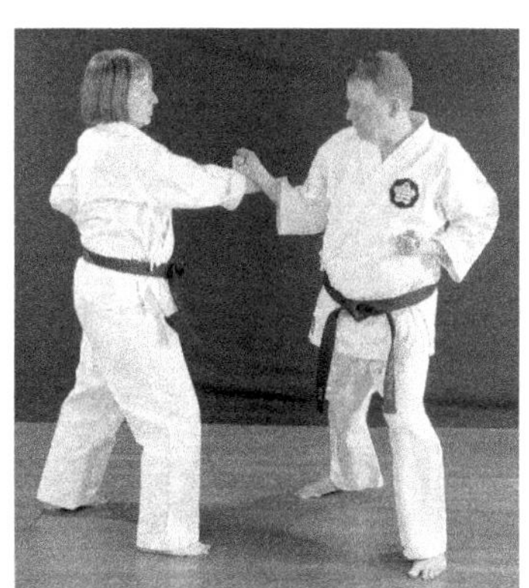
2. (Off - L): Step Forward, Jodan Zuki / (Def - R): Step Back to Side, Chudan Uchi Uke

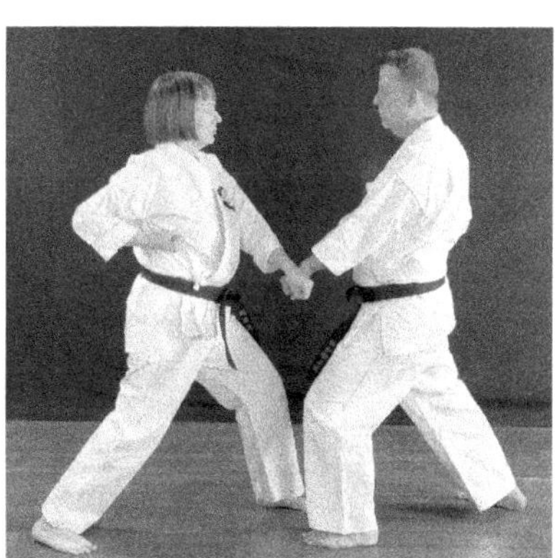
3. (Off - L): Step Forward, Gedan Zuki in Zenkutsu Dachi / (Def - R): Step Back, Gedan Shotei Barai in Zenkutsu Dachi

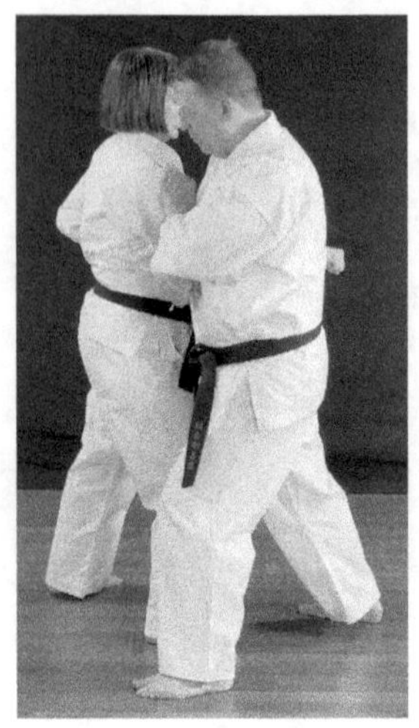

4. (Off - L): Step Forward, Chudan Zuki / (Def - R): Step to Side, Trap Opponent's Arm

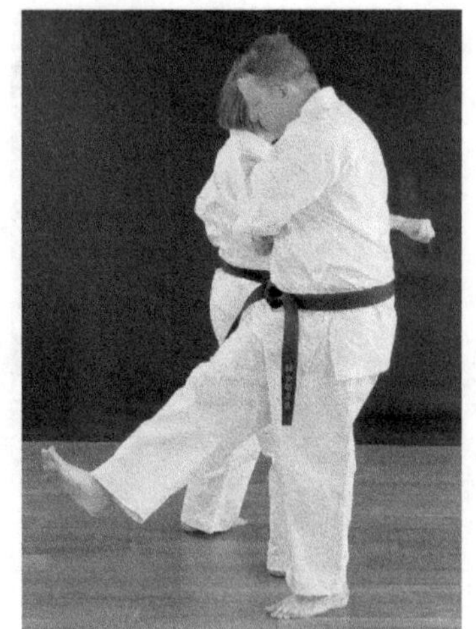

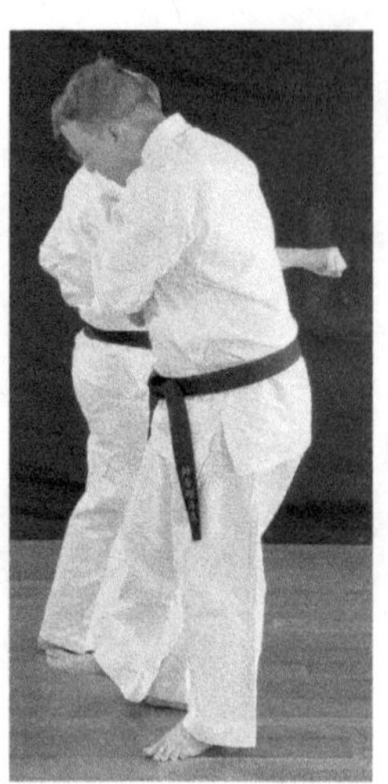

5. (Def - R): Osoto-gari

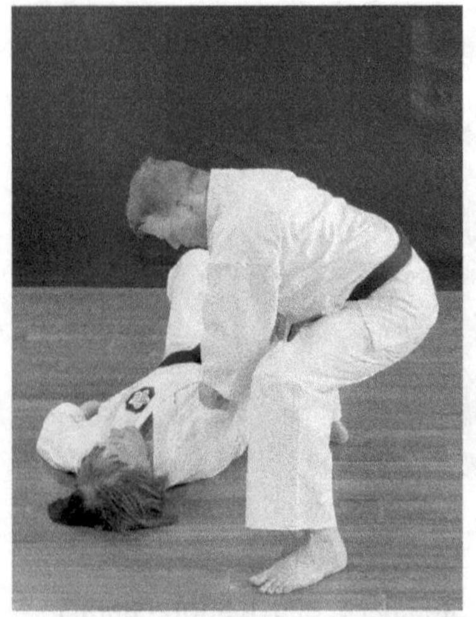

6. (Def - R): Arm Bar in Shiko Dachi (Kiai) as Opponent Goes to Ground

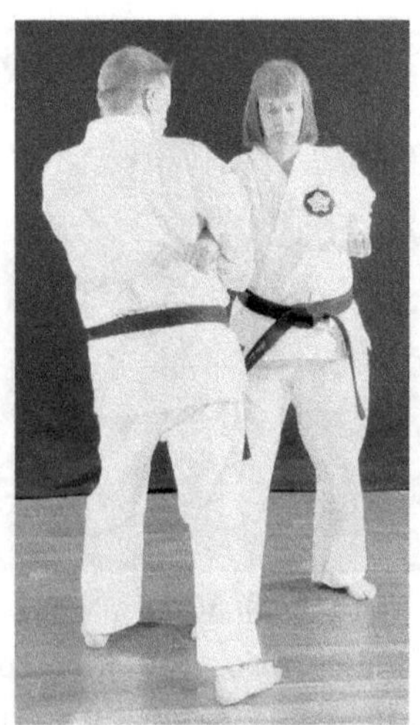

Front POV of Step 4

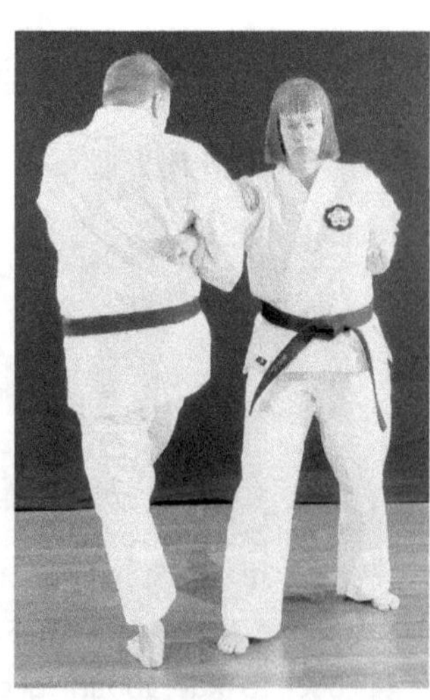

Front POV of Step 5

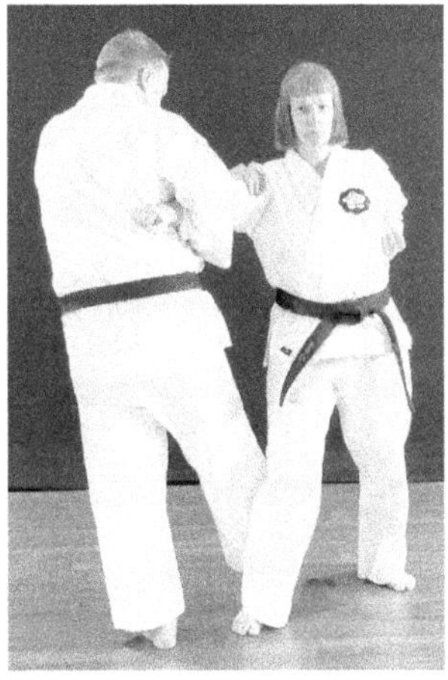

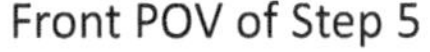

Front POV of Step 5

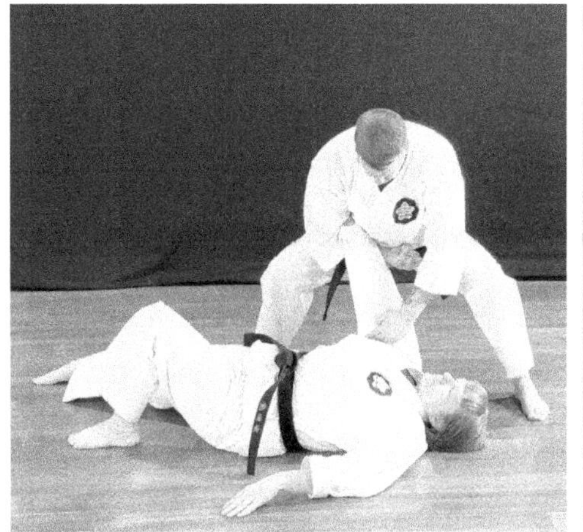

Front POV of Step 6

Repeat in Other Direction

Begin Counter 3

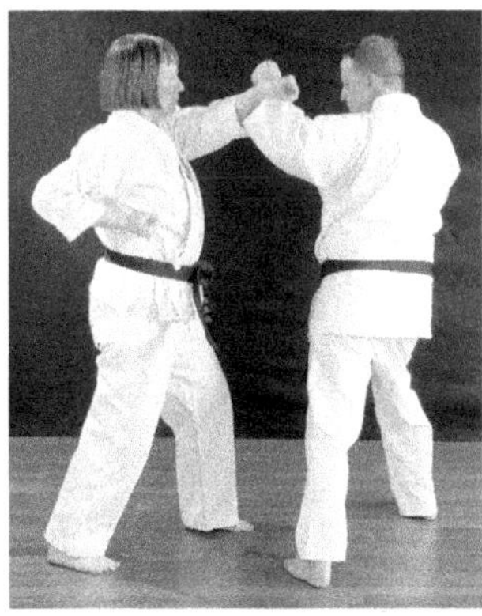

1. (Off - L): Step Forward, Jodan Zuki / (Def - R): Step Back to Side, Jodan Yoko Ko Uke

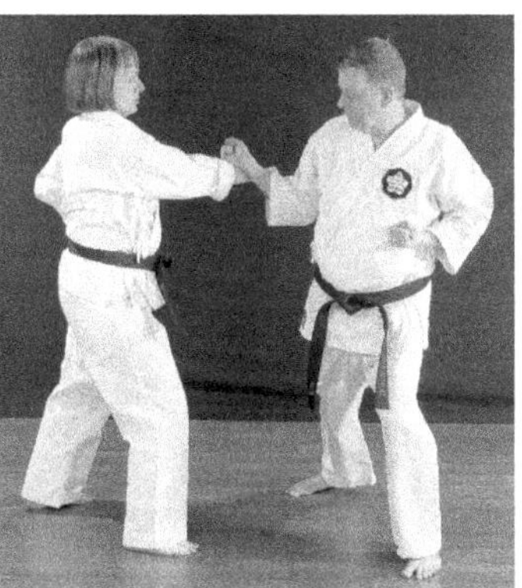

2. (Off - L): Step Forward, Jodan Zuki / (Def - R): Step Back to Side, Chudan Uchi Uke

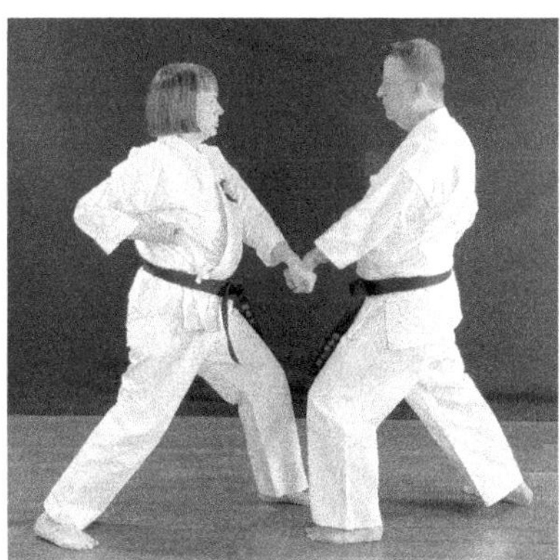

3. (Off - L): Step Forward, Gedan Zuki in Zenkutsu Dachi / (Def - R): Step Back, Gedan Shotei Barai in Zenkutsu Dachi

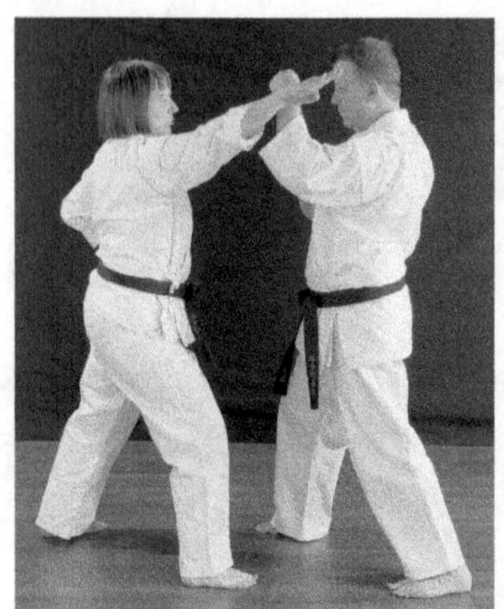

4. (Off - L): Step Forward, Right Jodan Haito Uchi / (Def - R): Jodan Yoko Ko Uke

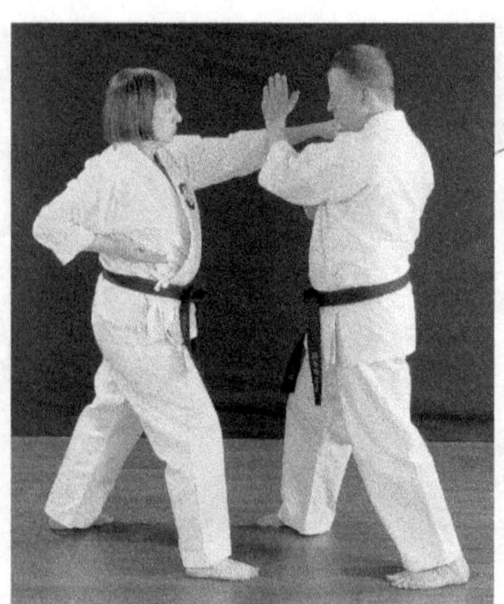

5. (Off - L): Left Jodan Haito Uchi / (Def - R): Jodan Shotei Oshi

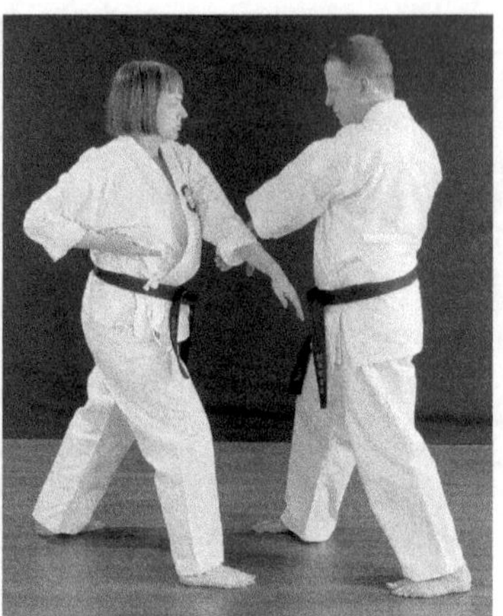

6. (Def - R): After Block, Continue Going Around Arm...

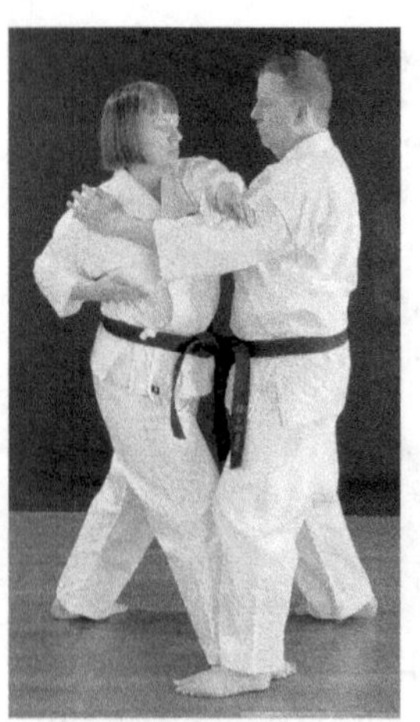

...Landing on Opponent's Right Shoulder while Stepping Forward

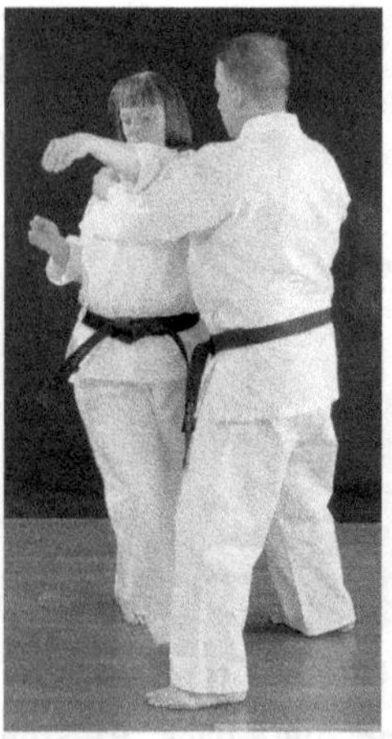

7. (Def - R): Right Shotei Oshi Behind Opponent's Left Shoulder in Tandem with Right Shoulder, Twisting Opponent, Using Right Leg as Leverage for Takedown

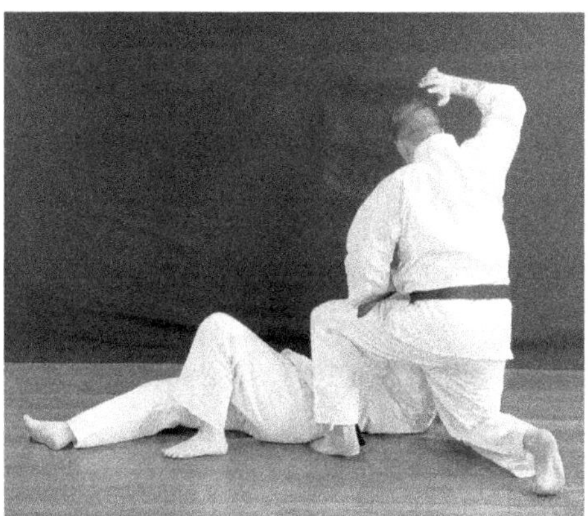

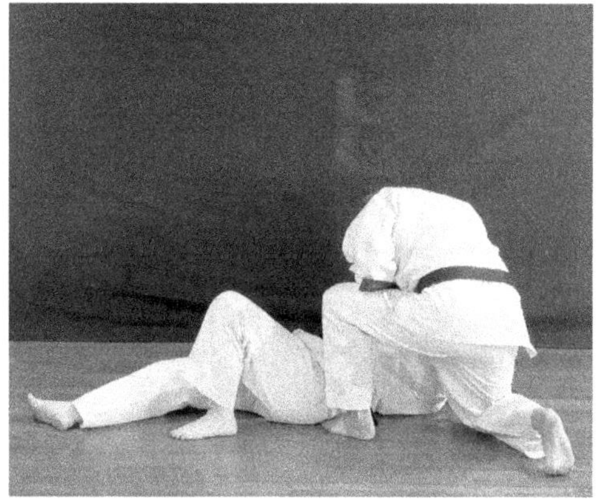

Repeat in Other Direction

8. (Def - R): Shuto Otoshi Uchi to Bridge of Nose (Kiai)

Begin Counter 4

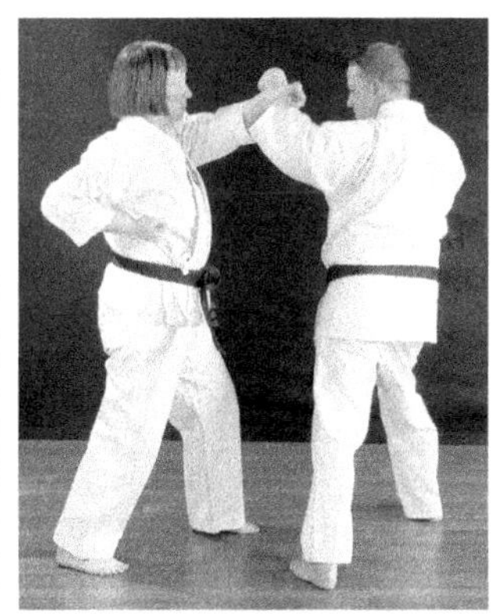

1. (Off - L): Step Forward, Jodan Zuki / (Def - R): Step Back to Side, Jodan Yoko Ko Uke

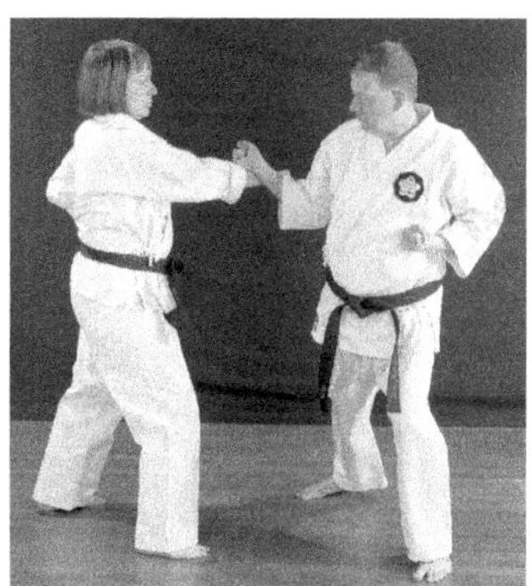

2. (Off - L): Step Forward, Jodan Zuki / (Def - R): Step Back to Side, Chudan Uchi Uke

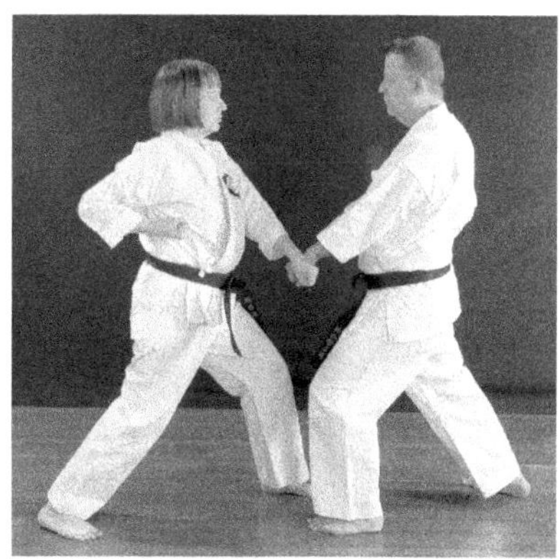

3. (Off - L): Step Forward, Gedan Zuki in Zenkutsu Dachi / (Def - R): Step Back, Gedan Shotei Barai in Zenkutsu Dachi

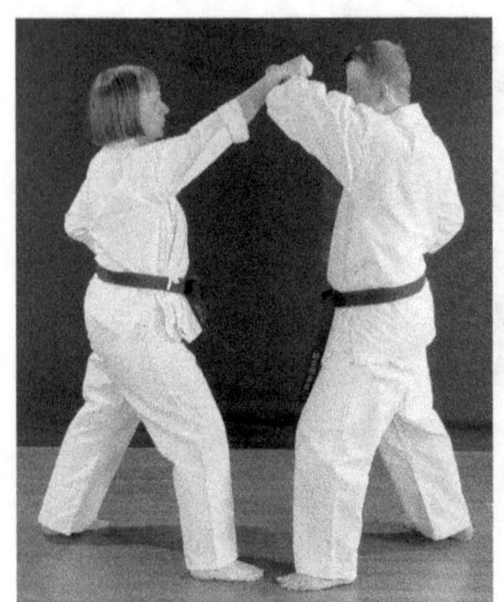

4. (Off - L): Step Forward, Jodan Zuki / (Def - R): Stutter Step Back, Jodan Age Uke

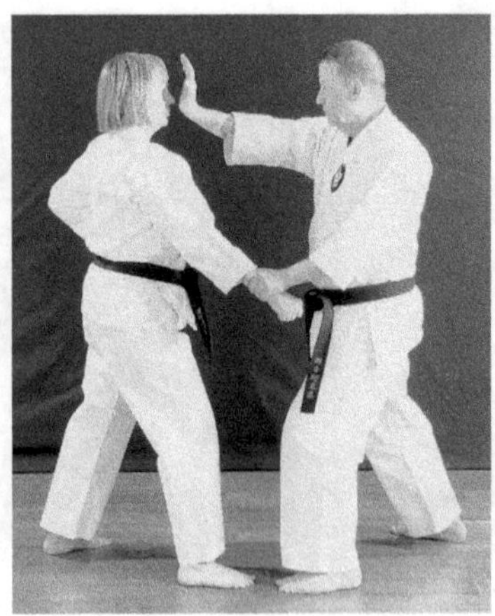

5. (Def - R): Jodan Shotei Uchi

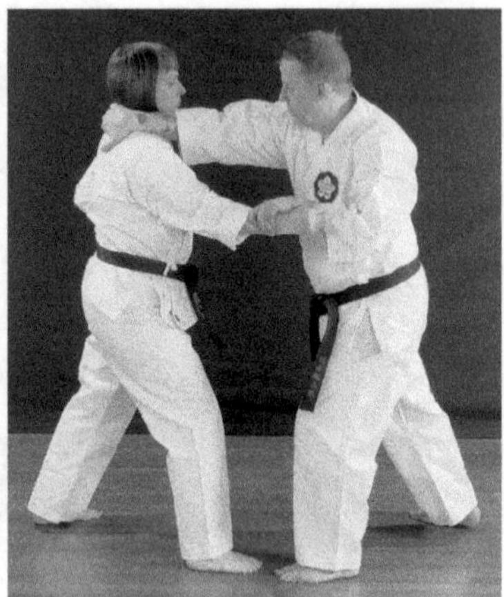

6. (Def - R): Reach Around Behind Neck

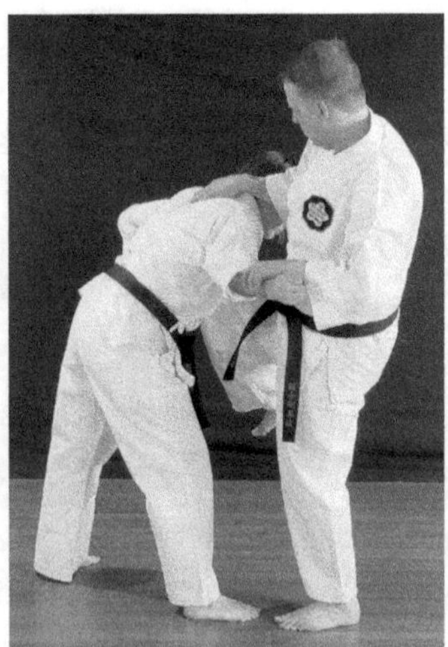

7. (Def - R): Pull Opponent Down into Hiza Uchi

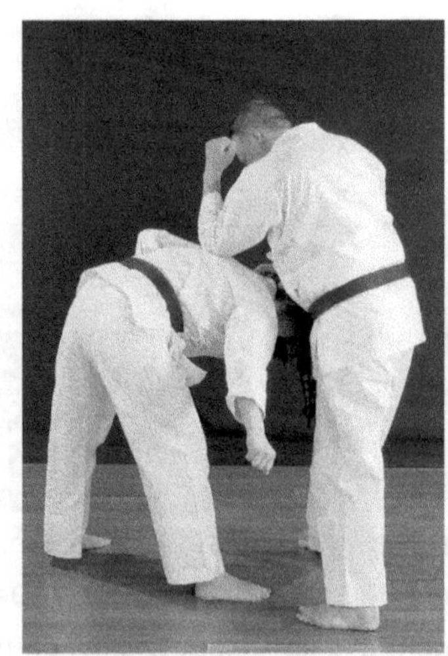

8. (Def - R): Empi Otoshi Uchi to Spine (Kiai)

Repeat in Other Direction

Begin Counter 5

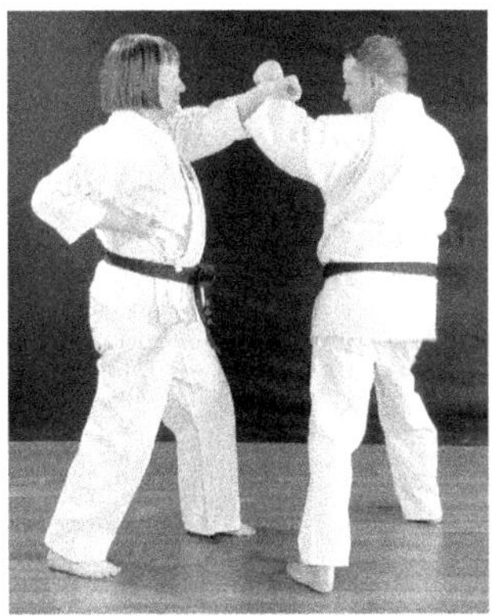

1. (Off - L): Step Forward, Jodan Zuki / (Def - R): Step Back to Side, Jodan Yoko Ko Uke

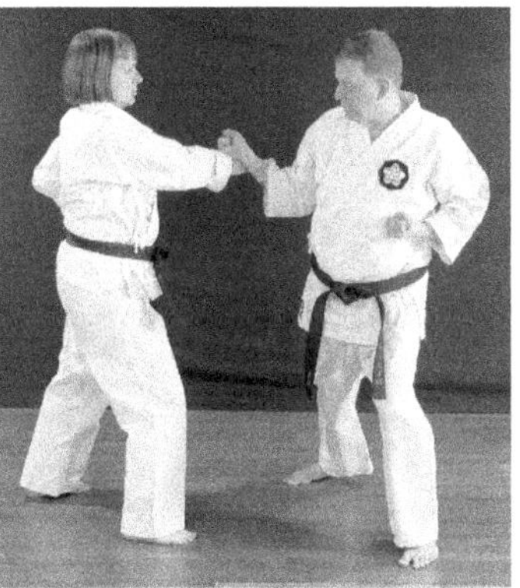

2. (Off - L): Step Forward, Jodan Zuki / (Def - R): Step Back to Side, Chudan Uchi Uke

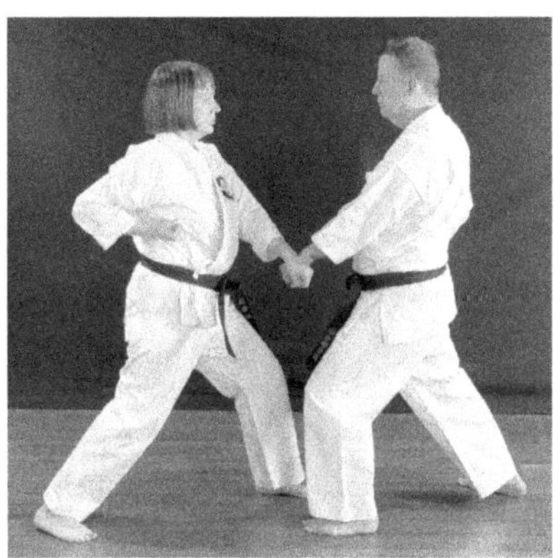

3. (Off - L): Step Forward, Gedan Zuki in Zenkutsu Dachi / (Def - R): Step Back, Shotei Gedan Shotei Barai in Zenkutsu Dachi

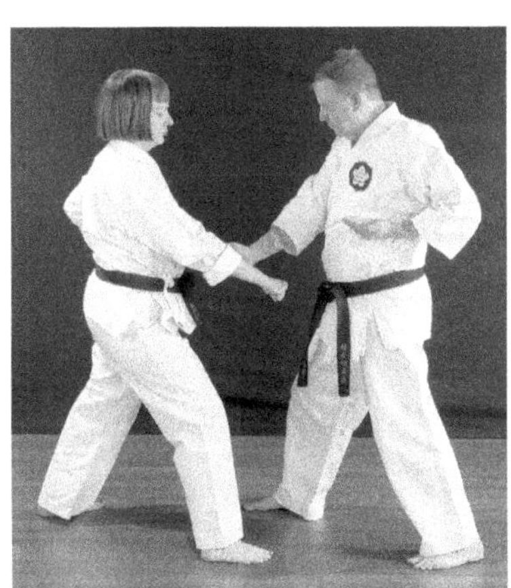

4. (Off - L): Step Forward, Right Gedan Zuki / (Def - R): Step Back, Right Gedan Nukite Uke

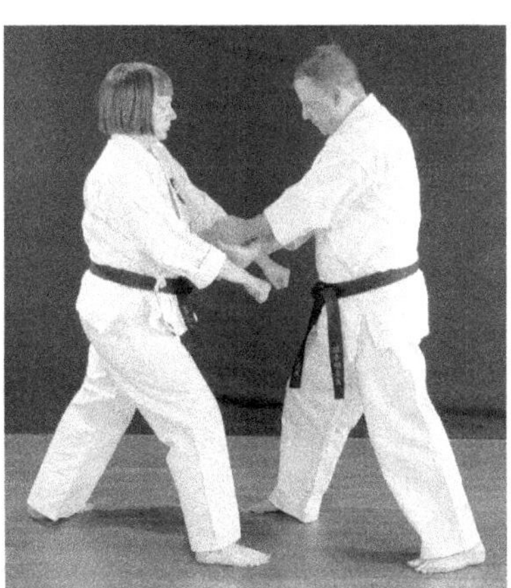

5. (Off - L): Left Gedan Zuki / (Def - R): Left Gedan Nukite Uke, Crossing Over Right Wrist

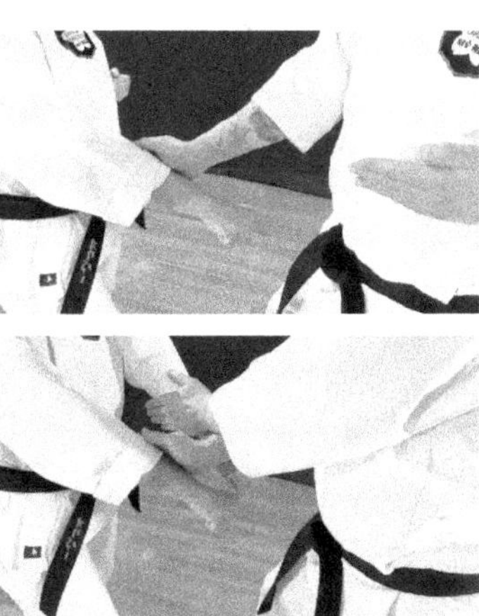

Closer POV of Steps 4 & 5

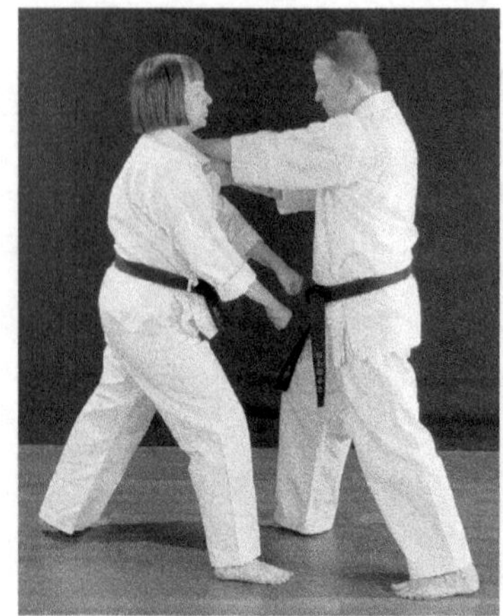

6. (Def - R): Slide Hands Up Collar

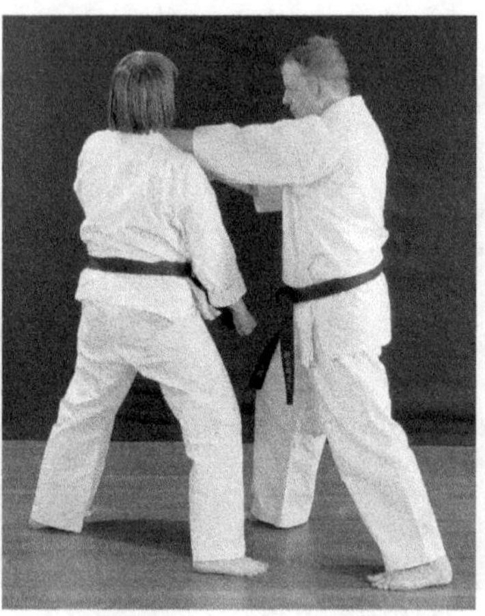

7. (Def - R): Pull with Right Hand, Push with Left Hand, Turning Opponent, Directing Opponent to Ground

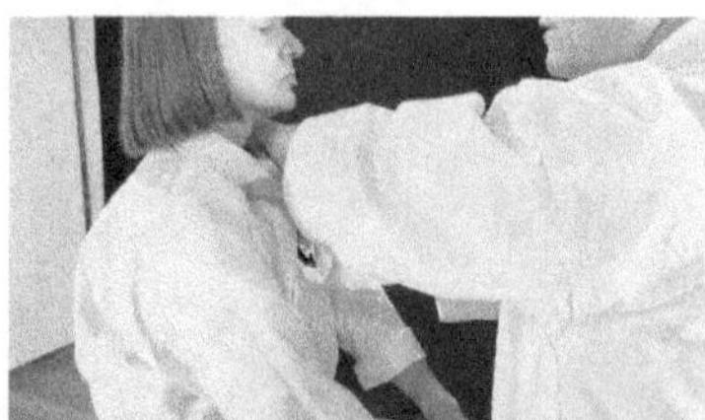

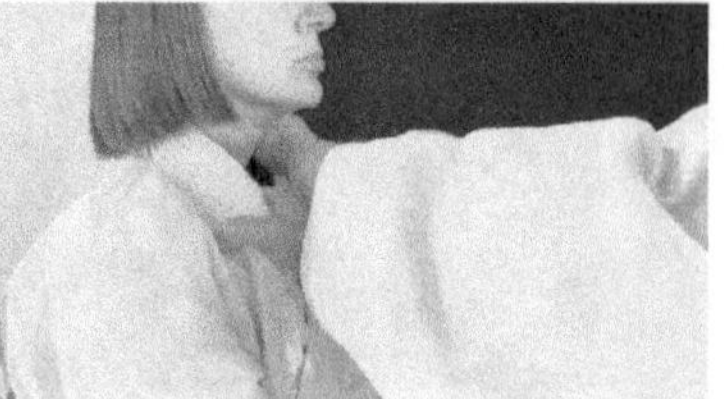

Closer POV of Step 7

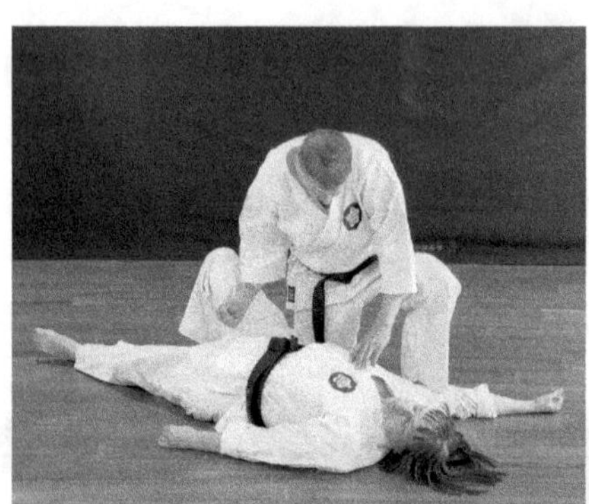

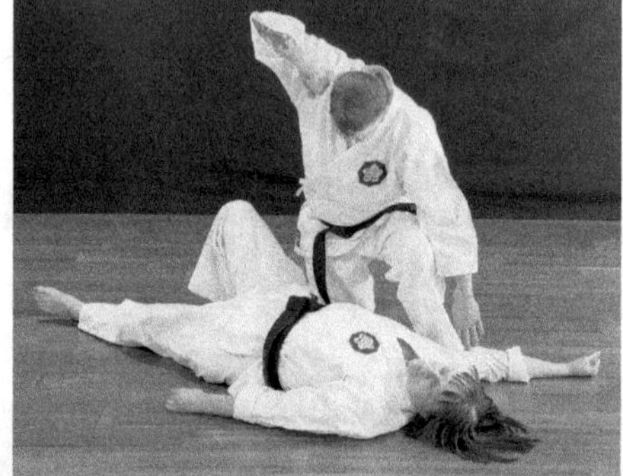

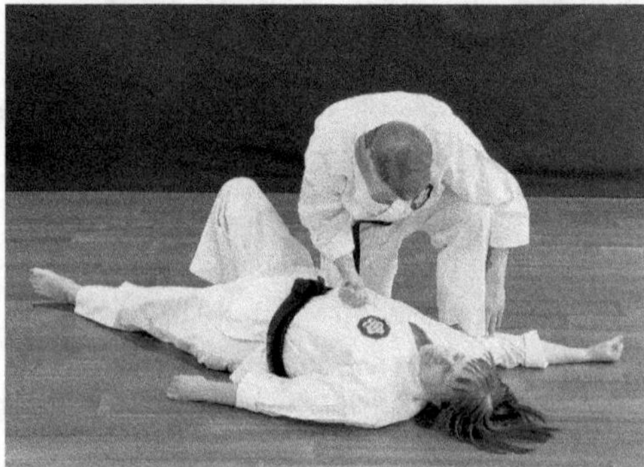

8. (Def - R): Tettsui Otoshi Uchi to Groin, then to Chest

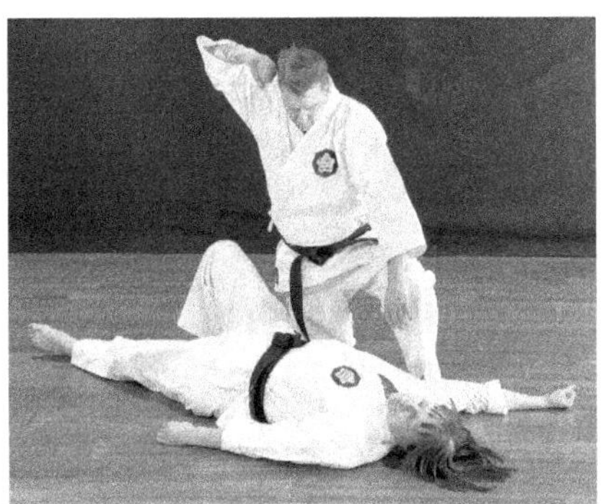

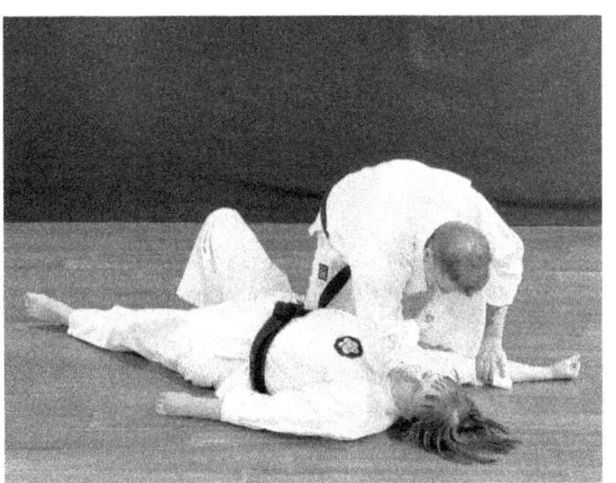

Repeat in Other Direction

9. (Def - R): Empi Otoshi Uchi to Jaw (Kiai)

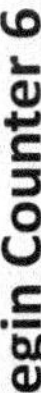

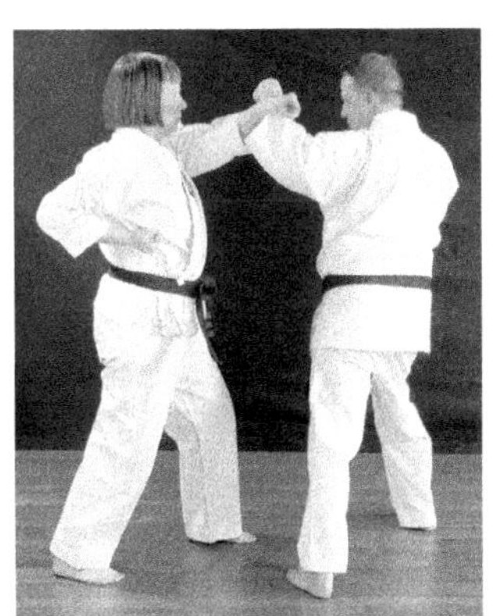

1. (Off - L): Step Forward, Jodan Zuki / (Def - R): Step Back to Side, Jodan Yoko Ko Uke

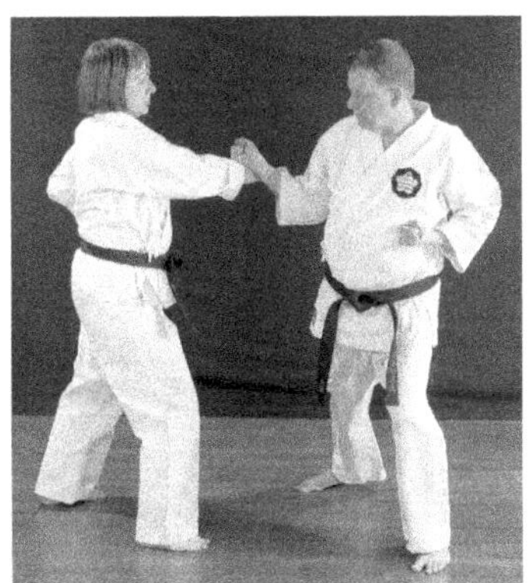

2. (Off - L): Step Forward, Jodan Zuki / (Def - R): Step Back to Side, Chudan Uchi Uke

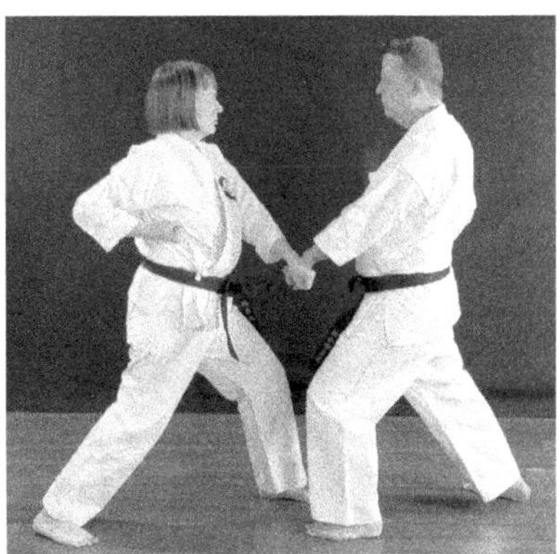

3. (Off - L): Step Forward, Gedan Zuki in Zenkutsu Dachi / (Def - R): Step Back, Gedan Shotei Barai in Zenkutsu Dachi

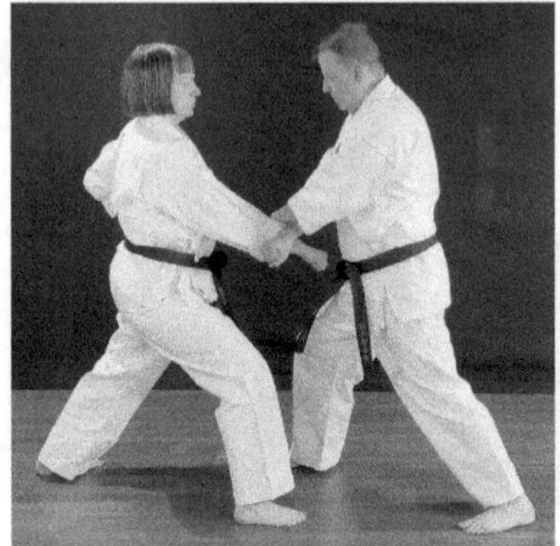

4. (Off - L): Step Forward, Gedan Zuki in Zenkutsu Dachi / (Def - R): Step Back, Juji Otoshi Uke in Zenkutsu Dachi

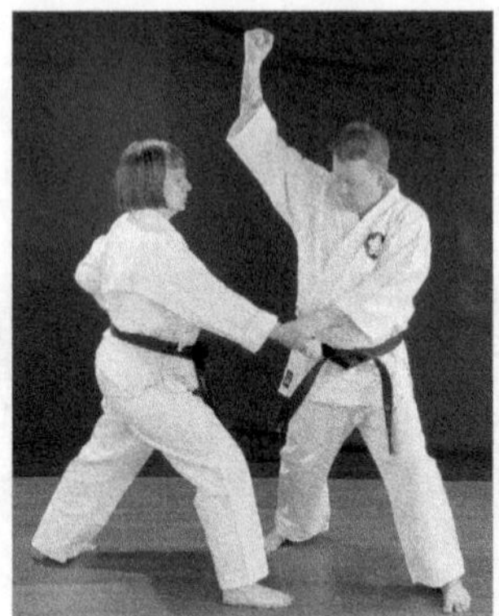

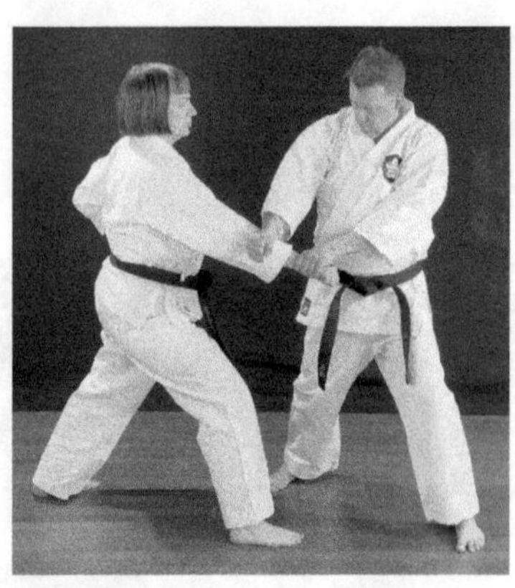

5. (Def - R): Pivot Left, Kote Otoshi Uchi to Opponent's Forearm

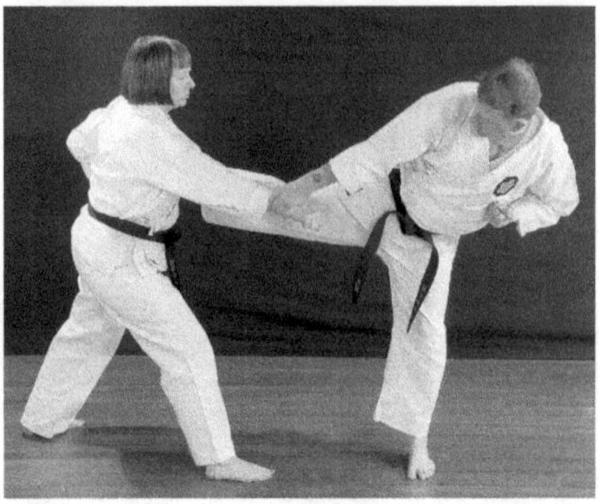

6. (Def - R): Mawashi Geri with Ball of Foot to Chest

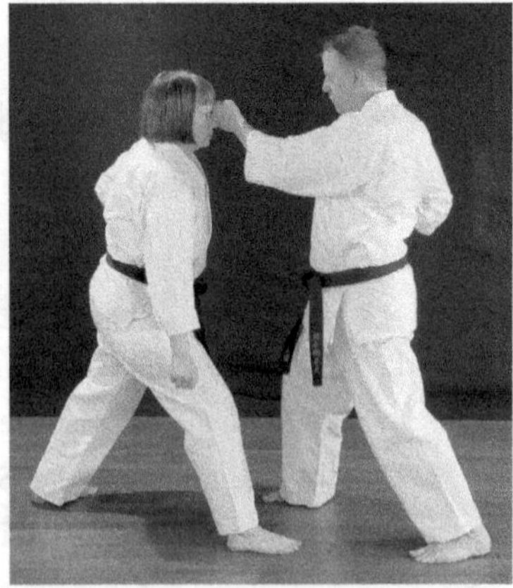

7. (Def - R): Left Jodan Tate Zuki

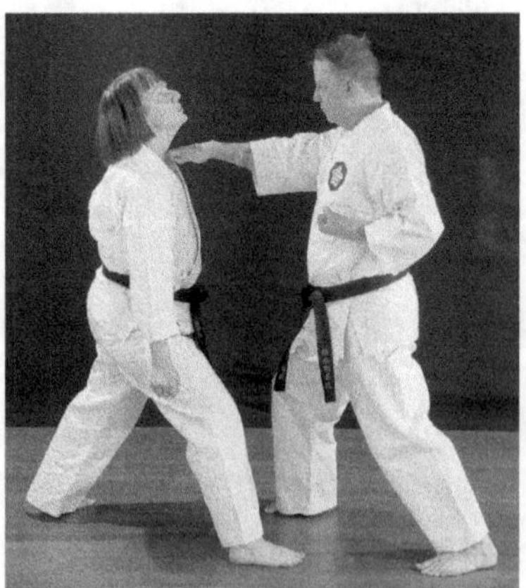

8. (Def - R): Right Hiraken Uchi to Throat (Kiai)

Repeat in Other Direction

Kumite Ku - Bag Work

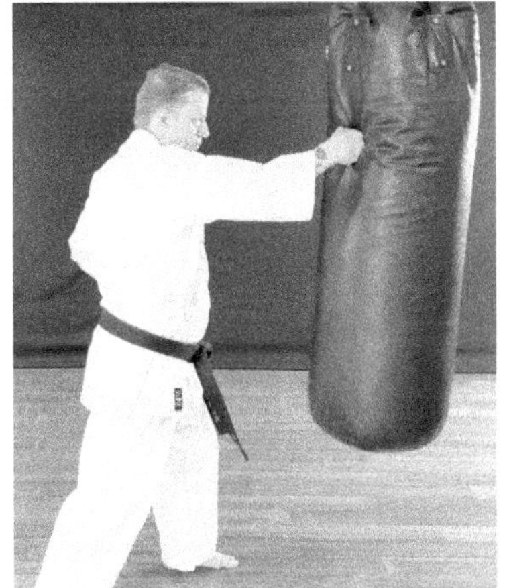

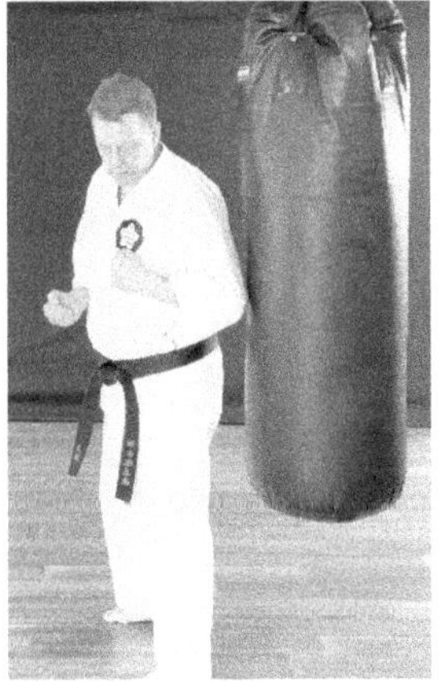

Counter 1: Tate Uchi (Top) & Ushiro Empi Uchi (Bottom)

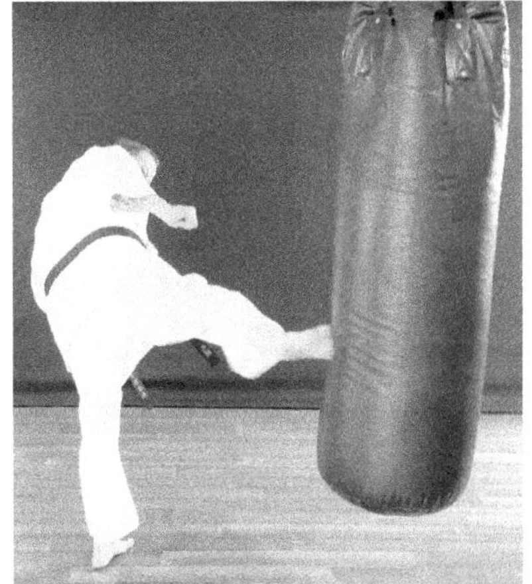

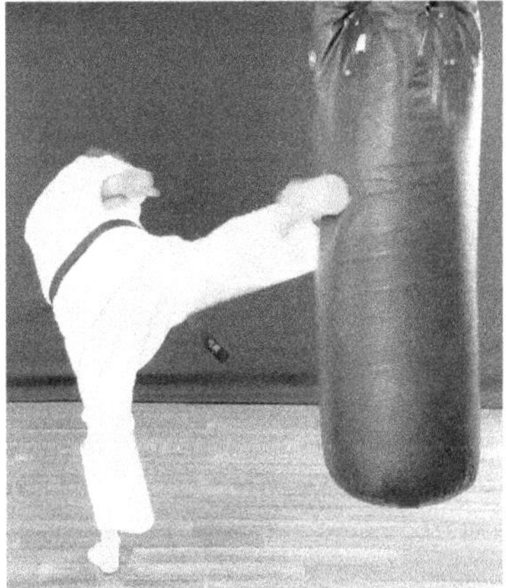

Counter 1: Mawashi Geri (Ball of Foot) (Top) & Mawashi Geri (Instep) (Bottom)

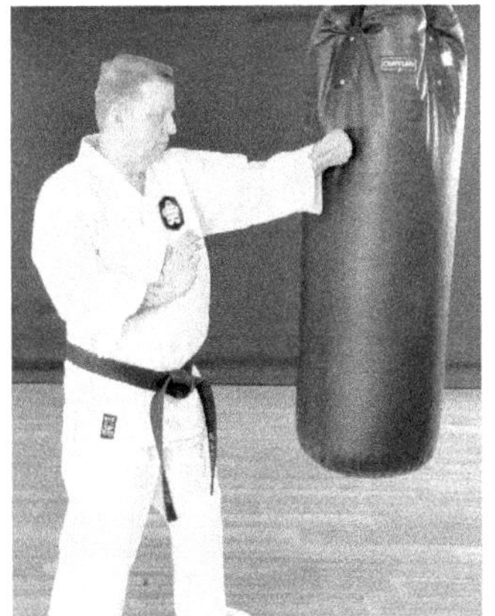

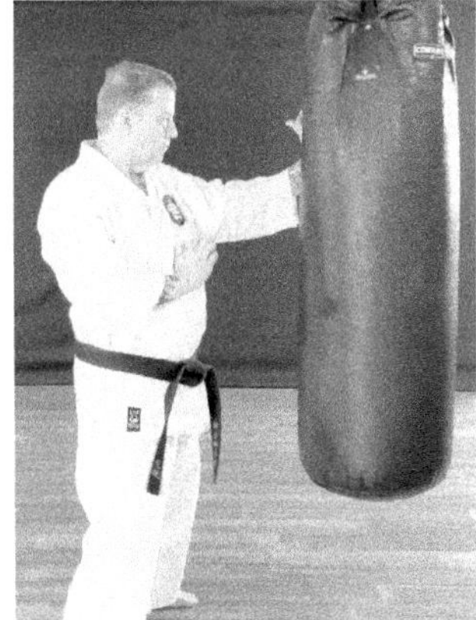

Counter 3: Jodan Yoko Ko Uke & Shotei Uchi

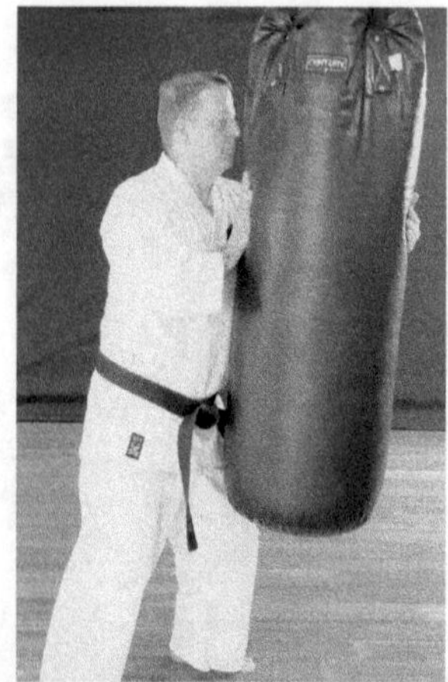

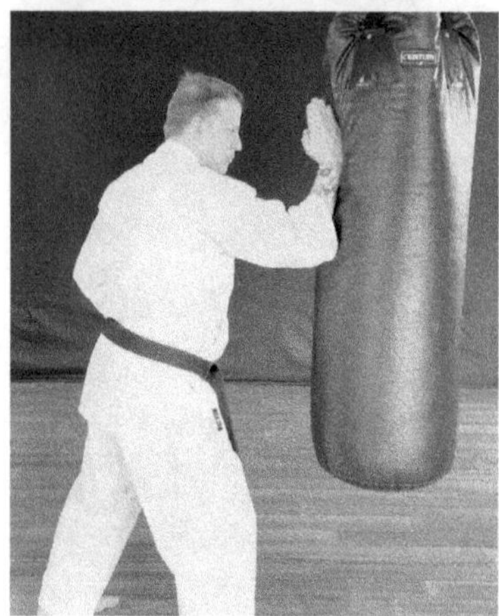

Counter 3: Morote Shotei Oshi (Top) & Shuto Otoshi Uchi (Bottom)

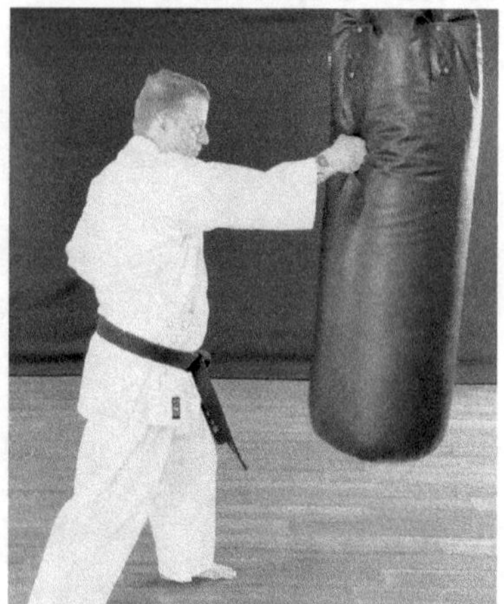

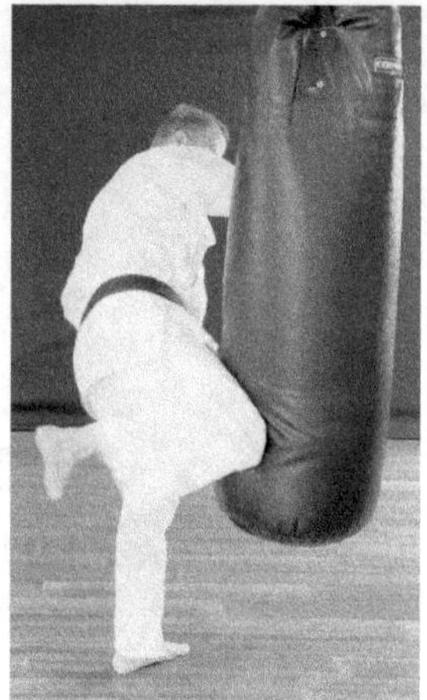

Counter 4: Tate Uchi (Top) & Hiza Uchi (Bottom)

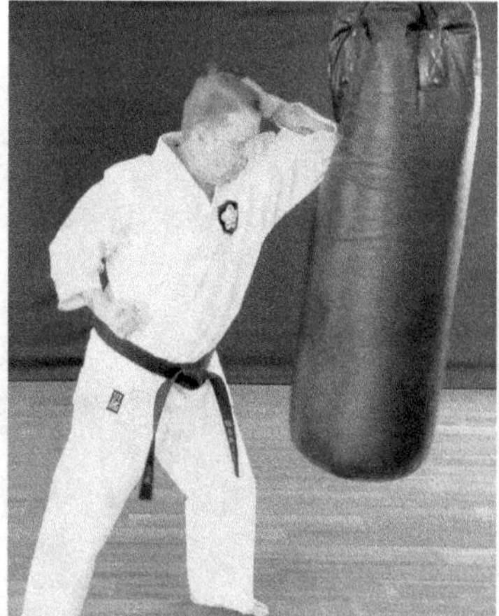

Counter 4: Empi Otoshi Uchi

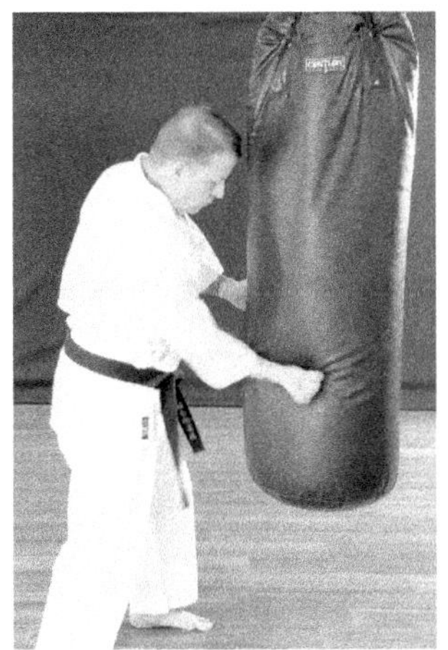
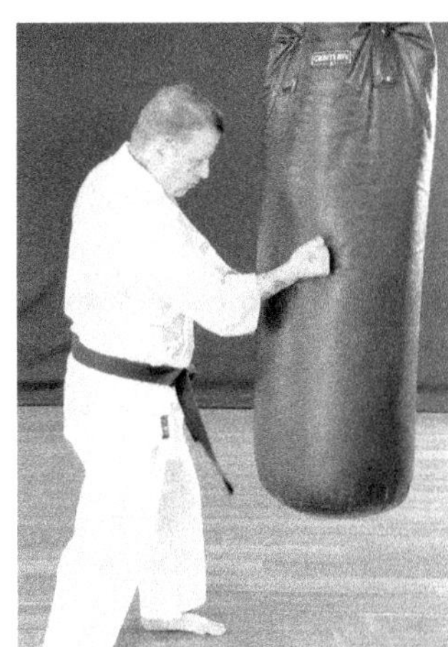

Counter 5: Gedan Tettsui Uchi & Chudan Tettsui Uchi

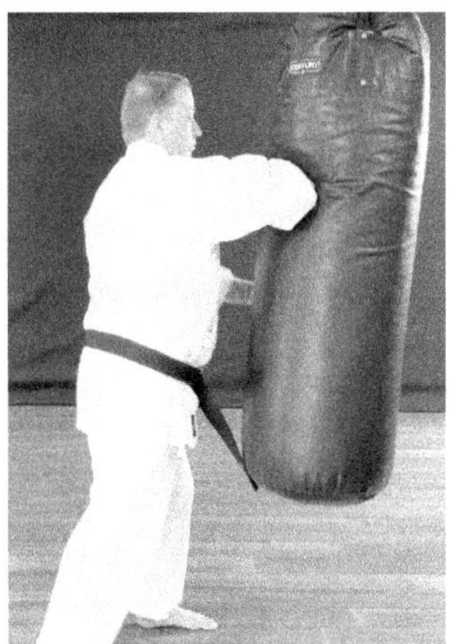

Counter 5: Jodan Mawashi Empi Uchi

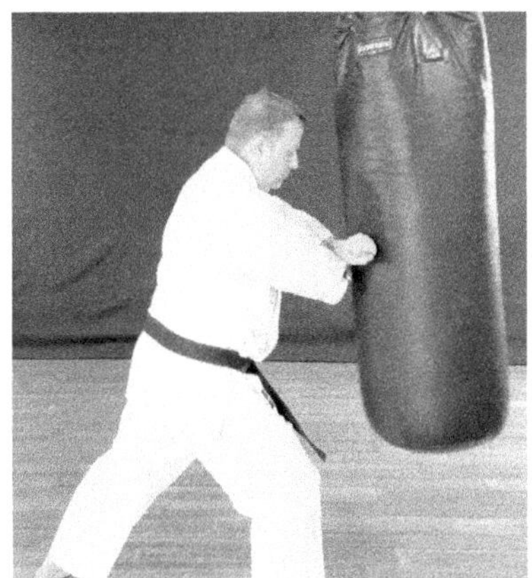
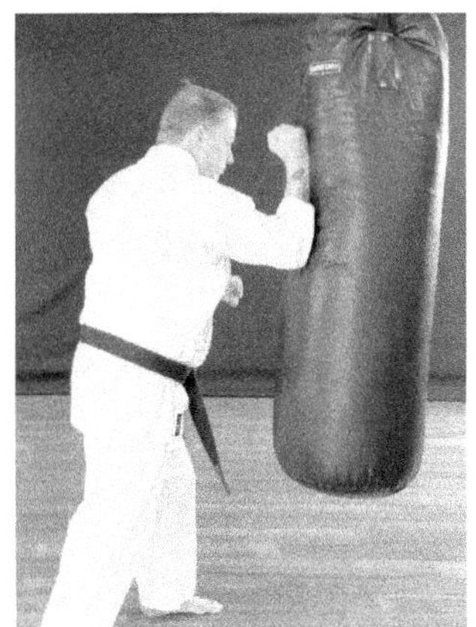

Counter 6: Juji Uke & Kote Uchi

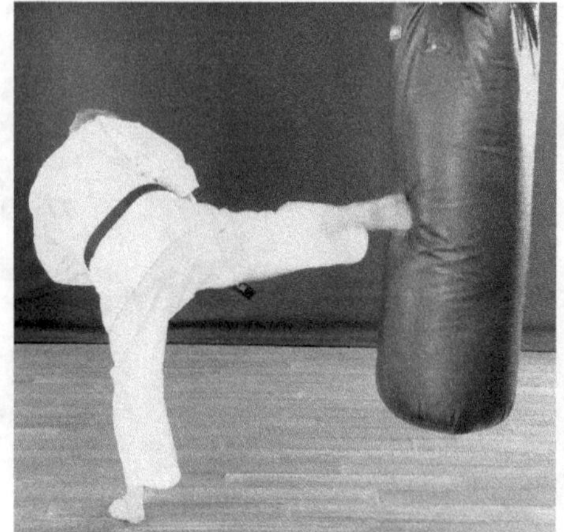
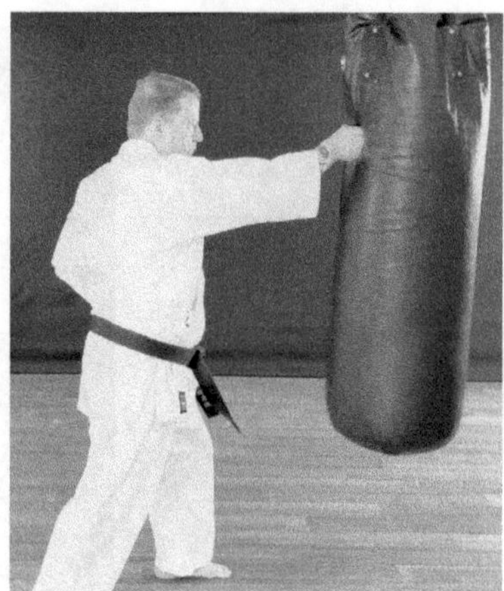
Counter 6: Mawashi Geri (Ball of Foot) & Tate Uchi

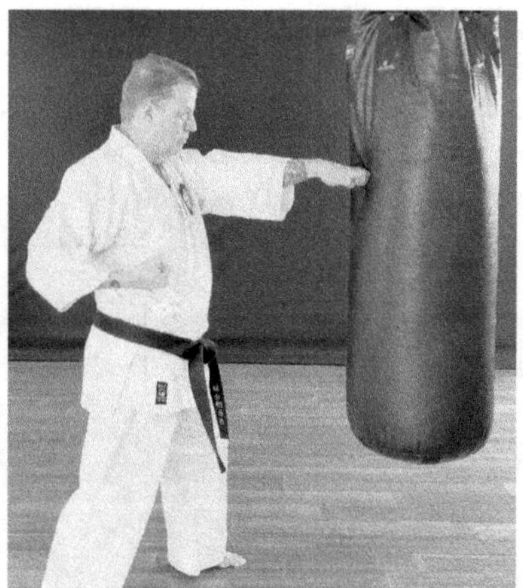
Counter 6: Hiraken Uchi

Sparring

Why we spar?

Practicing kata and perfecting techniques are extremely valuable elements of karate training, but without the experience of trying to strike someone who does not want to be struck—and who is trying to do the same thing—the concepts will remain theoretical or academic. The mental aspect of fighting should not be ignored. Of course, sparring, no matter how it is practiced, is not the same as a real fight or even true self-defense, and there is no way to replicate those situations perfectly. There are simply too many variables, many of them too dangerous to practice in a structured learning environment. However, sparring gives students a vital aspect of fighting and self-defense: the ability to stay calm in the face of danger, however relative that danger may be. If the mind is racing and out of control, self-defense will be sloppy and ineffective at best. One must be able to calm the mind while still evaluating the situation and keeping emotions in check. While it is true that muscle memory can "take over," the more control a person has over their emotions, the better equipped they will be to make proper decisions in the moment. Sometimes the proper decision is simply to do enough to escape.

Of course, 'Karate sparring' is not its own category of sparring. Sparring is defined by the rules and methodology of each school or organization. Martial arts schools must negotiate the balance between too much contact and not enough, but sparring should be hard enough to prepare a student's mind for the danger of a real fight while still maintaining an environment that allows for continuous training. Obviously, it would not be wise to risk a student's life or long-term health for the sake of preparing for a street situation that may never happen. At the same time, sparring should not be so safe that a student falls apart the first time they are punched in the face. Students should first be trained in techniques and be in reasonable physical condition before sparring, and sparring should gradually become more difficult as the student progresses. In time, students should reach a point where the fight appears to slow down, when in reality it is only slower in the student's perception. This is when the student learns one of the first major lessons of sparring: fight relaxed, but with vigilance.

In martial arts, sparring is a freestyle method of practical fight training. "Practical" because no style can legally replicate a real fight: no off-limits targets, possible weapons, multiple attackers, and the likelihood of serious injury or death. Different styles and dojos employ a variety of safety measures to keep fighters relatively safe. The purpose of sparring, at its core, is to practice techniques not only on a moving target, but on a target that wants to do the same thing in return. Boxing and kickboxing are obvious examples. Debates about the merits of sparring—and the shortcomings of particular forms of it—have existed as long as martial arts have existed, and likely always will. The accusations are endless: Is point sparring useless? Is light contact realistic enough? Is grappling a waste of time? Is knockout karate the toughest? But regardless of style, sparring should accomplish two things for the student:

- The student should learn what it feels like to be struck by another person. Many people never experience this until they are in a serious altercation, and much of the fear comes from the anxiety of getting hurt or feeling incredible pain.
- The student should develop the ability to stay calm in the middle of combative chaos. In the moment of truth, will the person stay composed and do what needs to be done, or panic?

It is difficult to judge how hard to strike someone if the mind is scattered. That difference can determine whether a situation ends in successful self-defense, an assault charge, or something worse.

In the heat of battle, the body and mind may have practiced hundreds of self-defense techniques and combinations, both with cooperative partners and in freestyle sparring, but still within the controlled confines of a training environment. In reality, the mind often narrows its focus to simple actions and falls back on what it truly believes will work. For example, the brain may not trust a spinning hook kick in a real fight. That does not mean such techniques are worthless, because no one truly knows what they will do until they face the situation. It is best to understand how the body functions, develop a committed sense of combat, cultivate survival instinct and confidence, and then let the situation dictate the response.

Methods

There are many ways to spar: full contact, light contact, points with rounds, points without rounds, boxing type points with continuous sparring, points where the action stops after every point, with or without grappling, with or without leg kicks, with or without face contact, with or without gloves, size of gloves, with or without groin strikes, take downs, sweeps, elbows, knees, head butts. Just name it and there is probably a rule set one can find to cater to a student's needs. And of course, there are pros and cons to all of it.

Sparring Techniques

Footwork for sparring completely depends on the rules being used. If groin strikes are allowed, a more sideways facing stance will be preferred. With leg kicks, a more half-sideways/half forward facing stance is advantageous in order to lift the front leg to check leg strikes. If the sparring style only uses hands, like boxing where there is no legal threat below the waist, a more forward facing stance makes the most sense. Since rules come and go, being able to switch stances is highly desirable. This also goes for being orthodox (left leg in front) or southpaw (right leg in front), where once again, being able to alternate sides will help against any opponent. Training to spar should emphasize fluidity, being ambidextrous as a fighter, with the ability to change for any occassion.

Irikumi Kumite

"Irikumi" refers to continuous engagement sparring. It is a free-style sparring format in which two participants continue exchanging techniques without stopping after a score is called. The concept emphasizes offensive and defensive strategy, with the goal of exploiting an opponent's mistakes during ongoing exchanges. In irikumi, it is not uncommon to absorb light contact in order to set up a more effective counterattack. In contrast, point fighting prioritizes timing, precision, and controlled entry; the first clean scoring technique typically stops the exchange and awards a point. Irikumi does not rely on this stop-start structure. Instead, it more closely resembles traditional kickboxing formats than modern Olympic-style point sparring.

16. Sparring Techniques (Waza)

Definition

Waza means "technique." Waza exercises are preparatory drills for sparring. Most students, when sparring for the first time, have no experience and are often unsure of what to do. Waza drills provide a structured introduction to fundamental actions and responses.

Purpose of Waza Drills

- Introduce basic tactical decision-making
- Provide scenarios for timing and distance training
- Build core sparring behavior prior to practicing actual free sparring

Stances

Yoko kumite dachi means "sideways fighting stance." This stance is used as a basic sparring position within systems that allow groin strikes, such as Ketsugo Goju-Ryu. The lateral hip alignment reduces exposure. From yoko kumite dachi, a fighter can effectively defend against:

- Backfist strikes
- Side kicks
- Hook kicks
- Roundhouse kicks
- Groin-level attacks

Mobility

In sparring, stances must remain mobile. A fighter should not become attached to any single position. Even when using yoko kumite dachi, fighters must be able to transition into other structures as needed, particularly when engaging straight-line attacks such as:

- Front kicks
- Straight punches

Sparring is characterized by continuous motion. Unlike self-defense, where structure may be momentary and decisive, sparring requires sustained adaptability over time. In sparring, a round is typically 2 to 5 minutes. During this time there is a lot of give and take, particularly in Irikumi style where fighters do not stop after each "point." In Irikumi, each fighter practices combinations, typically three strikes in one combination. For this type of sparring a fighter needs to stay mobile, changing stances as needed, but without losing power.

On the other end of the spectrum, point fighting, fighters may stay in a stance, usually sideways, but with the appearance of bouncing because they have to get in and out of combat quickly with minimal exposure. In this type of sparring, the object is to get the quickest point, not necessarily the best combination, therefore different approaches are used to prepare for point fighting.

Chambers and Blocks

When sparring, punches are not always going to start from the chamber position because in sparring, speed is key. When punching or striking, particularly from a forward facing stance, the non-striking hand should be up by the cheek to block counterstrikes to the head. However, with groin strikes, one hand may be ready to block the groin as well. Hip movement is important for low strikes as well. In other words, there is no static position; the body must be in motion when sparring and ready to deflect, counter, or block, ready for anything.

The following sequences are broken out into open and closed stance offensive combinations. Since these are primarily sparring techniques, they can be practiced with our without sparring gear. They can also be practiced outside of, or while sparring. Often it is best to practice in both scenarios.

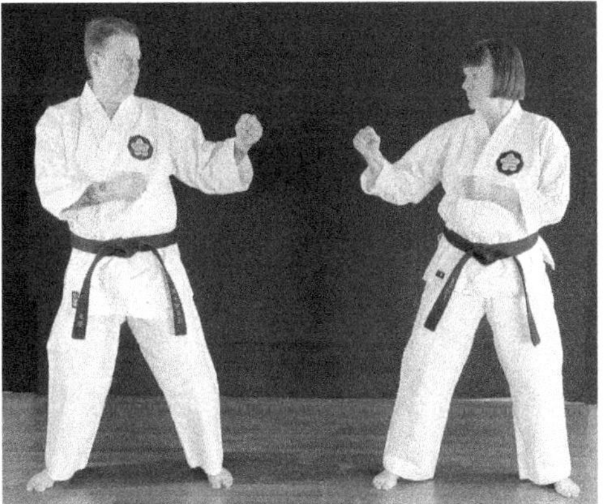

Open Stance - fighters face the same direction. "Open" does not necessarily mean the fighters have to be perfectly sideways, it just means that the opposite feet are facing the other fighter.

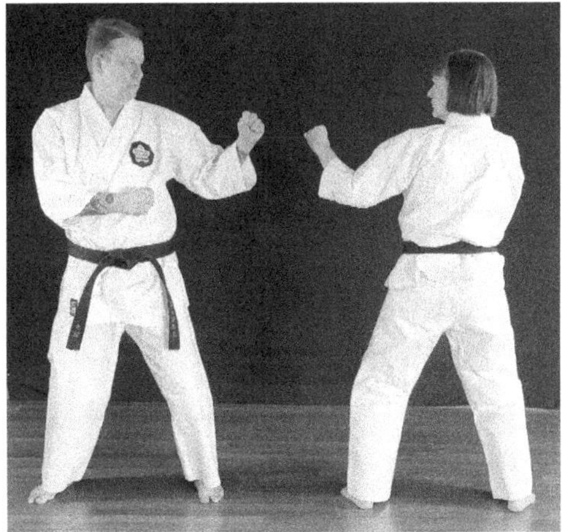

Closed Stance - fighters face opposite directions, meaning the same (right or left) feet are facing the other fighter.

From an Open Stance

1

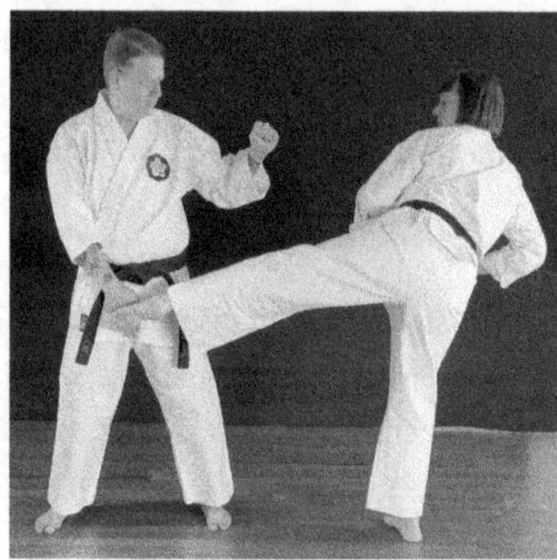

Rear Leg Round-
house Kick to Groin

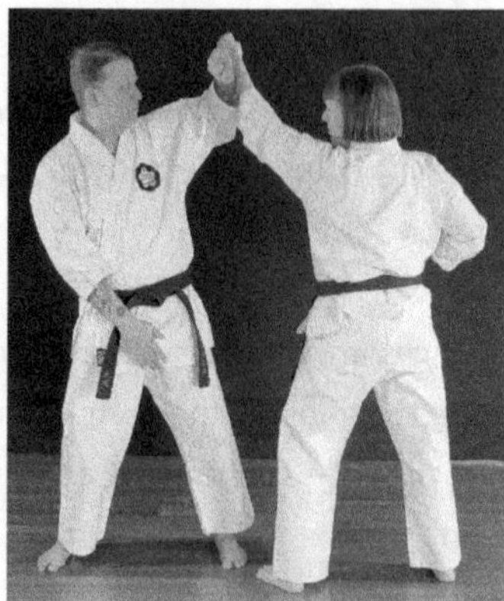

Backfist
Strike to Head

2

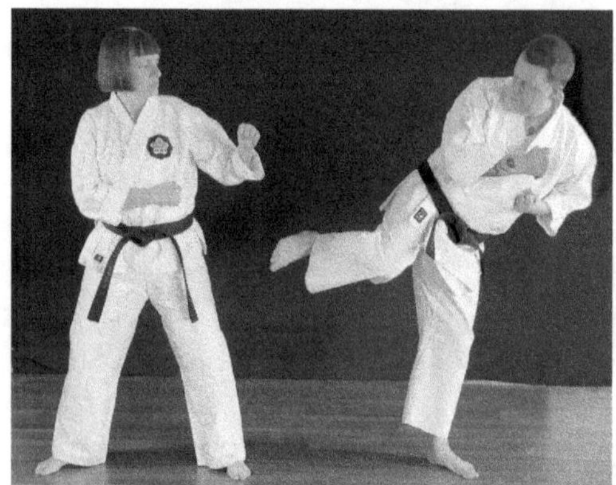

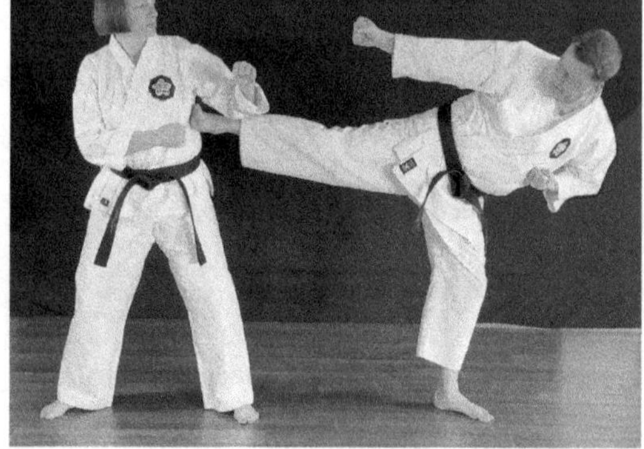

Hop Up Side Kick to Ribs Covered by
Backfist Strike to Head

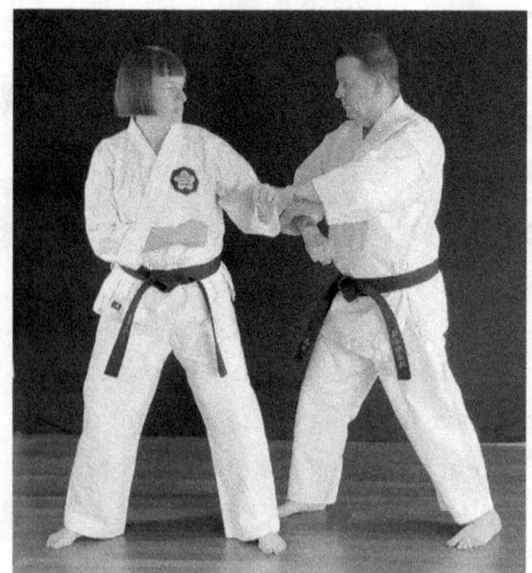

Cover Opponent's Lead
Hand with Back Hand

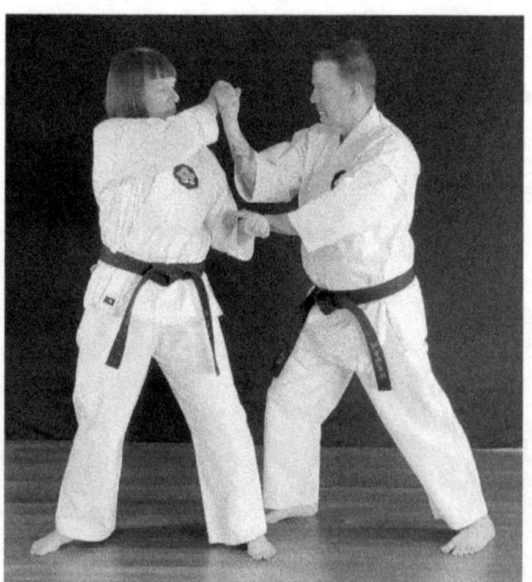

Rolling Backfist Strike to
Face with Lead Hand

3

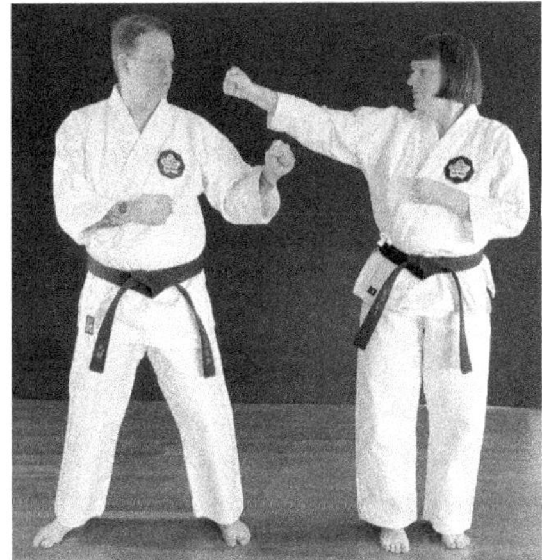

Slide Up, Backfist Strike to Head

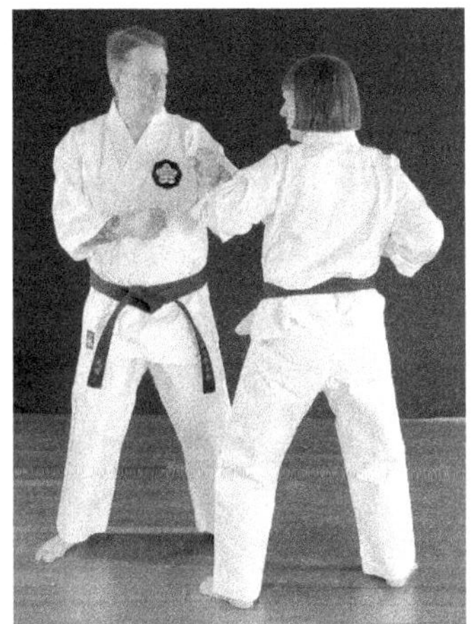

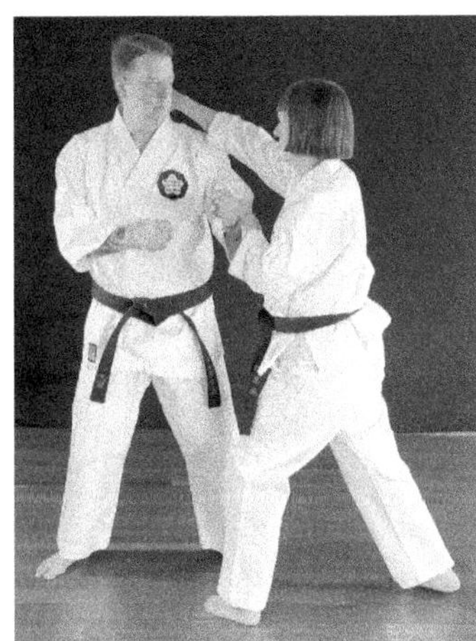

Spin for Ridge Hand Strike to Head Under Ear

4

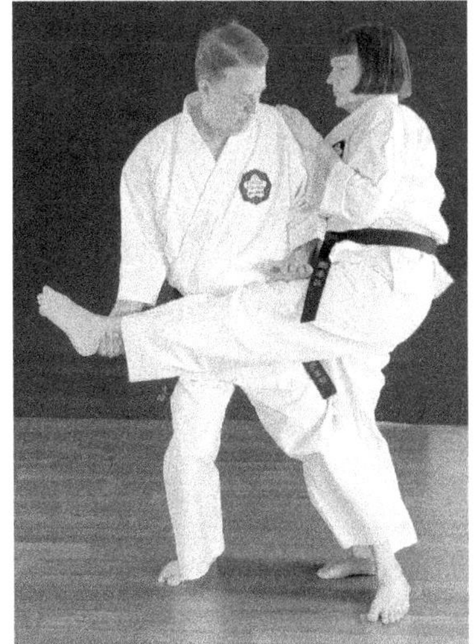

Offense: Front Snap Kick /
Defense: Step in, Trap Leg for
Takedown

5

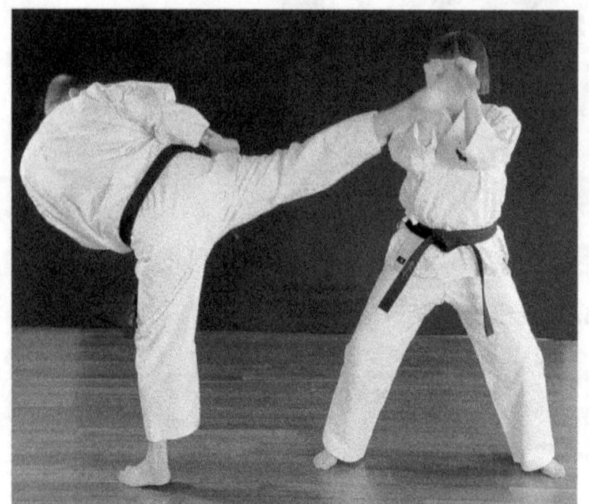

Offense: Rear Leg Round House Kick to Head / Defense: Double Forearm Block

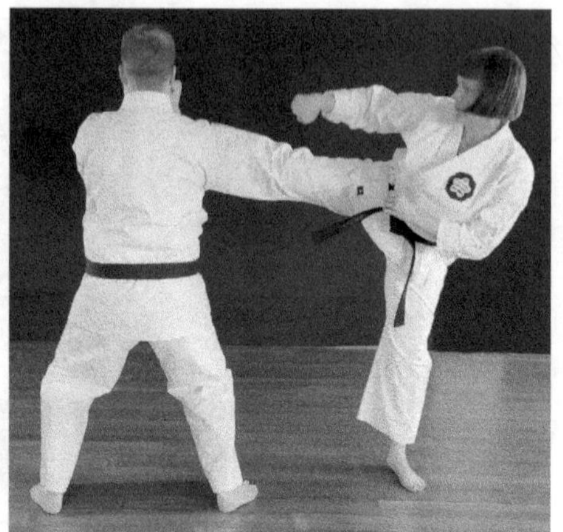

Defense: Double Forearm Block / Offense: Rear Leg Round House Kick to Head

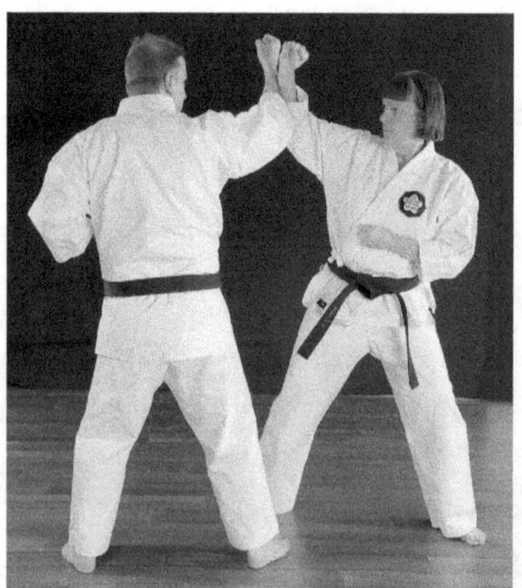

Offense: Backfist Strike to the Head / Defense: Rising Head Block

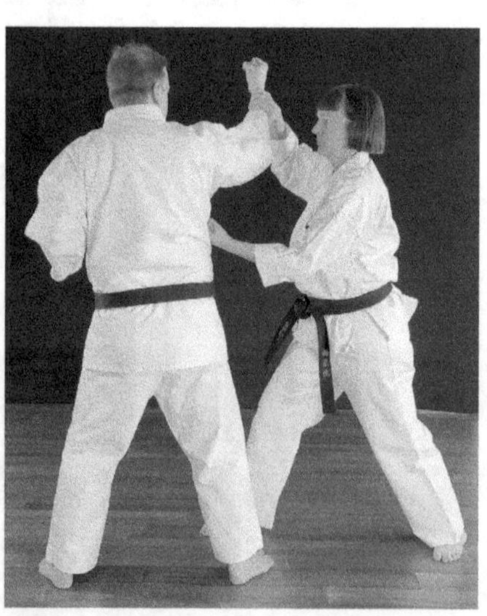

Defense: Grab Arm, Inverted Strike to Body

6

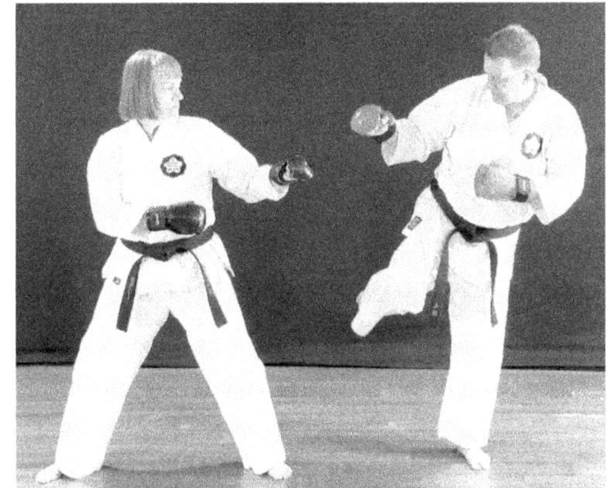

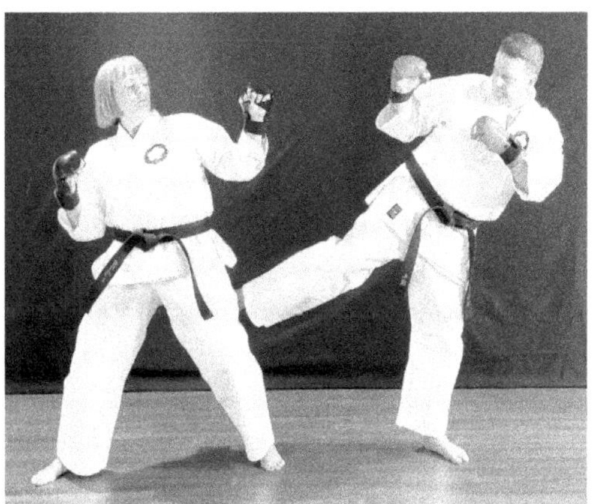

Double Kick (Low first to Off-balance Opponent)

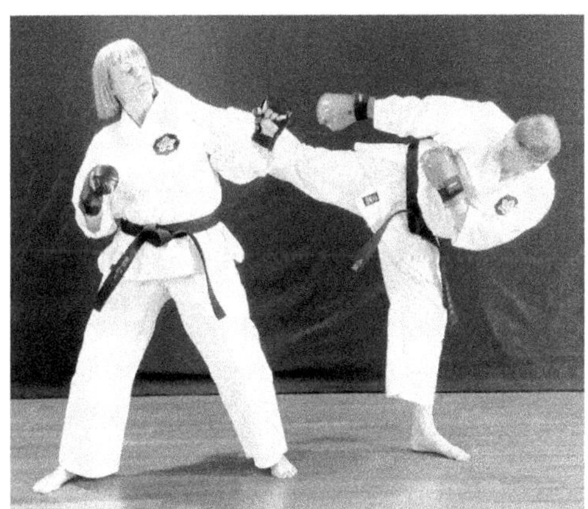

Double Kick (cont.) (High)

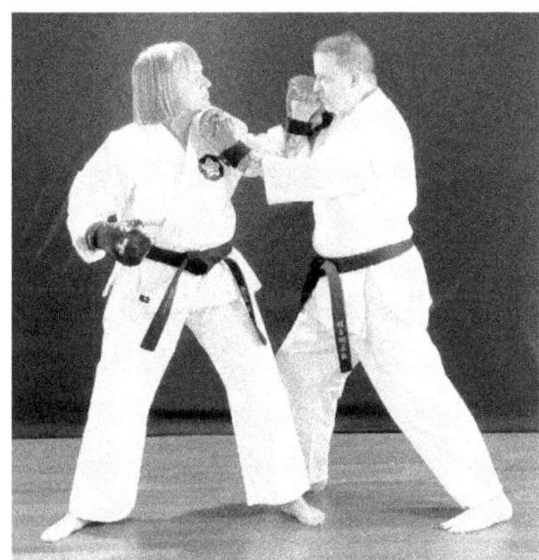

Land Behind Opponent, Blocking Opponent's Lead Hand, Upper Cut

7

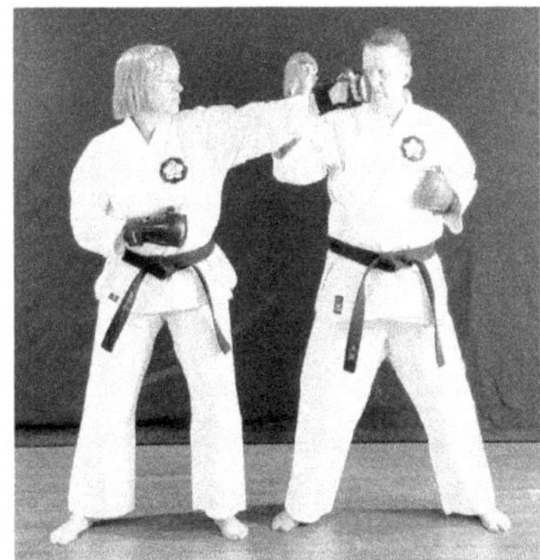

Backfist Strike to Raise Opponent's Guard

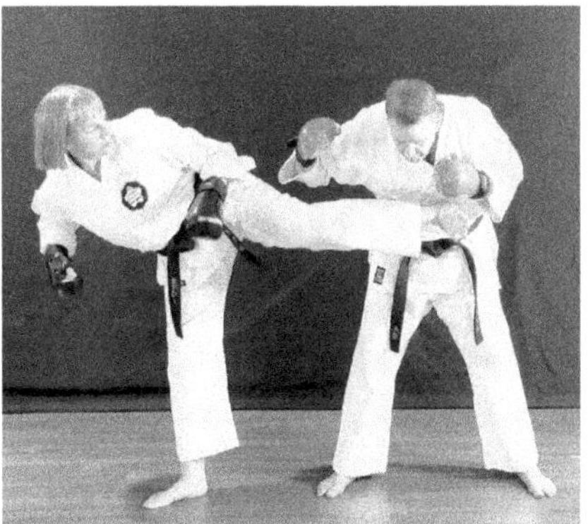

Hook Kick to Abdoment or Groin

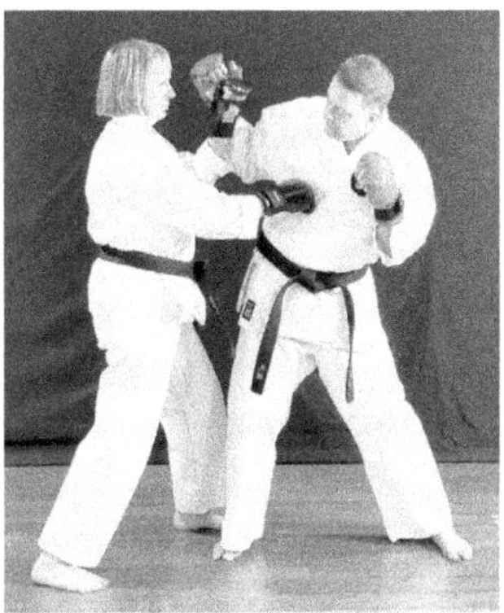

Land Behind Opponent, Reverse Punch

8

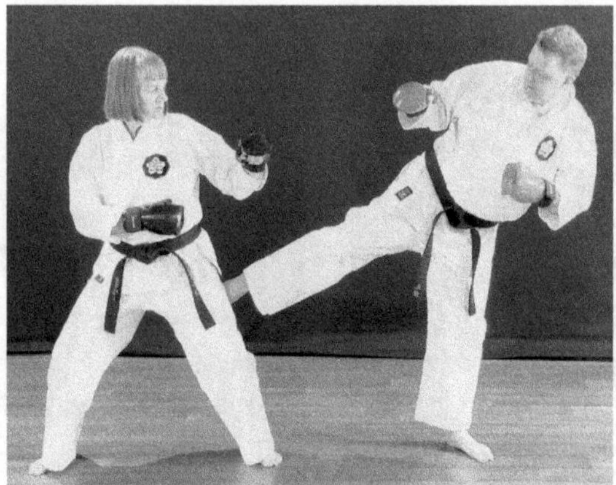

Low Kick to Off-balance Opponent

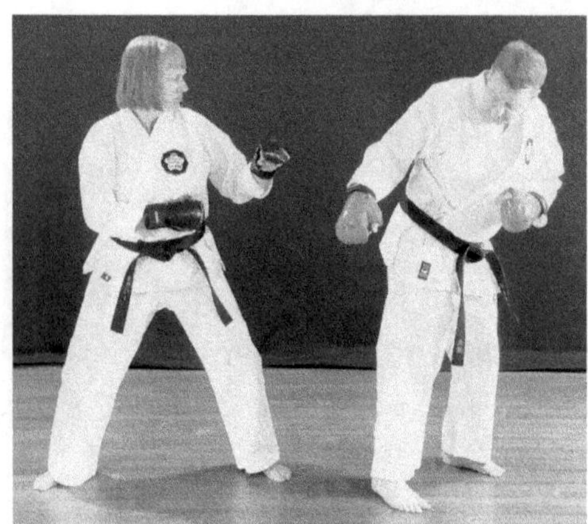

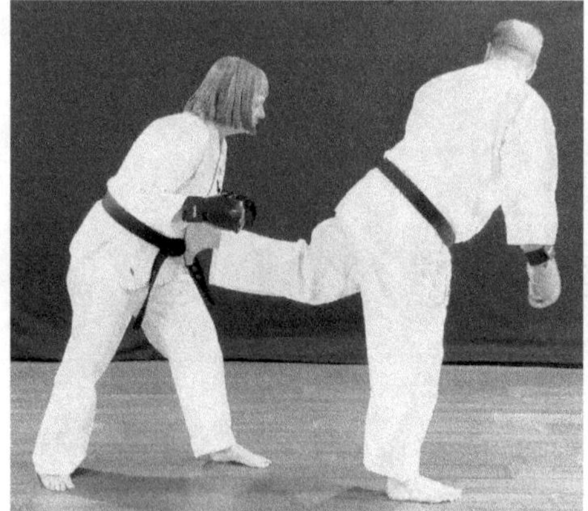

Land in Front of Opponent, Turn Kick or Back Heel Kick to Abdomen

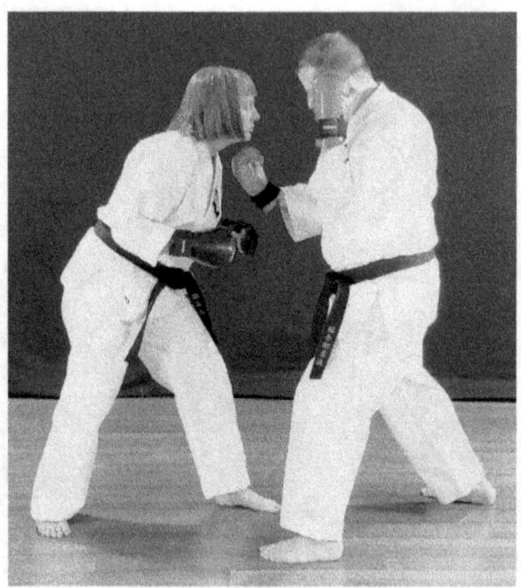

Upper Cut

9

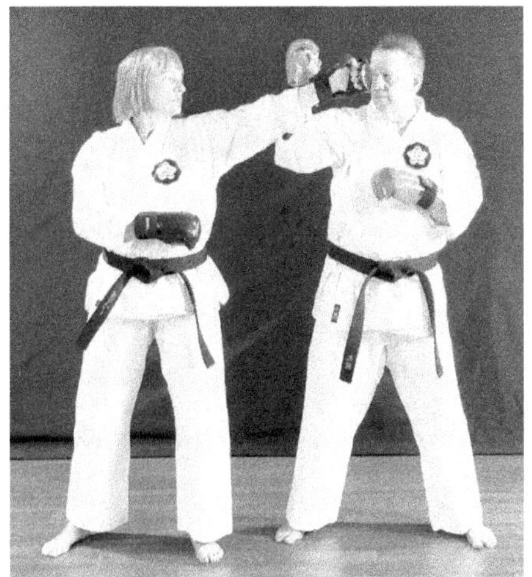
Slide Up Backfist Strike

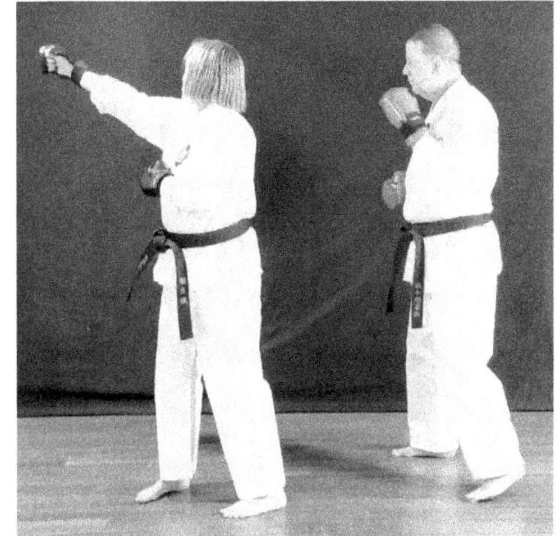
Quick Spinning Backfist Strike

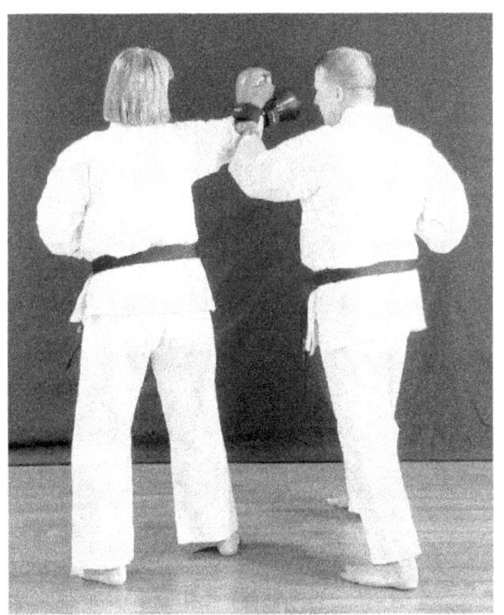
Spinning Backfist Strike (cont.)

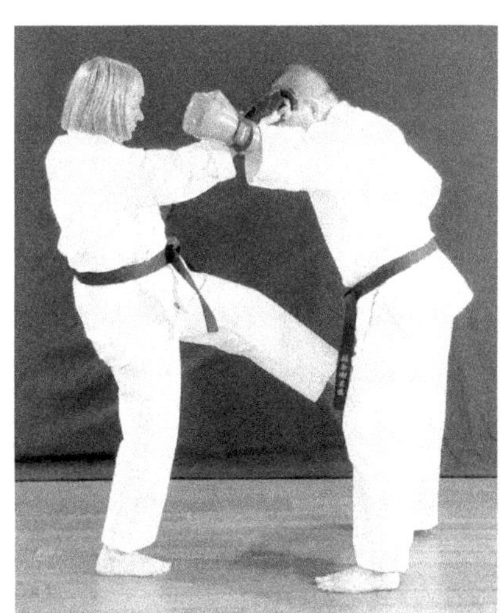
Groin Kick

From a Closed Stance

1

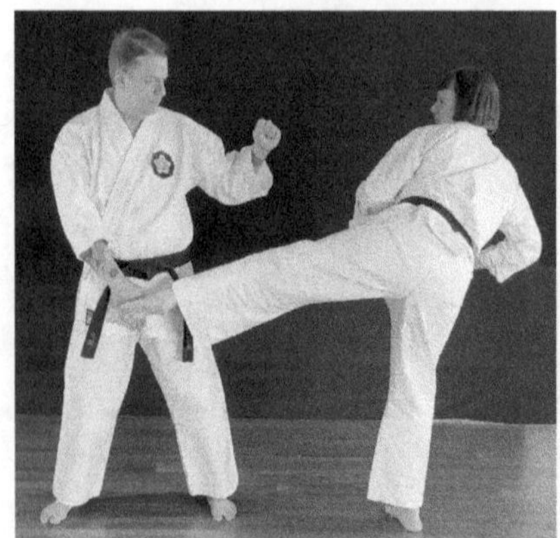

Hop Up Round-house Kick to Groin

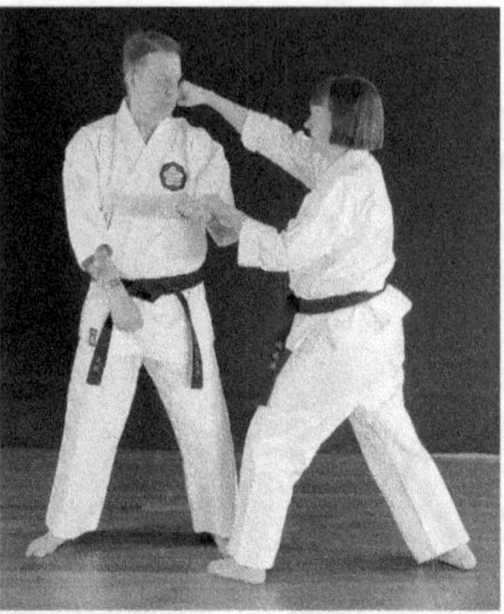

Control Opponent's Lead Arm, Punch to Head

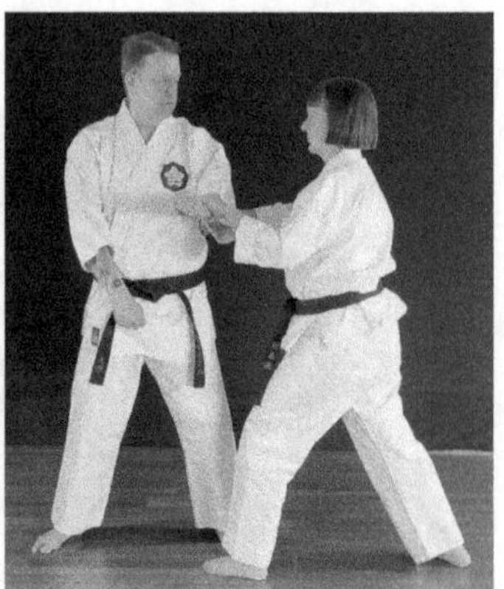

Follow Up Punch to Ribs

2

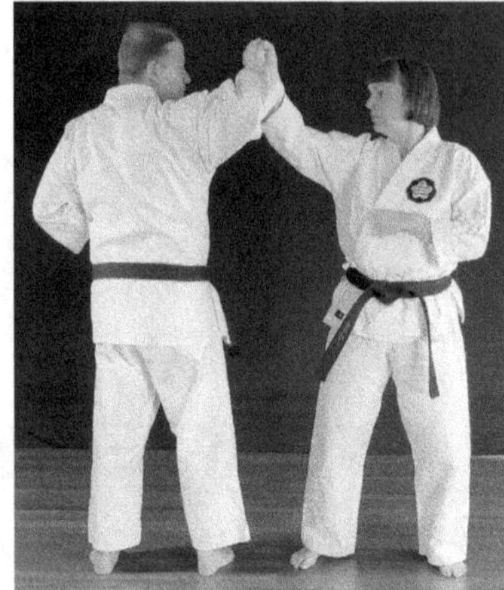

Backfist Strike to Head

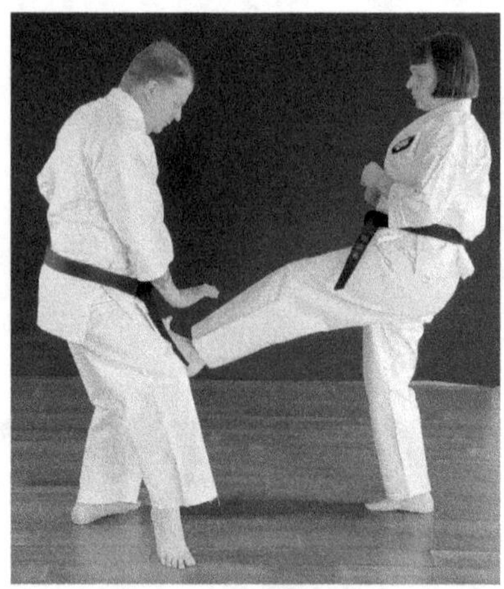

Offense: Front Snap Kick to Groin / Defense: Palm Heel Strike to Foot in Neko Ashi Dachi

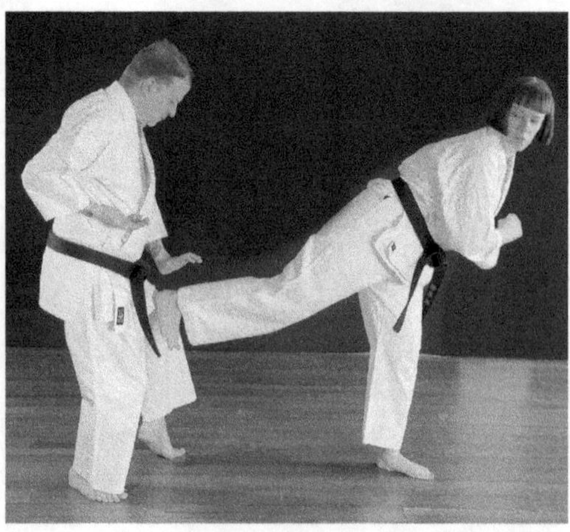

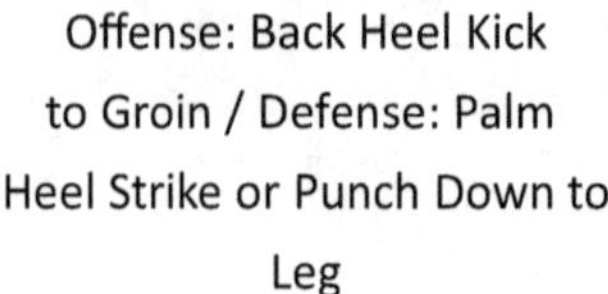

Offense: Back Heel Kick to Groin / Defense: Palm Heel Strike or Punch Down to Leg

3

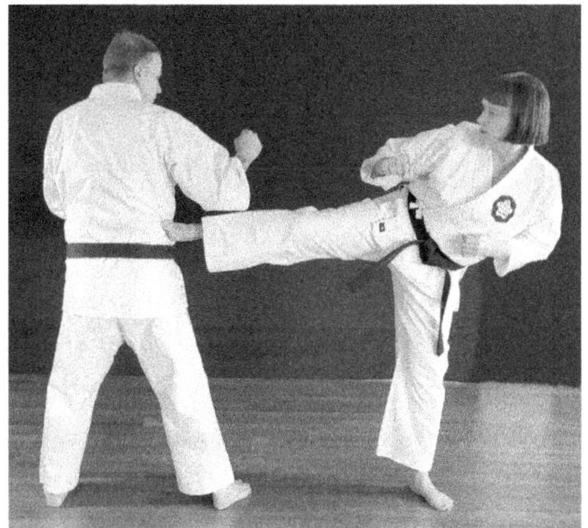

Hop Up Side Kick to Ribs (Faster Than Step Behind, Less Powerful)

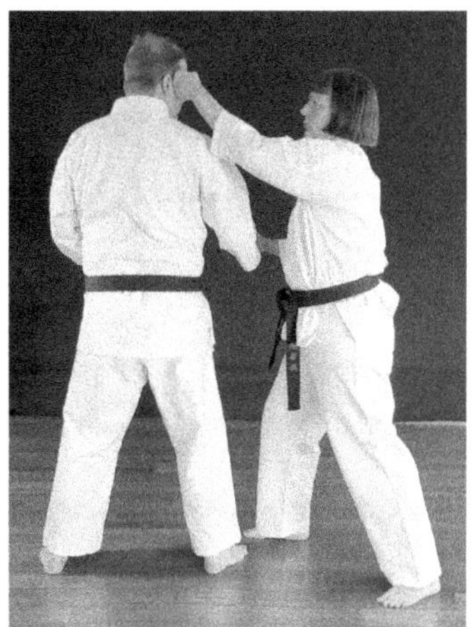

Control Opponent, Vertical Strike to Head

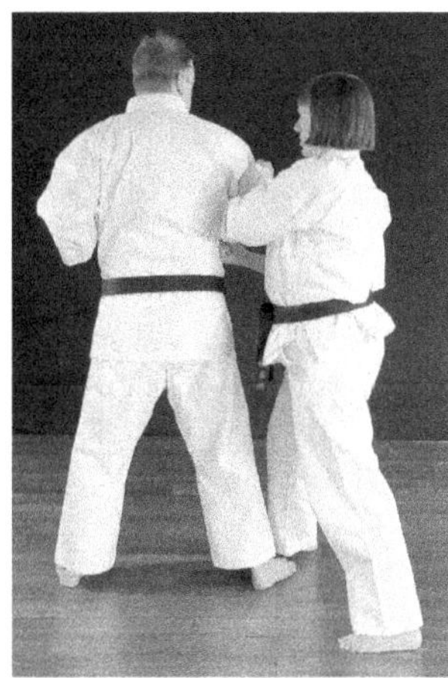

Step Around, Inverted Strike to Body

4

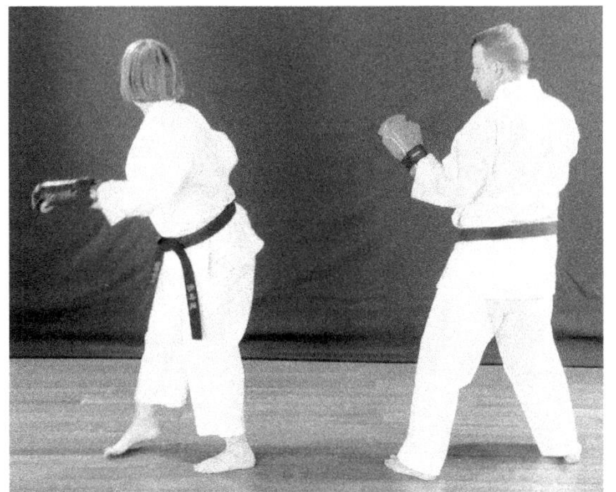

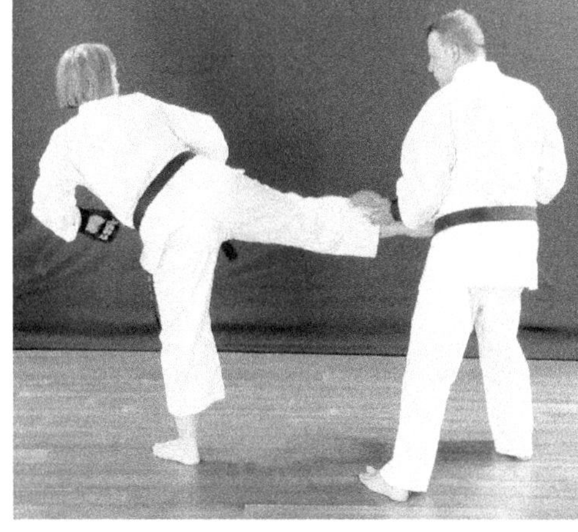

Turn Kick to Bring Opponent's Guard Down

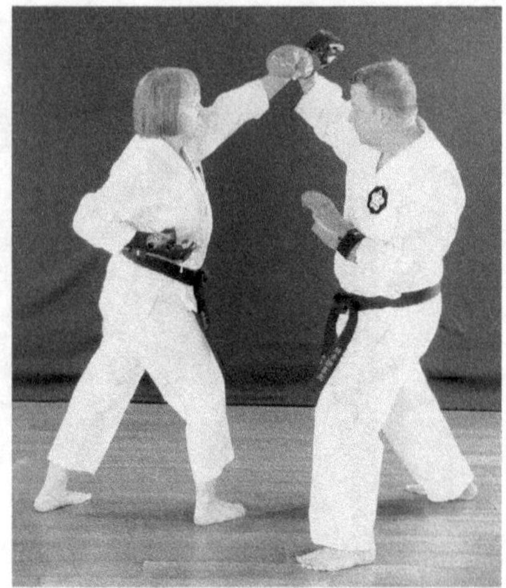
Ridgehand Strike to Head

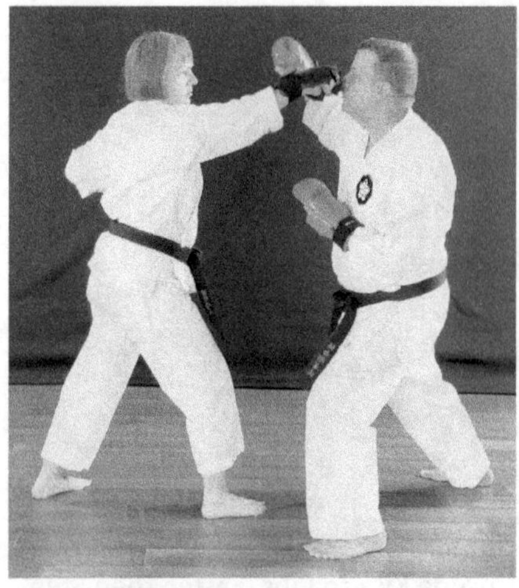
Quick Follow Up with Straight Punch

5

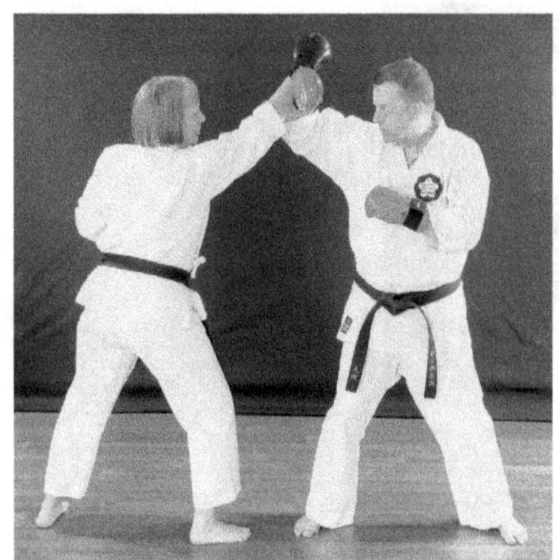
Backfist strike

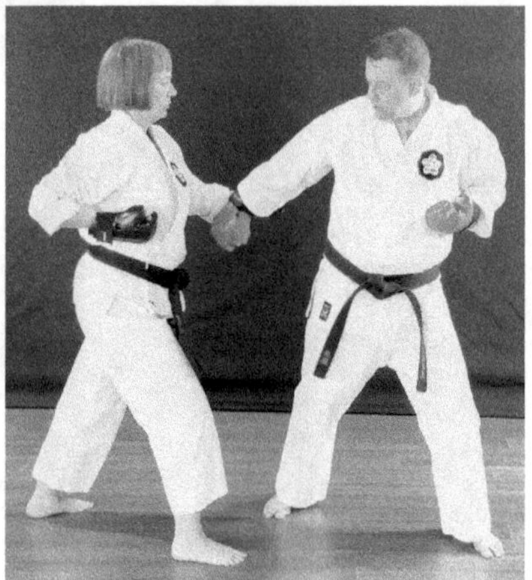
Inverted Strike

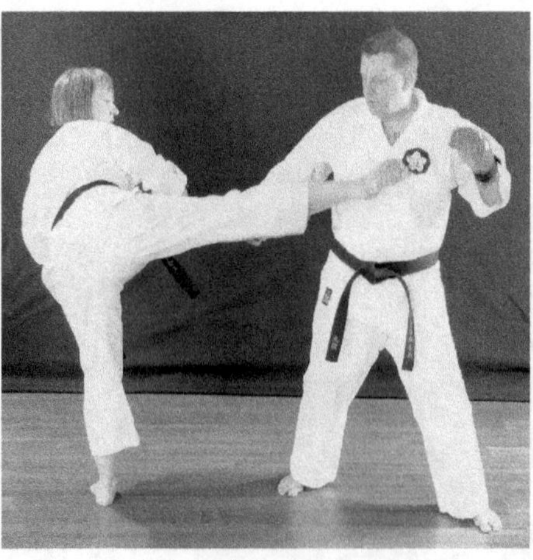
Roundhouse Kick

6

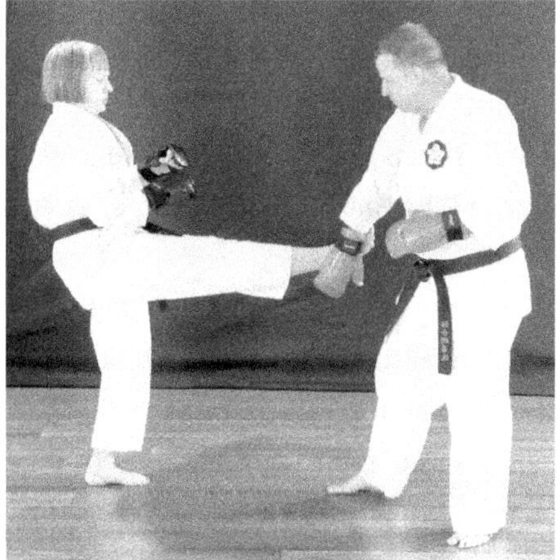

Front Snap Kick

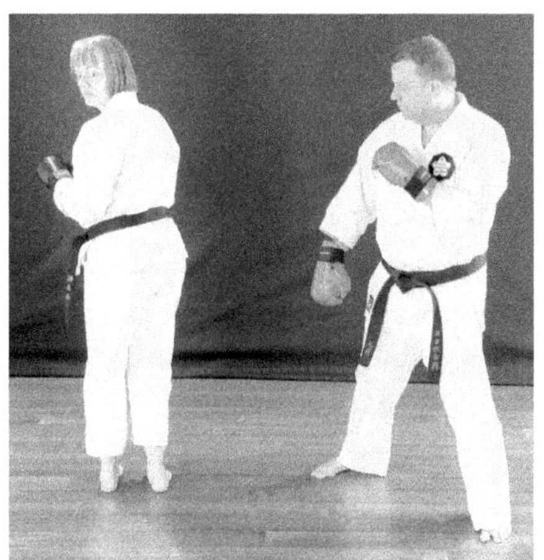

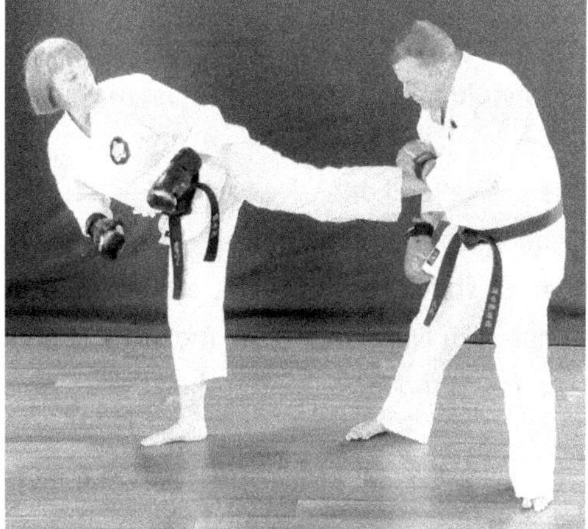

Turn Kick

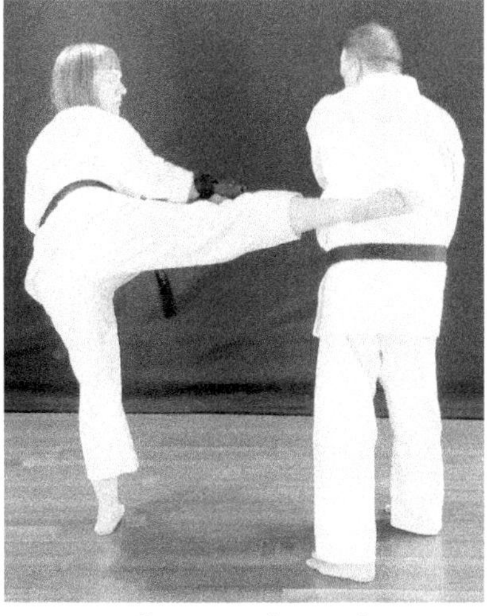

Roundhouse Kick to Kidneys

Defensive Sparring Techniques

There are those who argue that there is no such thing as "blocking" in karate, but this is really just semantics. At its core, blocking is just another way to keep one's self from getting struck, and is important when it comes to either self-defense or sparring. A defensive technique may resemble a strike, and that is no accident, but should always be followed by a counter strike as well.

Shodai taught his students to always fight in threes. When a fighter attacks, it should always be three strikes, never less. The assumption is that the defender may block the first two, but hopefully not the third. Along those lines, offensive strategy should not be three strikes to the same place. The plan should be to move the defenders guard. For example, if a fighter wants to punch the defender in the face, he must move the defender's hands out of the way so he has a clear shot. The strategy is, draw the hands away from where you want to strike.

For defense, one must anticipate the offensive strategy. Fighter B should not assume Fighter A will only strike once, but even so, Fighter B should not allow Fighter A to get off three clean strikes. Counter-striking after the first strike/block may disrupt or even eliminate the offensive strategy entirely. The point is, a fighter should never block a strike just to wait on another one, which only helps the attacker.

Another defensive (and offensive for that matter) strategy is to never fall into the trap of consistency, like always fighting with the dominant side in the back, or always starting an attack with the same combination of strikes. Beyond that, a fighter worst mistake is overthinking when it comes to sparring. Consider that each fighter is getting the same relative instructions and in the end, the winner will be the one who performs the moves better than the other, or faster, or with more impact.

For this section, instead of focusing on combinations, we will focus on basic defensive techniques. Something to consider when looking at these defensive techniques, they can be interchanged easily and may depend on how the fighter wants to counter-strike. And something not shown in the illustrations is the most perferred defensive move is moving just out of range. Not only is it the easiest defensive move, it keeps the fighter in range for a counter-strike.

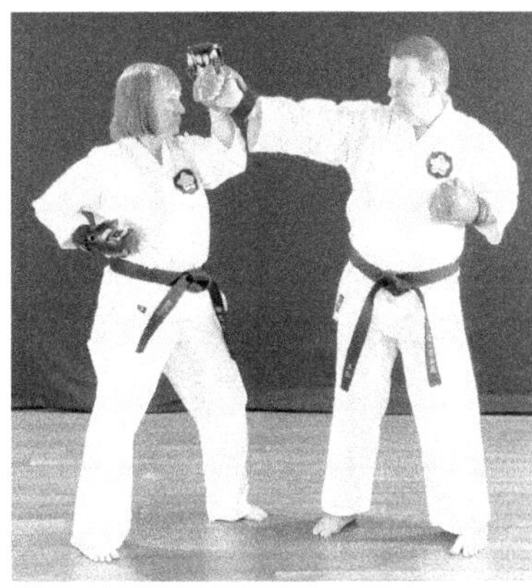

Offense: Backfist Strike
Defense: From the Outside, Slap Block with Lead Hand

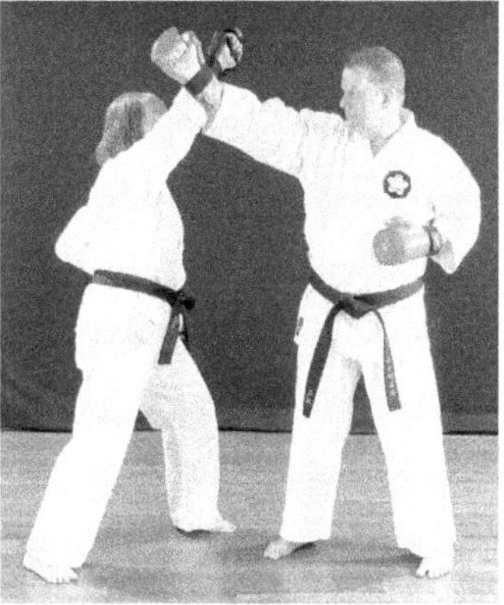

Offense: Backfist Strike
Defense: From the Outside, Rising Head Block with Back Hand

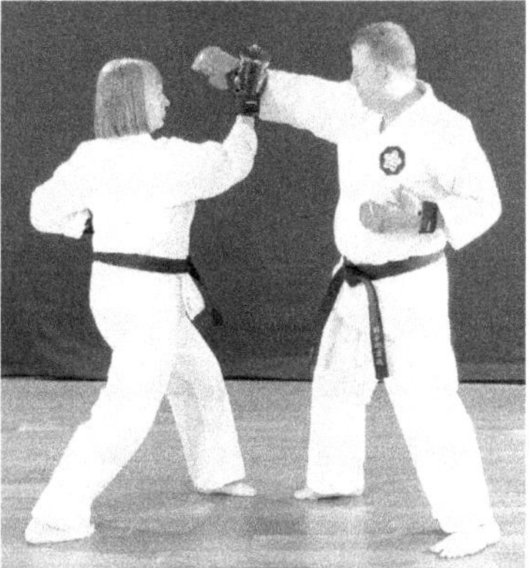

Offense: Ridgehand Strike (or Hook Punch, or Straight Punch)
Defense: From the Inside, Slap Block with Back Hand

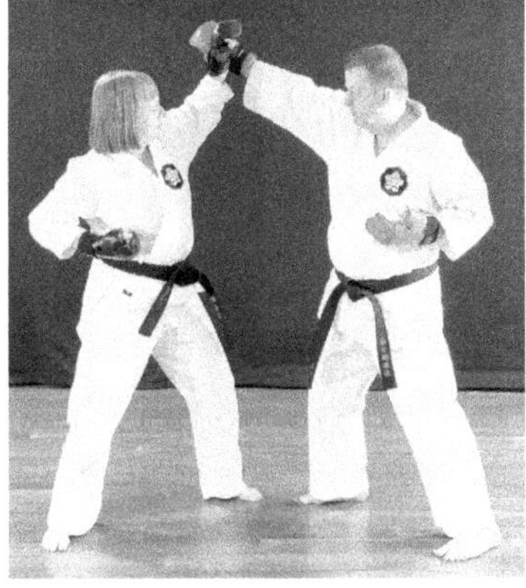

Offense: Ridgehand Strike (or Hook Punch, or Straight Punch)
Defense: From the Inside, Rising Head Block Out

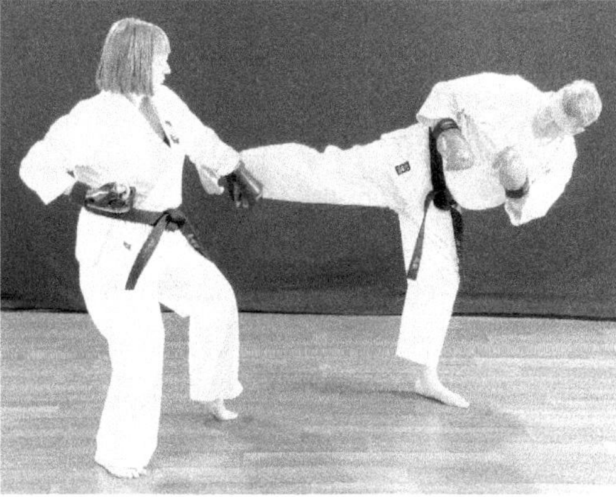

Offense: Side Kick
Defense: From the Inside, Hammer Fist Strike to the Leg, Directing the Opponent Outside

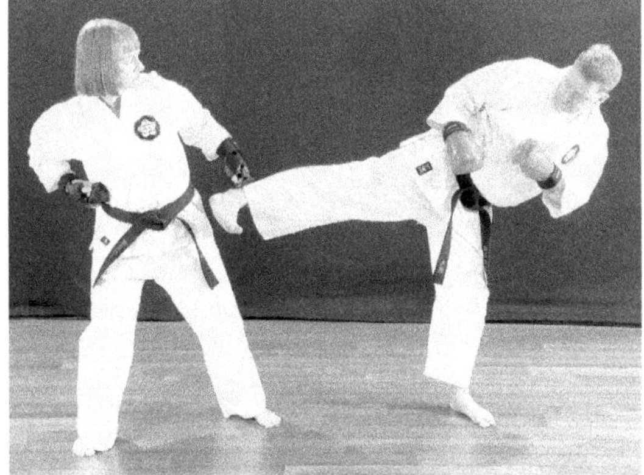

Offense: Side Kick
Defense: From the Inside or Outside, Strike Down to the Foot or Leg

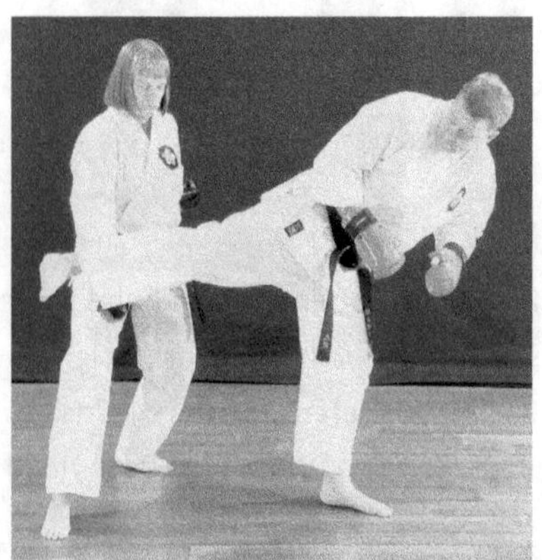

Offense: Side Kick
Defense: From the Outside,
Hammer Fist Strike to the Leg,
Direct Opponent Inside

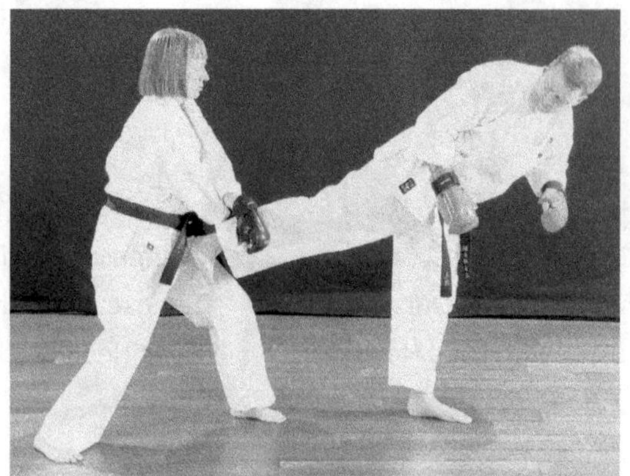

Offense: Side Kick
Defense: Downward X Block

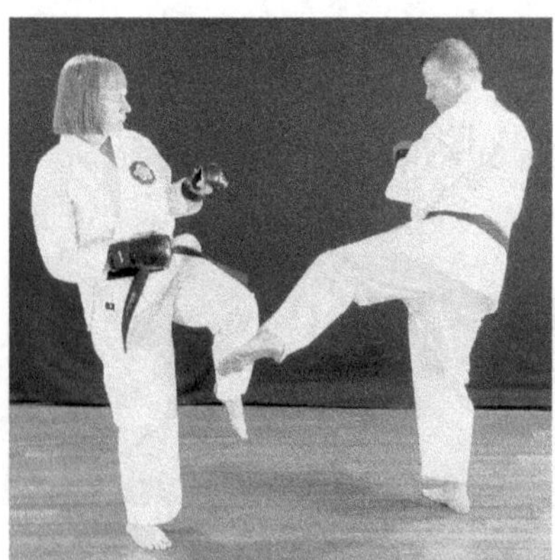

Offense: Roundhouse Kick
Defense: Raise Leg for Shin Block

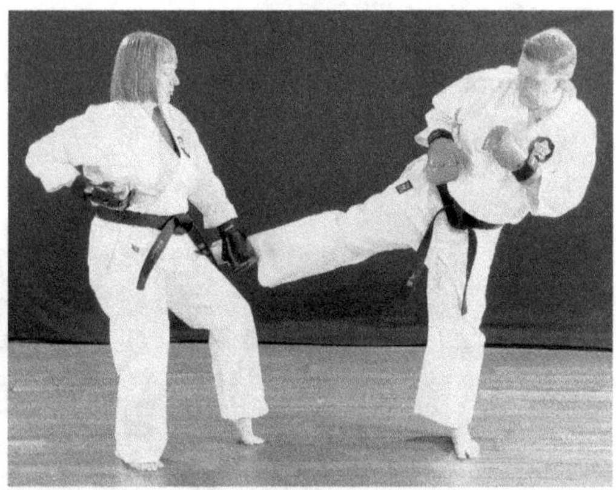

Offense: Roundhouse Kick
Defense: From the Inside, Hammer Fist Strike
to the Leg, Directing the Opponent Outside
(same as with Side Kick)

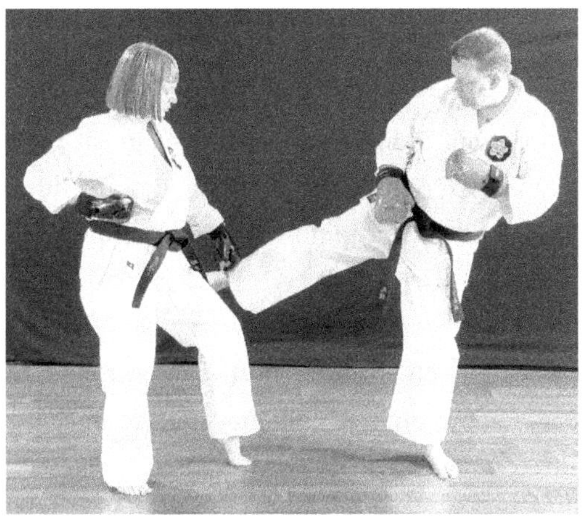

Offense: Roundhouse Kick
Defense: From the Inside or Outside, Strike Down to the Foot or Leg (same as with Side Kick)

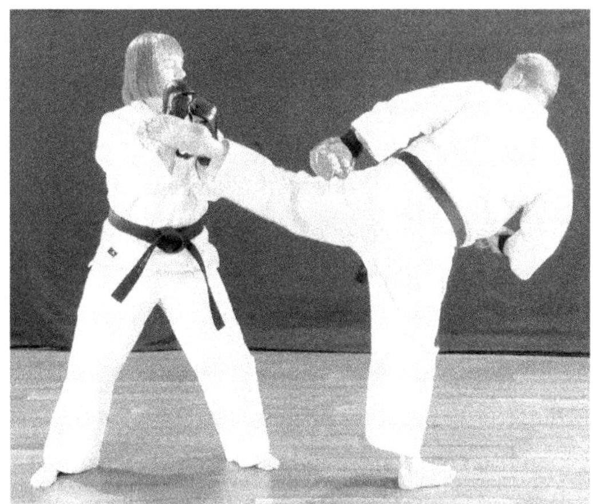

Offense: Roundhouse Kick
Defense: From the Inside or Outside, Double Forearm Block Outside

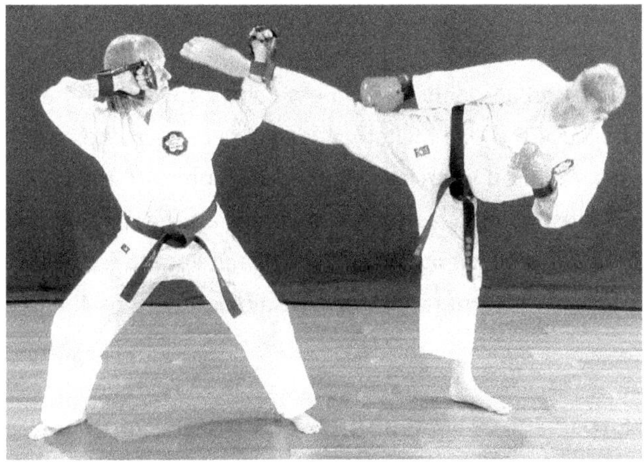

Offense: Roundhouse Kick
Defense: Back of Hand Strike

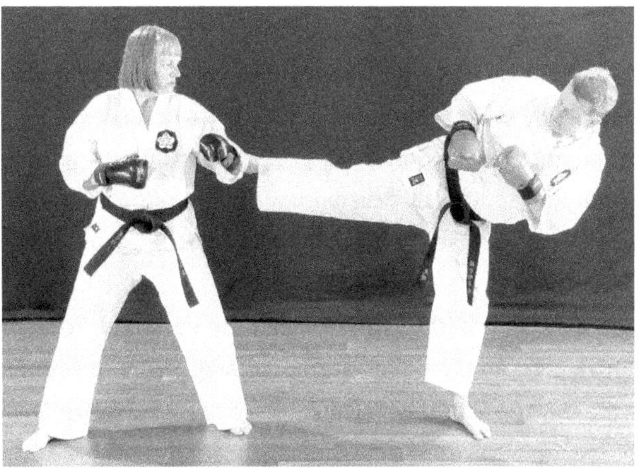

Offense: Mawashi Geri
Defense: Reverse Elbow Strike

17. Hojo Undo

Supplementary exercises exist in practically every physical activity. Training in karate is a similar process to training in a sport where the activity itself is generally the exercise trained. For the karate student, supplementary exercises exist to improve the core of karate. We do not jump rope, for example, simply for the sake of jumping rope.

Being in shape can make karate training easier because, if a person is not focused on controlling their breathing, that person can react with greater clarity. At the same time, it does not help to become so muscular that striking a precise target becomes difficult or speed is lost. There should, however, be enough strength to grip an opponent with authority, and offensive strikes should carry real power behind them. Without power, there would be no reason for an opponent to dodge or block. The ideal position is to develop strong technique, a rooted base, good grip strength, speed, power, durability, and the endurance necessary to train seriously in karate.

Chojun Miyagi wanted his students to do supplementary exercises to become more physically fit and improve their karate. Called Hojo Undo, they used mostly homemade equipment to accomplish this. In the 1950s, Seikichi Toguchi did not require the American students to do these things, except the heavy bag. It could have been a time issue or perhaps because the U.S. military students were presumed to be in shape already; even the makiwara was not a required exercise. Shodai and some of the other Americans learned how to use the makiwara, but most of the class time was spent on the main karate material: preparatory exercises (Daruma Taiso), kata, bunkai kumite, kiso kumite, and kumite (sparring). Shodai lifted weights on his own in Okinawa and later incorporated boxing training methods that he learned in Jacksonville Beach.

Traditional Hojo Undo typically refers to Chi Ishi, Ishi Sashi, Nigiri Game, Tan, and Kongoken. There are ways to obtain authentic versions of these tools, but there are also alternatives.

Chi Ishi looks like a dumbbell with the weight only on one end. For karate purposes, holding a dumbbell while performing punches and blocks can help develop strength and speed. Rotational benefits through controlled circular motions can also be gained by imitating the Chi Ishi with a dumbbell. Ishi Sashi are essentially stone kettlebells. Kettlebells can be used on the back of the hand when practicing open-hand techniques. Nigiri Game are gripping jars. These gripping jars can be left empty or filled with sand or water for additional resistance and are often held in each hand while walking in shiko dachi. As an alternative, adjustable grip trainers can be purchased at a fraction of the cost of gripping jars.

Tan is simply a barbell with a weight on each end. Traditional free weights are an easy alternative to the Tan. Kongoken is a metal or iron rectangular training implement in the shape of a closed frame. It is generally used for pushing and resisting movements. Once again, free weights can be used for similar purposes.

The key to getting stronger in karate is to practice karate with resistance. Performing kata with dumbbells or a weighted vest is a good way to develop speed and strength in kata performance. When practicing bunkai kumite or kiso kumite, students should provide appropriate resistance to their partner, thereby creating strength benefits for both participants. Kicking routines can also be performed using resistance bands or ankle weights. This may not look as "authentic" as using traditional metal geta, but the effect should be similar. We use many supplementary exercises, as shown below.

Makiwara

The makiwara is a traditional Okinawan training tool used to strengthen the wrists and develop precise striking placement and form. Unlike a heavy bag, the makiwara provides fixed resistance and then returns to its original position. A heavy bag can be used for similar benefits, but it does not replicate the same static resistance of the makiwara. Knuckle push-ups can also be used to strengthen the wrists.

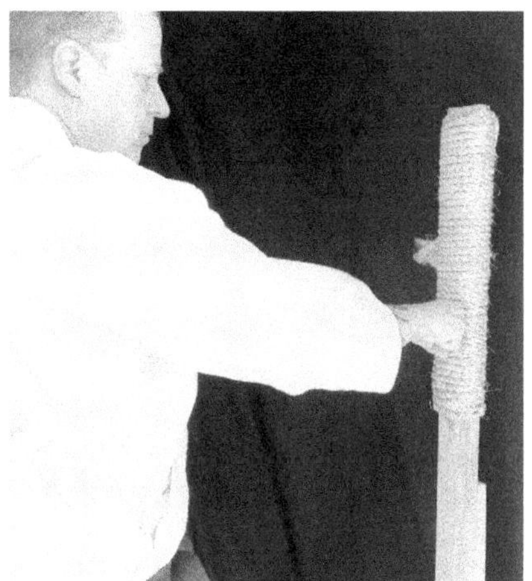

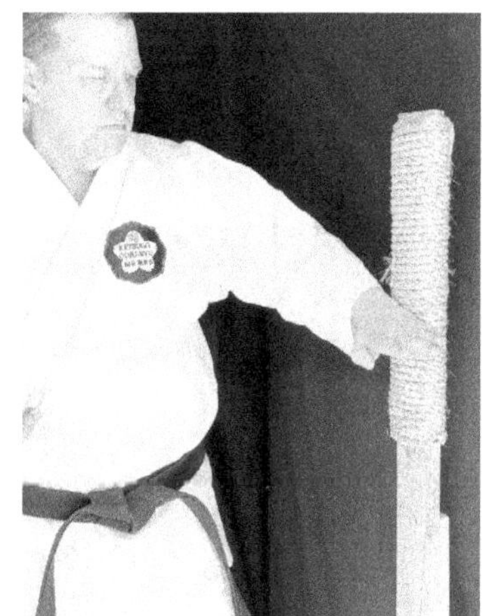

Double-End Bag

The double-end bag is suspended between the floor and ceiling by two cords and moves unpredictably when struck. Double-end bags improve hand-eye coordination, timing, speed, and accuracy. It can also be used for defensive movement drills to practice evading punches.

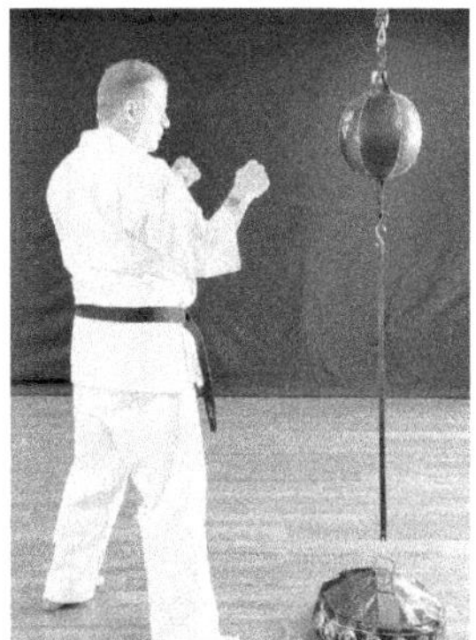

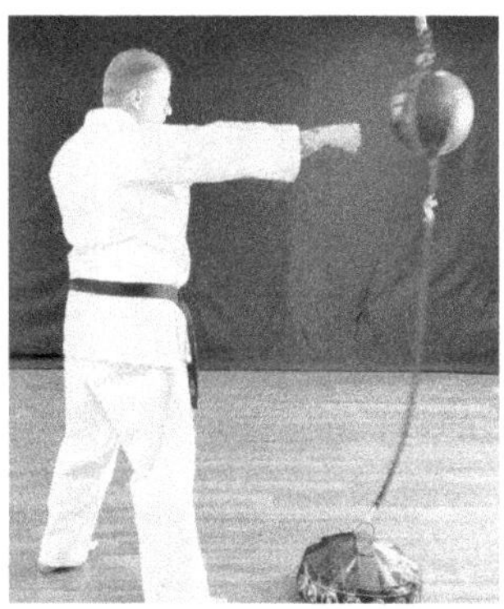

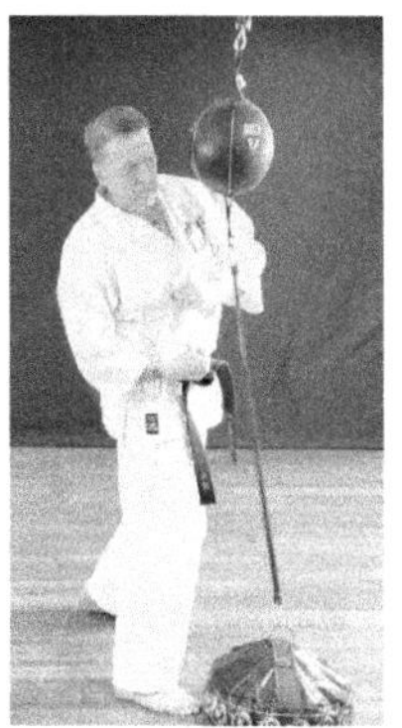

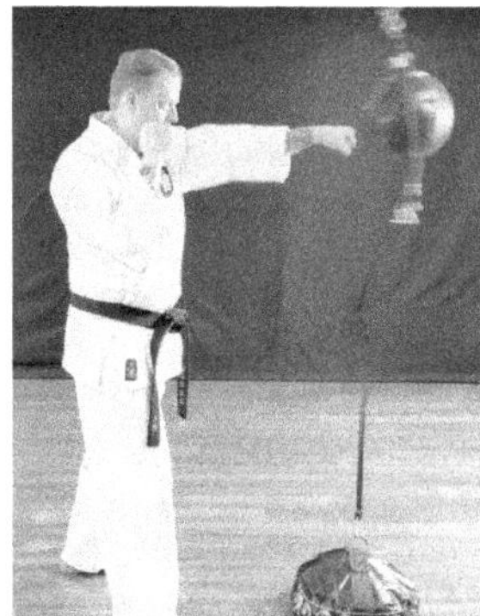

Heavy Bag

Heavy bag training is used to develop power, speed, distance control, and technical form. Many of the techniques introduced earlier as kiso kumite counters can also be practiced on the heavy bag, although nearly any striking technique can be applied to it.

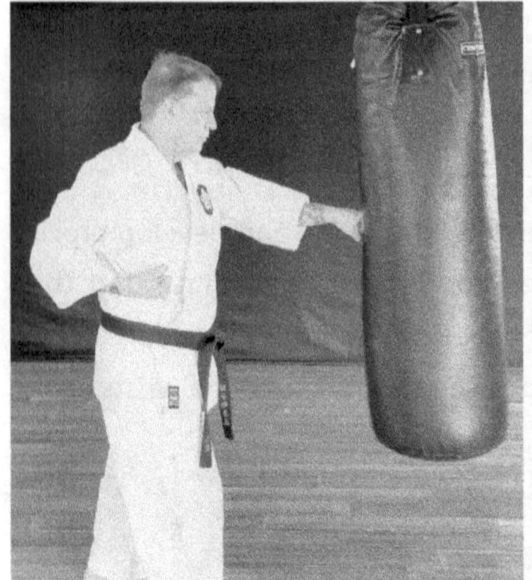

Gyaku Zuki

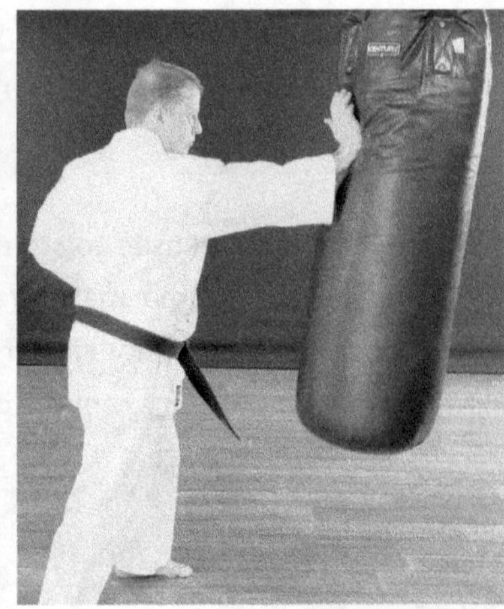

Shotei Uchi

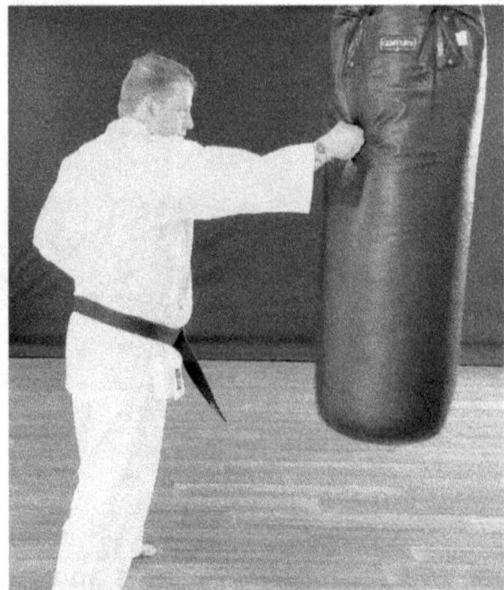

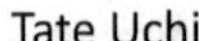

Tate Uchi

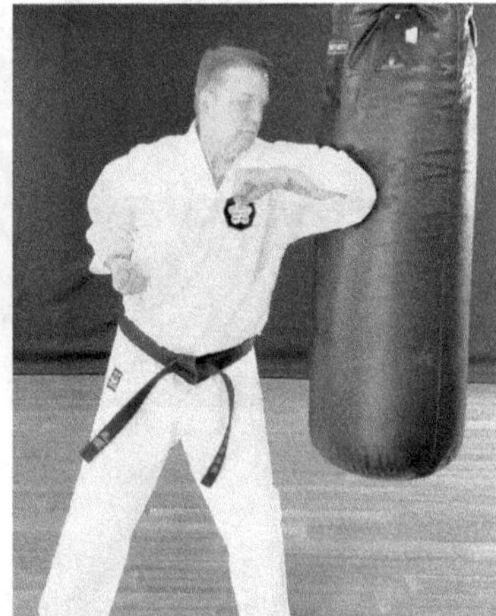

Yoko Empi Uchi

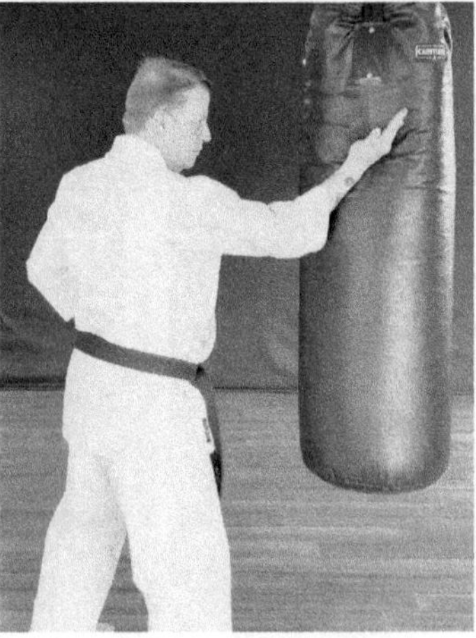

Mae Shuto Uchi

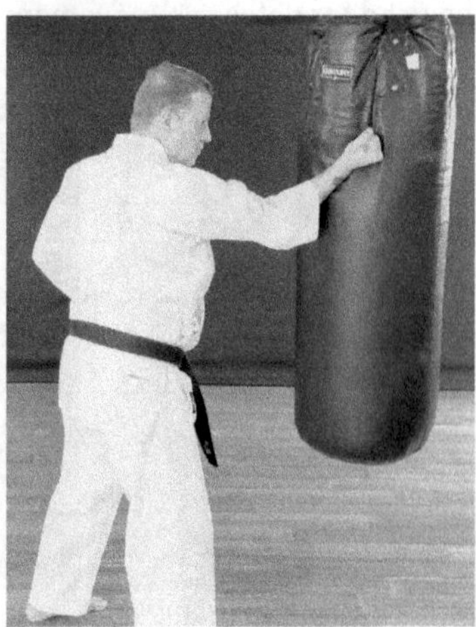

Mae Tettsui Uchi

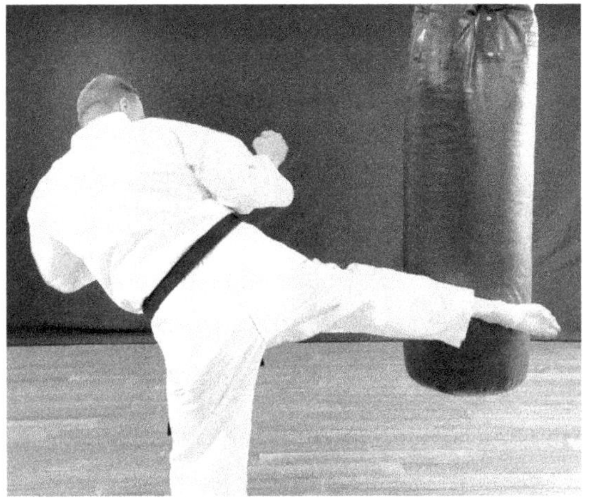

Mawashi Geri with Shin

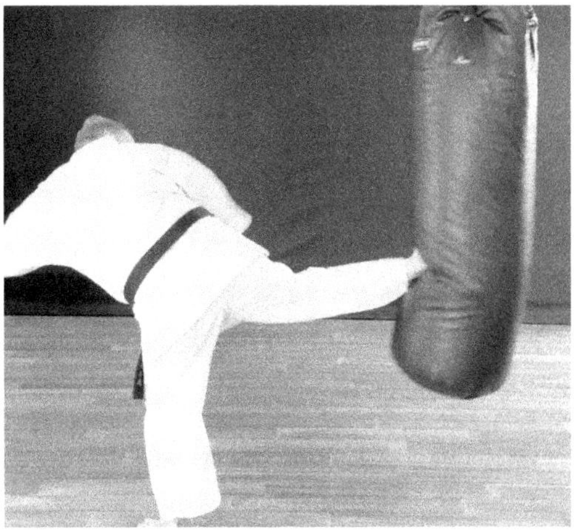

Yoko Geri

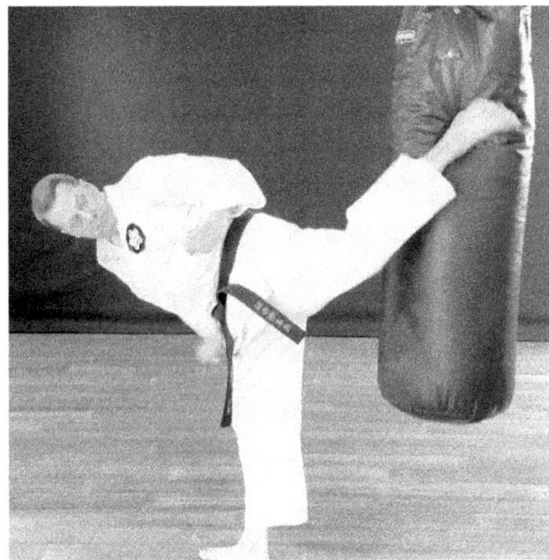

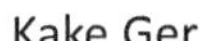

Kake Geri

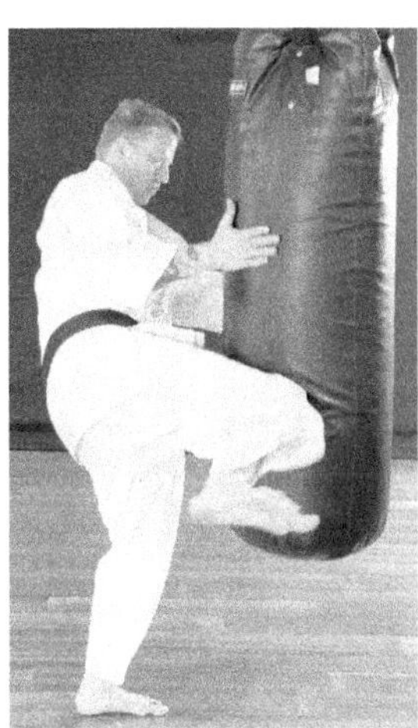

Hiza Uchi

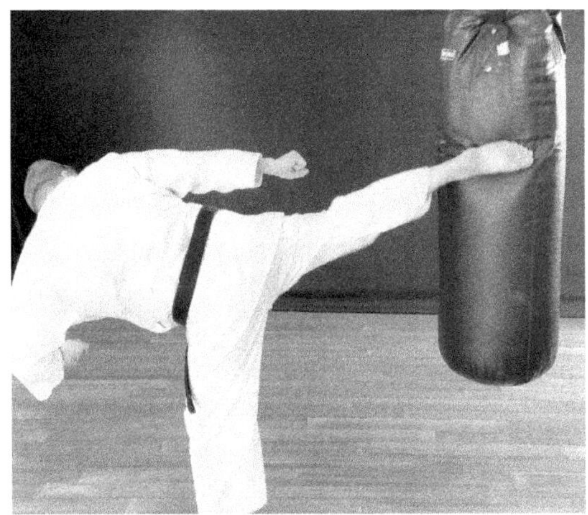

Mawashi Geri with Instep

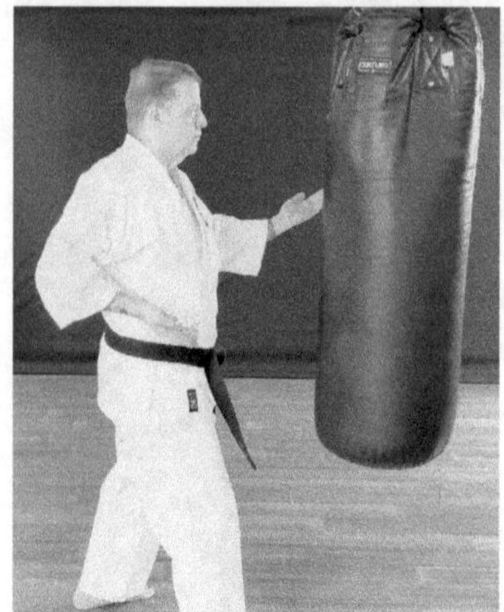
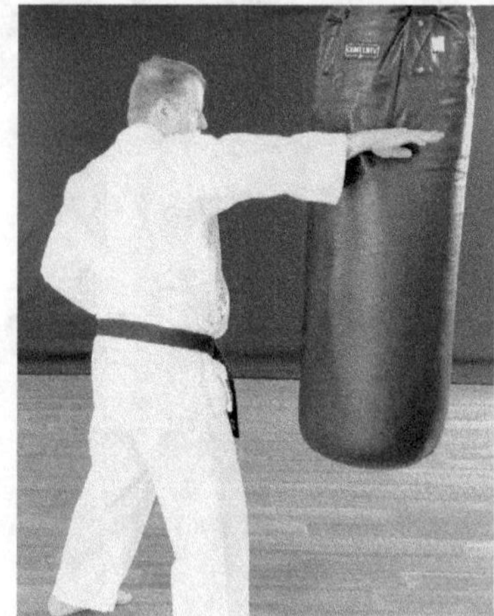

Haito Uchi

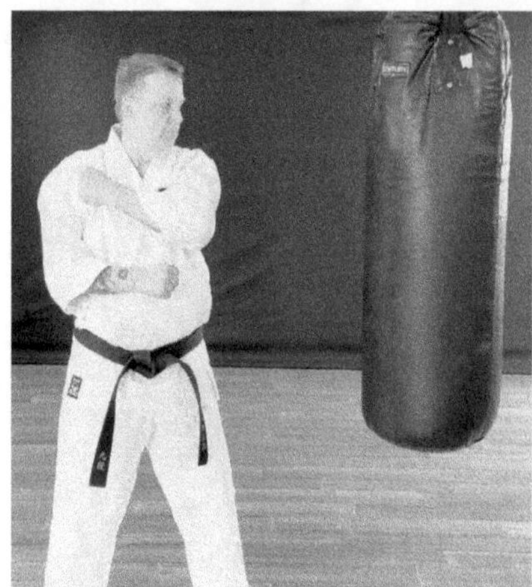
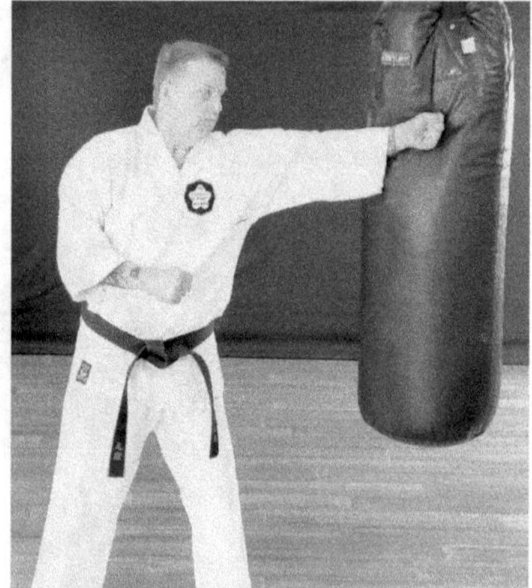

Yoko Uraken Uchi

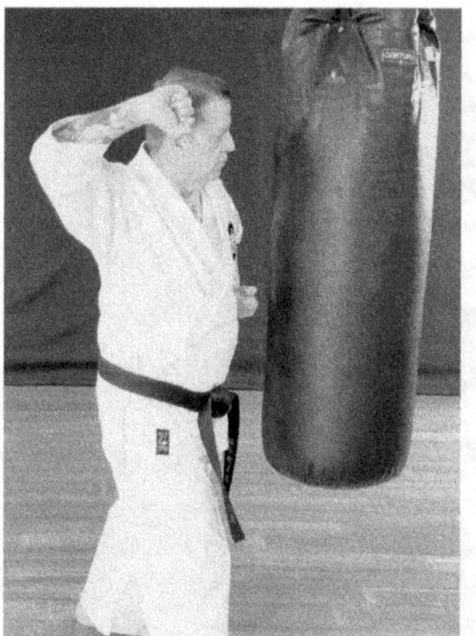
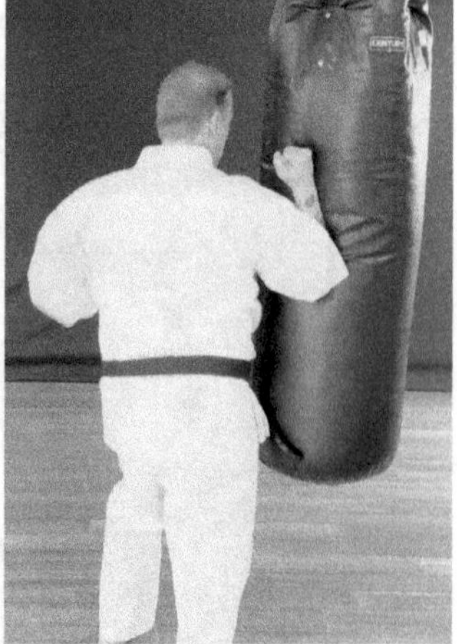

Soto Uke or Kote Uchi

Focus Mitts

Hand mitts are good for practicing sparring footwork (stepping with the front foot and dragging the back foot) along with basic punching combinations, including the jab, cross, uppercut, and hook. The student can also practice bobbing when the holder moves the pad over the puncher's head.

A good exercise is to move straight ahead while practicing combinations such as two jabs and a cross, two jabs and a hook, or two jabs and an uppercut. These drills should be practiced with both the left foot forward and the right foot forward, while also alternating which hand initiates the combination. Even if a student is not naturally ambidextrous, all drills should be practiced on both sides.

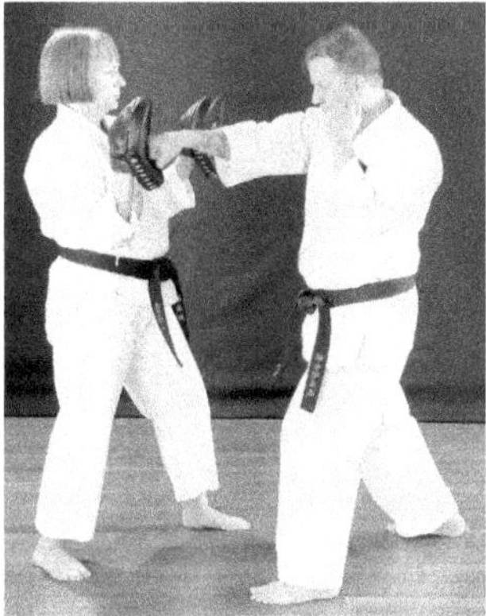

Jab and Cross
(Guard at the Cheek, Use the Hips for Power)

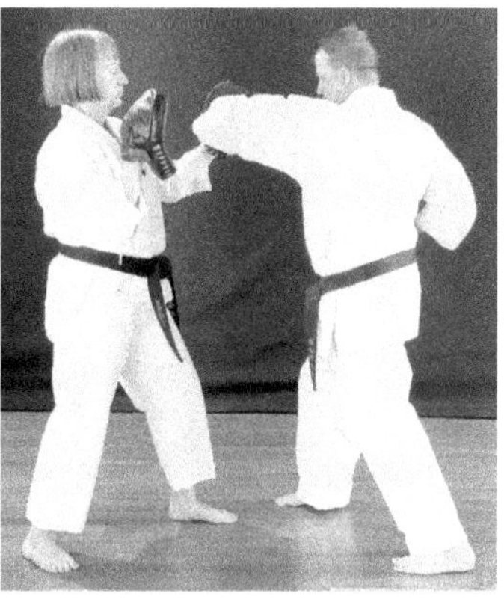

Hook Punch
(Keep Elbow and Forearm Parallel to the Floor)

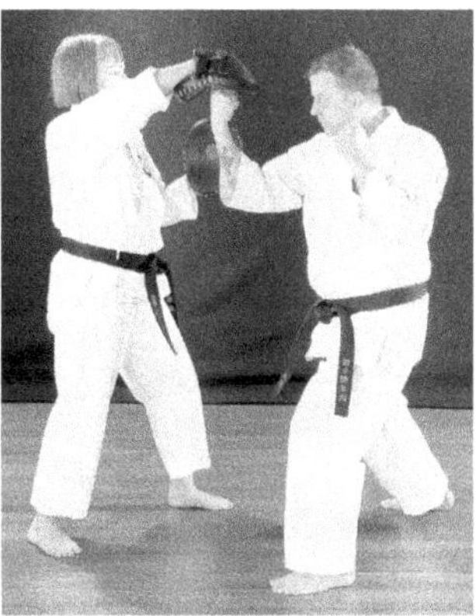

Uppercut
(Drive from the Legs and Punch Straight Up from Elbow)

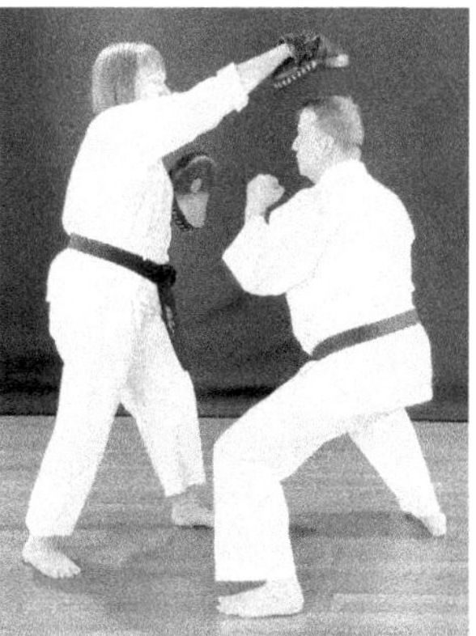

Bob
(Bend at the Knees, Not the Waist)

Forearm Shields

Forearm shields provide a larger target than focus mitts, which are better suited for hand techniques. Forearm shields are especially useful for kicking drills. Much like with hand mitts, one option is to practice moving straight ahead while attacking the person holding the shields. This teaches the student to continuously move forward while sparring.

In this drill, the person holding a shield on each forearm walks backward while the kicker advances, allowing the kicker to focus entirely on striking the target. Holding the pads at varying heights allows the kicker to practice without relying on a consistent pattern.

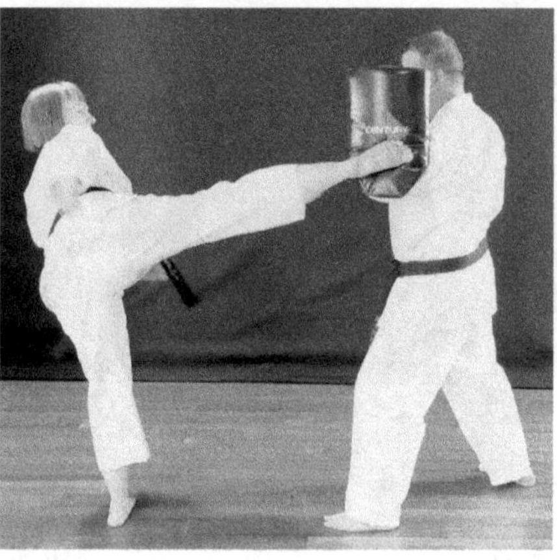

Body Shield

The body shield is the largest of the three types of focus pads and is generally used for practicing power kicks. Two options are to hold the pad either flat or sideways. When held flat (facing downward), students can practice front snap kicks or knee strikes. When held sideways, students can practice side kicks or back heel kicks.

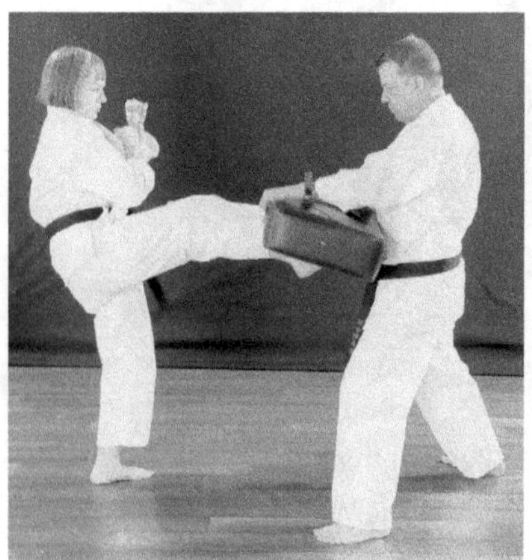

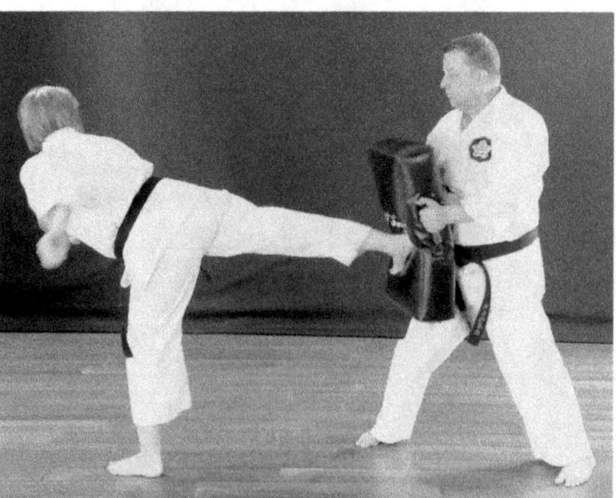

Medicine Ball

The medicine ball is a weighted ball that can be dropped or thrown into the receiver's stomach area to help condition the abdominal muscles. One good drill is to have the receiving partner lie on the floor with his legs extended and held six inches off the ground. Meanwhile, the other partner holds a medicine ball above the receiver's stomach and drops it. As the ball drops, the receiver tightens his abdominal muscles while exhaling, then throws the ball back to the partner holding it.

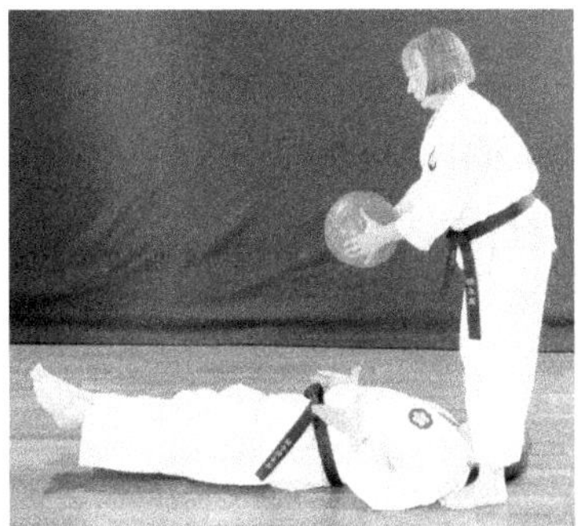

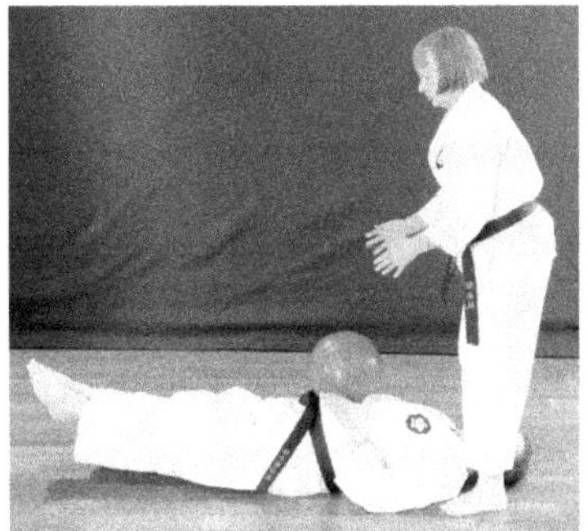

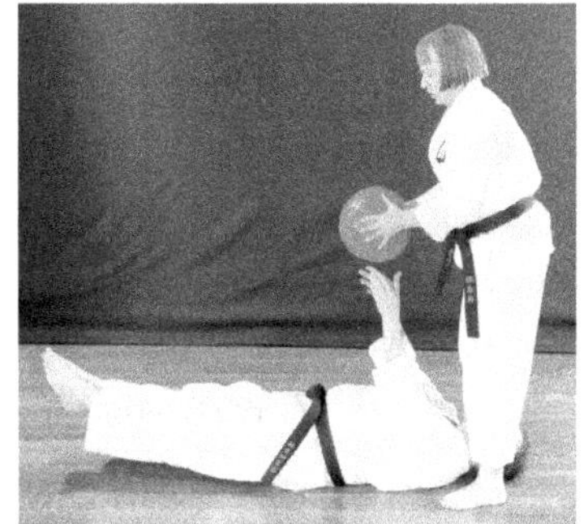

Speed Bag

The speed bag helps the student keep their hands up and develop hand-eye coordination. The typical routine is to hit the bag with the front of the fist, then roll the hand to the side. Other variations include using rolling backfist strikes, but virtually any combination of strikes can be used, including chops, ridgehand strikes, spearhand strikes, and more. The key is to develop a rhythm, keep both hands up, move while striking, and use both hands interchangeably.

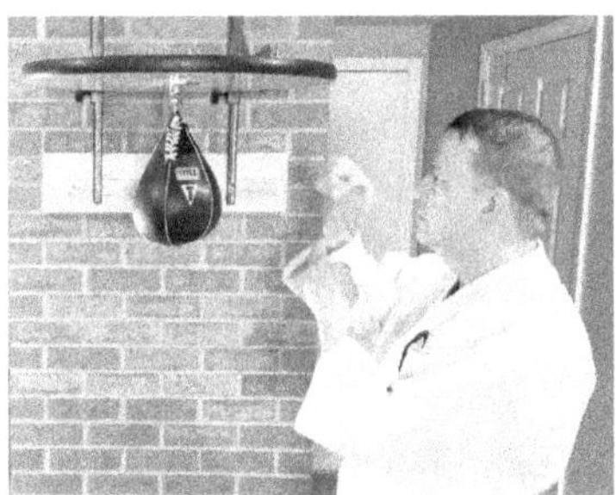

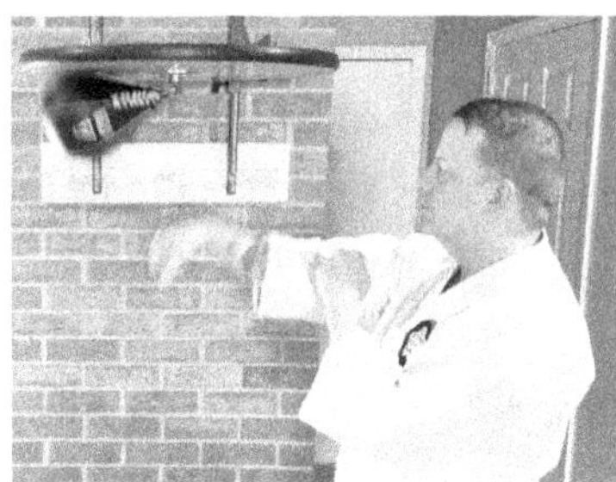

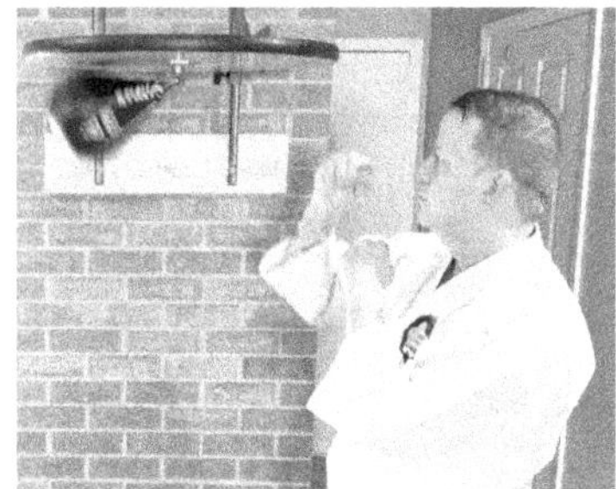

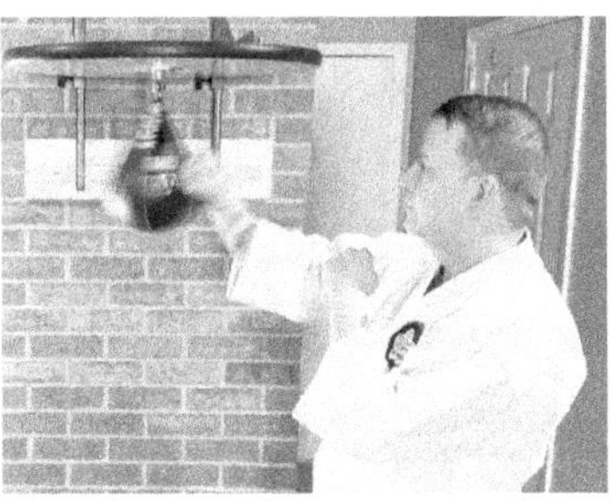

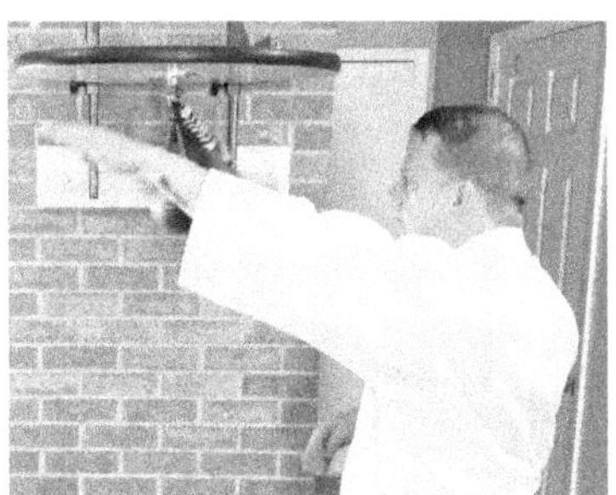

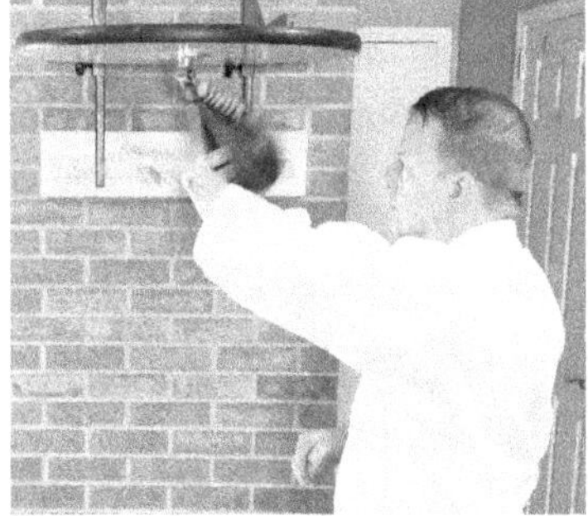

18. Stretching

Why we stretch

Practically every martial arts school utilizes stretching and places importance on it to some degree. Over time, stretching practices have changed significantly. When Shodai was in Okinawa, workouts in Seikichi Toguchi's dojo lasted four to five hours each night, and stretching comprised a significant portion of the first hour. The stretching routine was called Daruma Taiso. It is rooted in yoga and is primarily dynamic in nature. However, due to time constraints, Shodai modified Daruma Taiso so it could be performed in a reasonable amount of time for classes in America. Over time, he realized it still took too long for new students to perform effectively, so he made it an advanced stretching routine. With the help of one of his students, who was a doctor, he created a basic stretching routine. The basic routine is a combination of static and passive stretching.

Stretching can help improve flexibility, which helps maintain the joints' range of motion. Without it, muscles shorten and become tight. When we then call on those muscles for activity, they are unable to fully extend. This increases the risk of joint pain, strains, and muscle damage. We should stretch the muscles and joints that we routinely use in karate. Stretch in a smooth, controlled motion without bouncing. Breathe normally and hold each stretch for about 30 seconds. You should feel tension during stretching, not pain.

We use a dynamic warm-up, which involves performing karate movements or similar techniques at a low intensity. However, stretching does not eliminate the risk of injury, particularly overuse injuries. Stretching helps joints move through their full range of motion, allowing them to move more freely and helping muscles function more effectively. Warmed-up muscles stretch more easily and with a lower risk of injury. When a muscle is stretched, its tissue is extended to its full length. If that tension is held long enough, the muscle may remain slightly longer after relaxation.

Regular flexibility training causes connective tissues to stretch, which in turn allows them to loosen and elongate. When a muscle's connective tissue is weak, it is more likely to be damaged by overstretching or sudden, powerful muscular contractions. The likelihood of such injury can be reduced by strengthening the muscles supported by the connective tissue. Once a muscle has reached its absolute maximum length, attempting to stretch it further primarily stresses the ligaments and tendons and can place undue strain on them.

Static Stretch After a Workout

It is best to stretch after a workout when the muscles are warm. Static stretching of fatigued muscles helps increase flexibility, enhance muscular development, and reduce post-workout soreness. When muscles are fatigued, they retain a degree of swelling and become somewhat shortened. This results from repeated intense muscular activity that often moves the muscle through only part of its full range of motion. The "swollen" muscle contains lactic acid and other metabolic by-products. If the muscle is not stretched, it may retain this reduced range of motion, and the buildup of lactic acid can contribute to post-workout soreness. Static stretching helps return the muscle to its full range of motion. It also assists in clearing lactic acid and other waste products from the muscle.

Anatomy

Joints link bones together. Muscles surround joints and provide the force used to move them. The amount of tension in the muscles surrounding a joint is a key factor in determining its range of motion. Tendons are flexible cords of connective tissue that attach muscles to bones and make movement possible. When a joint moves, force generated by the muscle is transferred through the tendons, which then move the bones. Ligaments connect bone to bone, or bone to cartilage, at a joint. During stretching, we primarily work muscles and tendons rather than ligaments. Ligaments should not be stretched and are not designed to be elastic. A taut ligament provides the stability and support necessary for safe joint movement.

On a more microscopic level, muscle is composed of fascicles, which are composed of fasciculi (bundles of muscle fibers), which are composed of myofibrils capable of contracting, relaxing, and lengthening. Myofibrils are made up of sarcomeres. As a sarcomere contracts, the overlap between thick and thin myofilaments increases. As it stretches, this overlap decreases, allowing the muscle fiber to elongate. When all sarcomeres are fully extended, further stretching places force on the surrounding connective tissue. During stretching, the muscle fiber is lengthened sarcomere by sarcomere until the connective tissue begins to absorb additional tension. The overall length of a muscle depends on the number and length of its fibers; the more fibers that are stretched, the greater the total length achieved.

When a muscle is stretched, the muscle spindle is also stretched. The muscle spindle detects changes in muscle length and sends signals to the spinal cord, triggering the myotatic (stretch) reflex, which attempts to resist the change in length by causing the muscle to contract. The more sudden the change in muscle length, the stronger the resulting contraction. This mechanism helps maintain muscle tone and protect the body from injury. When a stretch is held, the muscle spindle gradually adapts to the new length and reduces its signaling, allowing the muscle to lengthen further over time.

The myotatic reflex has both dynamic and static components. The static component persists as long as the muscle is being stretched, while the dynamic component occurs briefly in response to the initial rapid change in muscle length. There are two types of intrafusal muscle fibers: nuclear chain fibers, which are responsible for the static component, and nuclear bag fibers, which are responsible for the dynamic component. Nuclear chain fibers lengthen steadily during a sustained stretch, while nuclear bag fibers respond to rapid changes in length, bulging at their center where the sensory nerve endings are located.

When muscles contract, they generate tension at the point where the muscle connects to the tendon, where the Golgi tendon organ is located. The Golgi tendon organ detects changes in tension and sends signals to the spinal cord. When this tension exceeds a certain threshold, it triggers the lengthening reaction, which inhibits further muscle contraction. This mechanism helps protect muscles, tendons, and ligaments from injury.

Types of Stretching

- Dynamic stretching consists of controlled movements that take the body through its full range of motion. In dynamic stretching, there are no bouncing movements.
  - Ballistic stretching involves attempting to force a part of the body beyond its normal range of motion using bouncing or rapid movements.

- Static stretching consists of stretching a muscle (or group of muscles) to its farthest point and then maintaining or holding that position.
  - Passive stretching involves a relaxed position in which an external force (either a person or an object) moves the joint through its full range of motion.
  - Isometric stretching is a type of static stretching that involves resisting a stretch through isometric muscle contractions (tensing the stretched muscles without movement).

Breathing

Proper breathing is important for an effective stretch. It helps relax the body, increases blood flow, and assists in the removal of lactic acid and other exercise by-products. Take slow, relaxed breaths while stretching, exhaling during the stretch. The proper breathing method is to inhale through the nose, expanding the abdomen rather than the chest, and exhale slowly through the mouth.

During inhalation, the diaphragm moves downward, increasing pressure on the abdominal cavity and influencing blood flow in the internal organs and associated vessels. During exhalation, pressure is reduced, allowing blood to circulate more freely through the abdomen and surrounding tissues. This rhythmic change in abdominal pressure contributes to overall circulation.

Increased blood flow to stretched muscles improves elasticity and supports more efficient removal of metabolic by-products such as lactic acid.

Daruma Taiso Stretching Routine

Daruma is the Japanese name for Bodhidharma, the Buddhist monk associated with Zen Buddhism and highly influential in the martial arts world. There are multiple written and online sources regarding Bodhidharma. The stretching routine, called Daruma Taiso, was created by Seikichi Toguchi, and all branches of his lineage include some variation of it. Shodai's version is presented here.

Most of the exercises resemble karate movements performed as stretches. Some of the movements also develop balance in addition to flexibility, similar in this respect to yoga. For example, the push-up variation incorporates movements similar to transitioning between downward-facing dog and upward-facing dog.

1. Toes & Ankles (Inside, Outside, Point & Flex, Rotate)
2. Knee Bends (Regular, Rotate, Alternate Right & Left)
3. Palm Heel Strikes (Overhead, Chest, Down, Behind)
4. Side to Sides
5. Shiko Dachi - Shoulder Stretch to Knee
6. Swoops (Right, Center, Left Center)
7. Shiko Dachi - Rise & Fall Breathing
8. Hip Throws (Alternate Right & Left)
9. Side Stretches (Regular & 45° Angle to Rear)
10. Touch Floor (3 Front, 3 Back - Feet Apart & Together)
11. Chop Strike (Single, Double, 4 Count)
12. Knuckle Wrap (Single & Double)
13. Arm Rotation (Forward & Reverse, Both Arms)
14. Neck Rotation (L & R, Up & Down, Side to Side)
15. Push Up (Push Up, Down, Legs, Back, Front, Up)
16. Frog x3 & Through - Touch 3, Slap & Back 3
17. Body Stretch
18. Leg Stretch

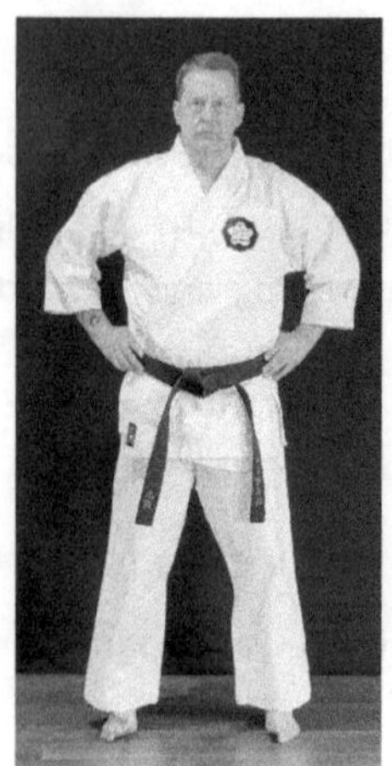
1a. Big Toes Up

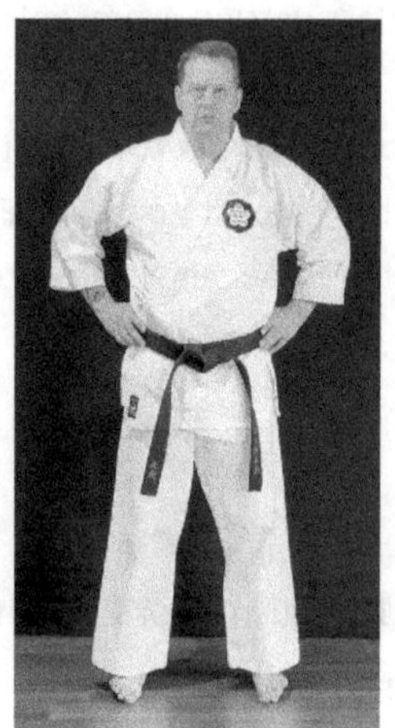
1b. Outside Up
(Repeat 1a-b, 5 to 10x)

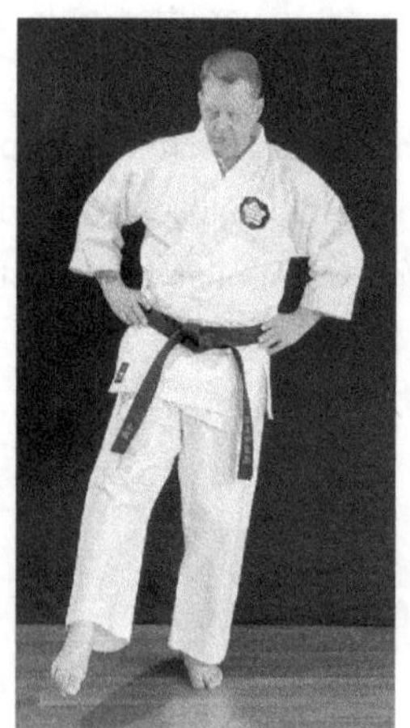
1c. Point Foot

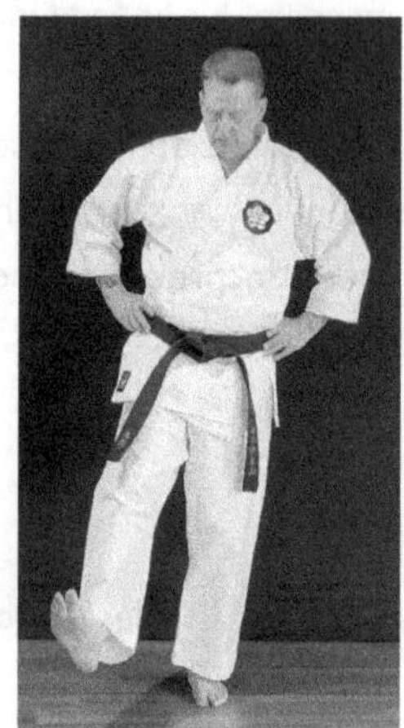
1d. Flex Back
(Repeat 1c-d, 5 to 10x)

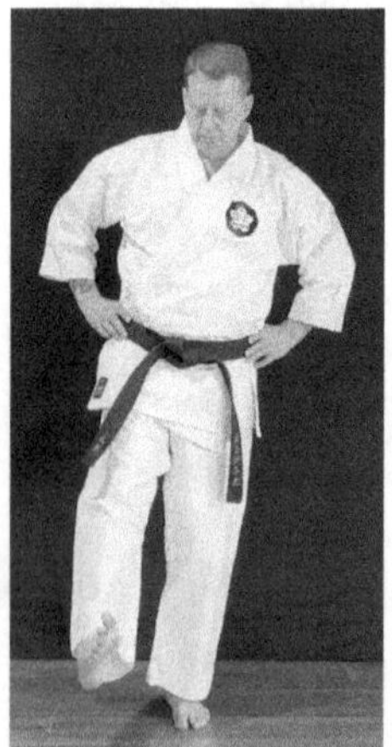

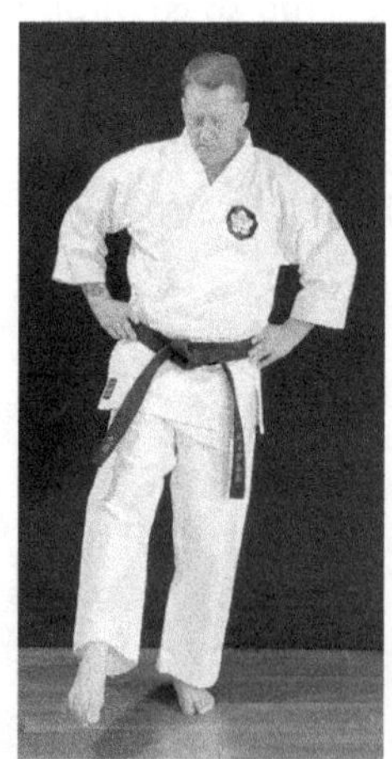
1e. Rotate Foot - Counter Clockwise

1e. Cont.
(Repeat 5 to 10x)

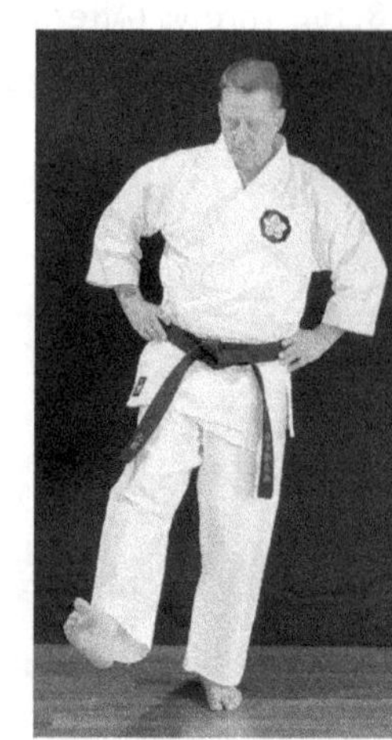
1f. Clockwise
(Repeat 5 to 10x)
(Repeat 1c-f with Other Foot)

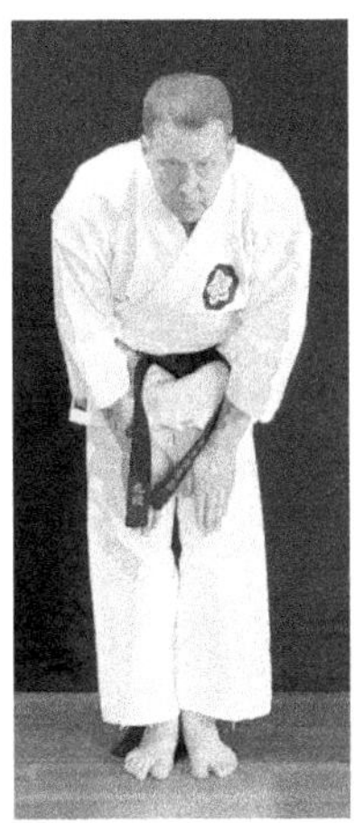
2. Feet Together, Hands on Thighs (Starting Position)

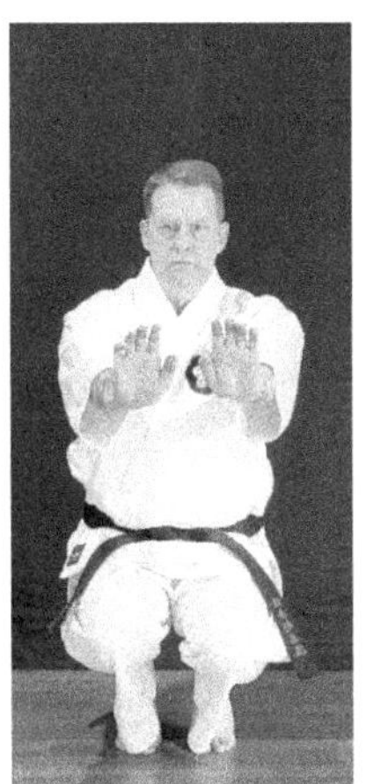
2b. Squat Down on Balls of Feet

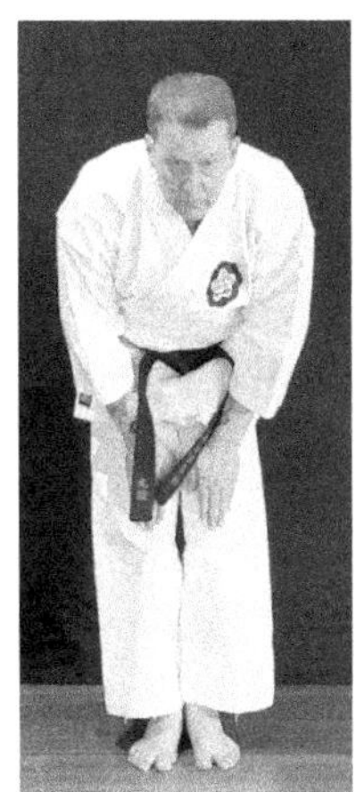
2c. Raise Up (Repeat Step 2b-c, 5 or 10x)

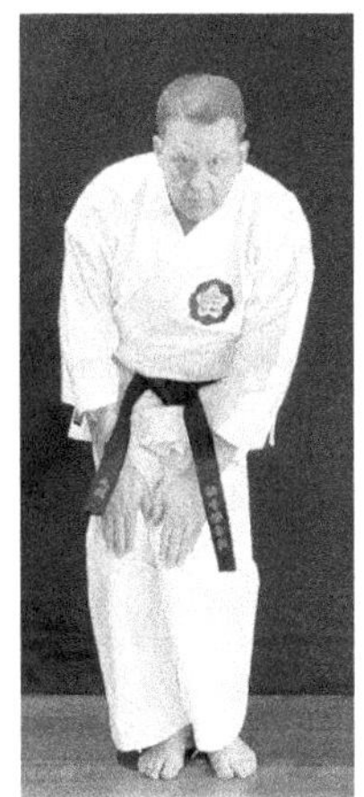
2d. Squat Down with Feet Flat, Rotate Legs Counter Clockwise

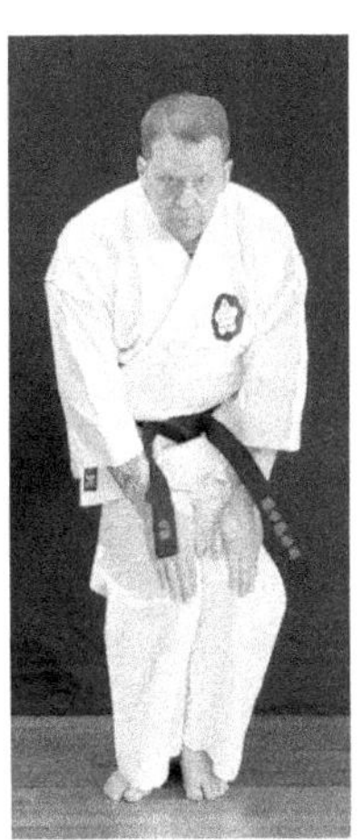
2d. Continue Rotating to Left

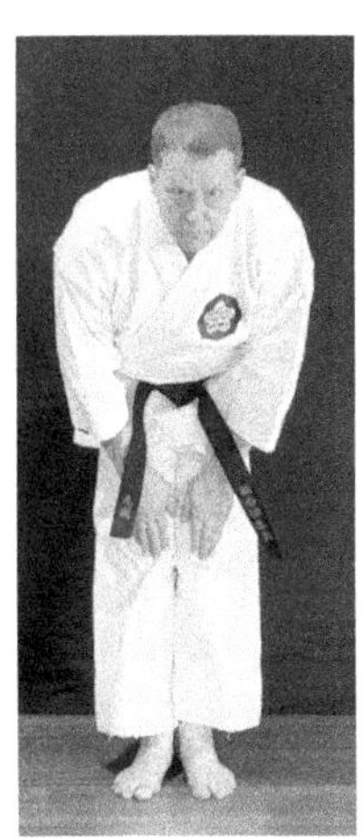
2d. Back to the Middle

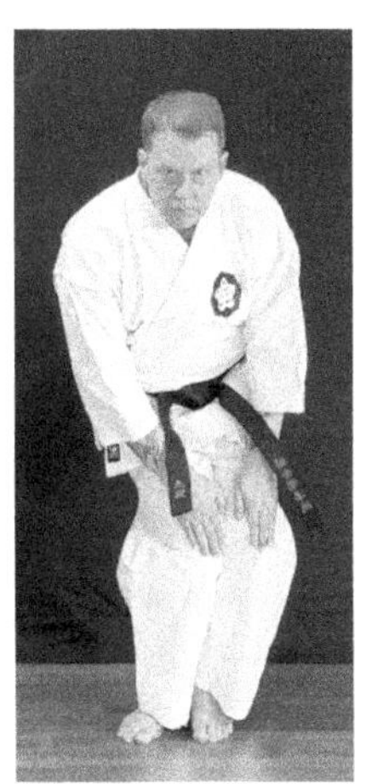
2e. Rotate Clockwise

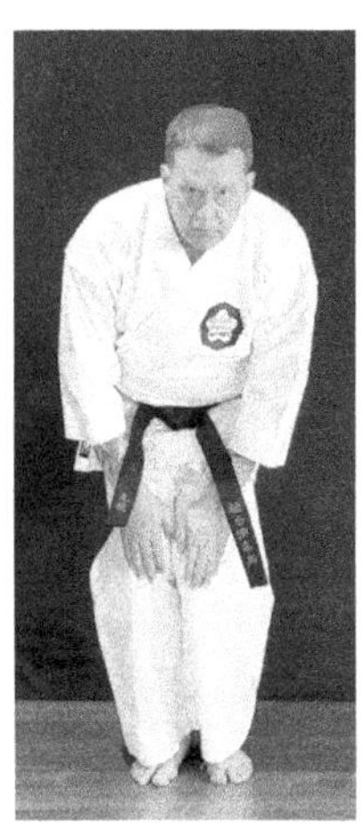
2e. Continue Rotating to Right

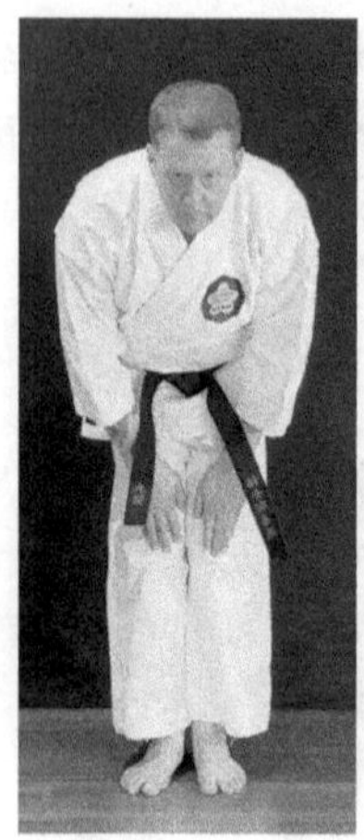

2e. Back to the Middle
(Repeat Step 2d-e,
5 or 10x)

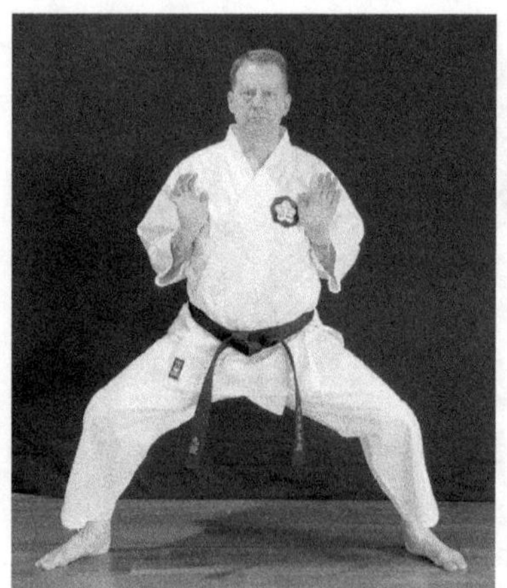

3. Palm Heel Strikes (Overhead, Chest, Down, Behind)
(Starting Position)

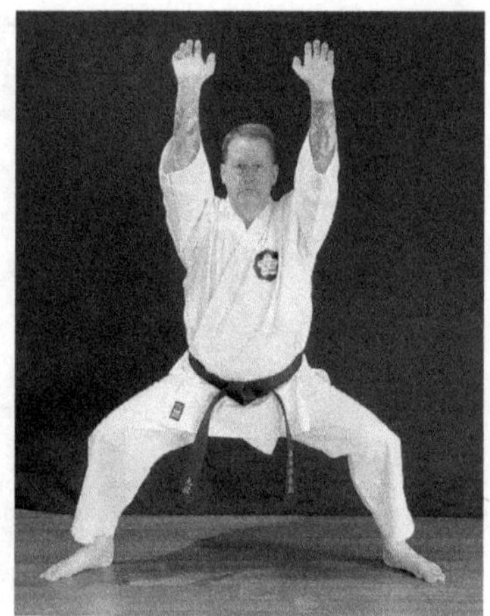

3a. Overhead
Sink Down, Push Arms Straight Up
(Repeat 5 or 10x)

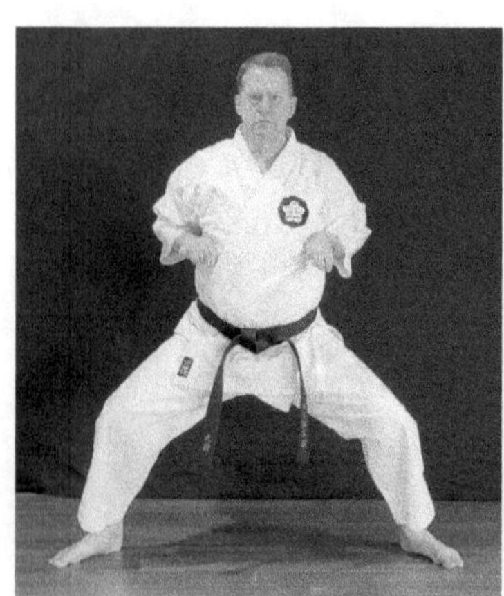

3. Palm Heel Strikes
(Starting Position)

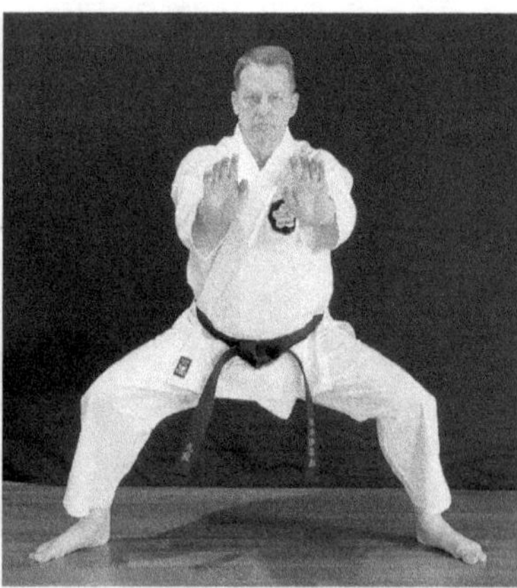

3b. Chest
Push Arms Straight Out
(Repeat 5 or 10x)

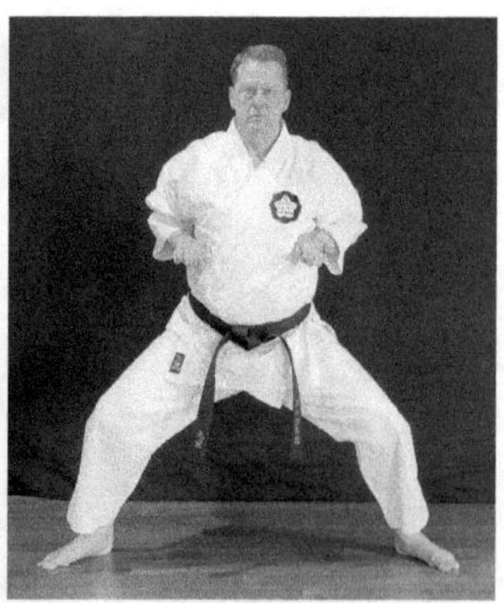

3. Palm Heel Strikes
(Starting Position)

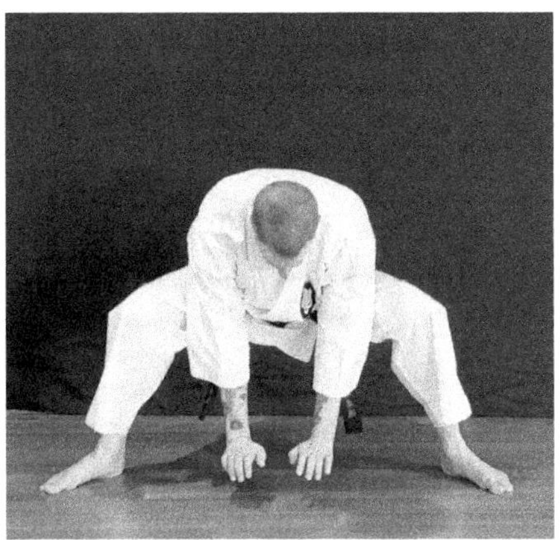

3c. Down
Push Arms Down to ground (Repeat 5 or 10x)

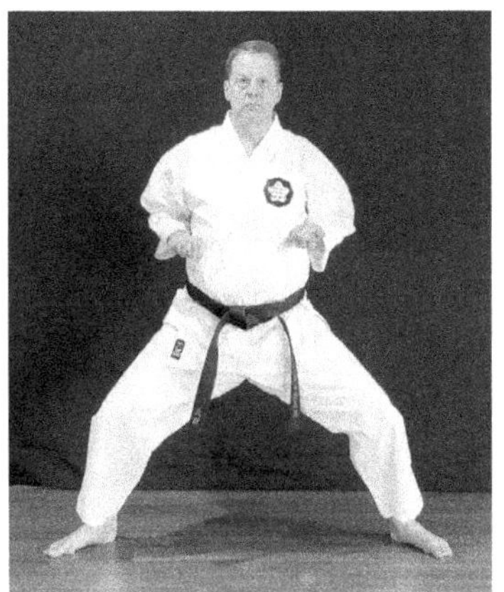

3. Palm Heel Strikes
(Starting Position)

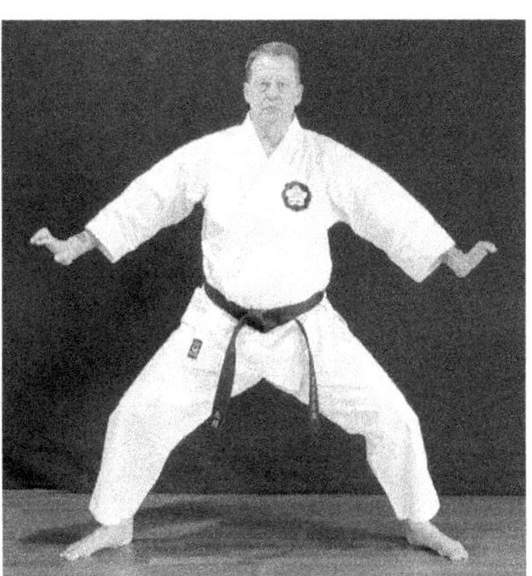

3d. Behind
Keeping Arms Straight, Simulate Palm Heel Strikes to Target Behind
(Repeat 5 or 10x)

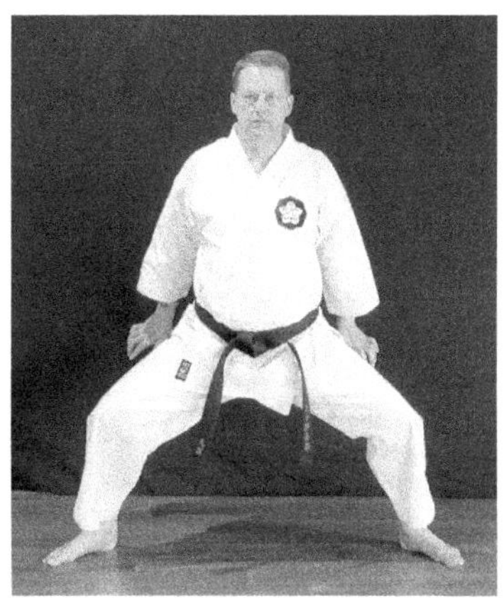

3d. Behind
(cont.)

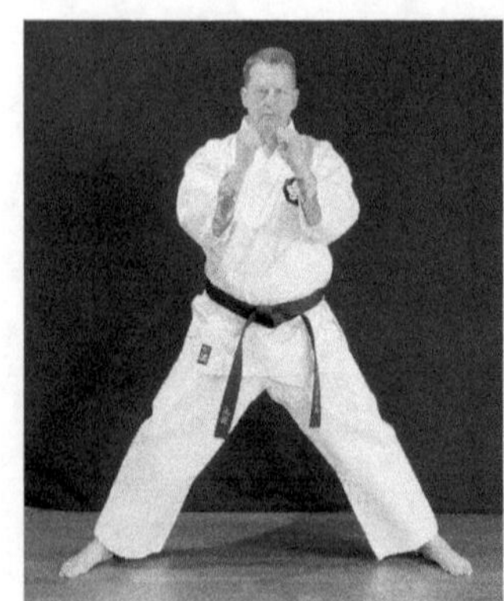

4. Side to Sides (Starting Position)

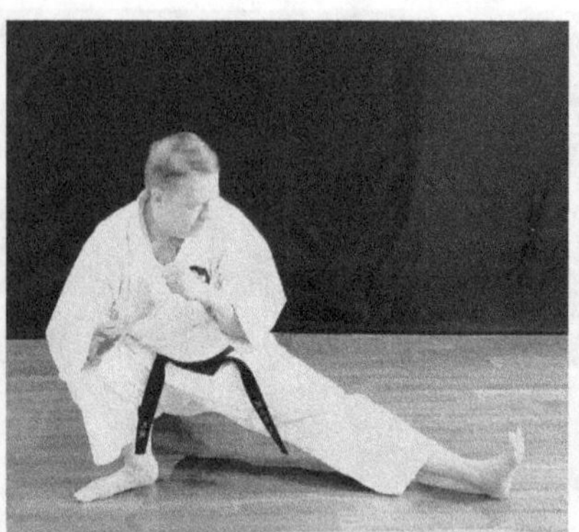

4a. Lower Down Over Right Leg Keeping Left Leg Straight

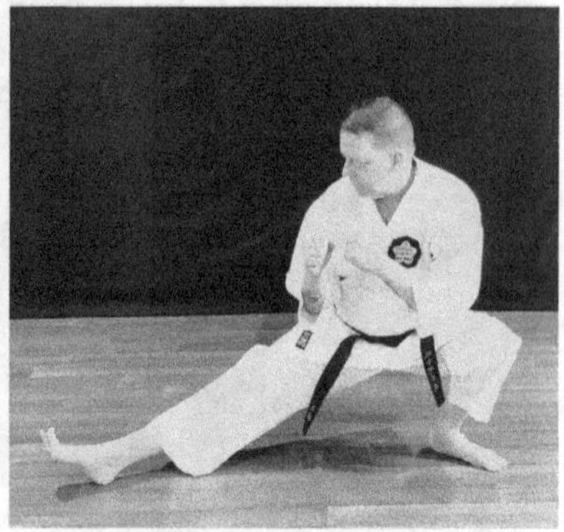

4b. Come Back Up and Lower Down Over Left Leg, Keeping Right Leg Straight

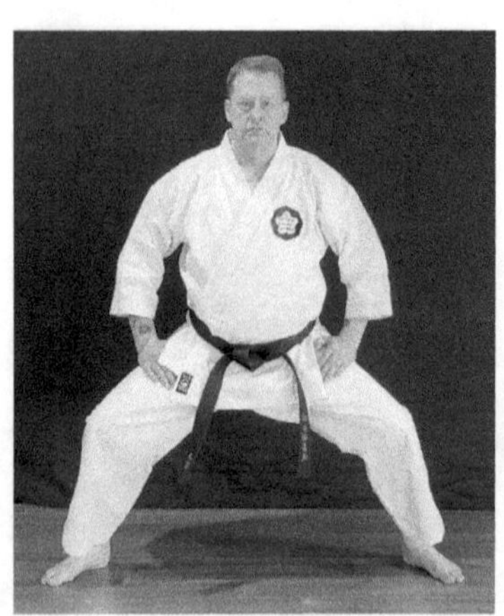

5. Shiko Dachi - Shoulder Stretch to Knee

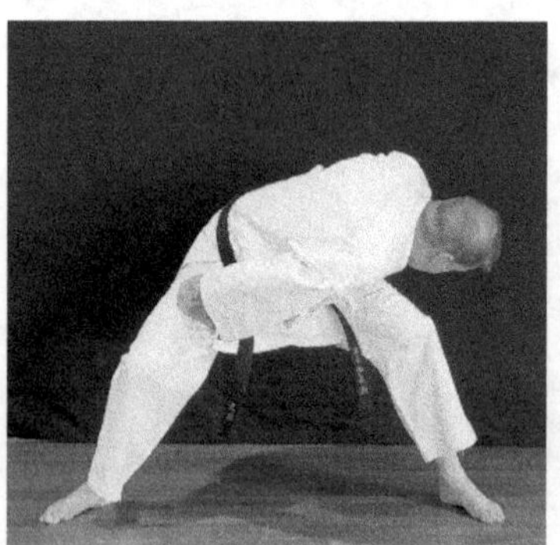

5a. Keeping Hands on Top of Thighs, Lean to Put Right Shoulder on Left Knee (3 count)

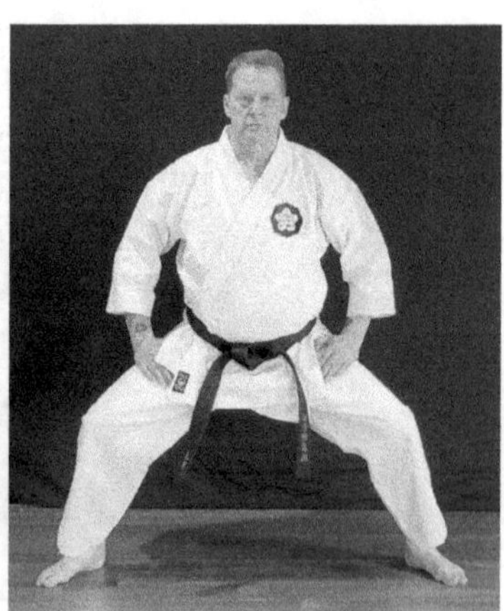

5a. Back Up to Starting Position

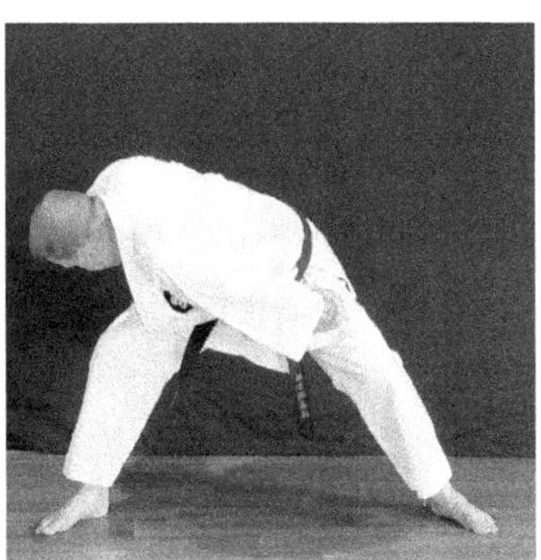

5b. Lean to Put Left Shoulder on Right Knee (3 count)

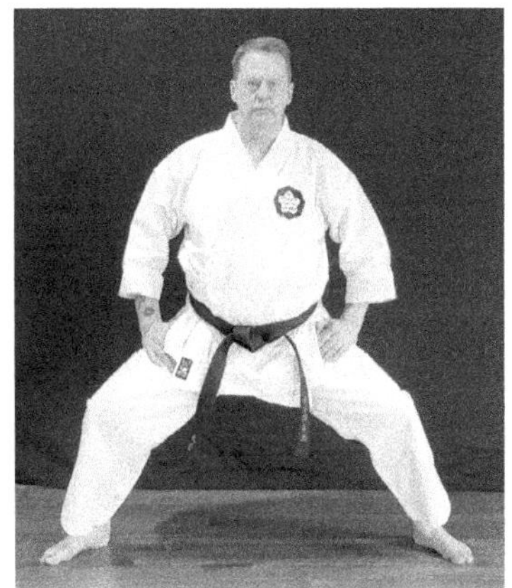

5b. Back Up to Starting Position (Repeat 5a-b, 5 or 10x)

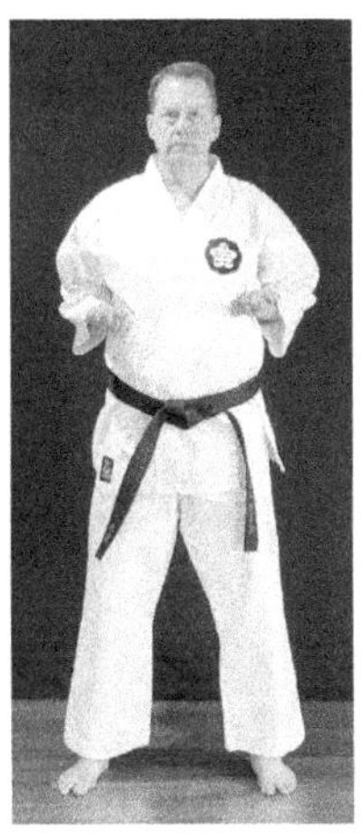

6. Swoops (Right, Center, Left, Center)

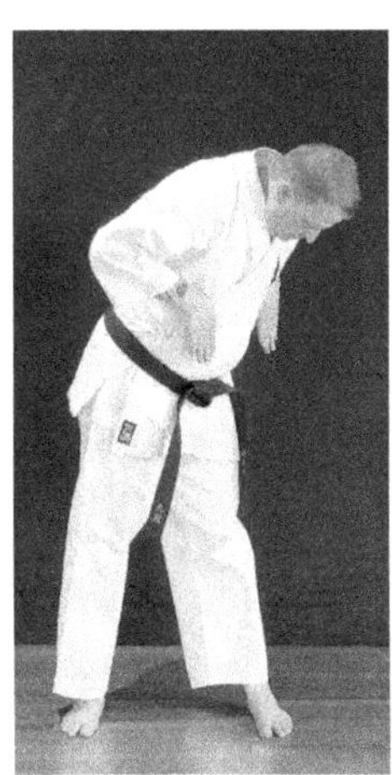

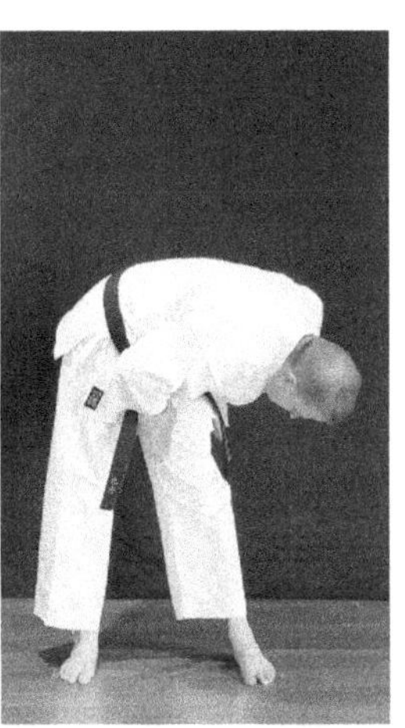

6a. Guide Palms Down, Side By Side, Along Left Leg

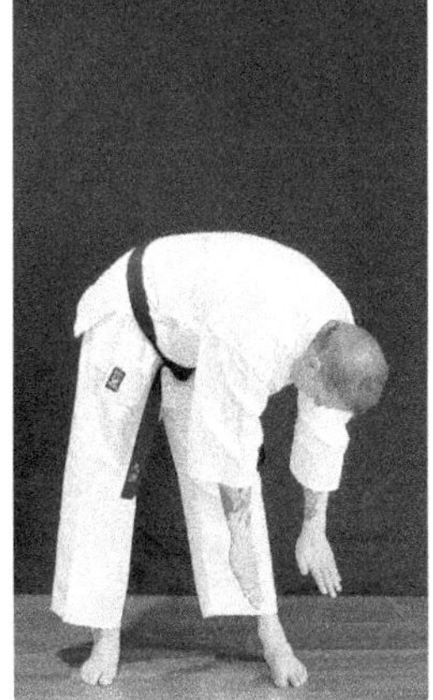

Palms Down Along Left Leg (cont.)

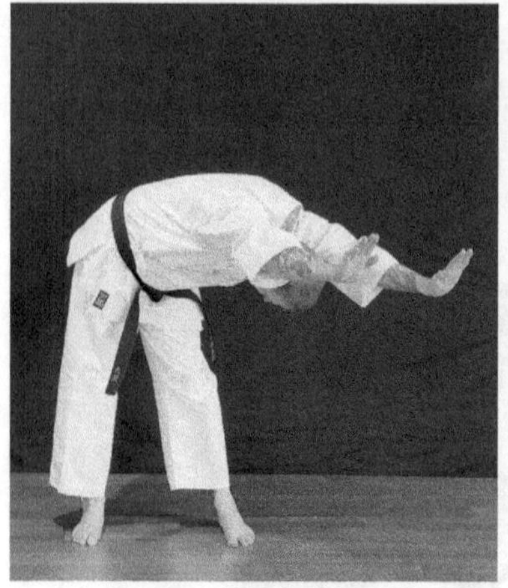

6a. Continue Down, Then Raise Arms Up As Far As Possible, Keeping Body Bent At Waist

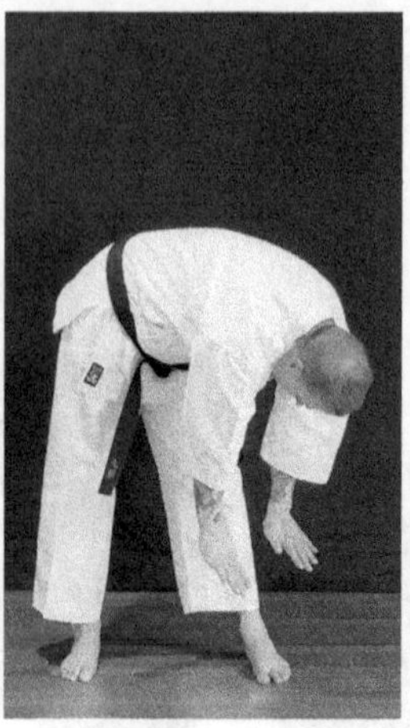

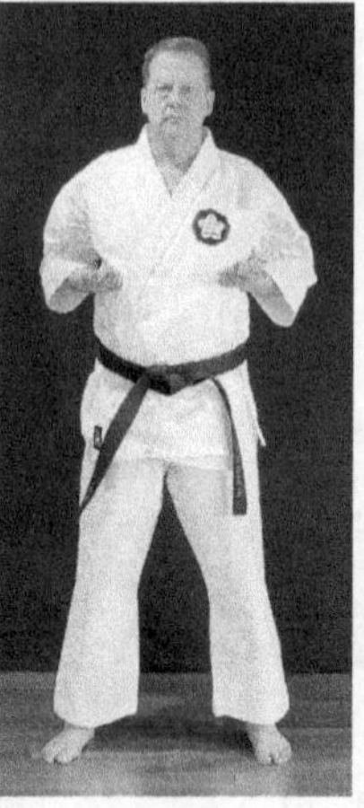

6a. Bring Hands Back Up Along Leg to Starting Position

6b. Repeat 6a in Middle

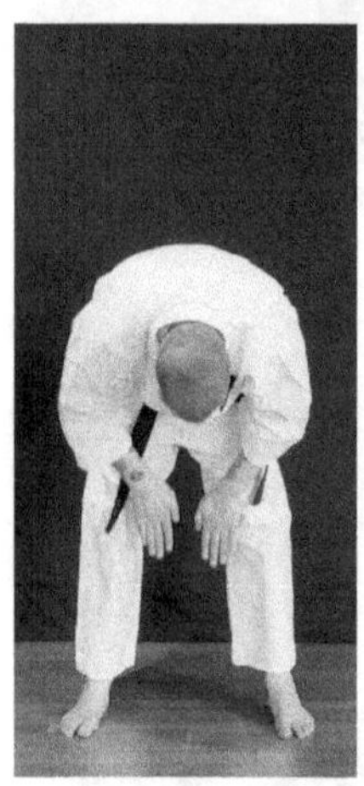

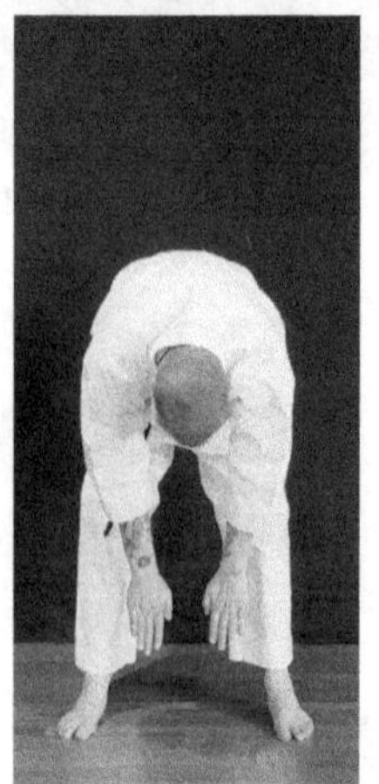

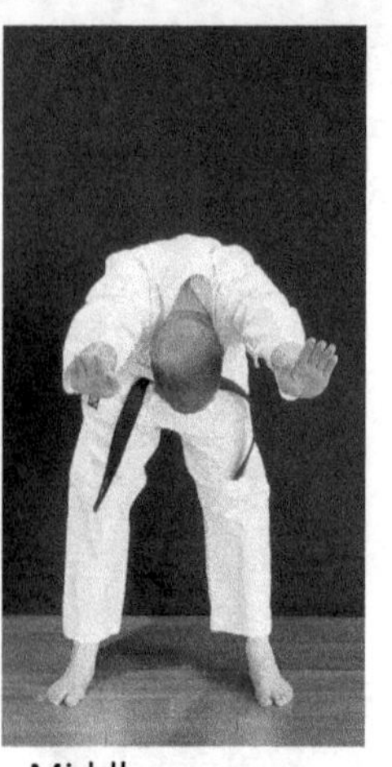

6b. Repeat 6a in Middle

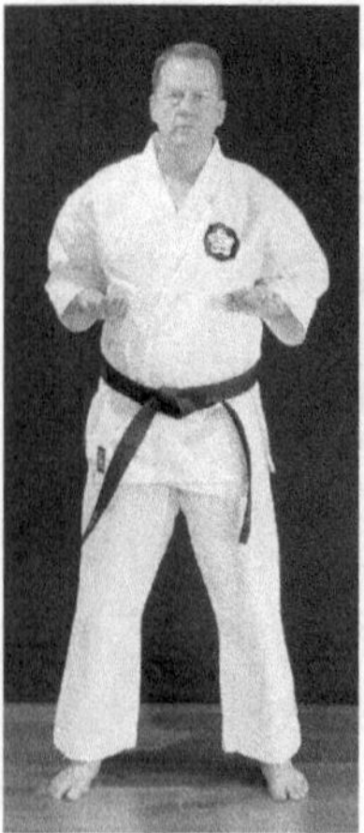

6b. Bring Hands Back Up to Starting Position

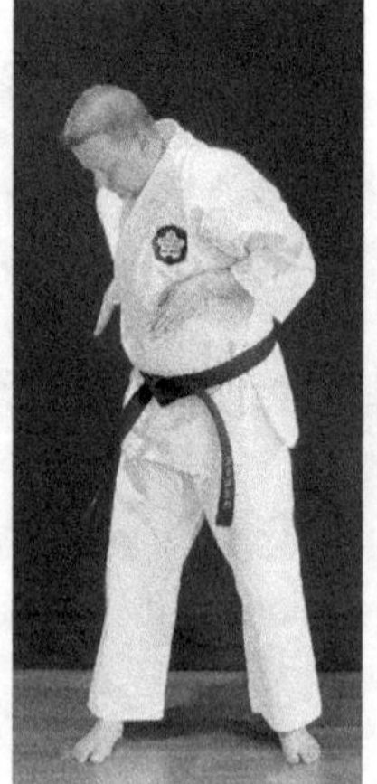

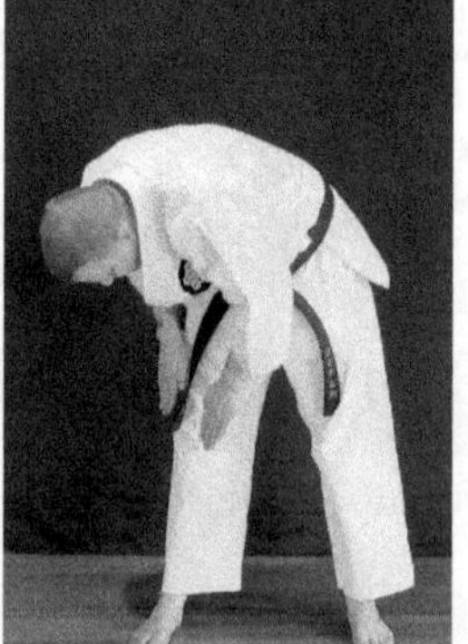

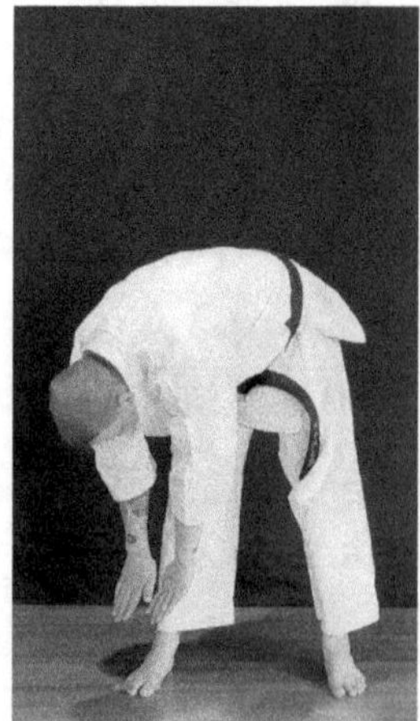

6c. Repeat 6a over Right Leg

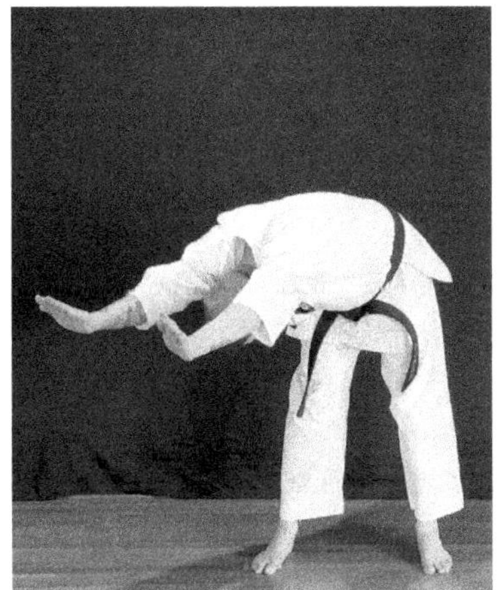
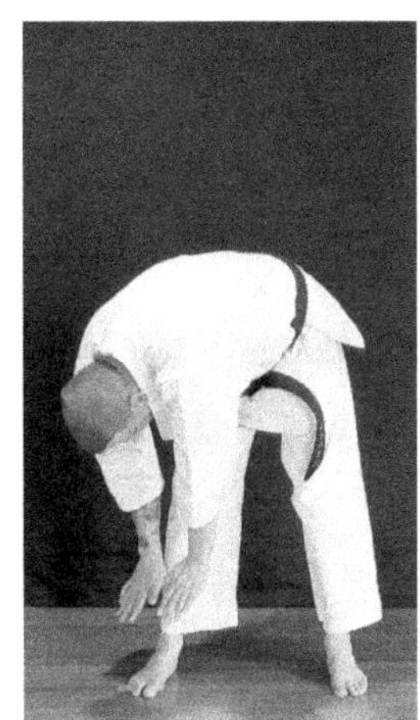

6c. Repeat 6a over Right Leg (cont.)

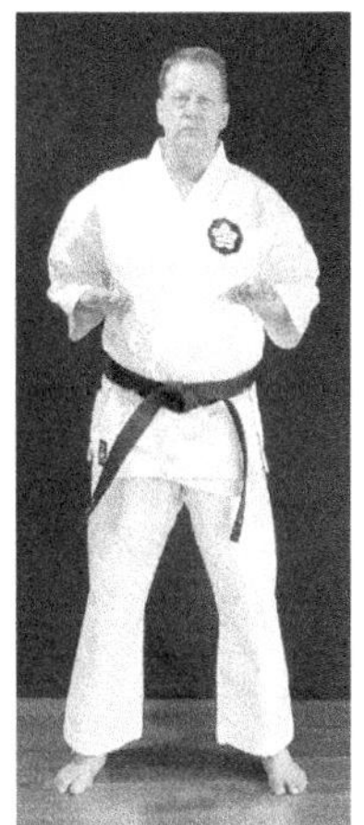

6c. Bring Hands Back Up to Starting Position

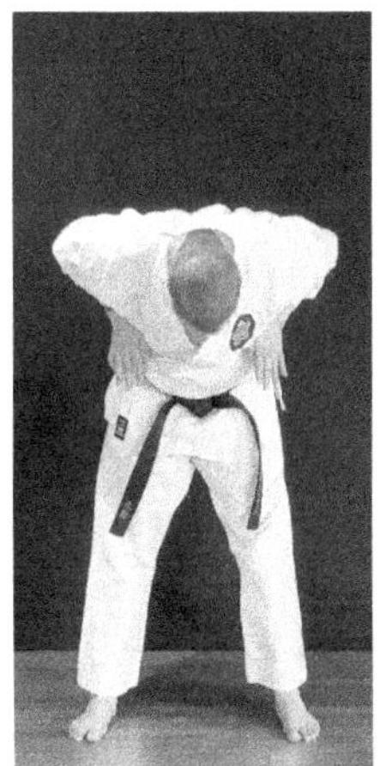
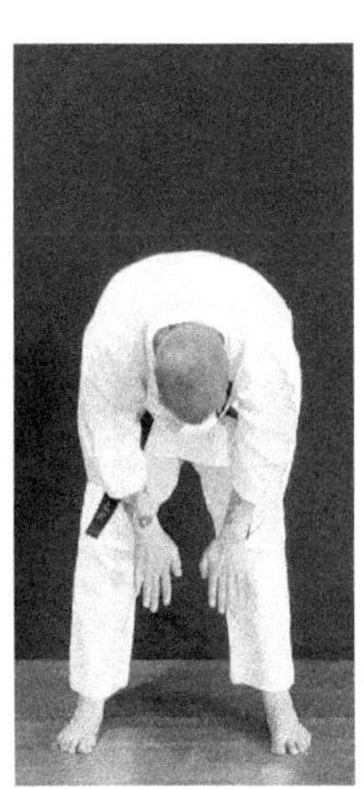
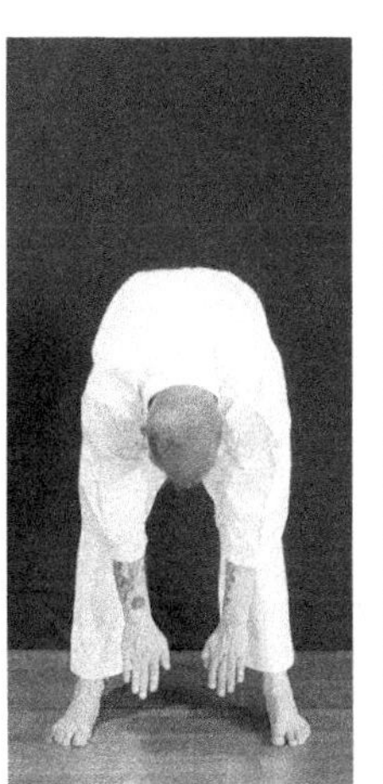
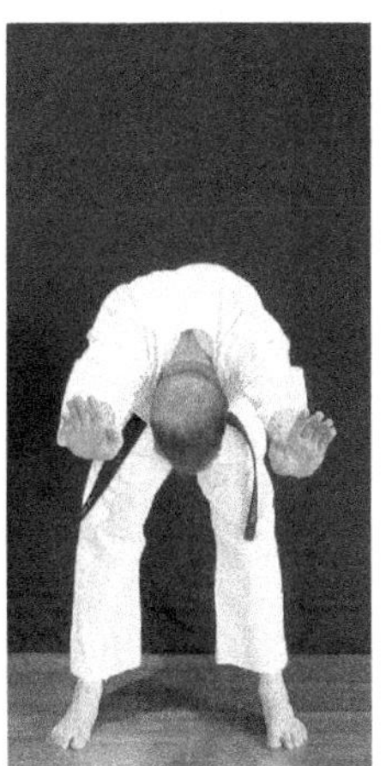
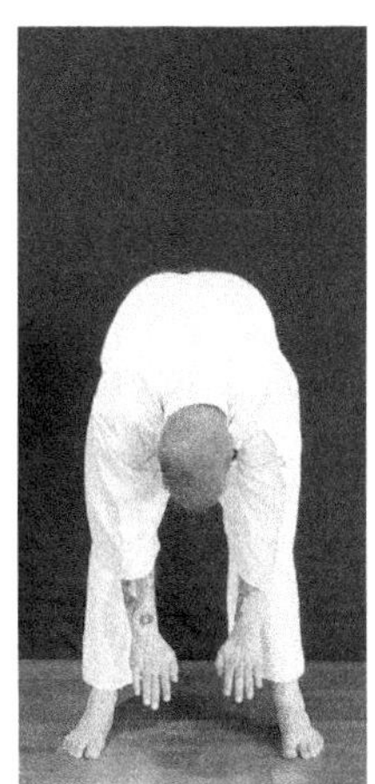

6d. Repeat 6a in Middle

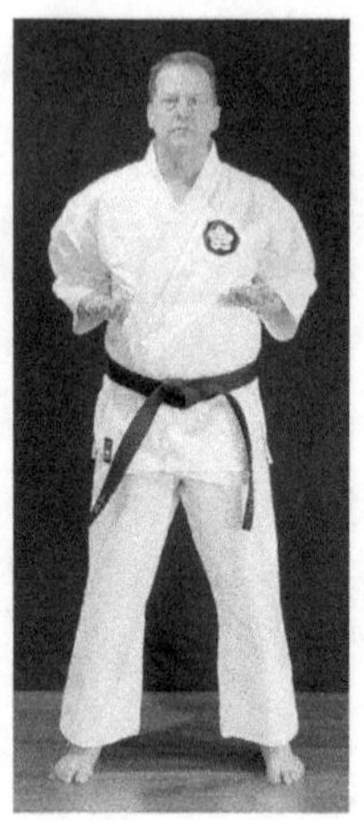

6d. Bring Hands Back Up to Starting Position (Repeat 6a-d, 5 or 10x)

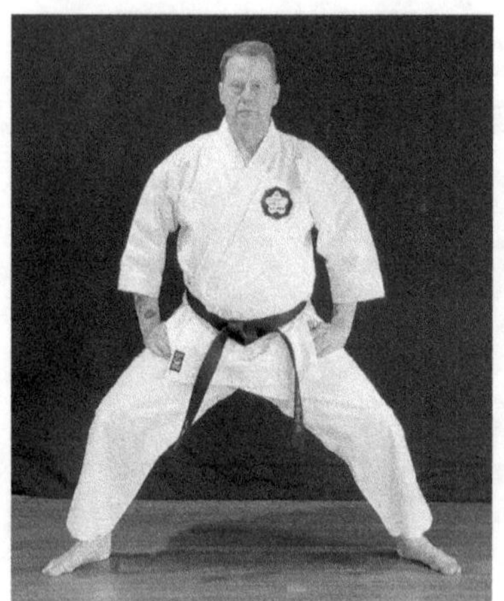

7a. Shiko Dachi - Rise & Fall Breathing
(Starting Position) - Inhale

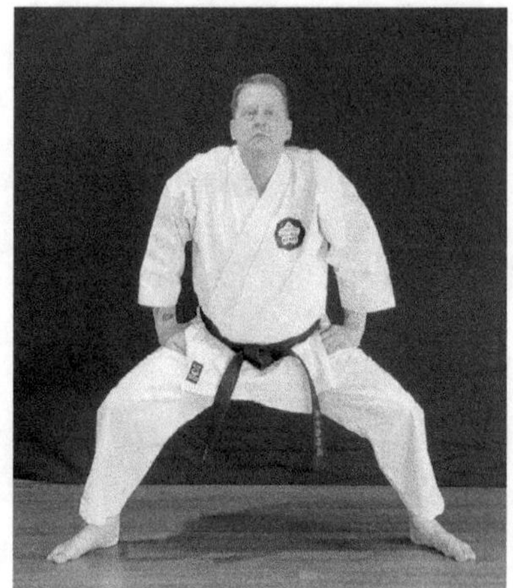

7b. Exhale while Sinking Head Between Shoulders
(Repeat 7a-b, 5 or 10x)

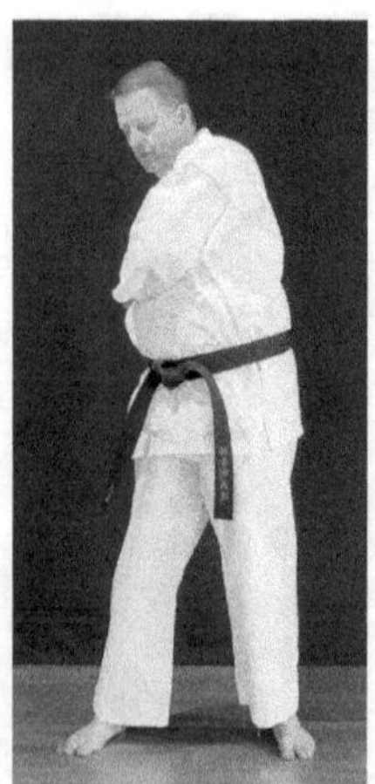

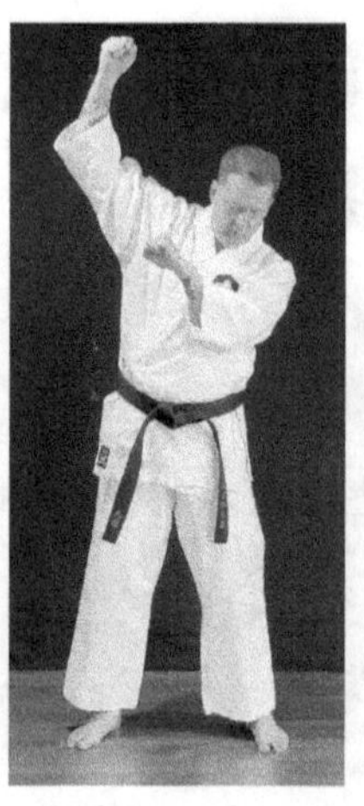

8a. Hip Throws
Reach Behind Right Rear Area, Move Hands to Left Front Area

8a. Left Front Area (3 count)

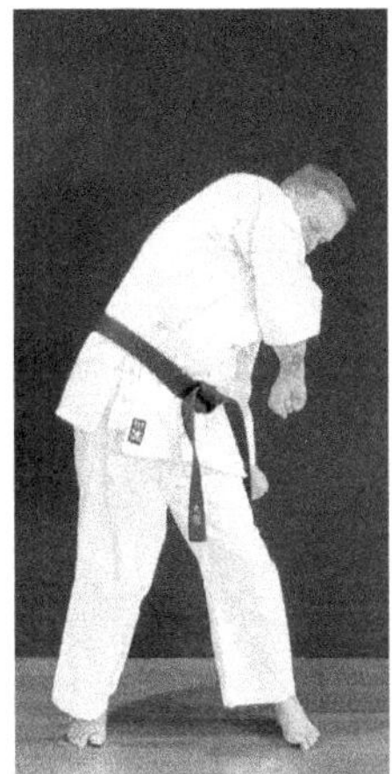

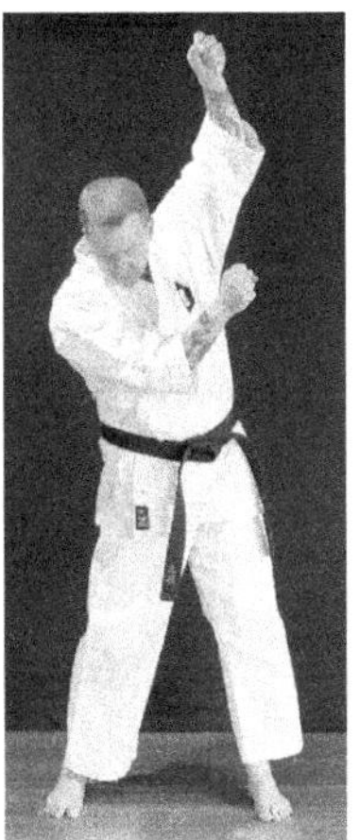

8b. Hip Throws
Reach Behind Left Rear Area, Move Hands to Right Front Area

8b. Right Front Area (3 count)
(Repeat 8a-b, 5 or 10x)

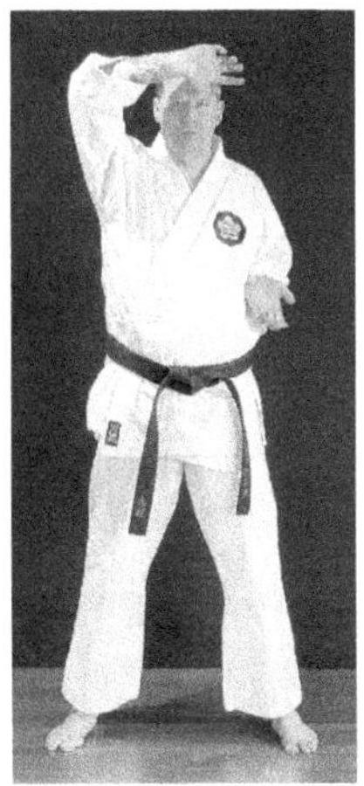

9a. Side Stretches (Regular) (Starting Position - One Hand on Forehead, One Hand at Side)

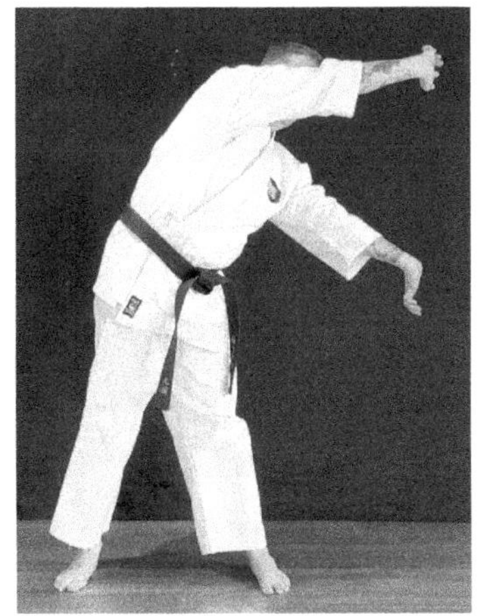

9a. Regular - Left
Push Both Hands Straight Out to Left Side (3 count)

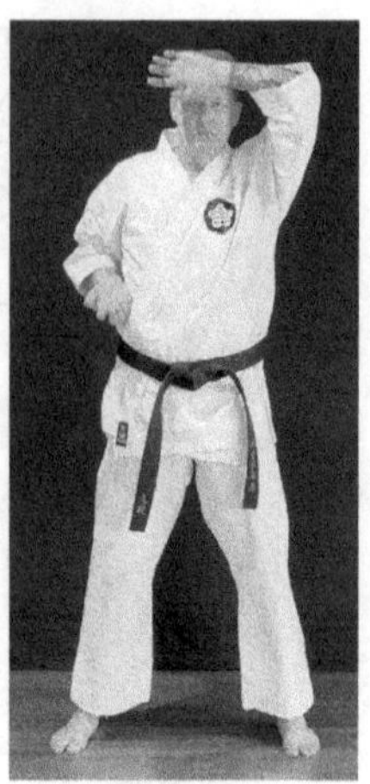

9b. Back to Starting Position With Hands in Opposite Positions

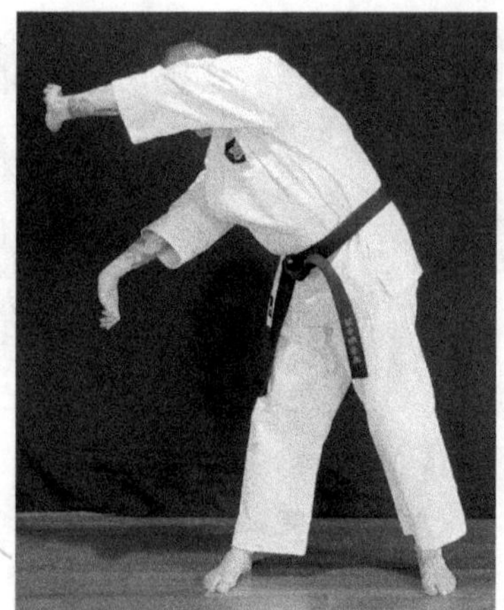

9b. Regular - Right
Push Both Hands Straight Out to Right Side (3 count)
(Repeat 9a-b, 5 or 10x)

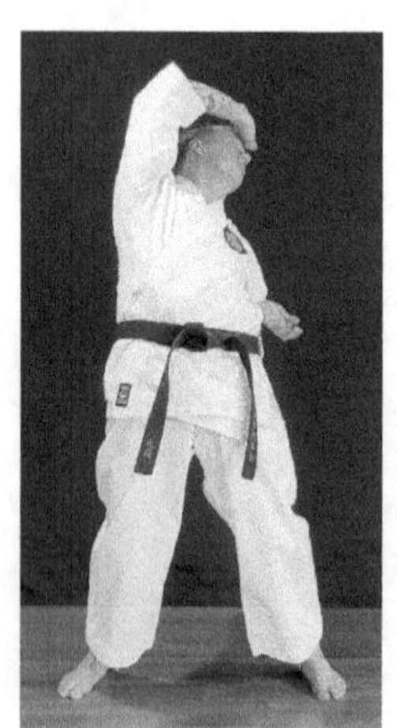

9c. Side Stretches (45° Angle to Rear) (Starting Position - One Hand on Forehead, One Hand at Side)

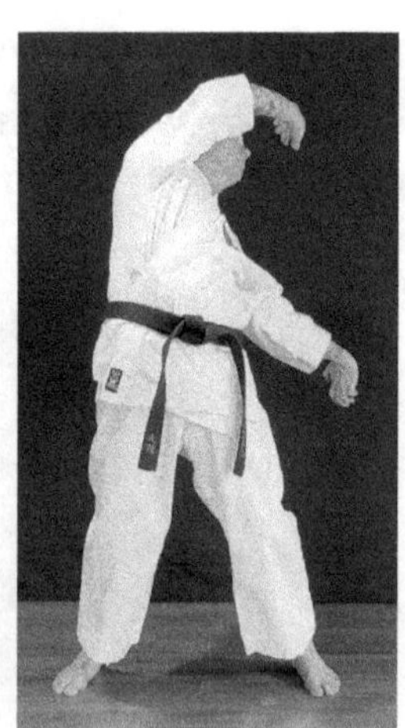

9c. 45° Angle - Left
Push Both Hands Straight Back to Left Side (3 count)

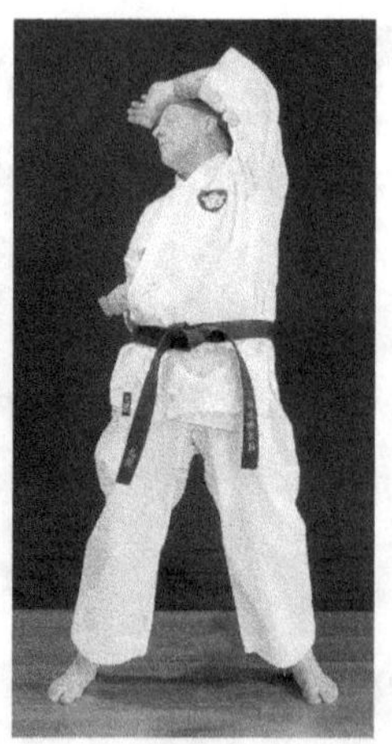

9d. Back to Starting Position With Hands in Opposite Positions

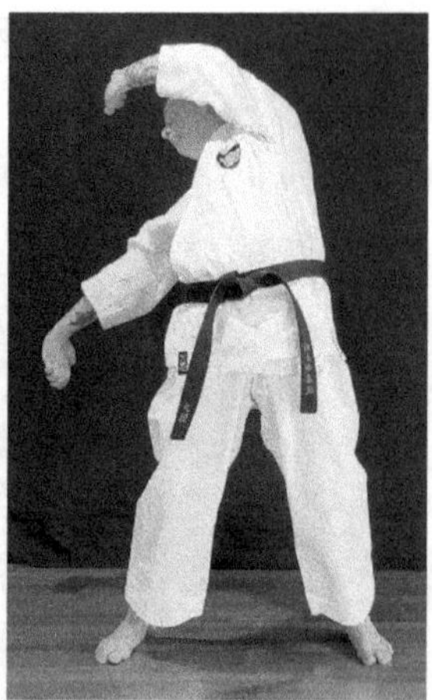

9d. 45° Angle - Right
Push Both Hands Straight Back to Right Side (3 count)
(Repeat 9c-d, 5 or 10x)

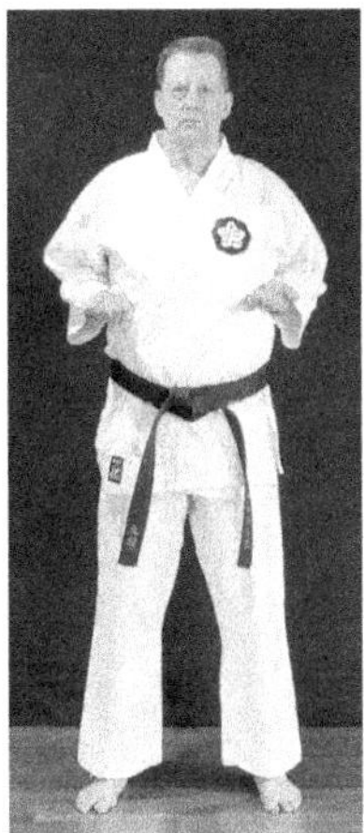

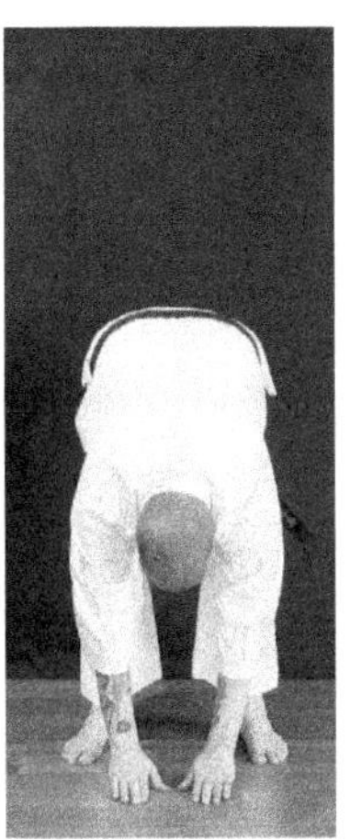

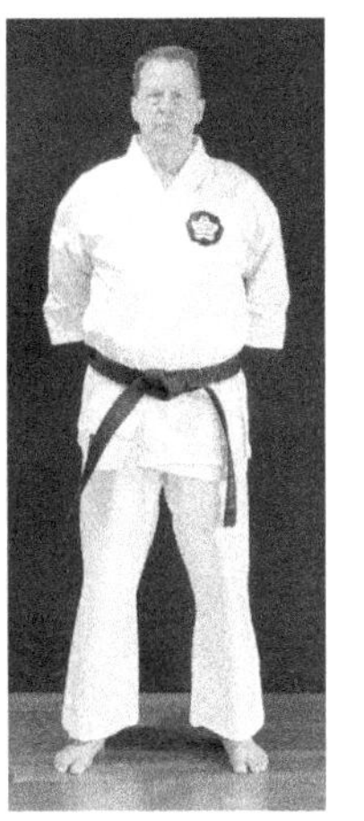

10a. Touch Floor
Feet Shoulder Width Apart, Palms Up at Side, Bend Down, Legs Straight, Touch Floor (3 count)

10b. Raise Up, Place Hands on Backside

10c. Bend Backwards (3 count) - Left Chin to Stretch Throat (Repeat 10a-b, 5 or 10x)

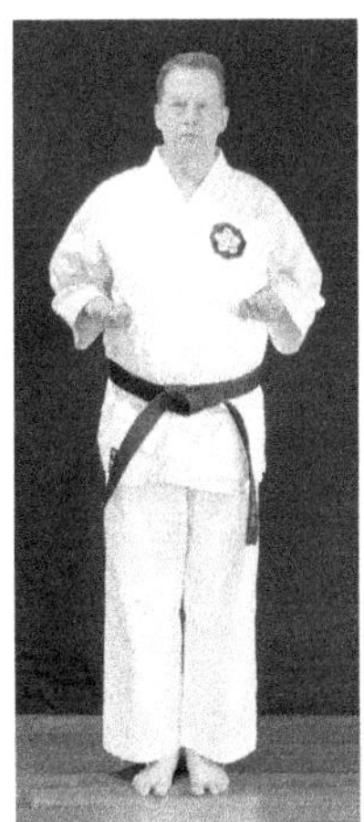

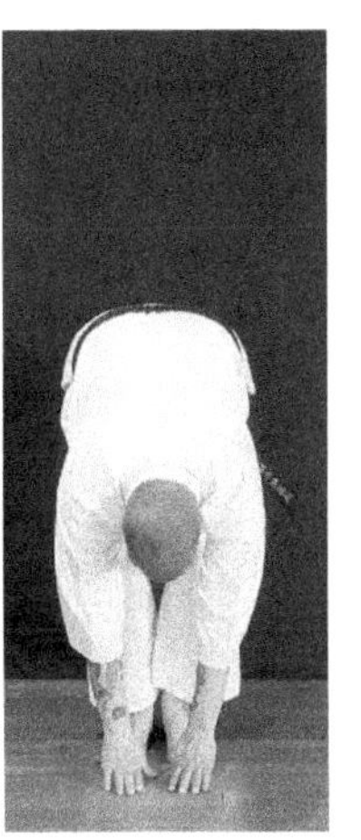

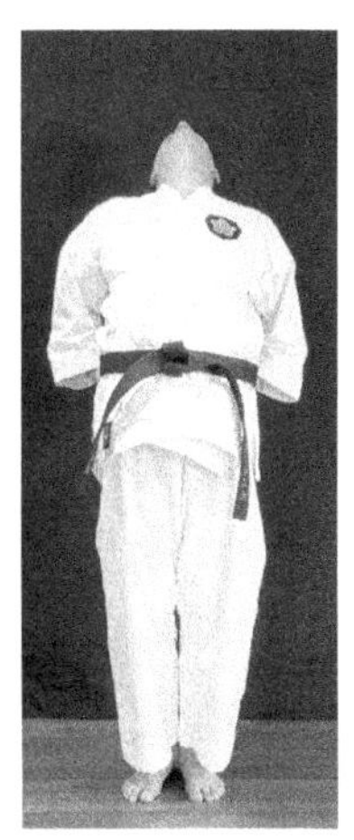

10d. Touch Floor
Feet Together, Palms Up at Side, Bend Down,
Legs Straight, Touch Floor (3 count)

10e. Raise Up, Place Hands on Backside

10f. Bend Backwards (3 count) - Left Chin to Stretch Throat (Repeat 10d-e, 5 or 10x)

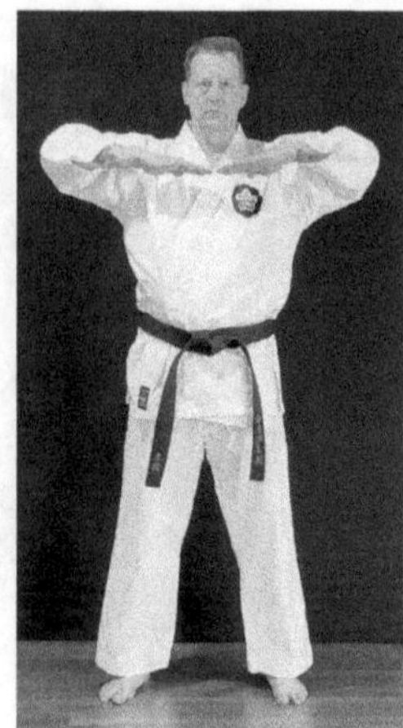

11a. Chop Strike (Single, Double, 4 Count)
Singles: Feet Shoulder Width Apart, Both Hands Open, Palms Down, Elbows Up

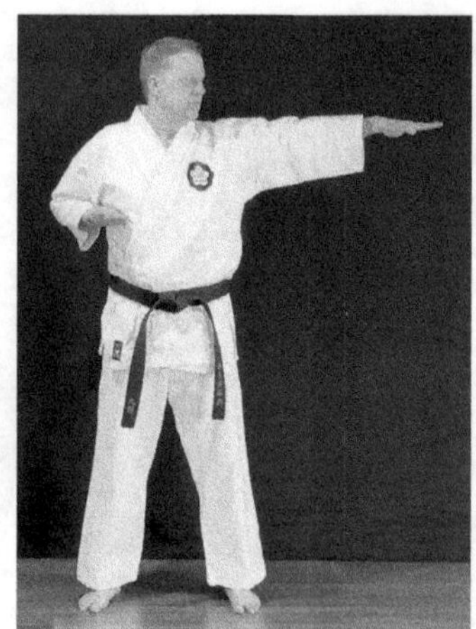

11b. Put Right Hand at Side of Body while Left Hand Goes Straight Out to Side (Stretch Pectoral Muscles)

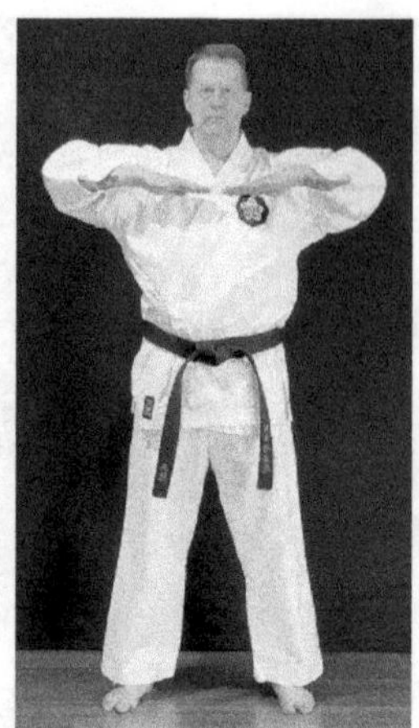

11c. Return Both Hands to Starting Position.

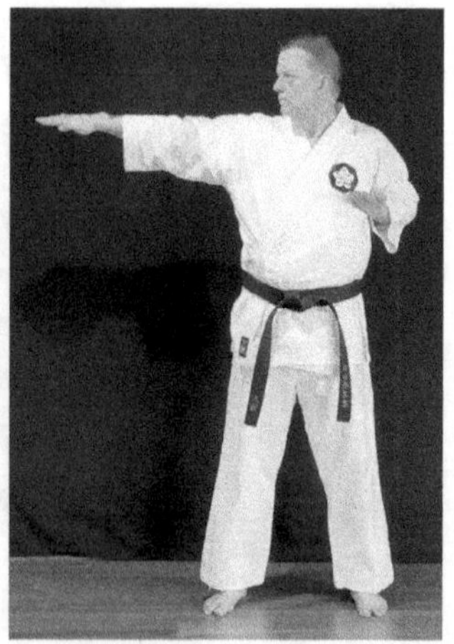

11d. Put Left Hand at Side of Body while Right Hand Goes Straight Out to Side (Stretch Pectoral Muscles)

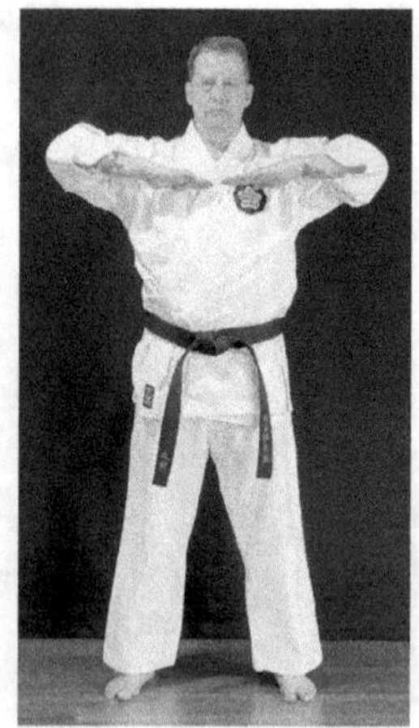

11e. Return Both Hands to Starting Position.
(Repeat 11a-d, 5 or 10x)

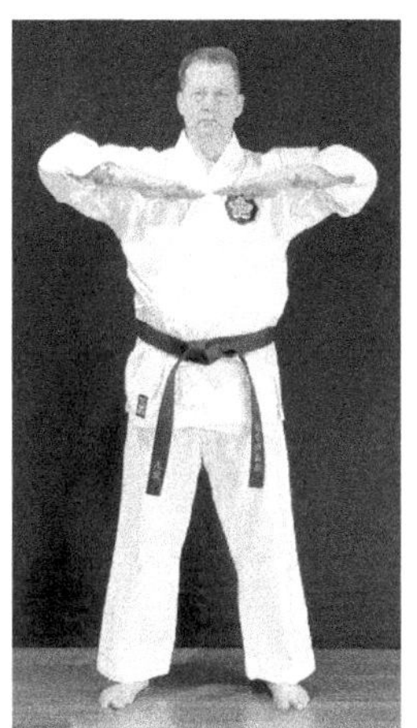

11f. Chop Strike (Double) Starting Position

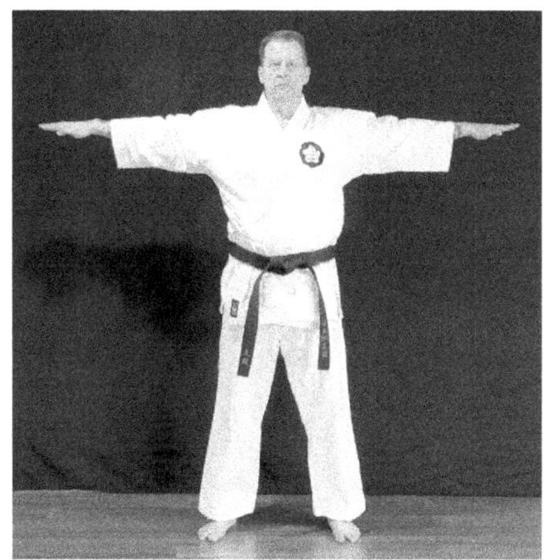

11g. Both Hand Go Straight Out to Side (Stretch Pectoral Muscles)

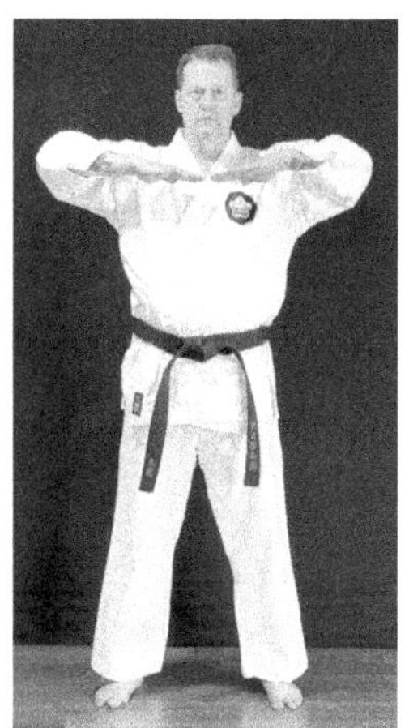

11h. Return Both Hands to Starting Position. (Repeat 11g-h, 5 or 10x)

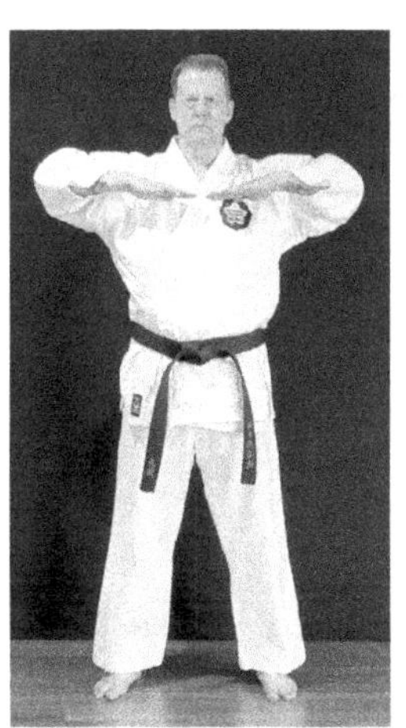

11i. Chop Strike (4 Count) Starting Position

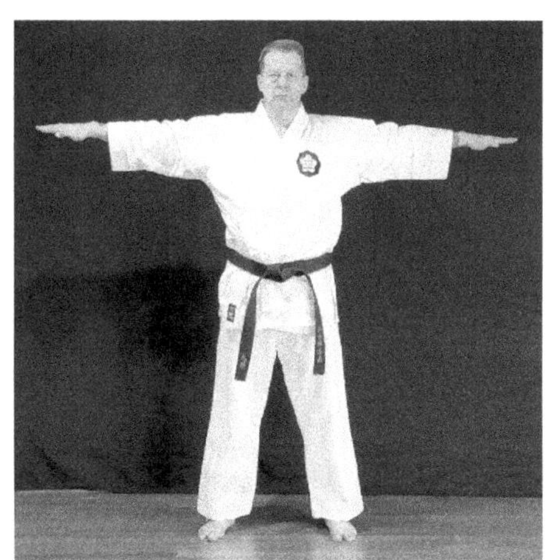

11j. Both Hand Go Straight Out to Side (Stretch Pectoral Muscles)

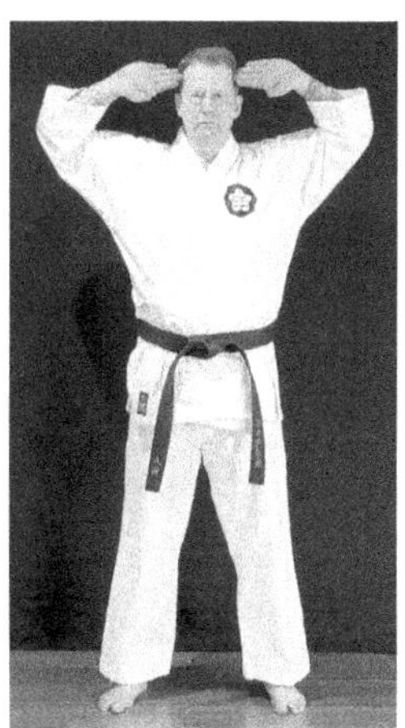

11k. Bring Both Hands Up to Head

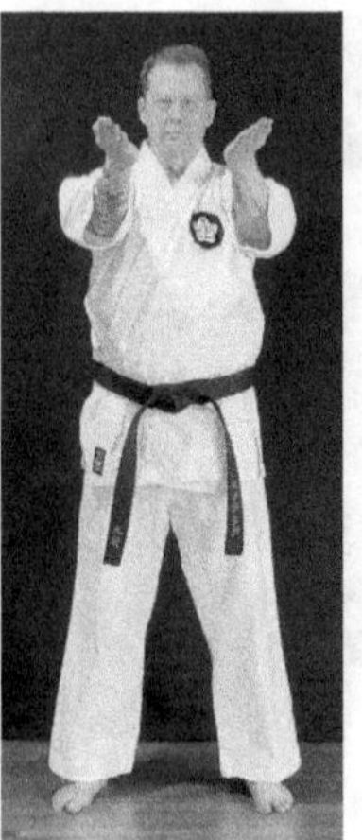

11l. Complete Front Chop with Both Hands

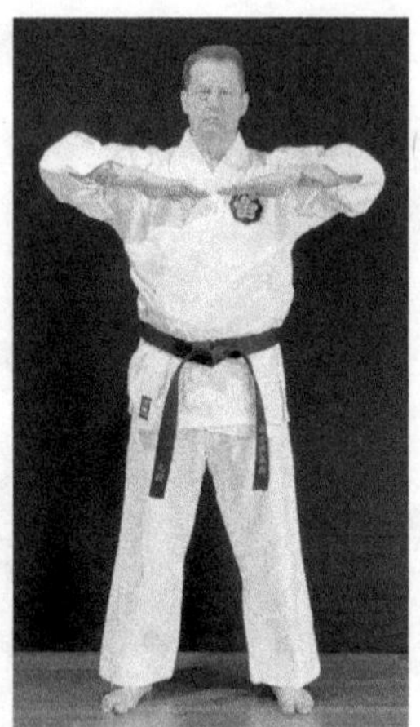

11m. Bring Both Hands Back to Starting Position
(Repeat 11i-m, 5 or 10x)

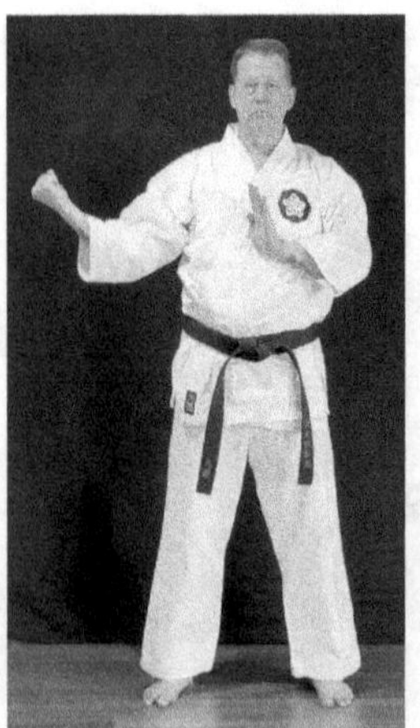

12a. Knuckle Wrap (Single)
Feet Shoulder Width Apart, Open Right Hand in Front of Chest, Right Hand Closed Out to Side

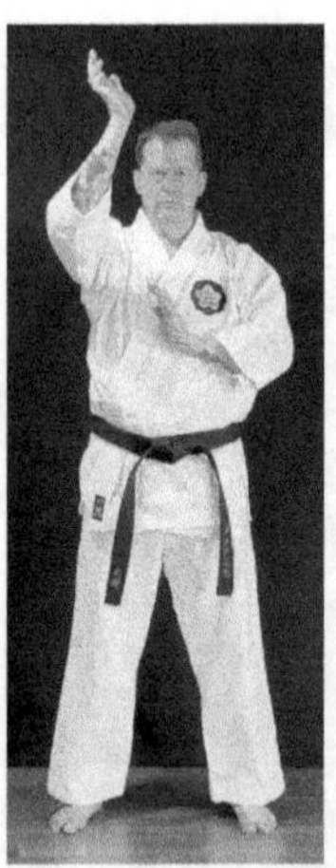

12b. Knuckle Wrap (Single & Double)
Open Right Hand, Bring Up and Around in
Front of Head, Drop Down while Left Hand Forms Fist...

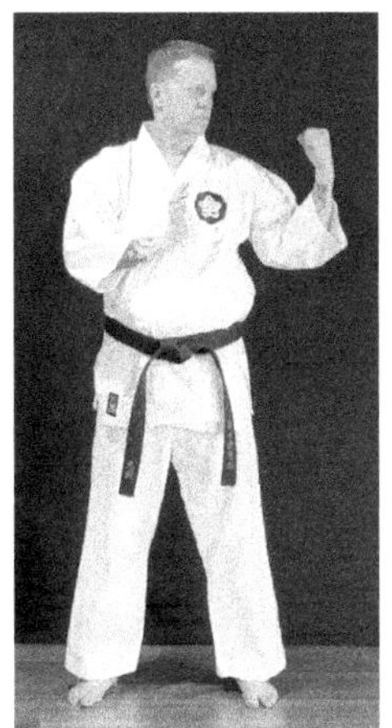

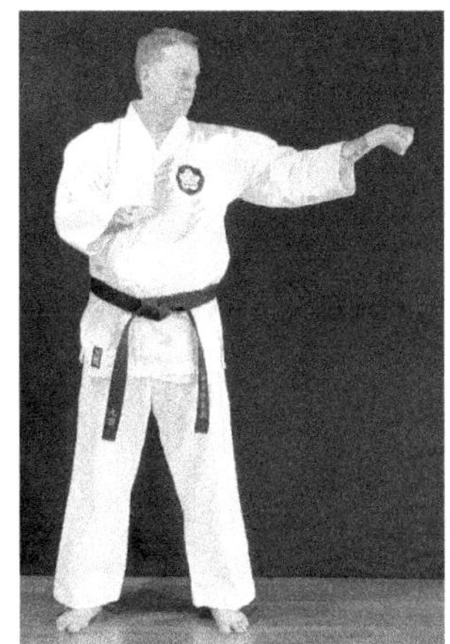

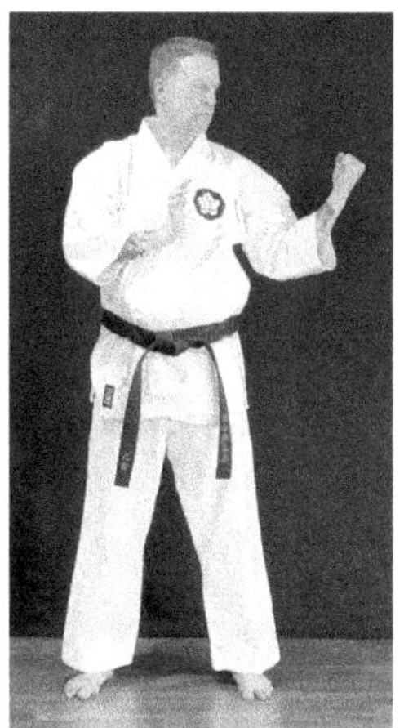

12c. Complete Left Backfist Strike While Allowing Wrist to Extend, Stretching Forearm. Repeat Other Side. (Repeat 12a-c, 5 or 10x)

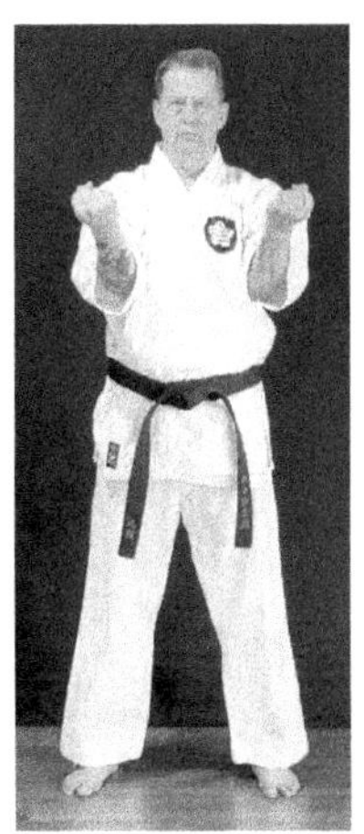

12d. Knuckle Wrap (Double) Feet Shoulder Width Apart, Hands in Fists, Arms Bent at Elbows

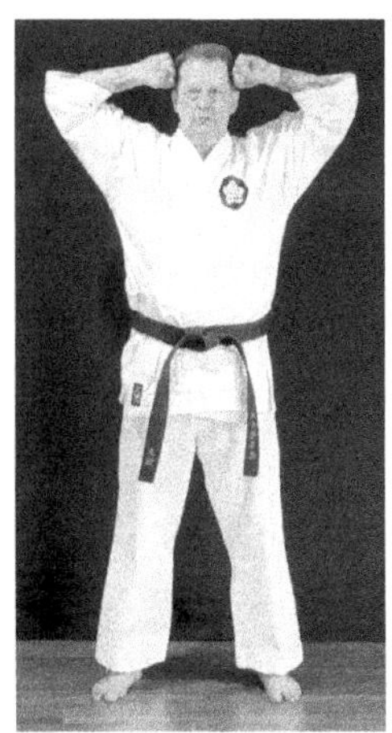

12e. Bring Both Fists Up to Head

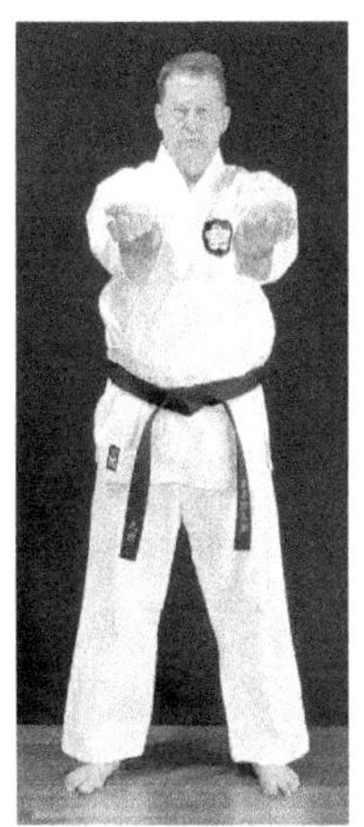

12f. Complete Foreword Backfist Strike with Both Hands

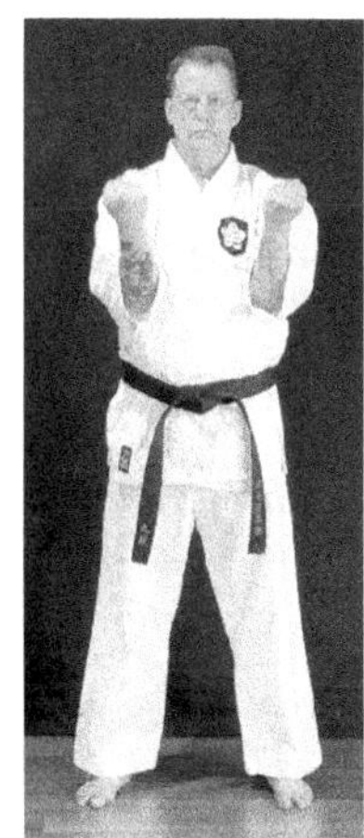

12g. Bring Both Hands Back to Starting Position (Repeat 12d-f, 5 or 10x)

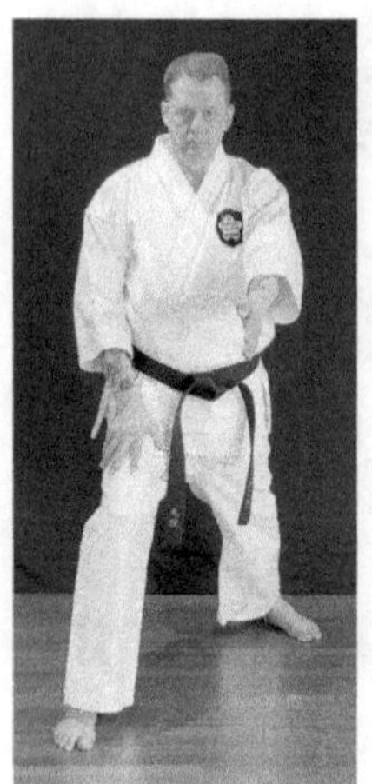
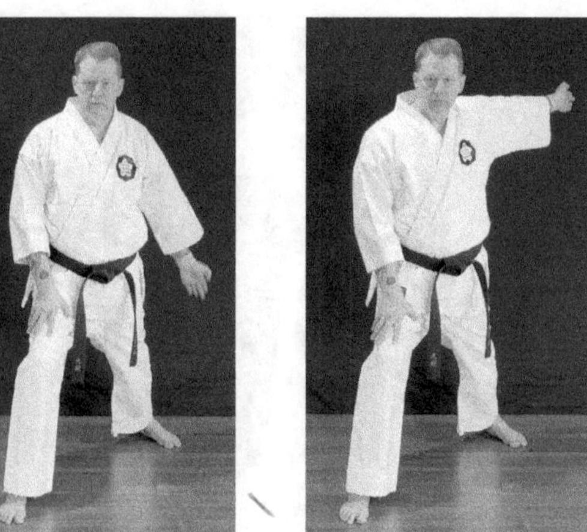

13a. Arm Rotation (Forward & Reverse, Both Arms)
Starting in Zenkutsu Dachi, One Hand on Thigh,
Rotate Left Arm One Direction

...Continue Rotating, Building Up Speed Comfortably, Working Rotator Cuff, Then Slow Down to a Stop

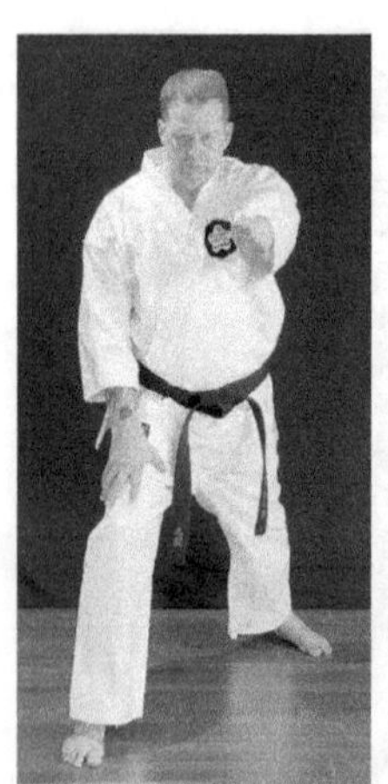
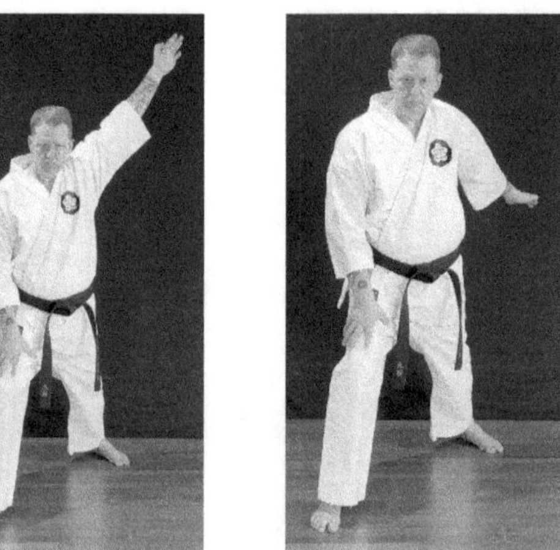
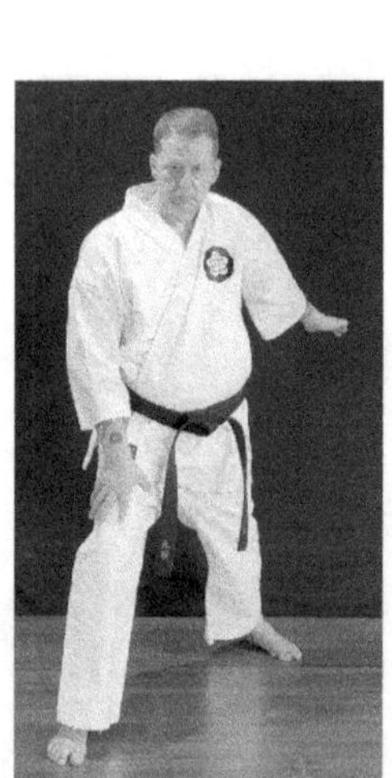
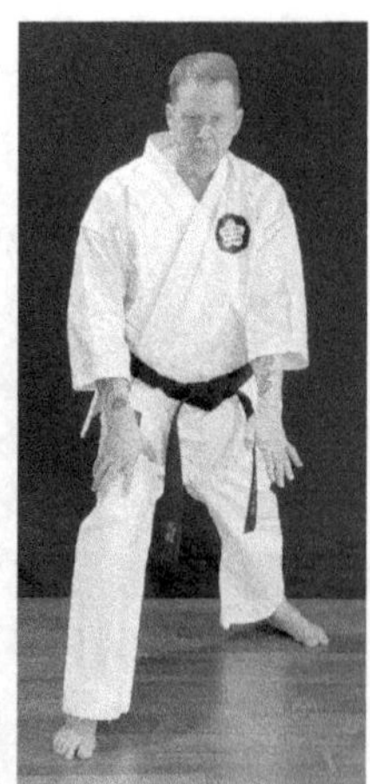

13b. Arm Rotation (Reverse)
Rotate Left Arm Other Direction

...Continue Rotating, Building Up Speed Comfortably, Working Rotator Cuff, Then Slow Down to a Stop
(Repeat Other Arm)

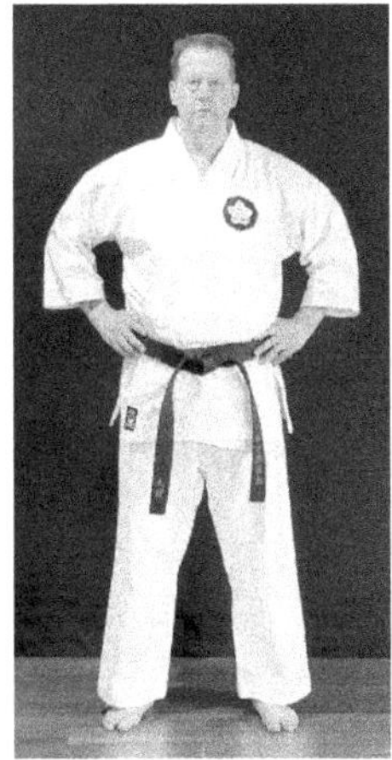
14a. Neck Rotation (Left & Right) Feet Shoulder Width Apart, Hands on Hips

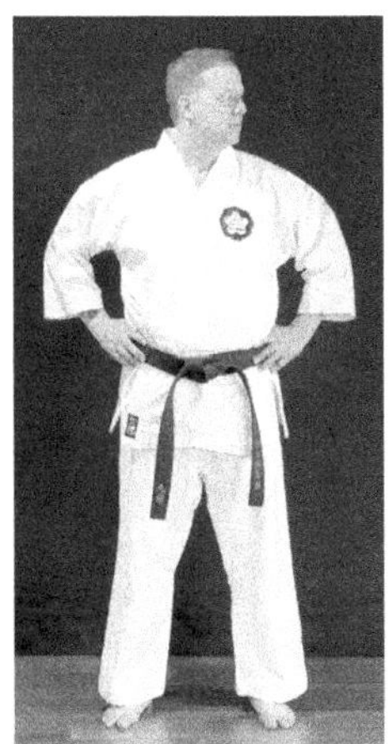
14b: Look Right (3 Count)

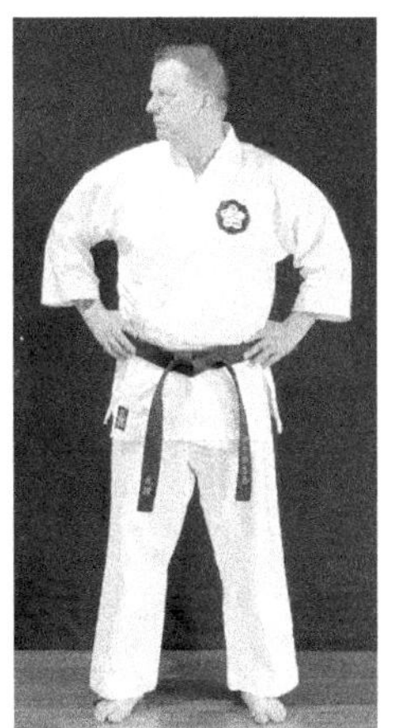
14c. Look Left (3 count) (Repeat 14a-b, 5 or 10x)

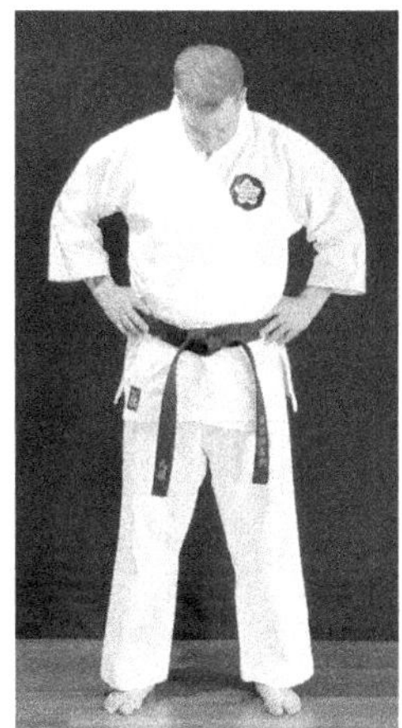
14d. Neck Rotation (Up & Down) Look Down (3 count)

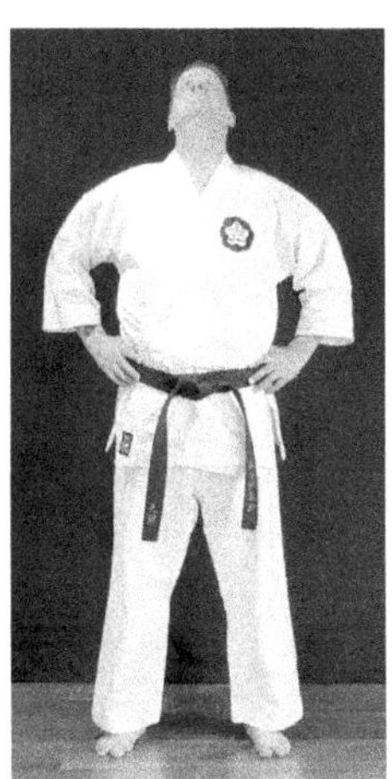
14e. Look Up (Stretch Throat) (3 Count) (Repeat 14d-e, 5 or 10x)

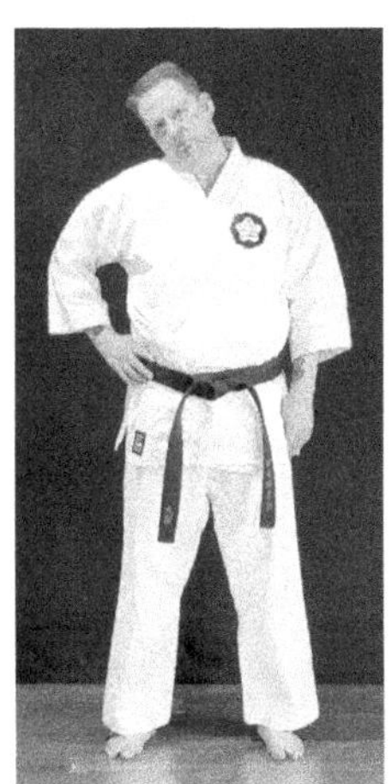
14f. Neck Rotation (Side to Side) Drop Left Shoulder, Stretch Right Ear Down to Right Shoulder (3 Count)

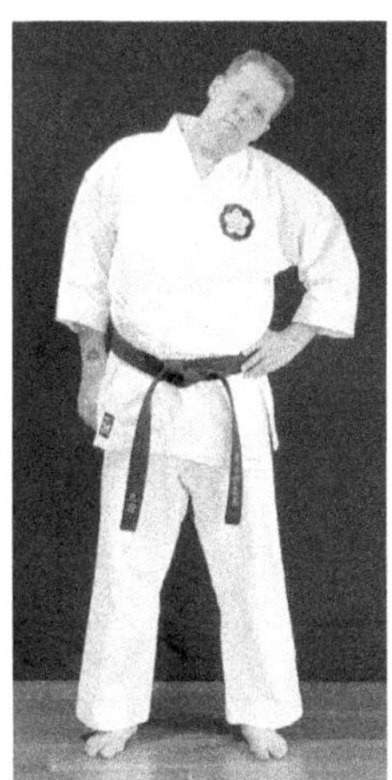
14g. Drop Right Shoulder, Stretch Left Ear Down to Left Shoulder (3 Count) (Repeat 14f-g, 5 or 10x)

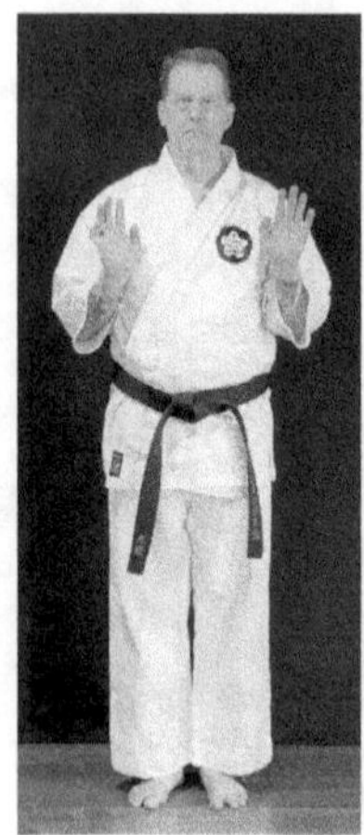
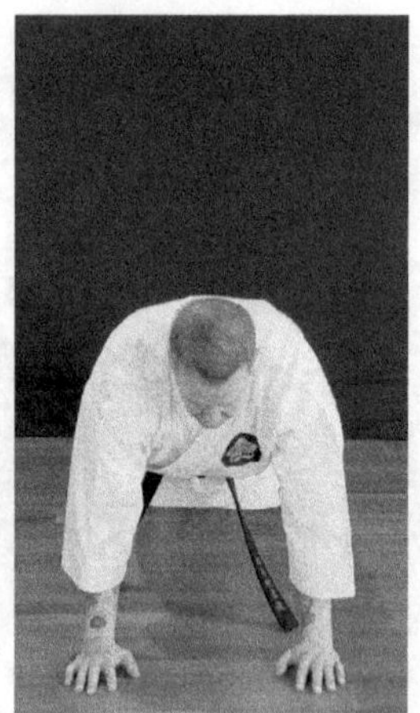
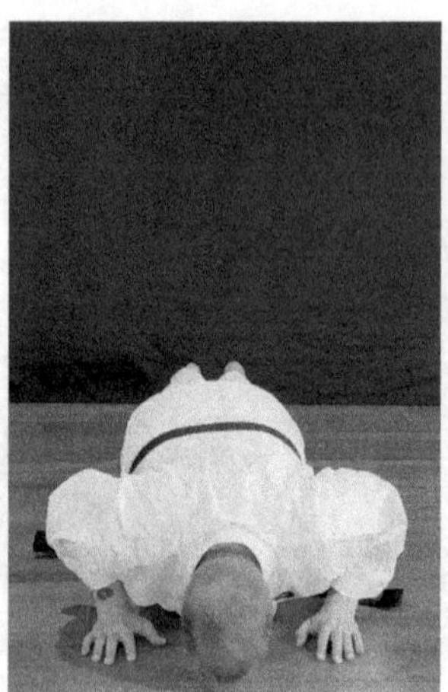

15. Push Up (Push Up, Down, Legs, Back, Front, Up)
With Feet Together and Hands Up at Chest Height, Fall Forward into Push Up Position (Can Also Do This From a Kneeling Position)

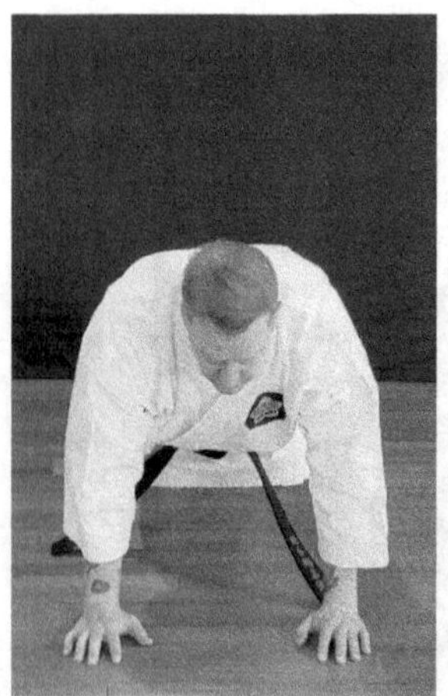
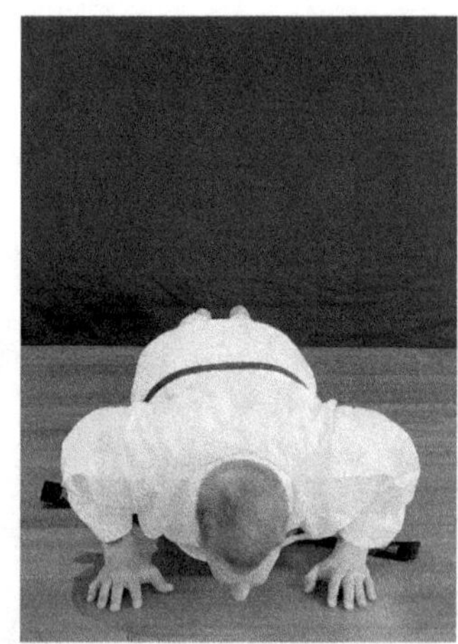
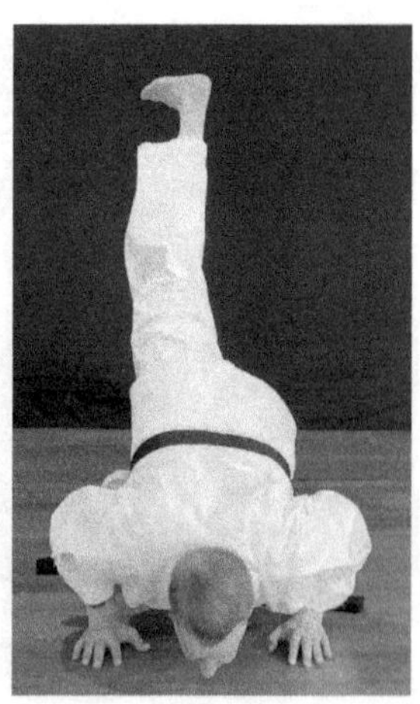

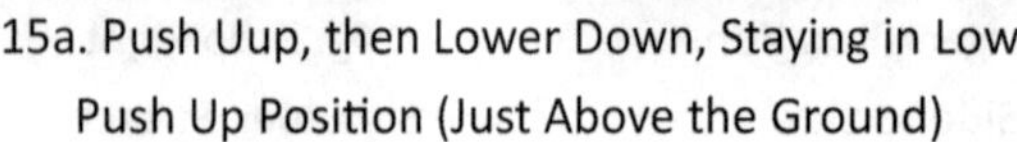
15a. Push Uup, then Lower Down, Staying in Low Push Up Position (Just Above the Ground)

15b. Lift Right Leg

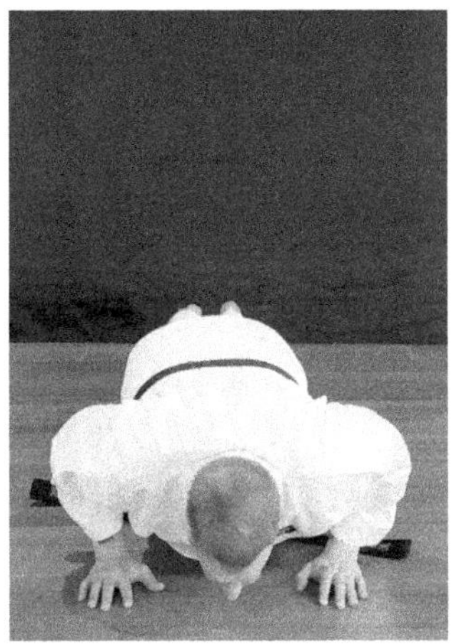

15c. Lower Right Leg

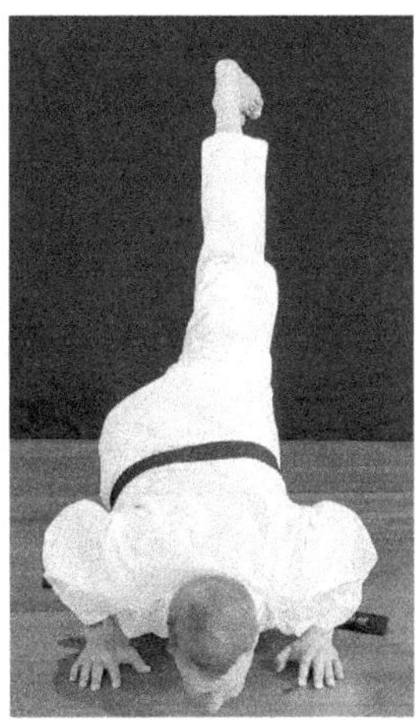

15d. Lift Left Leg

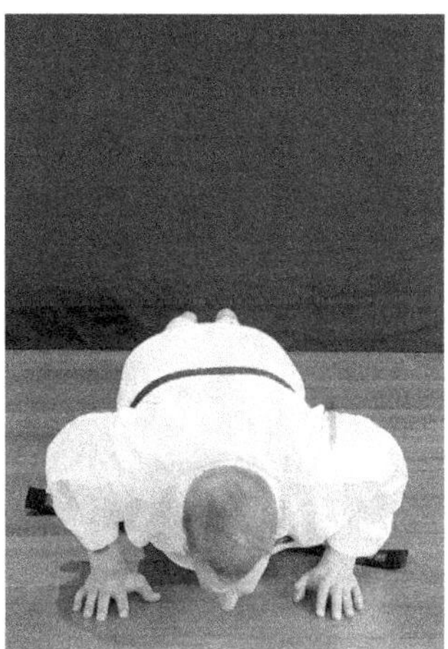

15e. Lower Left Leg

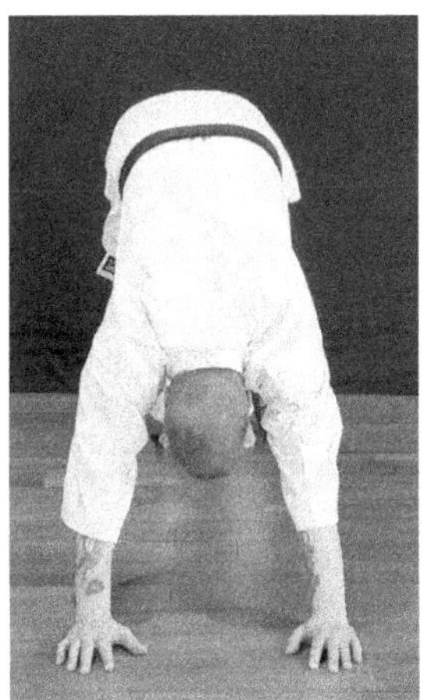

15f. Lift Hips in an "A" Frame (Arms and Legs Straight)

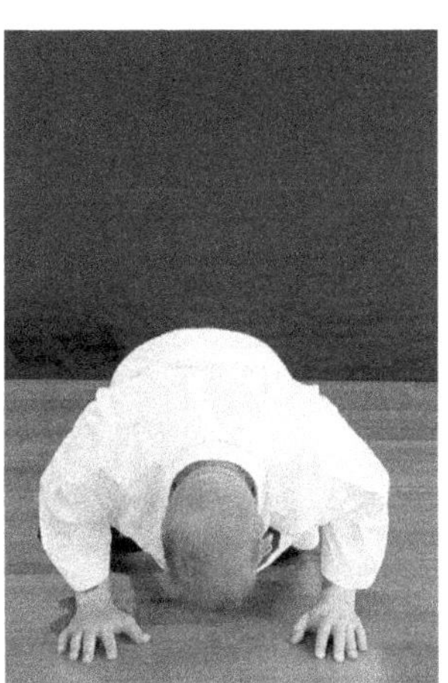

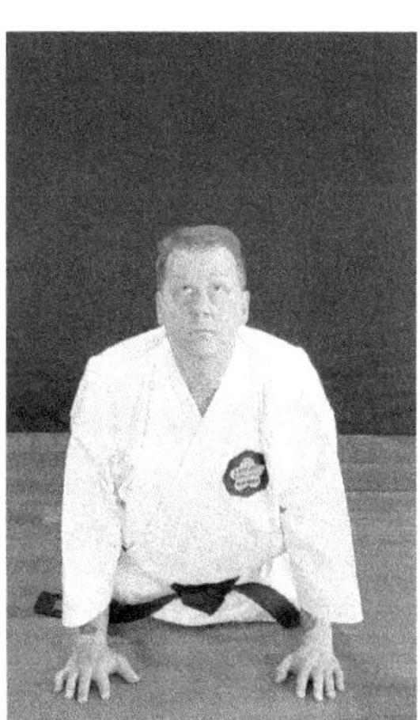

15g. Slowly Lower Head Down and Through, Dropping Hips and Legs, Lifting Chin, and Stretching Back.
Back to Push Up Position
(Repeat 15a-g, 5 or 10x)

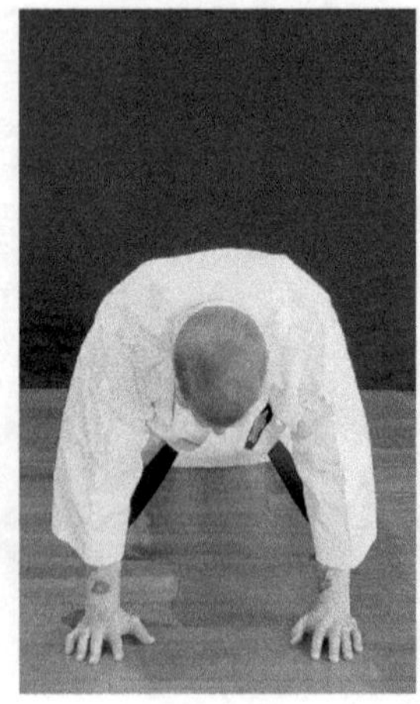
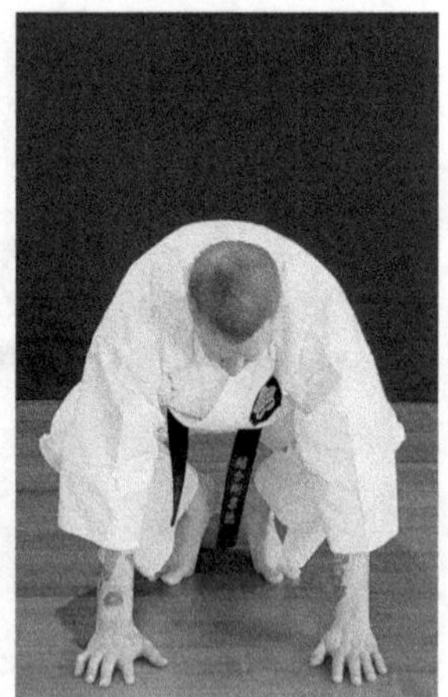
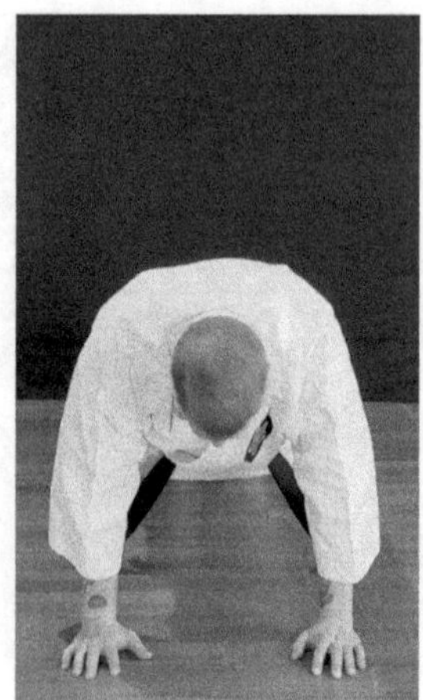

16a. Frog x3 & Through - Touch 3, Slap & Back 3
From Push Up Position, Bring Feet Up Under Hips (Small Bounce for 3 Count),
Bounce Feet Back to Push Up Position (Repeat 3x), Then Bring Feet Through to Sitting Position

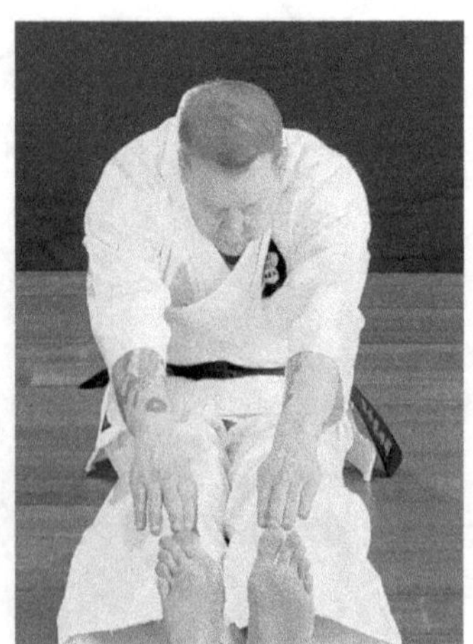
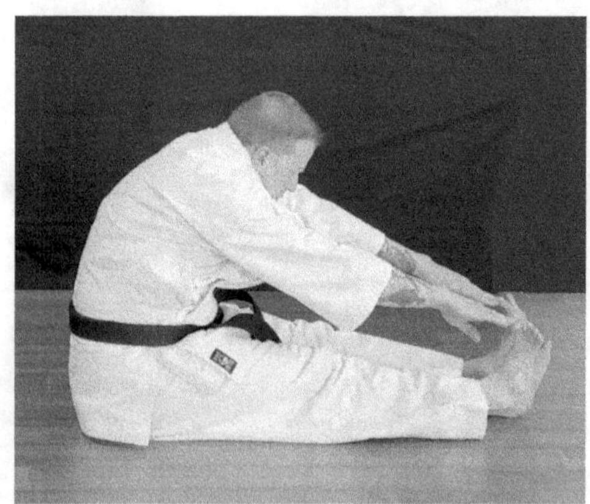

16b. From Sitting Position, Touch Toes for 3 Count

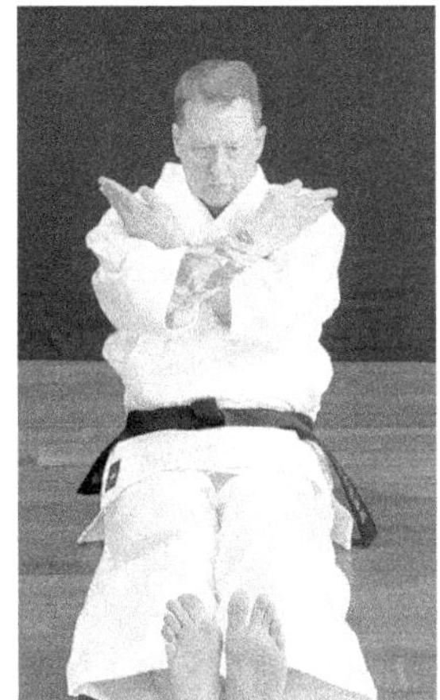

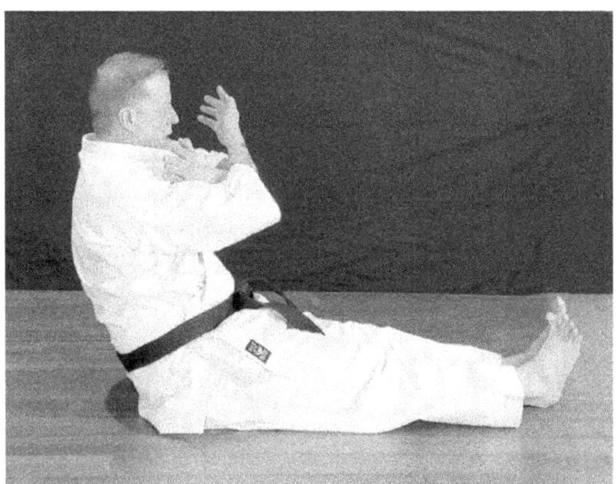

16c. Sit Up and Back, Bringing Crossed Hands to Chest

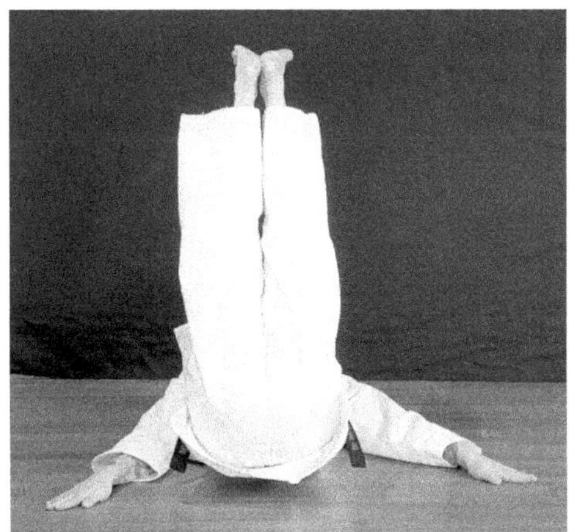

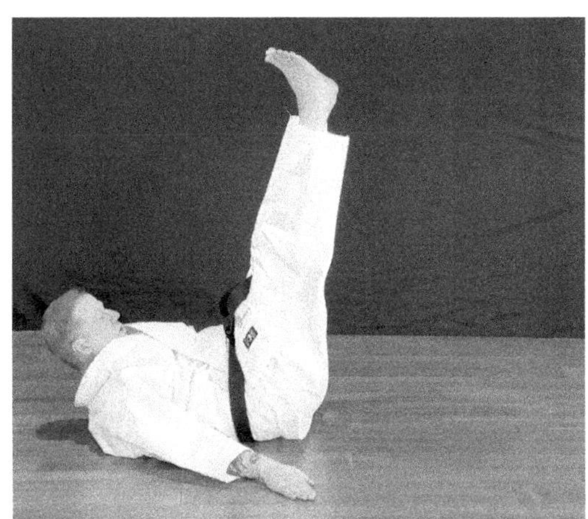

16d. Keep Feet Together and Legs Straight, Lift Legs Up
While Slapping Hands on the Floor Next to Hips

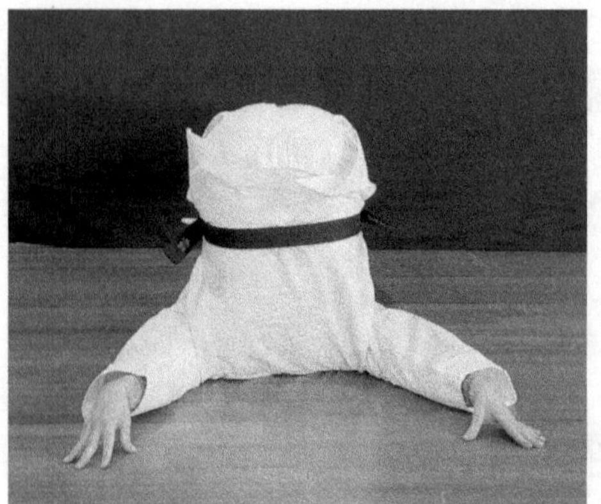
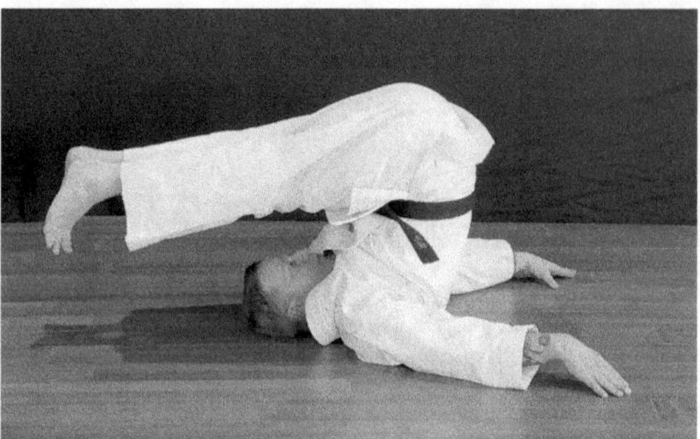

16e. Keep Arms Along Side Body, Chest and Shoulders on the Floor, Allow Legs to Fall Back Naturally for 3 Count. Bring Legs Back Down to the Floor in Front
(Repeat 16b-e, 5 or 10x)

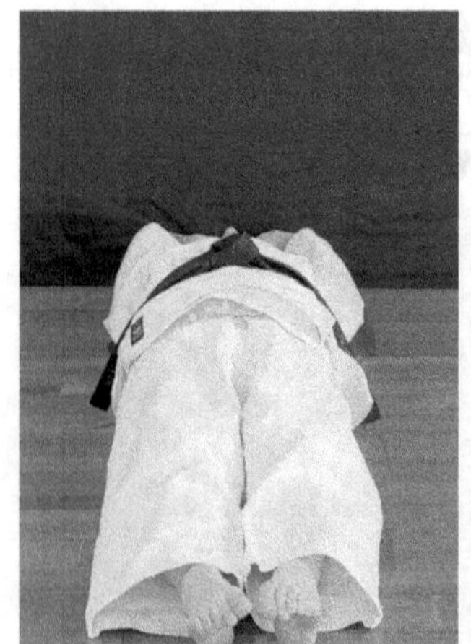
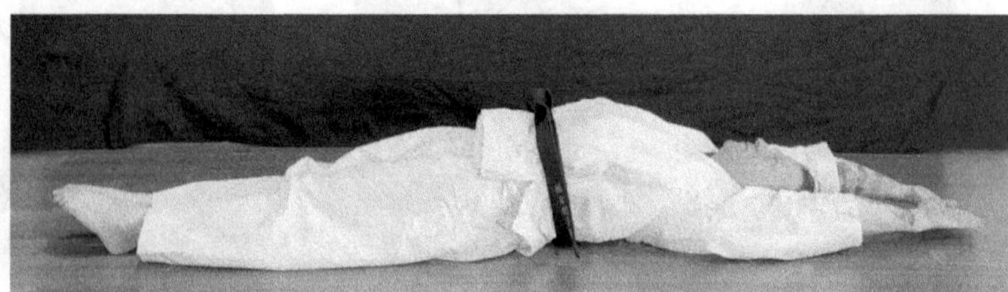

17. Body Stretch
Lying Out Completely, Point Toes and Stretch Out Arms, Inhale Deeply

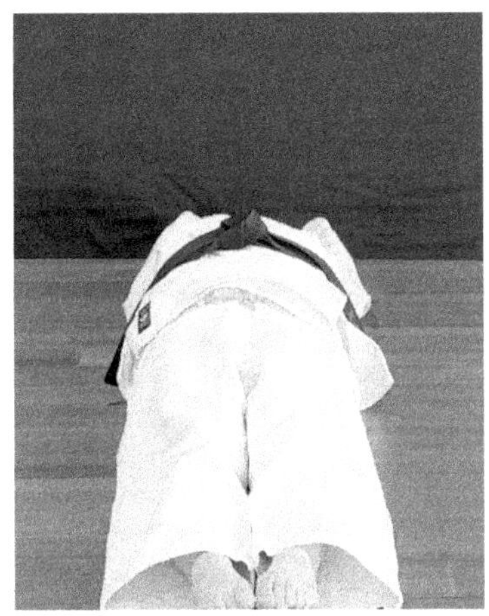

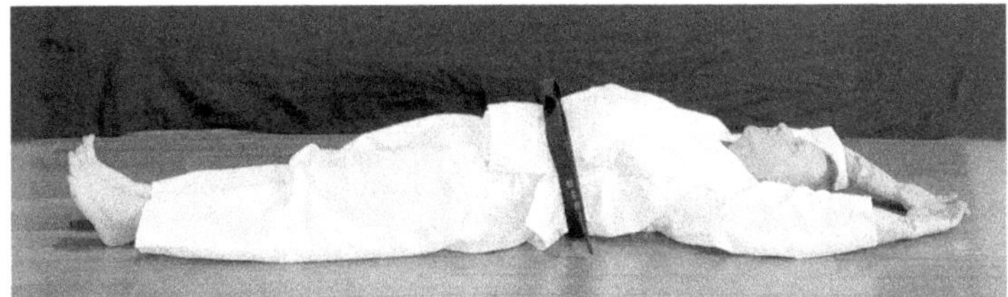

Exhale While Relaxing
(Repeat 17, 5 or 10x)

19. Appendix

Japanese to English Karate Terms

Directions

Heiko - parallel

Mae - front

Tate - vertical

Ushiro - rear (back)

Yoko - side

Motions

Age - rising

Barai - sweeping

Kake - hook

Mawashi - roundhouse

Mawatte - turn

Otoshi - downward

Sukui - scooping

Tobi - jumping

Targets

Chudan - middle level

Gedan - lower level

Jodan - upper level

Quantity

Morote - double

Classifications

Kihon - basic

Kumite - sparring

Chukyu - intermediate

Jokyu - advanced

Misc

Kiai - spirit shout

Stances

Dachi - stance

Hiza Geri no Kamae - knee kick stance

Juji - cross

Kamae - stance / ready posture

Stances (cont.)

Neko Ashi Dachi - cat leg stance

Renoji Dachi - L-stance

Shiko Dachi - straddle stance

Shuto Uchi no Kamae - knife hand striking posture

Yoko Shiko Dachi - side facing square stance

Zenkutsu Dachi - front stance

Numbers

Ichi - one

Ni - two

San - three

Shi - four

Go - five

Rokyu - six

Shichi - seven

Hachi - eight

Ku - nine

Ju - ten

Takedowns & Breakfalls

Ashi Kake Nage - leg hook takedown

Kibisu Gaeshi - heel/ankle takedown

Mae Mawari Ukemi - forward rolling breakfall

Mawari Ukemi - rolling breakfall

Osoto-gari - major outer reap

Seoi-nage - shoulder throw

Sukui-nage - scooping throw

Tai Otoshi - body drop throw

Te-nage - hand throw

Ukemi - breakfall

Ura Mawashi Ashi Barai - spinning leg sweep

Ushiro Mawari Ukemi - rear rolling breakfall

Ushiro Ukemi - backward breakfall

Yoko Ukemi - side breakfall

Body Parts

Ashi - leg

Empi - elbow

Japanese to English Karate Terms

Body Parts (cont.)

Hiza - knee

Kakato - heel

Ko - back of wrist

Kokyubu - throat

Shotei - palm heel

Shuto - knife hand

Uraken - backfist

Blocks

Chudan Sukui Uke - middle level scooping block

Chudan Uke - middle level block

Gedan Barai - low sweeping block

Gedan Shotei Barai - low palm heel sweeping block

Haiwan Uke - forearm block

Hiki Uke - pulling block

Jodan Age Ko Uke - upper level rising back of wrist block

Jodan Age Uke - upper level rising block

Jodan Juji Uke - upper level cross block

Jodan Yoko Age Uke - upper level side rising block

Jodan Yoko Ko Uke - upper level side crossed block

Juji Age Uke - rising cross block

Juji Otoshi Uke - downward cross block

Juji Uke - cross block

Morote Age Sukui Uke - double rising scooping block

Morote Shuto Uke - double knife hand block

Shotei Oshi - palm heel push

Shotei Otoshi Uke - downward palm heel block

Soto Uke - outside block

Sukui Uke - scooping block

Uchi Uke - inside block

Uke - receive/block

Ushiro Empi Uke - rear elbow block

Yoko Gedan Barai - side low sweeping block to side

Yoko Morote Shuto Uke - side double knife hand block

Leg/Knee/Foot Techniques

Age Hiza Uchi - rising knee strike

Chudan Mawashi Geri - middle level roundhouse kick

Fumikomi Geri - stomping kick

Gedan Hiza Uchi - low strike with the knee

Gedan Mae Geri - low front kick

Gedan Mawashi Geri - low roundhouse kick

Hiza Geri - kick to the knee

Hiza Uchi - strike with the knee

Jodan Mae Geri - upper level front kick

Jodan Mawashi Geri - upper level roundhouse kick

Jodan Tobi Mae Geri - upper level jumping front kick

Jodan Tobi Mawashi Geri - upper level jumping roundhouse kick

Jodan Yoko Geri - upper level side kick

Kakato Otoshi Geri - down heel kick

Kake Geri - hook kick

Keri/-Geri - kick

Kin Geri - groin kick

Mae Geri - front kick

Mawashi Geri - roundhouse kick

Mikazuki Geri - crescent kick

Sokuto Otoshi Geri - downward kick with the blade of foot

Soto Mikazuki Geri - outside crescent kick

Ushiro Kakato Geri - rear heel kick

Ushiro Ura Mawashi Geri - spinning heel kick

Yoko Geri - side kick

Arm/Elbow/Hand Techniques

Awase Zuki - U punch

Chudan Empi Uchi - middle level elbow strike

Chudan Tate Uchi - middle level vertical strike

Chudan Zuki - middle level punch

Empi Age Uchi - rising elbow strike

Empi Otoshi Uchi - downward elbow strike

Japanese to English Karate Terms

Arm/Elbow/Hand Techniques (cont.)

Gedan Morote Tate Shotei Uchi - low double vertical palm heel strike

Gyaku Zuki - reverse punch

Haishu Uchi - back of the hand strike

Haito Uchi - ridge hand strike

Hiraken Uchi - fore knuckle strike

Jodan Haito Uchi - upper level ridge hand strike

Jodan Mawashi Empi Uchi - upper level roundhouse elbow strike

Jodan Morote Shotei Tate Uchi - upper level double vertical palm heel strike

Jodan Shotei Oshi - upper level palm heel push

Jodan Tate Uchi - upper level vertical strike

Jodan Tettsui Uchi - upper level hammer fist strike

Jodan Ushiro Mawashi Uraken Uchi - upper level spinning backfist strike

Jodan Yoko Shuto Uchi - upper level side chop strike

Jodan Yoko Uraken Uchi - upper level side backfist strike

Jodan Zuki - upper level punch

Kote Uchi - forearm strike

Kubi Shuto Uchi - chop strike to the neck

Morote Mimi Uchi - double ear strike

Morote Oyayubi Ate - double thumb strike

Morote Yoko Kote Uchi - double side forearm strike

Nidan-zuki - double punch (one after the other)

Nodo Kaki - throat rip

Nukite Uchi - spear hand strike

Otoshi Shotei Uchi - downward palm heel strike

Shuto Otoshi Uchi - downward chop strike

Shuto Uchi - chop strike

Tate Uchi - vertical strike

Tettsui Otoshi Uchi - downward hammer fist strike

Tettsui Uchi - hammer fist strike

Tsuki/-Zuki - punch

Uchi - strike

Arm/Elbow/Hand Techniques (cont.)

Ura Zuki - inverted punch

Uraken Uchi - backfist strike

Ushiro Empi Uchi - rear elbow strike

Ushiro Mawashi Shuto Uchi - spinning chop strike

Ushiro Mawashi Uraken Uchi - spinning backfist strike

Ushiro Shuto Uchi - rear chop strike

Yoko Empi Uchi - side elbow strike

Yoko Otoshi Zuki - downward punch from the side

Yoko Shuto Uchi - chop strike from the side

Yoko Tettsui Otoshi Uchi - downward hammer fist strike from the side

Yoko Tettsui Uchi — hammer fist strike from the side

Yoko Uraken Uchi — backfist strike from the side

Ketsugo Goju-Ryu Dojos

Hombu Dojo (Home School)

Oliver Karate Academy
Colorado Springs, Colorado
(719) 581-3161
www.oliverkarate.com

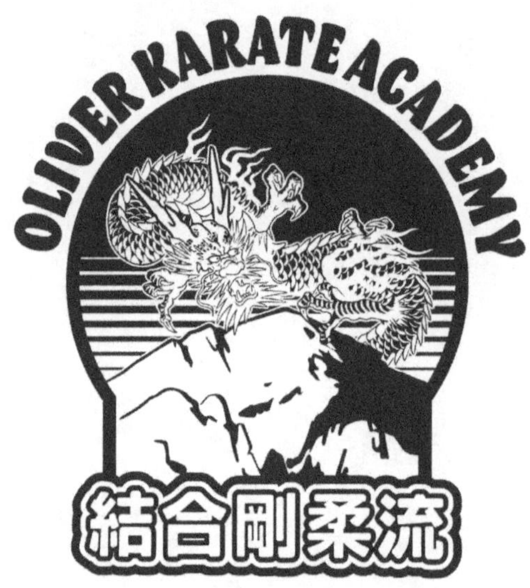

Branch Dojo

Bryant Karate Academy
North Richland Hills, Texas
(682) 325-9755
www.bryantkarateacademy.com

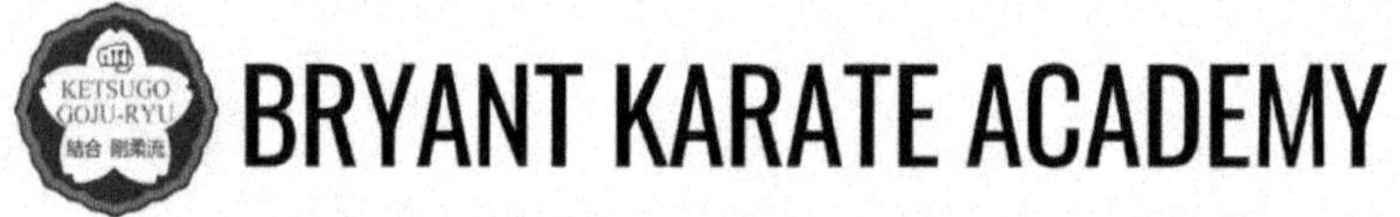

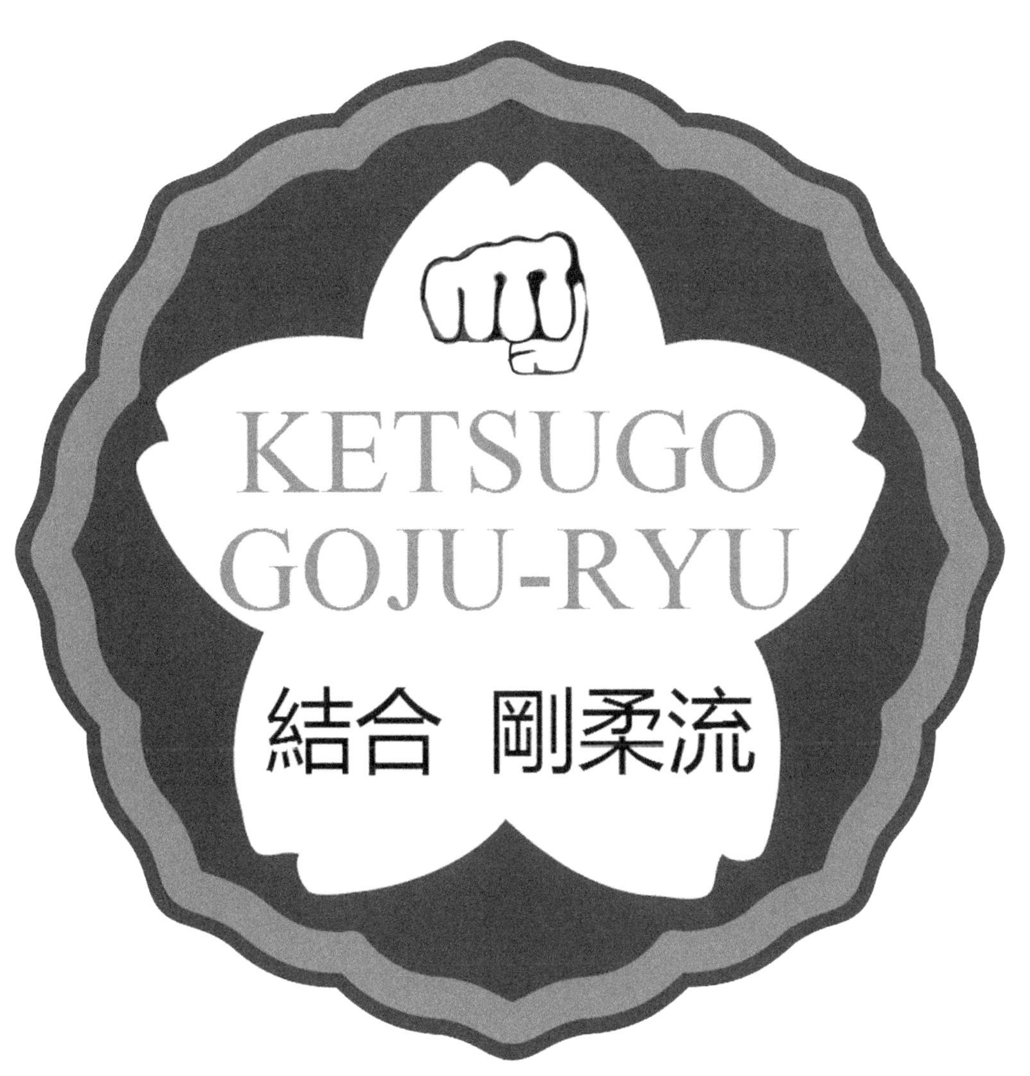
KETSUGO
GOJU-RYU
結合 剛柔流

Other Titles in the KGJKA Book Series:

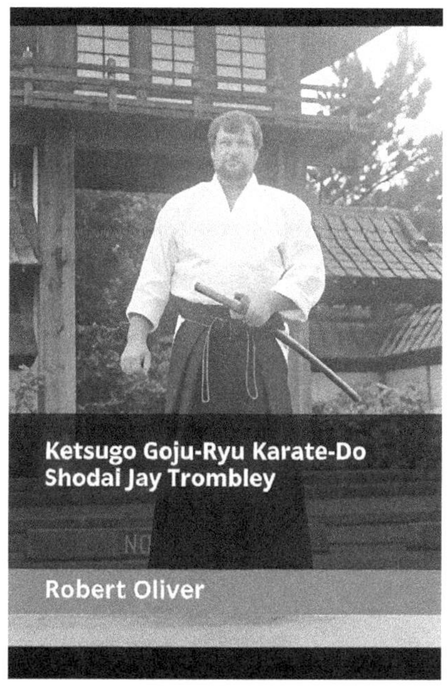

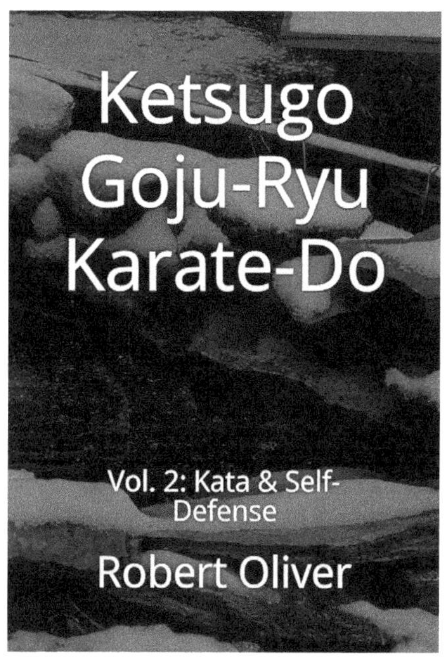

Ketsugo Goju-Ryu Karate-Do

Vol. 3: Kata Part 2

Robert Oliver

www.ingramcontent.com/pod-product-compliance
Lightning Source LLC
LaVergne TN
LVHW081323110826
845149LV00007B/1573

* 9 7 9 8 9 8 9 6 4 0 2 8 7 *